Advances in
Modern Environmental Toxicology

Series Editor, M.A. Mehlman, Ph.D.

**VOLUME XXI**

# Chemically-Induced Alterations in Sexual and Functional Development: The Wildlife/Human Connection

*edited by:*
*Theo Colborn and Coralie Clement*

Princeton Scientific Publishing Co., Inc.
Princeton, New Jersey

Printed and bound in the United States of America.

PRINCETON SCIENTIFIC PUBLISHING CO., INC.
P.O. BOX 2155
Princeton, New Jersey 08543
Tel: 609/683-4750
Fax: 609/683-0838

LIBRARY OF CONGRESS CATALOG NUMBER: 92-062331
ISBN: 0-911131-35-3

# TABLE OF CONTENTS

Acknowledgments

Preface

Acronyms

## BACKGROUND

This chapter represents the collective conclusions of 21 individuals who attended the Wingspread Work Session, most of whom have provided a chapter for this book. What follows is a collection of their thoughts, research, and review papers to support the Consensus Statement. The chapters are arranged in a somewhat orderly manner even though, in some cases, there is no intuitively obvious sequence for the material. To assist the reader, a short explanation is provided for why the chapter is included in the book.

Like the descriptive title Howard Bern selected for this chapter, he provides a concise overview of the discussions at the Wingspread Work Session. He describes the long-term changes reported in the reproductive tract and other compartments of the human and mouse endocrine system as the result of exposure in the womb to diethylstilbestrol (DES). With this as a model he conceptualizes the process of transgenerational loss of function preparing the reader for what follows.

In this chapter, Fred vom Saal and co-workers present an overview of sexual differentiation that is spiced with their most recent findings. They focus on the differentiation of the gonads and accessory reproductive organs in males and females as well as sexual differentiation of the brain and behavior. The chapter includes a discussion of vom Saal's findings that development in mouse and rat fetuses is altered as a result of exposure to different hormones transported to them from adjacent male vs. female siblings *in utero*. The intrauterine position phenomenon demonstrates the exquisite sensitivity of sexual development in both males and females to even small changes in the endocrine environment during fetal life.

The emphasis in this chapter shifts to the cellular level from the organismal level of the previous chapter. It is a comprehensive description of the processes that drive the morphological development of the urogenital tract. Although Cunha's research, like vom Saal's, falls in the realm of basic science, it provides a basis for comparison and a foundation for determining the mechanism of action of toxic chemicals. It adds to the data that supports the thesis of this book that the fetus is extremely vulnerable to exogenous influences.

In this chapter, John McLachlan reduces the discussion to the molecular level. His discussion of "orphan receptors" provides answers to some of the questions about the mechanism of action of chemicals like dioxin. These receptors appear to be the vehicles for turning on and off a cascade of events as the result of exposure to chemicals of this nature.

## WILDLIFE EVIDENCE

The Great Lakes hold 20% of the world's freshwater and following World War II became home for one of the largest industrial and agro-chemical complexes in North America. The Lakes also became the major disposal site for the wastes from these industries and other human activities that accompanied the growth in the region. Only because of the unique geo-physical characteristics of the Lakes, offering many isolated areas for large numbers of birds to nest, did the devastation among the nesting bird colonies become evident to field researchers. After eggshells thickened and mass mortality of wildlife abated as the result of regulatory actions in the 1970s, biologists began to recognize the other more insidious effects of endocrine disruptors, like DDT, in the environment. It is now well documented that the offspring of a large number of top-predator, fish-eating species in the Great Lakes and other regions of the Northern Hemisphere, are suffering a suite of anomalies associated with endocrine disruption—and that maternal exposure to contaminants in the fish and water does, indeed, affect the well-being of their progeny.

This chapter visits an aquatic system in Florida, USA, and describes the striking effect of a point-source release on a live-bearing sexually dimorphic fish species. Human activity that leads to single-point discharges has not traditionally been monitored for effects of this nature. Generally, regulatory agencies have used standards based on lethality to regulate point source pollution. In this case, as in so many instances, even though human activity is associated with the effect, the causal agent(s) has not been determined.

This chapter describes the widespread occurrence of endocrine disruption in fishes in the largest body of freshwater in the world, unlike the previous chapter that focussed on a discreet location. Here, John Leatherland discusses problems that have pervaded all five Great Lakes, as a result of the many industrial, agro-chemical, and land-use activities in the system, as well as long-range atmospheric transport of toxic chemicals into the system. Compared with the point-source situation in Chapter 6, tracing the source(s) of this widespread pollution is beyond the realm of practicality. In both situations, determining the causal agent(s) may be a much greater challenge.

Glen Fox was one of the first field biologists to report on the abnormal endocrine development of herring gulls and other bird species in the Great Lakes. In this chapter he uses ecoepidemiology to reveal the subtleties of abnormal sexual development in wildlife species. He describes research from three North American situations to make his point.

As persistent pollutants slowly move to the seas and oceans, one should logically expect to find health problems in marine mammals similar to those reported in animals of polluted inland aquatic systems. Peter Reijnder's earlier series of manuscripts on the reproductive problems in seals and in freshwater animals and humans exposed to endocrine disrupting chemicals are striking. In this overview, Reijnders and Brasseur reiterate the message of the pervasiveness of the problem of endocrine disruption by focussing on marine animals. The die-offs of dolphins, seals, and whales commencing in 1987 suggest that, indeed, the contaminants, moving slowly toward the oceans, have begun to reach concentrations of concern in the marine system as well. The marine mammals may be harbingers of the limit to which marine systems can handle the current terrestrial loading of contaminants.

# LABORATORY EVIDENCE

The findings of Dick Peterson and his coworkers in this paper read much like the results of Fred vom Saal's work on the feminization and demasculinization of male rats that had developed between two females *in utero*. This similarity between the results in vom Saal's and Peterson's research fueled the initiative to seek the funding for the Wingspread Work Session. When Peterson and vom Saal were asked if they had heard about each other's research, they said "No." In this case, two well executed studies with entirely different hypotheses and study designs, when considered together, provide powerful evidence concerning the sensitivity of the developing fetus to chemical perturbation.

This second paper from Dick Peterson's laboratory reveals again the importance of timing of exposure when determining risk. This paper also demonstrates the difference in sensitivity to contaminants among species. In this case Walker and Peterson use a wild species, the lake trout, and report the lowest-observed-adverse-level for dioxin (2,3,7,8-TCDD) leading to fry mortality.

Earl Gray's review provides evidence that a number of ubiquitous compounds can affect the endocrine system and via a wide variety of mechanisms yield a wide range of abnormalities in sexual development. Gray points out that the complexity of the endocrine system with its multiple paths of development, presents uncounted stages of vulnerability to bioaccumulative chemicals that are continually present in the developing animal or human.

Klaus Döhler and Barbara Jarzab present an overview of the literature intermingled with their research on the development of the neuroendocrine system. The complexity of sexual differentiation of the central nervous system is revealed. The influences of disturbances in timing and dose of endocrine and neuroendocrine mediators are discussed in depth.

# HUMAN EVIDENCE

In this chapter, Melissa Hines provides a comprehensive overview of the literature concerning neuroendocrine-related behavior in DES exposed individuals. The effects she discusses were not recognized in most cases until the subjects reached maturity. Hines provides an objective review of the information available and provides guidance for future research on estrogens and human neurobehavioral development.

The interrelationship between the endocrine and immune system has been reported elsewhere. Phyllis Blair summarized in 1981 on immunosuppression in mice neonatally exposed to diethylstilbestrol and later in 1988 reported on the susceptibility of women exposed to DES *in utero* to autoimmune disease. This and the next chapter are reports of her latest findings concerning this problem.

The work coming from Phyllis Blair's laboratory provides an example of the subtle effects of exposure to endocrine disruptors and emphasizes how difficult it is to link the effects with maternal exposure. As more chemicals are introduced into the environment, the difficulty of making links becomes greater. The cascade of effects as the result of exposure to a chemical is unpredictable. This chapter demonstrates that it has taken the greatest part of the lifetime of the DES exposed individuals to disclose the longterm immune effects that were initiated while they were in the womb.

Ana M. Soto and her coworkers have developed a tissue culture assay for estrogenicity (cell proliferation) using human breast cancer cells. In this assay, the proliferative effect of a compound is compared with estradiol, the most potent natural estrogen. This assay could serve as a relatively inexpensive and simple method for assessing the estrogenicity of chemicals as well as determining exposure. The paper also discusses structure activity relationships in an effort to define the chemical features responsible for estrogenicity.

"Do you have any evidence that there have been changes in human behavior as a result of endocrine disruptors in the environment?" is the first question many people ask when they hear for the first time about the topic of this book. Without doubt, this is the most difficult and controversial question addressed in this book. Pat Whitten courageously responds to this question in her analysis that dates back to the 1800s.

## EVIDENCE OF EXPOSURE

This section of the book addresses some practical questions concerning exposure, such as: What quantities and how many hormonally active compounds are in the environment? Were my children exposed in the womb? Was my exposure great enough to affect my children? Is there any way I can avoid exposure?

The authors reveal the difficulties encountered when seeking information on production and distribution of high-volume chemicals. Despite the proprietary nature of this information some conclusions can be inferred from the retrievable data.

Herbicides are now the highest volume chemicals deliberately released into the environment, not only by farmers but homeowners and professionals alike. In this chapter, the authors attempt to provide the reader with some insight into possible exposure pathways. Remembering from earlier chapters that length and timing of exposure are as important as dose, the reader is now introduced to the difficulties associated with determining exposure. The authors suggest that exposure is not merely possible, but probable. Comments on the adequacy of the pesticide registration process are provided.

The same chemicals that accumulate in wildlife and fish tissue also accumulate in human tissue. A number of surveys have shown an association between the concentrations of these chemicals in the tissues of individuals and the frequency with which they eat fish. In this chapter the authors provide an analysis of recent studies on commonly found endocrine disruptors in human tissue to emphasize the difficulty of measuring loss of function as the result of exposure to a potpourri of chemicals. As the Wingspread Consensus Statement concluded, we may have reached that point in time where we have released sufficient developmental toxicants in the environment that the tide must be turned before the drastic effects reported in offspring of exposed wildlife populations are manifested in our progeny.

# ACKNOWLEDGMENTS

We are indebted to the following individuals who reviewed manuscripts for this book: Dr. Carl Barrett, NIEHS, Research Triangle Park, NC; Dr. Charles Benbrook, Benbrook Consulting Services, Dickerson, MD; Dr. Geoffrey Birchard, George Mason University, Fairfax, VA; Dr. George Chrousos, National Institutes of Health, Bethesda, MD; Dr. Helen Daly, State University of New York, Oswego, NY; Dr. Stanley Dodson, University of Wisconsin, Madison, WI; Dr. Thomas Fox, Harvard Medical School, Boston, MA; Leonard Gianessi, Resources for the Future, Washington, DC; Mr. Michael Gilbertson, International Joint Commission, Windsor, Ontario; Dr. Stanley Glasser, Baylor College of Medicine, Houston, TX; Dr. Roger Gorski, UCLA School of Medicine, Los Angeles, CA; Dr. Mark Hahn, Woods Hole Oceanographic Institution, Woods Hole, MA; Dr. David Hoffman, US Fish and Wildlife Service, Laurel, MD; Dr. Polly Hoppin, World Wildlife Fund, Inc., Washington, DC; Mrs. Frances Irwin, World Wildlife Fund, Inc., Washington, DC; Dr. Allan Jensen, Danish Technological Institute, Taastrup, Denmark; Dr. William Kelce, The Johns Hopkins University, Baltimore, MD; Mr. Garrett Lahvis, University of Maryland, Baltimore, MD; Dr. George Lucier, NIEHS, Research Triangle Park, NC; Dr. Ian Nisbet, I.C.T. Nisbet and Co., Lincoln, MA; Dr. M. Olsen, Swedish Museum of Natural History, Stockholm, Sweden; Dr. Anne Palkovitch, George Mason University, Fairfax, VA; Dr. Stephen Safe, Texas A & M University, College Station, TX; Dr. Wayland Swain, ECO LOGIC, Ann Arbor, MI; Dr. Glen van der Kraak, University of Guelph, Guelph, Ontario; and Dr. Kim Wallen, Emory University, Atlanta, GA.

A number of authors also submitted their papers for review among their peers and within their institutions before submitting them to us for review and publication. In addition to preparing chapters for the book, many authors also spent a great deal of time internally reviewing each others papers. We thank them for sharing their time and expertise.

We would like to extend a special thanks to Mrs. Barbara Rodes, Director of Library Services and Research Librarian, and Ms. Carla Langeveld, Assistant Librarian, World Wildlife Fund, Inc., for their irreplaceable assistance and heartfelt interest throughout the project.

We are indebted to Dr. John Cairns, Jr. for serving as reader and encouraging the publication of this material.

This project was supported by the W. Alton Jones Foundation, Inc., the Charles Stewart Mott Foundation, Inc., the Joyce Foundation, the Keland Endowment Fund of The Johnson Foundation, and World Wildlife Fund, Inc.

# PREFACE

This book is devoted to information that led the individuals who attended a Work Session at the Wingspread Conference Center, Racine, Wisconsin, July 26 to 28, 1991, to arrive at the conclusions presented in Chapter 1. This meeting was attended by a multidisciplinary group of experts in fields relevant to the concern of the meeting, "Chemically Induced Alterations in Sexual Development: The Wildlife/Human Connection".

Interest for the Wingspread Work Session stemmed from a comprehensive review of the literature on adverse health effects in wildlife in the Great Lakes region of North America and Europe, and in marine mammals in the Northern Hemisphere. Encouragement for the Session came from lengthy conversations with biologists who had observed the anomalies in wildlife, with basic scientists who had demonstrated the sensitivity to perturbation of the developing endocrine system, with toxicologists who had reported on the results of exposing laboratory animals to endocrine system disrupting chemicals found in the environment, and with researchers who had documented the similarity in the anomalies in laboratory animals and humans exposed to diethylstilbestrol (DES) in the womb.

No attempt was made to synchronize the literary style of the chapters in this book. Each chapter stands alone, reflecting the discipline, research, and opinions of the author(s). The authors were requested to keep in mind the difficulty a reader might have grasping the jargon of unfamiliar disciplines. Several chapters are short and concise, describing the results of descriptive or manipulative research. Others are quite long, tutorial in nature, reviewing the basic science that provides the foundation for arriving at the Wingspread Work Session conclusions. Other chapters provide overviews to introduce the reader to the vast amount of literature already published on the subject and allow the reader to further explore topics of his or her liking. An acronym list is provided to assist the reader with the jargon from the assorted disciplines.

Following World War II, in the mid 1940s, a giant industrial complex emerged in the Great Lakes region of North America that released vast amounts of industrial and agricultural chemicals into the environment. For a number of years it was assumed that the bountiful water resources of the region were capable of assimilating these chemicals and maintaining the integrity of the system. However, reports started appearing in the scientific literature as early as 1950 indicating that all was not well within the wildlife community. Even today, after years of attempting to regulate the release of contaminants into the Great Lakes environment, top predator species including fish, birds, mammals, and reptiles are exhibiting reproductive problems and are unable to maintain stable populations. In some locations entire populations have been extirpated. Loss of fertility and early mortality in offspring contribute to these problems. The anomalies reported in the offspring that lead to premature death are the result of the offspring's indirect exposure, via the mother, to a mixture of chemicals that biomagnify in the food supply of the Great Lakes food web. We realize now that many chemicals once considered safe because they did not appear to be powerful carcinogens or mutagens and were not acute toxicants, have penetrated the Great Lakes and the organisms in that system, including man. Mass-balance studies reveal that in some instances, such as Lake Superior, long range atmospheric transport contributes more to the overall loading of certain contaminants in the Lake than point sources or agricultural run-off.

An extensive search of the global literature reveals that these chemicals have reached both the Arctic and Antarctic via the atmosphere as well. It also reveals that wildlife in other parts of the world were and are experiencing problems similar to those reported in the Great Lakes. The literature also provides associations between the levels of contaminant in the animals and the loading in the region where the troubled animals were found, and in some cases, shows dose-response relationships between incidences and expression of the effects. Unfortunately, it has taken over forty years, in the case of some chemicals, to come to the full realization of their toxic potential. It has now been determined that these chemicals, if present during critical stages of embryonic, fetal, and perinatal development can disrupt the growth and function of major physiological systems such as the endocrine, immune, and nervous systems, as well as interfere with metabolism. Most disturbing is the fact that, not one, but many chemicals that are produced in large quantities and widely dispersed, have this potential.

Recently a growing concern has been expressed by authors in the peer reviewed literature about the implications of the anomalies reported in wildlife offspring. Our Wingspread Work Session confirmed that the implications for human health are clear. Because of the fragmented and unreplicable nature of the research that has transpired in the past, scientists were unable to support their suspicions with the research from their disciplines alone. As a result when they were given the opportunity to attend the Wingspread Work Session to explore the topic from a multi-disciplinary perspective, to review the cross-discipline similarities, and test their hypotheses, they were delighted to participate. The Wingspread statement quickly emerged from the meeting and was written by individuals representing 17 disciplines. These individuals discussed the problems of endocrine disruption reported in wildlife, the concentrations at which the effects were being reported in the field and the laboratory, the many opportunities for exposure, and the effects reported in humans. The number of reports that paralleled across species and were biologically consistent and coherent added up to an overwhelming case that hormonally active chemicals in the environment pose a risk not only to wildlife, but to humans as well. The weight of evidence was too great to be ignored.

We could not ignore the fact that man-made chemicals in the environment can invade the pristine environment of the womb or the egg and permanently change the course of development and the potential of the developing individual. Nor could we ignore the insidious nature of those changes—changes that might not be recognized until the individual reached adulthood. So shocking was this revelation that no scientist could have expressed the idea using only the data from his or her discipline alone without losing the respect of his or her peers. However, the group speaking as one, gave life to the idea in the form of the Consensus Statement.

As you read this book, focus on the work outside of your discipline. By so doing, you will understand how the Wingspread Consensus Statement evolved.

T.C.

# ACRONYMS

| | |
|---|---|
| 2,4-D | 2,4-dichlorophenoxy acetic acid (herbicide) |
| 2,4-DB | 4-(2,4-dichlorophenoxy) butyric acid (herbicide) |
| 2,4-DP | 2-(2,4-dichlorophenoxy) proprionic acid: dichloroprop (herbicide) |
| 2,4,6-T | 2,4-D analog (herbicide) |
| $^3$H-T | radiolabelled testosterone |
| $^3$H-E$_2$ | radiolabelled estradiol |
| 3-MC | 3-methylcholanthrene |
| $^{125}$I-AFP | radiolabelled alphafetoprotein |
| AC | anterior commissure |
| ACT | American College Testing Scores |
| ACTH | adrenocorticotropin hormone |
| ADI | acceptable daily intake |
| Ah | arylhydrocarbon hydroxylase |
| AFP | alphafetoprotein |
| ai | active ingredient |
| AMP | adenosine monophosphate |
| AR | androgen receptor |
| ARCN | arcuate nucleus |
| As | arsenic |
| ATD | 1,4,6-androstatriene-3,17-dione |
| B[a]P | benzo[a]pyrene |
| b-FGF | basic fibroblast growth factor |
| BLE | bladder epithelium |
| BLS | bladder stroma |
| BPH | benzo[a]pyrene hydroxylase |
| BSRI | Bem Sex Role Inventory |
| BUG | bulbourethral gland |
| CA | cyproterone acetate |
| CB | chlorobiphenyl |
| CBG | corticosteroid binding globulin |
| CCC | chlormequat chloride |
| CDFBS | charcoal-dextran fetal bovine serum |
| CDHuS | charcoal-dextran stripped human serum |
| CMA | Chemical Manufacturers Association |
| CNS | central nervous system |
| CP | cytochrome P-450 |
| CP-450 | cytochrome P-450 |
| DAS | delayed anovulatory syndrome |
| DCBA | Dacthal: dimethyl tetrachlorobenzoic acid (herbicide) |
| DCPA | Dacthal: dimethyl tetrachloroterephthalate (herbicide) |
| DBCP | dibromochloropropane |
| DDD | 1,1-Dichloro-2,2-bis(p-chlorophenyl) ethane: TDE |
| DDE | dichloro diphenyl dichloroethylene (insecticide) |

| | |
|---|---|
| DDT | dichloro diphenyl trichloroethane (insecticide) |
| DES | diethylstilbestrol |
| DESAD | diethylstilbestrol adenosis |
| dioxin | 2,3,7,8-tetrachloro-$p$-dioxin: TCDD |
| DHT | 5 alpha-dihydrotestosterone |
| DME | Dulbecco's modification of Eagle's Medium |
| DMSO | dimethylsulfoxide |
| DNA | deoxyribonucleic acid |
| DZ | dizygotic |
| $E_2$ | estradiol |
| EB | estradiol benzoate |
| EBDC | ethylenebisdithiocarbamate (fungicide) |
| ED50 | statistically estimated dose at which 50% of a tested population produces a specific effect |
| EGF | epithelial growth factor |
| ER | estrogen receptor |
| EROD | ethoxyresorufin $O$-deethylase |
| ETU | ethylene thiourea |
| FASE | Foundation for the Advancement of Science and Education |
| FBS | fetal bovine serum |
| FIFRA | Federal Insecticide, Fungicide, Rodenticide Act |
| FSH | follicle-stimulating hormone |
| g | gram |
| gm | gram |
| GC-MS | gas chromatography-mass spectrometry |
| GnRH | gonadotropin-releasing hormone |
| GX | gonadectomized |
| GZTS | Guilford Zimmerman Temperament Survey |
| HAL | health advisory levels |
| HCB | hexachlorobenzene |
| HCG | human chorionic gonadotropin |
| HCH | hexachlorocyclohexane |
| HPLC | high powered liquid chromatography |
| HSDB | hazardous substance data base |
| HxCdd | hexachlorodibenzo-$p$-dioxin |
| HxCDF | hexachlorodibenzofuran |
| IgA | immune globulin A |
| IgG | immune globulin G |
| IgM | immune globulin M |
| INAH | interstitial nuclei of the anterior hypothalamus |
| i.p. | intraperitoneally |
| IU | international unit |
| KGF | keratinocyte growth factor |
| KME | kraft mill effluent |
| LD50 | lethal dose at which 50% of subjects die |
| LH | luteinizing hormone |

| | |
|---|---|
| LHRH | luteinizing hormone releasing hormone |
| LOAEL | lowest-observable-adverse-effect-level |
| M | molar |
| MAN | medial amygdaloid nucleus |
| MAO | monoamine oxidase |
| MCL | maxium contaminant level |
| MeHG | methylmercury |
| $MgCL_2$ | magnesium chloride |
| MIS | Mullerian inhibiting substance |
| mgd | milligrams per day |
| mg/kg/d | milligrams per kilogram per day |
| ml | milliliter |
| mM | millimolar |
| MPN | medial preoptic area |
| mRNA | messenger ribonucleic acid |
| MSG | monosodium glutamate |
| NaCL | sodium chloride |
| ND | N-demethylase |
| ng/L | nanograms per liter: parts per trillion |
| NK | natural killer white blood cells |
| nM | nanomolar |
| NOEL | no-observed-effect-level |
| MW | molecular weight |
| OC | optic chiasma |
| o,p'-DDD | ortho, para prime DDD (insecticide) |
| o,p'-DDT | ortho, para prime DDT (insecticide) |
| OPP | Office of Pesticide Programs (USEPA) |
| OTS | Office of Toxic Substances (USEPA) |
| PADI | provisional acceptable daily intake |
| PBB | polybrominated biphenyl |
| PBDD | polybrominated dibenzo-dioxin |
| PBDF | polybrominated dibenzofuran |
| PCB | polychlorinated biphenyl |
| PCDD | polychlorinated dibenzo-$p$-dioxin |
| PCDF | polychlorinated dibenzofuran |
| p-CPA | para-chlorophenyl-alanine |
| PCT | porphyria cutanea tarda |
| PE | proliferative effect |
| PeCB | pentachlorobiphenyl |
| PeCDD | pentachlorodibenzo-$p$-dioxin |
| PeCDF | pentachlorodibenzofuran |
| PG | prostaglandin |
| pg/ml | picograms per millimeter: parts per trillion |
| pM | picomoles |
| POA | preoptic area (in hypothalamus) |
| PO-AHA | preoptic-anterior hypothalamic area |

| | |
|---|---|
| ppb | parts per billion |
| p,p'-DDE | para, para prime DDE (insecticide) |
| ppt | parts per trillion |
| PVC | persistent vaginal cornification |
| RBC | red blood cell |
| RfD | reference dose |
| RFF | Resources for the Future |
| RPE | relative proliferative effect |
| RPP | relative proliferative potency |
| SADS-L | Schedule for Affective Disorders and Schizophrenia, Life-time Version |
| sc | subcutaneous |
| SCN | suprachiasmatic nucleus |
| SDN | sexually dimorphic nucleus |
| SDN-POA | sexually dimorphic nucleus of the preoptic area |
| Se | selenium |
| SEM | standard error of the mean |
| SL | standard length |
| SRY | sex determining region of the Y chromosome in human genes |
| Sry | sex determining region of the Y chromosome in mice genes |
| SV | seminal vesicle |
| SVIB | Strong Vocational Interest Blank |
| SVM | seminal vesicle mesenchyme |
| T | testosterone |
| $T_3$ | triiodothyronine |
| $T_4$ | thyroxine |
| Tam | tamoxifen |
| TBT | tributyltin (molluscicide, anti-foulant) |
| TCB | tetrachlorobiphenyl |
| TCBT | tetrachlorobenzyltoluenes (PCB substitute) |
| TCDD | dioxin: 2,3,7,8-tetrachlorodibenzo-$p$-dioxin |
| TCDF | furan: 2,3,7,8-tetrachlorodibenzofuran |
| $T_D$ | the time interval in which an exponentially growing culture doubles its cell number |
| TDF | testis determining factor |
| TEC | TCDD equivalent concentration |
| TEF | toxic equivalency factor |
| TEQs | toxicity equivalents |
| Tfm | testicular feminization |
| THC | tetrahydrocannabinol |
| TP | testosterone propionate |
| TRI | toxic release inventory |
| ug | microgram |
| UGM | urogenital sinus mesenchyme |
| UGS | urogenital sinus |
| URE | ureter epithelium |

| | |
|---|---|
| USDA | United States Department of Agriculture |
| USEPA | United States Environmental Protection Agency |
| USFS | United States Forest Service |
| V | third ventricle |
| VE | vaginal epithelia |
| VMN | ventro medial nucleus |
| VS | vaginal stroma |
| WAIS | Wechsler Adult Intelligence Scale |
| WISC | Wechsler Intelligence Scale for Children |

## STATEMENT FROM THE WORK SESSION ON

## CHEMICALLY-INDUCED ALTERATIONS IN SEXUAL DEVELOPMENT: THE WILDLIFE/HUMAN CONNECTION

### THE PROBLEM

Many compounds introduced into the environment by human activity are capable of disrupting the endocrine system of animals, including fish, wildlife, and humans. The consequences of such disruption can be profound because of the crucial role hormones play in controlling development. Because of the increasing and pervasive contamination of the environment by compounds capable of such activity, a multidisciplinary group of experts gathered in retreat at Wingspread, Racine, Wisconsin, 26-28 July 1991 to assess what is known about the issue. Participants included experts in the fields of anthropology, ecology, comparative endocrinology, histopathology, immunology, mammalogy, medicine, law, psychiatry, psychoneuroendocrinology, reproductive physiology, toxicology, wildlife management, tumor biology, and zoology.

The purposes of the meeting were:

1. to integrate and evaluate findings from the diverse research disciplines concerning the magnitude of the problem of endocrine disruptors in the environment;
2. to identify the conclusions that can be drawn with confidence from existing data; and
3. to establish a research agenda that would clarify uncertainties remaining in the field.

### CONSENSUS STATEMENT

The following consensus was reached by participants at the workshop.

1. *We are certain of the following:*

    • A large number of man-made chemicals that have been released into the environment, as well as a few natural ones, have the potential to disrupt the endocrine system of animals, including humans. Among these are the persistent, bioaccumulative, organohalogen compounds that include some pesticides (fungicides, herbicides, and insecticides) and industrial chemicals, other synthetic products, and some metals.[1]

---

[1]Chemicals known to disrupt the endocrine system include: DDT and its degradation products, DEHP (di(2-ethylhexyl)phthalate), dicofol, HCB (hexachlorobenzene), kelthane, kepone, lindane and other hexachlorocyclohexane congeners, methoxychlor, octachlorostyrene, synthetic pyrethroids, triazine herbicides, EBDC fungicides, certain PCB congeners, 2,3,7,8-TCDD and other dioxins, 2,3,7,8-TCDF and

- Many wildlife populations are already affected by these compounds. The impacts include thyroid dysfunction in birds and fish; decreased fertility in birds, fish, shellfish, and mammals; decreased hatching success in birds, fish, and turtles; gross birth deformities in birds, fish, and turtles; metabolic abnormalities in birds, fish, and mammals; behavioral abnormalities in birds; demasculinization and feminization of male fish, birds and mammals; defeminization and masculinization of female fish and birds; and compromised immune systems in birds and mammals.

- The patterns of effects vary among species and among compounds. Four general points can nonetheless be made: (1) the chemicals of concern may have entirely different effects on the embryo, fetus, or perinatal organism than on the adult; (2) the effects are most often manifested in offspring, not in the exposed parent; (3) the timing of exposure in the developing organism is crucial in determining its character and future potential; and (4) although critical exposure occurs during embryonic development, obvious manifestations may not occur until maturity.

- Laboratory studies corroborate the abnormal sexual development observed in the field and provide biological mechanisms to explain the observations in wildlife.

- Humans have been affected by compounds of this nature, too. The effects of DES (diethylstilbestrol), a synthetic therapeutic agent, like many of the compounds mentioned above, are estrogenic. Daughters born to mothers who took DES now suffer increased rates of vaginal clear cell adenocarcinoma, various genital tract abnormalities, abnormal pregnancies, and some changes in immune responses. Both sons and daughters exposed *in utero* experience congenital anomalies of their reproductive system and reduced fertility. The effects seen in *in utero* DES-exposed humans parallel those found in contaminated wildlife and laboratory animals, suggesting that humans may be at risk to the same environmental hazards as wildlife.

2. *We estimate with confidence that:*

- Some of the developmental impairments reported in humans today are seen in adult offspring of parents exposed to synthetic hormone

---

other furans, cadmium, lead, mercury, tributyltin and other organo-tin compounds, alkyl phenols (non-biodegradable detergents and anti-oxidants present in modified polystyrene and PVCs), styrene dimers and trimers, soy products, and laboratory animal and pet food products.

disruptors (agonists and antagonists) released in the environment. The concentrations of a number of synthetic sex hormone agonists and antagonists measured in the US human population today are well within the range and dosages at which effects are seen in wildlife populations. In fact, experimental results are being seen at the low end of current environmental concentrations.

- Unless the environmental load of synthetic hormone disruptors is abated and controlled, large scale dysfunction at the population level is possible. The scope and potential hazard to wildlife and humans are great because of the probability of repeated and/or constant exposure to numerous synthetic chemicals that are known to be endocrine disruptors.

- As attention is focused on this problem, more parallels in wildlife, laboratory, and human research will be revealed.

3. *Current models predict that:*

- The mechanisms by which these compounds have their impact vary, but they share the general properties of (1) mimicking the effects of natural hormones by recognizing their binding sites; (2) antagonizing the effect of these hormones by blocking their interaction with their physiological binding sites; (3) reacting directly and indirectly with the hormone in question; (4) by altering the natural pattern of synthesis of hormones; or (5) altering hormone receptor levels.

- Both exogenous (external source) and endogenous (internal source) androgens (male hormones) and estrogens (female hormones) can alter the development of brain function.

- Any perturbation of the endocrine system of a developing organism may alter the development of that organism: typically these effects are irreversible. For example, many sex-related characteristics are determined hormonally during a window of time in the early stages of development and can be influenced by small changes in hormone balance. Evidence suggests that sex-related characteristics, once imprinted, may be irreversible.

- Reproductive effects reported in wildlife should be of concern to humans dependent upon the same resources, e.g., contaminated fish. Food fish is a major pathway of exposure for birds. The avian (bird) model for organochlorine endocrine disruption is the best described to date. It also provides support for the wildlife/human connection because of similarities in the development of the avian and mammalian endocrine systems.

4.  *There are many uncertainties in our predictions because:*

-   The nature and extent of the effects of exposure on humans are not well established. Information is limited concerning the disposition of these contaminants within humans, especially data on concentrations of contaminants in embryos. This is compounded by the lack of measurable endpoints (biologic markers of exposure and effect) and the lack of multi-generational exposure studies that simulate ambient concentrations.

-   While there are adequate quantitative data concerning reduction in reproductive success in wildlife, data are less robust concerning changes in behavior. The evidence, however, is sufficient to call for immediate efforts to fill these knowledge gaps.

-   The potencies of many synthetic estrogenic compounds relative to natural estrogens have not been established. This is important because contemporary blood concentrations of some of the compounds of concern exceed those of internally produced estrogens.

5.  *Our judgment is that:*

-   Testing of products for regulatory purposes should be broadened to include hormonal activity *in vivo*. There is no substitute for animal studies for this aspect of testing.

-   Screening assays for androgenicity and estrogenicity are available for those compounds that have direct hormonal effects. Regulations should require screening all new products and by-products for hormonal activity. If the material tests positive, further testing for functional teratogenicity (loss of function rather than obvious gross birth defects) using multigenerational studies should be required. This should apply to all persistent, bioaccumulative products released in the past as well.

-   It is urgent to move reproductive effects and functional teratogenicity to the forefront when evaluating health risks. The cancer paradigm is insufficient because chemicals can cause severe health effects other than cancer.

-   A more comprehensive inventory of these compounds is needed as they move through commerce and are eventually released to the environment. This information must be made more accessible. Information such as this affords the opportunity to reduce exposure through containment and manipulation of food chains. Rather than separately regulating contaminants in water, air, and land, regulatory agencies should focus on the ecosystem as a whole.

• Banning the production and use of persistent chemicals has not solved the exposure problem. New approaches are needed to reduce exposure to synthetic chemicals already in the environment and prevent the release of new products with similar characteristics.

• Impacts on wildlife and laboratory animals as a result of exposure to these contaminants are of such a profound and insidious nature that a major research initiative on humans must be undertaken.

• The scientific and public health communities' general lack of awareness concerning the presence of hormonally active environmental chemicals, functional teratogenicity, and the concept of transgenerational exposure must be addressed. Because functional deficits are not visible at birth and may not be fully manifested until adulthood, they are often missed by physicians, parents, and the regulatory community, and the causal agent is never identified.

6. *To improve our predictive capability:*

• More basic research in the field of developmental biology of hormonally responsive organs is needed. For example, the amount of specific endogenous hormones required to evoke a normal response must be established. Specific biologic markers of normal development per species, organ, and stage of development are needed. With this information, levels that elicit pathological changes can be established.

• Integrated cooperative research is needed to develop both wildlife and laboratory models for extrapolating risks to humans.

• The selection of a sentinel species at each trophic level in an ecosystem is needed for observing functional deficits, while at the same time describing the dynamics of a compound moving through the system.

• Measurable endpoints (biologic markers) as a result of exposure to exogenous endocrine disruptors are needed that include a range of effects at the molecular, cellular, organismal, and population levels. Molecular and cellular markers are important for the early monitoring of dysfunction. Normal levels and patterns of isoenzymes and hormones should be established.

• In mammals, exposure assessments are needed based on body burdens of a chemical that describe the concentration of a chemical in an egg (ovum) which can be extrapolated to a dose of the chemical to the embryo, fetus, newborn, and adult. Hazard evaluations are needed that repeat in the laboratory what is being seen in the field. Subsequently, a gradient of doses for particular responses must be determined in the laboratory and then compared with exposure levels in wildlife populations.

• More descriptive field research is needed to explain the annual influx to areas of known pollution of migratory species that appear to maintain stable populations in spite of the relative vulnerability of their offspring.

• A reevaluation of the *in utero* DES-exposed population is required for a number of reasons. First, because the unregulated, large-volume releases of synthetic chemicals coincide with the use of DES, the results of the original DES studies may have been confounded by widespread exposure to other synthetic endocrine disruptors. Second, exposure to a hormone during fetal life may elevate responsiveness to the hormone during later life. As a result, the first wave of individuals exposed to DES *in utero* is just reaching the age where various cancers (vaginal, endometrial, breast, and prostatic) may start appearing if the individuals are at a greater risk because of perinatal exposure to estrogen-like compounds. A threshold for DES adverse effects is needed. Even the lowest recorded dose has given rise to vaginal adenocarcinoma. DES exposure of fetal humans may provide the most-severe-effect model in the investigation of the less potent effects from environmental estrogens. Thus, the biological endpoints determined in *in utero* DES-exposed offspring will lead the investigation in humans following possible ambient exposures.

• The effects of endocrine disruptors on longer-lived humans may not be as easily discerned as in shorter-lived laboratory or wildlife species. Therefore, early detection methods are needed to determine if human reproductive capability is declining. This is important from an individual level, as well as at the population level, because infertility is a subject of great concern and has psychological and economic impacts. Methods are now available to determine fertility rates in humans. New methods should involve more use of liver-enzyme-system activity screening, sperm counts, analyses of developmental abnormalities, and examination of histopathological lesions. These should be accompanied by more and better biomarkers of social and behavioral development, the use of multigenerational histories of individuals and their progeny, and congener-specific chemical analyses of reproductive tissues and products, including breast milk.

Work Session participants included:

Dr. Howard A. Bern
Prof. of Integrative Biology
(Emeritus) and Research
Endocrinologist
Dept. of Integrative Biology and,
Cancer Research Lab
University of California
Berkeley, CA

Dr. Phyllis Blair
Prof. of Immunology
Dept. of Molecular and Cell Biology
University of California
Berkeley, CA

Sophie Brasseur
Marine Biologist
Dept. of Estuarine Ecology, Research
Institute for Nature Management
Texel, The Netherlands

Dr. Theo Colborn
Senior Fellow
World Wildlife Fund, Inc., and W.
Alton Jones Foundation, Inc.
Washington, DC

Dr. Gerald R. Cunha
Developmental Biologist
Dept. of Anatomy
University of California
San Francisco, CA

Dr. William Davis*
Research Ecologist
U.S. EPA
Environmental Research Lab
Sabine Island, FL

Dr. Klaus D. Döhler
Director Research
Development and Production
Pharma Bissendorf Peptide GmbH
Hannover, Germany

Mr. Glen Fox
Contaminants Evaluator
National Wildlife Research Center
Environment Canada
Quebec, Canada

Dr. Michael Fry
Research Faculty
Dept. of Avian Science
University of California
Davis, CA

Dr. Earl Gray*
Section Chief
Developmental and Reproductive
Toxicology Section
Reproductive Toxicology Branch
Developmental Biology Division
Health Effects Research Laboratory
U.S. EPA
Research Triangle Park, NC

Dr. Richard Green
Prof. of Psychiatry in Residence
Dept. of Psychiatry/NPI
School of Medicine
University of California
Los Angeles, CA

Dr. Melissa Hines
Asst. Prof. in Residence
Dept. of Psychiatry/NPI
School of Medicine
University of California
Los Angeles, CA

Mr. Timothy J. Kubiak
Environmental Contaminants
Specialist
Dept. of Interior
U.S. Fish and Wildlife Service
East Lansing, MI

Dr. John McLachlan
Director, Div. of Intramural Research
Chief, Laboratory of Reproductive and
Developmental Toxicology
National Institute of Environmental
Health Sciences
National Institute of Health
Research Triangle Park, NC

Dr. J.P. Myers
Director
W. Alton Jones Foundation, Inc.
Charlottesville, VA

Dr. Richard E. Peterson
Prof. of Toxicology and
Pharmacology
School of Pharmacy
University of Wisconsin
Madison, WI

Dr. P.J.H. Reijnders
Head, Section of Marine Mammalogy
Dept. of Estuarine Ecology
Research Institute for Nature
Management
Texel, The Netherlands

Dr. Ana Soto
Associate Prof.
Dept. of Anatomy and Cellular
Biology
Tufts University School of Medicine
Boston, MA

Dr. Glen Van Der Kraak
Asst. Prof.
College of Biological Sciences
Dept. of Zoology
University of Guelph
Ontario, Canada

Dr. Frederick vom Saal
Prof.
College of Arts and Sciences
Division of Biological Sciences
University of Missouri
Columbia, MO

Dr. Pat Whitten
Asst. Prof.
Dept. of Anthropology
Emory University
Atlanta, GA

## ACKNOWLEDGEMENT

Funding was provided by the Charles Stewart Mott Foundation, W. Alton Jones Foundation Inc., The Keland Endowment Fund of The Johnson Foundation and World Wildlife Fund.

* Although the research described in this article has been supported by the USEPA, it does not necessarily reflect the views of the Agency and no official endorsement should be inferred. Mention of trade names or commercial products does not constitute endorsement or recommendation for use.

# THE FRAGILE FETUS

**Howard A. Bern**
Department of Integrative Biology and Cancer Research Laboratory
University of California, Berkeley, California

*This chapter underlines the particular sensitivity of the developing organism to exposure to estrogens in the induction of long-term changes in the reproductive tract and elsewhere. It also emphasizes that agents which are weakly estrogenic by postnatal criteria may have major developmental effects especially during a critical period. Exposure of pregnant women and animals to environmental estrogens may pose a threat parallel to that occurring after similar exposure to diethylstilbestrol (DES).*

## INTRODUCTION

As a part of the consideration of the possible effects of environmental agents (Bason and Colborn, Clement and Colborn, Thomas and Colborn herein) on human and animal populations, the action of such agents during embryonic/fetal development demands extensive attention. The issue involved is not only the possible occurrence of birth defects but also the possible long-term effects which in humans may not manifest themselves until adolescence and even much later in life. These effects may result in structural, reproductive, endocrinological, metabolic, immunological, neurological, behavioral, dysplastic, and neoplastic changes, and so the search for the consequences on the offspring of exposure during intrauterine life must be stringent and diversified (see Takasugi and Bern, 1988, Fig. 1). Especially should it be recognized that cryptic (occult) changes may occur, which are difficult to detect and whose consequences may be unpredictable.

This chapter will attempt to outline briefly some of the possibilities in regard to long-term (persistent) effects that require consideration and is based upon experience involved in the analysis of the human "DES syndrome" and in utilizing the neonatal mouse model as an indicator of possible long-term consequences of exposure to estrogens. Two compendia of the results from both human and animal studies are available (Herbst and Bern, 1981; Mori and Nagasawa, 1988), and these volumes and a recent summary article (Bern, 1992) can be consulted for detailed references.

## HUMAN DES SYNDROME AND ITS
## NEONATAL MOUSE MODEL

For a period of about 25 years, the synthetic estrogen diethylstilbestrol (DES) was administered in some countries, including the United States, to pregnant

1. Corresponding Author: Howard A. Bern, Department of Integrative Biology and Cancer Research Laboratory, University of California, Berkeley, CA, 94720.

women threatening premature birth. This orally-effective estrogen was prescribed in various doses and for various periods of time. In 1970, Herbst related several cases of vaginal clear-cell carcinoma in young women to the ingestion of DES by their mothers during the first trimester of pregnancy. It has been estimated that as many as 2-3 million pregnant women may have taken DES during this period, meaning that as many as 1.5 million women offspring, and an equal number of men, may have been exposed to the drug during development.

In the early 1960s, it was found that treatment of neonatal mice with estrogenic steroids or DES led to pathological changes in the female tract, beginning with persistent vaginal stratification and cornification and developing into a variety of dysplastic and possibly neoplastic lesions. If the amounts of estrogen administered in the first few days after birth were large enough, the changes persisted even after ovariectomy, and thus, once induced, were estrogen-independent. The neonatal mouse was thus a preexisting model for the human DES syndrome when the latter was delineated a decade later.

From the analysis of the human syndrome and of its mouse model have emerged several important aspects:

1.   Exposure to estrogen early in embryonic or fetal life can lead to the development of major structural changes in the genital tract (vom Saal et al., on mice herein), including neoplasia.

2.   There are critical periods for such exposure (e.g., human vaginal clear cell carcinoma before the end of the first trimester; murine persistent vaginal and uterine epithelial dysplasias before the 4th postnatal day). The state of development of the human genital tract toward the end of the third month of pregnancy is roughly equivalent to that of the neonatal mouse. Thus, the neonatal mouse can serve as a model for the early prenatal human in regard to reproductive tract development.

3.   Early exposure may not lead to readily recognizable changes at the time of birth. Thus, the type of alteration characteristic of the DES syndrome is not encompassed by the term "birth defect." The consequences, especially neoplastic, of exposure during development may not manifest themselves until adolescent, adult and even senescent life. Studies which report on the presence or absence of congenital anomalies in offspring after exposure of mothers during pregnancy to a particular agent are concerned with only one aspect of the possible consequences. The occurrence of delayed long-term effects must also be considered. Clinical studies using progestins to prevent premature birth, for example, need to consider the experience associated with the use of DES for the same purpose. In a recent report (Green et al., 1991) on children of patients who received mutagenic chemotherapeutic agents in their youth, the absence of congenital anomalies was noted. However, the question of long-term consequences can only be ascertained by lifelong tracking of these children.

4.   From the first observations on mice (Takasugi et al., 1962), it was implied that the postnatal and adult disorders ensuing upon early exposure to estrogen were a consequence of a teratogenic process. In the case of ovary-independent persistent vaginal cornification, the selection of a cell population that would have disappeared normally from the vagina was postulated as the source of the abnormal epithelium (Takasugi, 1976). This kind of thinking also underlies the suggestion that vaginal adenosis in the human DES syndrome arises from the retention of Müllerian epithelium in the upper vagina, an epithelium which normally should not persist in that locale as development proceeds. To these ideas should now be added the possibility that it is not the ectopic epithelium itself that may persist but an underlying ectopic stroma that "instructs" the epithelium in its abnormal differentiation (Cunha et al., herein).

5.   Estrogens vary in potency depending in part upon the assay system used for their assessment. Natural plant estrogens (phytoestrogens such as coumestrol present in alfalfa and other plants or zearalenone which is a mycotoxin) are generally considered to be weak estrogens in assays using immature or mature rodents. However, it may be fallacious to extrapolate the potency of an agent as indicated by postnatal measurements to that which it may demonstrate during development.

6.   The fact that DES-associated vaginal cancer appears only after puberty strongly suggests that exposure to hormones during adolescence may be required. Thus, ovarian estrogens may play a secondary synergistic role in the full expression of changes induced early in development. Studies on mice support this concept of a postnatal contribution from hormones in increasing the severity of abnormal genital tract changes (e.g., Ostrander et al., 1985; Newbold et al., 1991; Mori et al., 1992). Environmental estrogens could obviously serve such a "promoting" role in the origin of adult disorders including neoplasia, and if it is recommended that exogenous estrogens be avoided when possible by DES daughters, the same strictures should apply to contact, generally unintended and unknown, with estrogenic materials in the environment including the diet.

## ADDITIONAL  CONSIDERATIONS

Vertebrates other than humans and mice also prove to be a valuable source of information relevant to the developmental effects of exposure to various agents (see Gray, Peterson et al., vom Saal et al., on rats; Reijnders and Brasseur on marine mammals; Fox on birds; Davis and Bortone, Leatherland, Walker and Peterson on fishes—all herein).

Antiestrogens are so called because they may compete with natural estrogens in binding to estrogen receptor(s) in cells. Most antiestrogens when administered alone are themselves weakly estrogenic. Exposure to such "weak" estrogens may protect the individual by competing for receptors with stronger estrogens, but at higher dose levels the antiestrogens themselves can have major effects, especially during early development. The neonatal mouse reacts to antiestrogens such as tamoxifen and clomiphene in a manner similar to its response to DES or estradiol.

The basis for a greater susceptibility of developing tissues than of postnatal tissues to a particular estrogen, or to weak estrogens (phytoestrogens and antiestrogens), or to agents little related to steroidal estrogens, can only be speculated upon at this juncture. The answer may lie in the concept of "orphan receptors" (McLachlan herein) and/or in the concept of a more "primitive" and less specific type of sex hormone receptor during ontogeny. If the latter phenomenon be correct, the undiscriminating receptor may "see" organic structures as estrogens which the mature receptor would not bind or bind only weakly. The neonatal mouse, for example, reacts similarly to androgens and to progestins as it does to estrogens (steroidal and nonsteroidal) in regard to the induction of genital tract pathology. There is no ready explanation as yet for this promiscuity of responsiveness. What is needed is detailed study of the nature and development of the steroid receptor family during embryogenesis and fetal life—a challenging task which the existence of appropriate molecular probes may facilitate undertaking.

Although the focus of this conference was on reproductive effects, neonatal exposure to sex hormones and related agents has many other, often less dramatic, effects. Even limiting consideration to direct and indirect influences on reproduction, a variety of systems and processes may be implicated, including the hypothalamo-hypophysio-gonadal axis, the central and peripheral nervous systems and behavior (Döhler and Jarzab, Hines, Whitten herein), the immune system (Blair, Blair et al., Bason and Colborn herein), hepatic enzymes, sex ducts and accessory glands (e.g., epididymis, prostate), secondary sex characteristics (e.g., mammary gland), etc. All of these have been shown in the mouse to be affected by neonatal sex hormone exposure. Other systems, including skeletal (e.g., Iguchi et al., 1988) and muscular, may also be influenced. In DES-exposed human offspring, effects on fertility, genital ducts, the immune system, and possibly behavior and "intelligence" have been reported.

There are additional cryptic effects which can be detected in the neonatally DES-exposed mouse. Our laboratory has been particularly concerned with changes in receptor levels, and Table 1 summarizes these studies. Most of the effects are evident only with higher doses of DES. Receptor levels may be upregulated ($\uparrow$) or downregulated ($\downarrow$) depending on the receptor and the target organ. The differential responses of the progestin receptor in the vagina and the uterus and of the estrogen receptor in the prostate and the seminal vesicle clearly demonstrate that generalization without specific experimentation is not justifiable. The relation between receptor changes and hormone sensitivity in these structures requires clarification.

**TABLE 1.    Response of Receptors (R) to Perinatal Exposure of Mice to DES**

Vagina: ↓ estrogen-R; ↑ progestin-R; ↓ EGF-R
Uterus: ↓ estrogen-R; ↓ progestin-R
Mammary Gland: ↓ estrogen-R; ↑ progestin-R

Prostate: ↓ estrogen-R; ↓ androgen-R; ↓ prolactin-R
Seminal Vesicle: ↑ estrogen-R; ↓ androgen-R; ↓ prolactin-R

Examination of epithelial cell cultures derived from the postnatal vagina and prostate indicate changes in growth patterns and in sensitivity to hormones and growth factors as a consequence of neonatal DES exposure. In addition, there are many changes in protein patterns (gene expression—see Newbold et al., 1989) if the vaginal epithelium or the vaginal stroma from neonatally DES-exposed and unexposed adult mice are compared (Uchima et al., 1990; Takamatsu et al., 1992).

The fact that a host of natural and man-made chemicals in the environment may disrupt the neuroendocrine system related to reproduction raises the issue of their estrogenicity. A standard method of assay of such agents for estrogenic activity (such as that proposed by Soto et al. herein) would aid greatly in initial screening. The relative developmental potency of such agents, however, may not be predictable from such an assay system. Thus, after determining potential estrogenicity, *in vivo* testing using the neonatal mouse system may be essential to gauge possible long-term effects. Although many months may be required for the full spectrum of dysplastic, preneoplastic and neoplastic genital lesions to become evident, there are other potentially predictive criteria that can be detected in mice shortly after neonatal exposure: morphological features such as persistent vaginal cornification and its precedent in the form of EGF-positive subepithelial nodules (Ozawa et al., 1991), vaginal fornical adenosis (the heterotopic columnar epithelium of Forsberg), and polyovular follicles; possible receptor and protein pattern alterations. Efforts need to be directed to the formulation of a practical and sensitive system for systematic (routine) testing for long-term developmental effects.

## IMPORTANCE OF CONTINUING DES STUDIES

The two major reasons why concern with the human DES syndrome cannot be allowed to abate derive from (1) the possibility that even though DES is no longer prescribed as an "antiabortive" agent, the large population (particularly in the U.S.A. and in the Netherlands) exposed *in utero* to DES is only now reaching the age of maximal risk for a variety of neoplastic and dysplastic genital disorders, and (2) the possibility of exposure from therapeutic and contraceptive procedures, from ingestion in foodstuffs, and from contact in the environment to substances either which are frank estrogens, steroidal or nonsteroidal, or which possess estrogenic bioactivity. Such agents may have developmental effects that will parallel the DES syndrome and may have adult effects that will promote the emergence of severe consequences of early exposure either to these agents themselves or to DES. These effects are in addition to the reproduction-associated effects generally which are discussed in this volume. It seems evident that epidemiological, histopathological, biochemical and behavioral studies on human and animal populations and experimental analyses *in vivo* and *in vitro* must continue in order to allow potentially disastrous problems to be defined and confronted. Only by the application of results from such studies can "the fragile fetus" be protected.

## ACKNOWLEDGMENTS

Many collaborators have contributed to the studies on the neonatal mouse referred to herein (see Bern, 1992). Dr. Marc Edery has been especially important in the receptor studies. Aided by longtime support from the NIH (grants CA-05388 and CA-09044).

## REFERENCES

Bern, H.A. (1992). Diethylstilbestrol (DES) syndrome: present status of animal and human studies. In *Hormonal Carcinogenesis*, (ed). J. Li, S. Nandi, and S.A. Li. Springer-Verlag, New York. (in press).

Green, D.M., Zevon, M.A., Lowrie, G., Seigelstein, N., and Hall, B. (1991). Congenital anomalies in children of patients who received chemotherapy for cancer in childhood and adolescence. *N. Engl. J. Med.*, **325**, 141-146.

Herbst, A.L. and Bern, H.A. (eds). (1981). *Developmental Effects of Diethylstilbestrol (DES) in Pregnancy*. Thieme-Stratton, New York.

Iguchi, T., Irisawa, S., Uchima, F.-D.A., and Takasugi, N. (1988). Permanent chondrification in the pelvis and occurrence of hernias in mice treated neonatally with tamoxifen. *Reprod. Toxicol.*, **2**, 127-134.

Mori, T., Mills, K.T., and Bern, H.A. (1992). Sensitivity of the vagina and uterus of mice neonatally exposed to estrogen or androgen to postnatal treatment with estrogen or androgen. *Proc. Soc. Exper. Biol. Med.*, **199**, 466-469.

Mori, T. and Nagasawa, H. (eds). (1988). *Toxicity of Hormones in Perinatal Life*. CRC Press, Boca Raton, FL.

Newbold, R.R., Bullock, B.C., and McLachlan, J.A. (1991). Uterine adenocarcinoma in mice following developmental treatment with estrogens: a model for hormonal carcinogenesis. *Cancer Res.*, **50**, 7677-7681.

Newbold, R.R., Pentecost, B.T., Yamashita, S., Lum, K., Miller, J.V., Nelson, P., Blair, J., Kong, J., Teng, C., and McLachlan, J.A. (1989). Female gene expression in the seminal vesicle of mice after prenatal exposure to diethylstilbestrol. *Endocrinology*, **124**, 2568-2576.

Ostrander, P.L., Mills, K.T. and Bern, H.A. (1985). Long-term responses of the mouse uterus to neonatal diethylstilbestrol treatment and later sex hormone exposure. *J. Nat. Cancer Inst.*, **74**, 121-135.

Ozawa, S., Iguchi, T., Sawada, K., Ohta, Y., Takasugi, N., and Bern, H.A. (1991). Postnatal vaginal nodules induced by prenatal diethylstilbestrol treatment correlate with later development of ovary-independent vagina and uterine changes in mice. *Cancer Letters, 58,* 167-176.

Takamatsu, Y., Iguchi, T., and Takasugi, N. (1992). Effects of neonatal exposure to diethylstilbestrol on protein expression by vagina and uterus in mice. *In Vivo,* **6**, 1-8.

Takasugi, N. (1976). Cytological basis for permanent vaginal changes on mice treated neonatally with steroid hormones. *Int. Rev. Cytol.,* **44**, 193-224.

Takasugi, N. and Bern, H.A. (1988). Introduction: abnormal genital tract development in mammals following early exposure to sex hormones. In *Toxicity of Hormones in Perinatal Life*, ed. T. Mori and H. Nagasawa. CRC Press, Boca Raton, FL, pp. 1-7.

Takasugi, N., Bern, H.A., and DeOme, K.B. (1962). Persistent vaginal cornification in mice. *Science,* **138**, 438-439.

Uchima, F.D.A., Vallerga, A.K., Firestone, G.L., and Bern, H.A. (1990). Effects of early exposure to diethylstilbestrol on cellular protein expression by mouse vaginal epithelium and fibromuscular wall. *Proc. Soc. Exper. Biol. Med.,* **195**, 218-224.

# SEXUAL DIFFERENTIATION IN MAMMALS

**Frederick S. vom Saal**
Division of Biological Sciences and John M. Dalton Research Center,
University of Missouri, Columbia, Missouri

**Monica M. Montano**
Division of Biological Sciences and John M. Dalton Research Center,
University of Missouri, Columbia, Missouri

**Ming Hseng Wang**
Division of Biological Sciences and John M. Dalton Research Center,
University of Missouri, Columbia, Missouri

## INTRODUCTION

The period of differentiation of the gonads and accessory reproductive organs varies from species to species. In long-gestation mammals, such as humans and pigs, differentiation of reproductive organs occurs primarily during prenatal life, although some aspects of sexual differentiation may occur after birth. For example, in swine, where pregnancy lasts about 115 days, masculinization (the induction of male traits) begins during the fourth week of fetal life in males in response to the secretion of testosterone by the testes (Ford et al., 1980), but the loss of the capacity to exhibit both female sexual behavior and the cyclic release of gonadotropins (defeminization) occurs in male pigs between 3-4 months after birth as a result of the pubertal rise in testosterone (Ford and D'Occhio, 1989).

In species with a very short gestation length, such as the mouse (18-19 days) and rat (21-23 days), gonadal and secondary sexual differentiation begins during the middle of gestation (Schlegel et al., 1967; Warren et al., 1973) and continues into the neonatal period, which is the transition period from prenatal to postnatal life; in humans this term is used for the first two weeks after birth and in rodents the first few days after birth (Gorski, 1986; Shima et al., 1990). There is evidence is that in rats, there is also a temporal separation of masculinizing and defeminizing effects of gonadal hormones, with masculinization of the brain occurring earlier (beginning during prenatal life) in development than defeminization. Defeminizing effects of gonadal steroids appear to occur primarily after birth, immediately after the dramatic drop in gonadal steroid concentrations of maternal and placental origin (Davis et al., 1979; Nordeen and Yahr, 1983). The ferret offers an interesting contrast to the rat in this regard (Baum, 1979; Baum et al., 1990).

The determination of gonadal sex in mammals involves direct effects of genes and is typically dependent on the presence within species of different sex

---

1. Corresponding Author: Frederick S. vom Saal, 205 Lefevre Hall, Division of Biological Sciences, University of Missouri, Columbia, MO 65211.

chromosomes in males and females. In lower vertebrates (fish, amphibians and reptiles), what is remarkable is the degree of diversity found in the process of primary (gonadal) sex determination in species which are not phylogenetically very distant from each other. For example, in reptiles, such as lizards and turtles, temperature acts to regulate sex determining genes, although the effect of temperature in these two reptiles is opposite: in lizards, high temperatures result in males, while in turtles, high temperatures result in females (Bull, 1980; Janzen and Paukstis, 1991). Even in closely related species, the male can be found to be the heterogametic sex (i.e., produces gametes with different sex chromosomes, for example, X or Y) in one species while the female is the heterogametic sex in the other (Witschi, 1959; Becak, 1983). Alternatively, some lower vertebrates show no chromosomal differences between the sexes (Ohno, 1967).

In fish, the most primitive class of vertebrates, there is true hermaphroditism, i.e., the presence of functional oocyte-containing and spermatocyte-containing gonads and thus the capacity to fertilize and be fertilized. The hermaphroditic organism may be capable of self fertilization and/or cross fertilization (Harrington, 1961). While this is the typical perception of hermaphroditism, sequential hermaphroditism also occurs in which first the gonads function as one sex and then at a later time function as the other sex. For example, in fish referred to as protandrous, the gonads produce sperm when the organism is young and then at an older age, the gonads differentiate into ovaries and produce oocytes. Alternatively, in fish referred to as protogynous, the gonads produce oocytes when the fish is young and then at an older age, the gonads metamorphose and begin producing sperm; this reproductive strategy insures that only the most fit of the species survive to reproduce as males.

In vertebrates other than fish, hermaphroditism typically occurs due to errors in development and is thus rare (McKelvie et al., 1987). Situations in which the gonads contain both ovarian and testicular tissues occur, but the organism is always sterile (Becak, 1983). More common in mammals is pseudohermaphroditism, where external appearance is discordant with gonadal sex and, typically, the rest of the internal genitalia as well (Imperato-McGinley, 1979; Baker, 1980).

Gonadal sex determination in mammals is not influenced by environmental events and is referred to as syngamic. However, the genetic basis of sex determination may differ from that of most mammals in a few selected species of rodents and monotremes, which are primitive, reptile-like mammals (Fredga, 1983; Byskov and Hoyer, 1988). Prior to the twentieth century, the environment was presumed to determine sex in mammals as well as other animals. The observation by Painter (1923) that there were different chromosomes in men and women led to the hypothesis that, similar to drosophilia, the number of X chromosomes (in relation to autosomes) determined sex. Subsequently, the critical role of the Y chromosome in sex determination in mammals was revealed

(Page et al., 1987; Bianchi, 1991). Specifically, a gene on the Y chromosome interacts with genes on other chromosomes to produce a signal that leads to the development of the testes, irrespective of the number of X chromosomes (e.g., XY, XXY, XXXY, XXXXY, etc.).

The time in development at which differentiation of the gonads in male and female mammals occurs is typically quite different. While the germ cells migrate into the indifferent gonad at the same time in male and female embryos, the onset of morphological differentiation of the ovary in females begins considerably later (around the third to fourth month of fetal life in humans) than gonadal differentiation in males (during the second month of gestation). This temporal difference in the differentiation of testes and ovaries led to speculation that the main action of sex determining gene(s) was to regulate the rate of gonadal development (Mittwoch et al., 1969; Mittwoch, 1973). The secretion of testosterone coincident with morphological differentiation by the male gonad would then also render other aspects of sexual differentiation asynchronous in males and females (Fox, 1987).

Witschi proposed the concept of cortico-medullary antagonism to explain the differential development of the cortex and medullary region of the female and male embryonic gonad (Chang and Witschi, 1956). This idea stemmed from observations of amphibian larvae which were fused together. For example, in frogs, the presence of the testes partially interfered with development of the ovaries, while in salamanders, the testes completely inhibited ovarian differentiation (Burns, 1961; Witschi, 1967).

In birds, females are the heterogametic sex and actively differentiate in response to hormonal stimulation (similar to male mammals); the basic developmental program is followed by the homogametic sex while active processes are involved in the differentiation of sexual phenotype in the heterogametic sex. There may be communication between the two gonads in birds: the left gonad may suppress development of the right gonad in genetic females. For example, in chickens (Gallinaceae), if the normally-developed left ovary is removed prior to twenty days after hatching, the right rudiment enlarges and becomes a sperm producing testis; however, since there would be no duct system to transport the sperm, the animal is sterile. Along with testis development from the rudimentary right gonad after removal of the left ovary, the female develops male secondary sexual characteristics, such as a comb, plumage, and male copulatory behaviors. Estrogens secreted by the left ovary have been found to be involved in the suppression of the right gonad (Burns, 1961). An interesting aspect of humans which show true hermaphroditism (although they are sterile) is that the ovarian tissue is typically located in the left gonad while testicular cords are more commonly found in the right gonad, although either gonad might also contain both cortical and medullary structures typical of the female and male gonad, respectively (van Niekirk, 1974).

The pioneering work of Jost (1972, 1985) showed that in mammals, differentiation of the testes in males was a necessary prerequisite to masculinization of the accessory reproductive organs and external genitalia. This finding led to studies which demonstrated the critical role of testosterone, the primary androgen secreted by testes in fetuses as well as adults, in masculinizing not only the reproductive organs and external genitalia, but enzyme systems in other tissues, such as the liver, kidney and brain (De Moor et al., 1973; Einarsson et al., 1973; Colby, 1980; Bardin and Catterall, 1981). During fetal life these tissues express androgen receptors (which bind testosterone or its 5α-reduced metabolite, 5α-dihydrotestosterone, DHT) or estrogen receptors (which bind the aromatized metabolite of testosterone, estradiol). Masculinization of these tissues thus occurs in response to high levels of testosterone in the systemic circulation, intracellular reduction or aromatization of testosterone, binding of testosterone or one of its metabolites to receptors, and the activation of gene transcription (Pelliniemi and Dym, 1980; Bardin and Catterall, 1981; Wilson et al., 1981; Jost, 1985; Rories and Spelsberg, 1989).

The concept that during development testosterone exerts an organizing (irreversible) action on neuroendocrine function in males (Pfeiffer, 1936; Harris and Jacobson, 1952; Barraclough and Leathem, 1954) was extended to the study of the differentiation of behaviors relating to reproduction (Harris, 1964; Young et al., 1964). However, in contrast to the organizing effects of steroids on the structure and functioning of organs, most sexually dimorphic behaviors are not viewed as being irreversibly organized. Even though the hormonal milieu of a developing male or female may influence the animal's behavior after birth, postnatal social factors also have profound effects which can override hormonal influences during early life. There is thus considerably greater plasticity in terms of hormonal influences during early life on behavior than had initially been appreciated (vom Saal, 1983a, 1989a; Gorski, 1986). It is unclear at this time what role genotype, hormones, and postnatal social factors play in the development of human gender identity (the perception of oneself as male, female or inbetween) and sexual orientation (which sex one is attracted to). But, once established, sexual orientation does not appear to be easily altered (Baker, 1980; Ehrhardt and Meyer-Bahlburg, 1981; Hines and Green, 1991), contradicting the suggestion that reversal of sexual identity and orientation at puberty can readily occur (Imperato-McGinley et al., 1979).

Since mammalian sexual differentiation (other than gonadal sex) is regulated by hormones, sexual phenotype (morphology, physiology and behavior) is inherently variable. Considerable individual variability in plasma steroid concentrations is typically reported in studies of fetuses (humans: Reyes et al., 1974; Monkeys: Resko, 1975; rats: Weisz and Ward, 1980; mice: vom Saal and Bronson, 1980; vom Saal, 1989a). There is also considerable variability in the responsiveness of organs in different individuals to the same blood concentrations of hormones; steroid metabolizing enzymes and numbers of hormone receptors in tissues determine the capacity for tissues to respond to hormones, and both steroid metabolizing enzymes and steroid receptor numbers are regulated by genes as well as steroid hormones (Meyer et al., 1975; Gower and Cooke, 1983; Hall, 1988; Nonneman et al., 1992).

In litter-bearing species: rats (unpublished observation), mice (vom Saal, 1989a) and gerbils (Clark et al., 1991), the sex of adjacent fetuses influences the blood concentrations of sex steroids within a fetus, since steroids pass between fetuses via diffusion through the amniotic fluid across the fetal membranes surrounding each fetus (Even et al., 1992; vom Saal and Dhar, 1992). In single-birth species, there is also considerable variability in plasma sex steroid levels in fetuses (Reyes et al., 1974; Resko, 1975), but, as yet, the etiology of this variability (maternal ovaries, placentae, fetal gonads, differential rates of metabolism) remains unknown. However, the consequence of exposure to high vs. low levels of testosterone (and other hormones) is likely to be similar in all mammals, regardless of whether the source of the variability in hormone levels is of unknown origin in humans or due to the number of adjacent male fetuses or other variables, such as maternal stress, in mice (vom Saal et al., 1990).

It has been argued that variability in sexual phenotype, itself, may be adaptive (vom Saal, 1984). It is possible that natural selection operated in higher vertebrates to have hormones regulate sexual differentiation due to the fact that blood levels of hormones are influenced by a wide range of factors (maternal environment, sex of adjacent fetuses, etc.) and are thus highly variable. Increased variability would be particularly adaptive in situations in which a parent produces many offspring in a constantly changing environment (Real, 1980); the more variability in phenotype, the more likely that at least some of an individual's offspring might successfully reproduce and thus propagate one's genes, since there would be no one optimum phenotype for all possible environments which might be encountered by one's offspring.

## DETERMINATION OF GONADAL SEX

### Differentiation of the Testes

At the beginning of the fourth week after fertilization in humans, movement of the primordial germs cells from the yolk sac endothelium toward tissue bordering the dorsal part of the coelomic cavity begins (Moore, 1982; Figure 1). By the sixth week of gestation the germ cells have migrated into one of two masses of tissue which project into the coelomic cavity, referred to as the genital ridges (previously, these were referred to as germinal ridges due to confusion concerning the site of origin of the germ cells). These tissue masses consist of mesenchyme (the medullary area of the embryonic gonad) with a surface covering of coelomic epithelium (the cortex of the embryonic gonad). The first morphological sign of differentiation of the embryonic gonad into a testis is the aggregation of mesenchyme cells into seminiferous (testicular) cords surrounding invading germ cells in the medullary area of the genital ridge (Figure 2). The seminiferous cords have been variously proposed to be derived from coelomic epithelium,

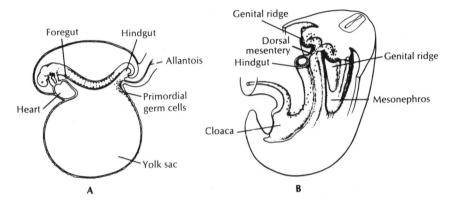

**FIGURE 1.** Schematic drawings showing (A) the location of primordial germ cells in a 3-week human embryo in the yolk sac at the caudal end of the embryo and (B) the path of their migration around the gut and dorsal mesentery and into the genital ridge, during which time they are undergoing mitotic divisions. (From Ham and Veomett, 1980, p. 575).

mesenchyme or from the mesonephric tubules (Pelliniemi and Dym,1980; Byskov and Hoyer, 1988). During the time of migration of the germ cells they undergo rapid mitotic divisions, so that whereas there are only a few hundred primordial germ cells in the yolk sac endoderm, in humans there are many hundreds of thousands at the time they migrate into the genital ridges.

The seminiferous cord mesenchyme differentiates into Sertoli cells, which form intimate contact with, and both support and regulate, the undifferentiated germ cells. The seminiferous cords eventually become surrounded by connective tissue, which likely is secreted by the Sertoli cells. A critical early function of the Sertoli cells is the synthesis and secretion of Müllerian inhibiting substance (MIS), which is also known as antiMüllerian hormone (Josso, 1986; Byskov and Hoyer, 1988; Rabinovici and Jaffe, 1990). The seminiferous cords do not develop a central canal (at which time they are referred to as seminiferous tubules) prior to sexual maturation and the onset of fertility associated with puberty.

Between the seventh and eighth week of gestation, stromal tissue derived from mesenchyme differentiates into the steroid secreting Leydig cells, which are located in the interstitial area between the seminiferous cords (Pelliniemi and Niemi, 1969; Byskov and Hoyer, 1988; Rabinovici and Jaffe, 1990). The Leydig cells rapidly begin secreting testosterone, which is responsible for initiating subsequent events referred to as secondary sexual differentiation.

In mammals, the Y chromosome carries a gene whose product is referred to as the testis determining factor (TDF), even though this factor does not, by itself, mediate the series of developmental events described above which result in the differentiation of the indifferent gonad into a testis; how many other genes are

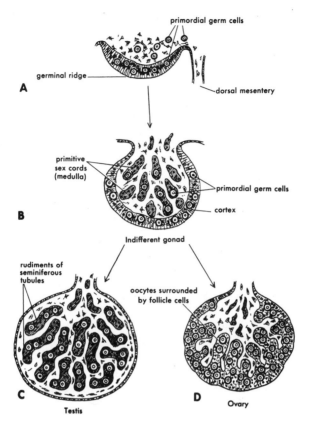

**FIGURE 2.** Diagram showing development of gonads in higher vertebrates. (A) Genital ridge stage (previously referred to as the germinal ridge); primordial germ cells partly embedded in epithelium of the ridge and located partly in the adjacent mesenchyme. (B) Indifferent gonad; germ cells in the cortex and in primary sex (seminiferous) cords. (C) Gonad differentiating as testis; cortex reduced; germ cells in sex cords (future seminiferous tubules). (D) Gonad differentiating as ovary; primary sex cords reduced; proliferating cortex contains the germ cells (From Balinsky, 1975, p. 432).

involved, and the chromosomes on which they are located, remains to be determined. Also unclear at this time is the cell population in which TDF expression is critical for testis formation, although it is assumed that the Sertoli cells, but definitely not the germ cells, play a critical role in the induction of testicular differentiation (McLaren, 1991). Gonads in embryos lacking a Y chromosome (for example with XO, XX, XXX, XXXX, XXXXX sex chromosomes) develop into ovaries. While the presence of a Y chromosome leads to masculinization of the gonads, all other aspects of the masculine and feminine phenotype are mediated through differential exposure of males and females to gonadal (and other) hormones (Jost, 1985).

Two repeated sequences of DNA on the long arm of the Y chromosome in humans account for about 70% of DNA in the Y chromosome (Cook et al., 1983). Based on an examination of 3 men with XX sex chromosomes and 1-XX intersex patient, Palmer et al., (1989) suggested that the TDF should be within segment 1A1 of the short arm of the Y chromosome (Yp). Based on detailed maps of segment 1A1, a gene called SRY (sex determining region of the Y chromosome) was cloned in humans (Sinclair et al., 1990), and its equivalent, Sry, in mice was also found (Gubbay et al., 1990). When the Sry, but not SRY, was introduced into XX female mouse embryos, it was able to initiate testis formation and, subsequently, lead to full phenotypic sex reversal in the XX transgenic adults (Koopman et al., 1991). Therefore, this genomic DNA fragment appears to contain the entire TDF (i.e., Sry) and includes all regulatory elements required for appropriate embryonic expression of the mouse testis (McLaren, 1991).

Structural homologies between the X and Y chromosomes have been proposed to be the basis for pairing of X and Y chromosomes during meiosis; they also provide evidence for a common evolutionary ancestor for both chromosomes (Goodfellow, 1983). One hypothesis concerning the evolution of differences in X and Y chromosome morphology is that an inversion led to the prevention (at least partial) of crossing over and thus the isolation of the two chromosomal units from each other. Mutation of genes would then lead to different sex determining traits (Becak, 1983). Models concerning situations in which selection could operate to produce extreme sex chromosome heteromorphism have been described (Bull, 1983, p. 249).

*Differentiation of the Ovaries*
Organization of the mammalian ovary into its adult form occurs later in embryonic life than does differentiation of the testes in males. However, in humans, but not all mammals, prior to organization of the primordial follicles, hormones are secreted which can influence ovarian differentiation as well as other aspects of sexual differentiaton (Wilson et al., 1981; Josso, 1986; Byskov and Hoyer, 1988; Vigier et al., 1989).

After invasion of the genital ridge by germ cells, there are mitotically active germ cells associated with mesenchymal cells in the medullary area of the ovary as well as clusters of germ cells in the cortical area. Oocytes which remain in the medullary area of the developing gonad degenerate or migrate with associated cells (proposed to be of mesonephric rete origin; Byskov and Hoyer, 1988) into the cortical region. In the differentiated ovary, primordial follicles consist of an oocyte surrounded by a single layer of follicular cells in the cortical area of the gonad, while the medullary area of the ovary consists of stromal tissue (connective tissue, blood vessels, nerves, lymphatics, etc.). Whether all follicular cells in primordial follicles differentiate from coelomic epithelium or are also of mesonephric origin remains controversial (Pelliniemi and Dym, 1980; Byskov and Hoyer, 1988; Rabinovici and Jaffe, 1990).

The greatest population of oocytes is achieved during embryonic life (in most species) or by early postnatal life (Zuckerman and Baker, 1977). The formation of primordial follicles (and the initiation of meiosis) in the cortical region of the ovary occurs over many months in humans, with maximal rates of formation of follicles occurring around the fifth month of fetal life. After peak numbers of primordial follicles are reached in mammals (about 6 million total for both ovaries in humans), there then begins a rapid depletion of follicles and the oocytes in them (by 6 months after birth, only 1 million remain), but the rate of decline is not constant throughout life (vom Saal and Finch, 1988).

Most follicles become atretic (undergo degenerative changes), and relatively few are selected for continued growth into mature follicles. Some follicles begin the early phase of growth during fetal life while others remain as primordial follicles until midlife. However, the continuation of growth into mature follicles can only occur between puberty and reproductive senescence with appropriate hormonal control, which is not present prior to puberty. Why some follicles are selected to begin further development during fetal life while others remain as primordial follicles until midlife remains unknown, although it has been proposed that the origin of the follicular cells (cortex or mesonephric rete cells) may be a factor (Byskov and Hoyer, 1988). The production-line hypothesis proposed that follicles containing oocytes which began meiosis earliest in fetal life were the first to be selected for development. However, at least in short-lived mammals, the evidence does not support this hypothesis (Speed and Chandley, 1983; vom Saal and Finch, 1988).

The total (mice: Gosden et al., 1983; women: Richardson et al., 1987) or near total (rats: Sopelak and Butcher, 1982) depletion of oocytes, which results in menopause in women and signals the end of fertility in all mammals, typically occurs long before the maximum lifespan. Reproductive senescence signals the absence of sufficient follicular cells to secrete a sufficient amount of estradiol to stimulate target tissues, such as the breast, vagina, uterus, etc. These organs begin to involute, thus reversing many of the changes that occurred at puberty when an increase in estradiol secretion leads to growth of estrogen-sensitive tissues. The fate of germ cells and hormone-secreting follicular cells in ovaries thus differs dramatically from that of germ cells and Leydig cells in the testes. Testicular germ cells maintain a stem cell population which, in healthy males, continues to provide mature spermatozoa throughout the lifespan (vom Saal and Finch, 1988).

Oogonia enter the first meiotic division during fetal life even in short gestation rodents such as rats and mice (Borum, 1966). However, this occurs shortly after birth in hamsters, which have the shortest gestation length (16 days) of any mammal (Challoner, 1974). Meiosis is then arrested during the first meiotic prophase. While there are species differences in the timing of the reinitiation of meiosis, in the majority of mammals this is coupled with the preovulatory surge in luteinizing hormone (LH), and the final stages of meiosis are completed only after fertilization (Baker, 1972; vom Saal and Finch, 1988).

Gonadotropins may have an organizing effect on the process of follicular growth and atresia, although the requirement for, and effects of, hormonal stimulation during early follicular development is controversial (Challoner, 1975; vom Saal and Finch, 1988; Rabinovici and Jaffe, 1990). For example, in mice and rats plasma, follicle stimulating hormone (FSH) levels are significantly higher in females (levels reach those observed in ovariectomized adult females) than in males during the first few weeks after birth. Plasma LH levels are also somewhat elevated in females, but only slightly above adult diestrus levels (Goldman et al., 1971; Stiff et al., 1974; Dullaart et al., 1975). Estrogens and MIS may also play a role in oocyte and follicular maturation during this early critical period in some species (Reiter et al., 1972; Angelova and Jordanov, 1986; Josso, 1986; Mazur and Younglai, 1986; Byskov and Hoyer, 1988; Vigier et al., 1989; Miller, 1990; Rabinovici and Jaffe, 1990).

The presence of two X chromosomes in females, while males have only one X chromosome, was initially puzzling. Compensation for an extra chromosome (dosage compensation) is thought to be required for the homogametic sex. The finding by Lyon (1970) that the Barr body was an inactivated X chromosome provided an answer to this problem for mammals, but the mechanisms of dosage compensation in other vertebrates remain to be determined (Becak, 1983; Hodgkin, 1990). In mammals, inactivation of the extra X chromosome in females occurs in all cells during early embryonic life. The inactivated X then begins replicating out of phase with the rest of the chromosomes. In premeiotic germ cells (oogonia), one X chromosome is still inactive, but with the onset of meiosis, reactivation occurs. In women with XO genotype, the absence of two functional X chromosomes in the oocyte may be similar to the lethal effect of autosomal monosomy (the complete absence of one of a pair of homologous chromosomes due to nondisjunction). Secondary to the death of oocytes in XO women is gonadal dysgenesis (complete loss of the gonad). Reactivation of the extra X in XXY men (Kleinfelder's syndrome) may also occur during meiosis, which may produce effects similar to tetrasomy for autosomes; men with Kleinfelder's syndrome also experience gonadal dysgenesis (Schellhas, 1974).

## HORMONAL REGULATION OF SEXUAL DIFFERENTIATION

While the determination of gonadal sex is mediated by genes in mammals, the differentiation of all of the other aspects of an organism's morphology, physiology and behavior, which distinguish males from females within a species, is mediated by hormones produced by the gonads acting in conjunction with hormones and a variety of "factors" produced in other tissues. In mammals, shortly after the onset of differentiation of the embryonic gonads into testes, testosterone is secreted at a high rate into the circulation (and also possibly into the embryonic ducts located near the gonad) by Leydig cells (Tapanainen et al.,

1981, 1984; Huhtaniemi, 1985). Testosterone is clearly the hormone which serves to initiate the process of masculinization and some aspects of defeminization. Müllerian inhibiting substance mediates the loss (defeminization) of the Müllerian ducts in male fetuses; after the onset of differentiation of organs, such as the testes, the developing organism is typically referred to as a fetus rather than an embryo (Moore, 1982).

Testosterone, or its metabolites, can act directly in target tissues to regulate cell proliferation and protein synthesis. However, many actions of testosterone are likely to be indirect, with the high levels of testosterone secreted by the fetal testes inducing a cascade of endocrine changes. Many specific aspects of sexual differentiation may thus be mediated by other hormones, growth factors, neuropeptides, glucocorticoids, etc., which are different in male and female fetuses due to the initial action of testosterone (Gupta, 1988; Rabinovici and Jaffe, 1990; vom Saal et al., 1990; Montano et al., 1991).

Establishment of the female phenotype normally proceeds only in the absence of secretion of high levels of testosterone and MIS from the testes. Whether differentiation in females is independent of ovarian control, as suggested by Jost (1985) remains controversial. However, there is evidence for active effects of estrogen of ovarian and extra-ovarian origin on ovarian as well as psychosexual differentiation (Reiter et al., 1972; Döhler et al., 1984a; Angelova and Jordanov, 1986; vom Saal, 1989a; Rabinovici and Jaffe, 1990). In some mammals, including humans, the ovaries secrete estrogen during the time of sexual differentiation, which occurs prior to the organization of primordial follicles (George et al., 1979; Wilson et al., 1981; George and Wilson, 1987).

Estrogen may be necessary for normal phenotypic development. In both the male and female fetal circulation there are high levels of estradiol and other estrogens (see below). In the mouse, there is no detectable estradiol during the last few days of pregnancy in the fetal ovaries (unpublished observation). The fetal ovaries are able to synthesize estrogen *in vitro* with supplemental FSH and co-factors in some species (George et al., 1979; Terada et al., 1984; Weniger, 1989). Since rat and mouse placentae secrete progesterone and androgen, but not estrogen, the various sources of the high level of estrogen in fetal blood in rats and mice are not clear (Gibori and Sridaran, 1981; Soares and Talamantes, 1982, 1983; Jackson and Albrecht, 1985). However, the maternal ovaries contribute to estrogen in the fetal circulation in rats (Jackson and Albrecht, 1985; Bassett and Pete, 1987; Sridaran and Gibori, 1987). The placenta is the primary source of estrogen in the fetal circulation in primates (Diczfalusy, 1968; Resko et al., 1975), although the fetal ovaries also contribute to estradiol in the fetal circulation (George and Wilson, 1987).

Progesterone is the primary gestagen in that it is required for the maintenance of pregnancy. Progesterone levels are quite high during pregnancy in both maternal and fetal plasma (Tulchinsky et al., 1972; Resko, 1975; vom Saal and Bronson,

1980; Weisz and Ward, 1980). Progesterone can exert an antiandrogenic effect on developing fetuses, and progesterone has been proposed to modulate the action of testosterone in target tissues in rats and monkeys (Resko, 1975; Shapiro et al., 1976; Bardin and Catterall, 1981). The ratio of testosterone to progesterone in plasma may thus be important rather than the individual concentrations of each steroid.

*Critical Periods vs. Sensitive Periods in Brain Development*
The critical period hypothesis of sexual differentiation of behavior was proposed many years ago (Harris, 1964). Although there is overwhelming evidence refuting this hypothesis for many behaviors (Beach, 1975; vom Saal, 1983a), it is still commonly regarded as applying broadly to the development of behaviors which differ between males and females. Specifically, the concept of critical periods in development, which applies to differentiation of embryonic tissues (such as formation of the seminal vesicles and vas deferens from the Wolffian ducts) was applied to the differentiation of areas of the brain mediating sexual behavior and neuroendocrine function relating to LH secretion. For example, it is clear that if the embryonic Wolffian ducts are not induced to differentiate by testosterone during a brief period during early fetal life, then these ducts will degenerate due to programmed cell death. Differentiation of Wolffian ducts at a subsequent time could thus not possibly occur. There is a similar critical period during which Müllerian ducts respond to MIS, while exposure after the critical period is without effect (Burns, 1961). However, the evidence is that the differentiation of many behaviors relating to reproduction (such as mounting and intermale aggression) and LH secretion in rodents is not restricted to an absolute critical period in development (vom Saal, 1983a; Gorski, 1986; vom Saal and Finch, 1988).

While some specific morphological features, such as cell density, in specific brain regions can only be modified during critical periods, no definitive behavioral correlate of any sex difference in brain morphology has, as yet, been found in mammals (Gorski et al., 1978; Arnold, 1980; Commins and Yahr, 1984; Jacobson et al., 1985; Baum et al., 1990; LeVay, 1991). Rather, the brain areas which work together to mediate specific behaviors are characterized by plasticity. A dramatic example is individuals with hydrocephalis who may show gross structural abnormalities in the brain but whose behavior may be relatively normal. Similarly, the dramatic recovery of brain function, including behavior, which can occur following brain damage is in marked contrast to most other organs; this occurs even though neurons in mature mammals are unable to undergo mitosis (with the exception of the olfactory epithelium). This plasticity may reflect the tremendous redundancy of function in the mammalian brain.

A permanent, organizational change in brain function induced by gonadal steroids is generally thought to only be possible during a restricted critical period during the first few days after birth in rats or during prenatal life in long-gestation species (Young et al., 1964; Harris and Levine, 1965). In contrast, exposure to gonadal steroids after the presumed critical period was only thought to result in transient activational effects; when a specific hormone was present an effect would be observed, but when the hormone was withdrawn, the effect would disappear. Animals are typically gonadectomized and administered hormones to order to distinguish the sex differences that are permanent (due to differences in hormone exposure during the critical period in development) and the sex differences which are only observed in response to differences in plasma levels of hormones.

In contrast to the hypothesis that organizational effects of hormones only can occur during a restricted critical period in development, there is direct experimental evidence for permanent (organizational) effects of gonadal steroids on the brain as well as reproductive organs throughout life (vom Saal and Finch, 1988). For example, guinea pigs have a long gestation period (9-10 weeks) relative to rats and mice (about 3 weeks). Contrary to initial reports that the organization of sexual behavior was restricted to prenatal life in guinea pigs (Phoenix et al., 1959), treatment with the synthetic estrogen, estradiol dipropionate, after birth increased male sex behavior in adulthood in female guinea pigs (Feder and Goy, 1983). The loss of the capacity to show female sexual behavior and defeminization of the female pattern of LH release in male swine has also been related to the pubertal rise in testosterone, not sex differences in gonadal hormones during fetal life (Ford and D'Occhio, 1989). Brawer et al. (1978) have shown that a single injection of another synthetic estrogen, estradiol valerate, to an adult female rat quickly leads to anovulatory sterility and the absence of cyclic changes in sexual receptivity. In addition, prolonged exposure of adult female mice to the synthetic estrogen, ethynyl estradiol, resulted in permanent changes in the functioning of the vaginal epithelium (Jesionowska et al., 1990).

With regard to behavior, two different developmental processes have been identified (vom Saal, 1983a). First, aggression in mice provides an example of the process of sensitization rather than organization of brain areas during early life by testosterone. Aggression in mice was initially presumed to be organized during a critical period after birth in males, such that in adulthood, only animals exposed to high levels of testosterone during the critical period of organization of the brain would exhibit aggressive behavior when again exposed to testosterone in adulthood (vom Saal, 1983a). However, this hypothesis was refuted by the finding that female mice would exhibit aggression when treated with testosterone only in adulthood, but these normal females had to be administered testosterone for a longer period of time than was the case for females previously treated with testosterone during early life. Females administered testosterone during early life were thus simply rendered more sensitive to subsequent exposure to testosterone, no prior organization was involved (vom Saal, 1979, 1983a; Simon and Whalen, 1987).

The above findings thus refuted the hypothesis that exposure to high levels of testosterone during a critical period in development is an absolute requirement for the activation of aggressive behavior by testosterone in adulthood; there is no organized difference in the brain with regard to aggression in mice. The distinction between the process of sensitization as opposed to organization was initially made by Beach (1945). The capacity for steroids to sensitize the brain to subsequent exposure to the same steroid may change with age, but the capacity for steroids to exert sensitizing effects does not stop at the end of a defined critical period (vom Saal, 1983a).

The second process involves organizing effects of steroids on behaviors which do not require subsequent exposure to specific gonadal steroids to be observed in adulthood. These behaviors include play behaviors in infant monkeys (Young et al., 1964; Harlow et al., 1966) and adult urination patterns in dogs (Beach, 1975), which are different in males and females even when they have their gonads removed at birth. Prenatal treatment with testosterone also increases the frequency of male-like behavior in females without any subsequent exposure to testosterone. These permanently organized behaviors are thus in marked contrast to aggression in adult mice, where a threshold level of testosterone in the blood is required for aggression to be elicited by another mouse, which must also have circulating testosterone to provide the pheromonal stimulus which elicits an attack (vom Saal, 1983a). The results of most studies show that sexual behaviors (mounting and intromission in males and lordosis in females) are organized during perinatal (fetal/neonatal) life in short-gestation rodents (Yahr, 1988), although there are some findings contradicting this hypothesis. Specifically, the inability for male rats to show lordosis in response to treatment with estradiol was thought to reflect the permanent loss of this capacity due to the defeminizing action of testosterone (via aromatization to estradiol) during the perinatal period of sexual differentiation. However, Sodersten et al. (1983) have reported that with a specific injection regime of estradiol, adult male rats show lordosis.

*Differentiation of Accessory Reproductive Organs and External Genitalia*
Prior to gonadogenesis, both male and female embryos develop a dual, bilateral ductal system: mesonephric ducts and paramesonephric ducts. The mesonephric ducts develop from the pronephric ducts (or remnants of this tissue located in the dorso-posterior region of the abdomen near the eventual position of the adult kidney) prior to differentiation of the paramesonephric ducts (Figure 3). The mesonephric ducts extend caudally to the urogenital sinus and are also referred to as the Wolffian ducts. Development of each paramesonephric (Müllerian) duct then begins as an evagination from the pronephros or, in some species, from coelomic epithelium derived from the pronephros. The paramesonephric ducts lie just lateral to the mesonephric ducts and open cranially into the coelomic cavity via funnel-shaped ends. Caudally, the two paramesonephric ducts fuse in the midline prior to entering the urogenital sinus (Figure 4). The metanephric duct, which differentiates into the ureter, begins as a bud off of the caudal portion of

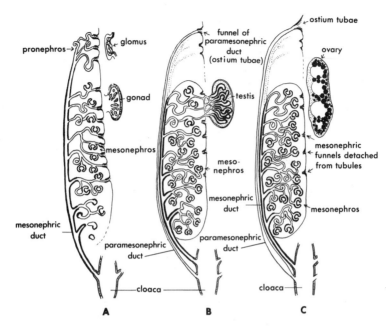

**FIGURE 3.** Diagram showing the transition from the indifferent stage of the urogenital system (A) into the male condition (B) and the female condition (C) in frogs. (From Balinsky, 1975, p. 435).

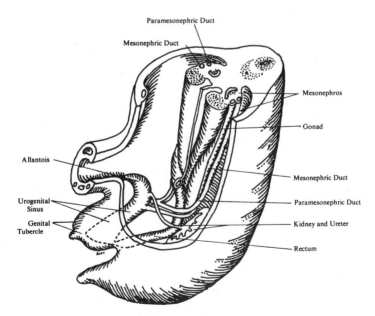

**FIGURE 4.** Genital ducts prior to differentiation. Drawing of a human embryo at about 42 days of age with the upper half and left body wall cut away to demonstrate the gonad, mesonephros and associated ducts, and urogenital sinus. The gut and its mesentery have also been removed. (From Allan, 1960, p. 119).

the mesonephric duct and then extends cranially until it comes in contact with the differentiating kidney. The absence of a Wolffian duct will result in the absence of the ipsilateral Müllerian and metanephric ducts, suggesting an inducing action of the Wolffian duct (Balinsky, 1975, p. 423).

*External genitalia.* External genitalia are derived from a tissue mass called the genital eminence, which is composed of a genital tubercle flanked by a pair of labiosacral swellings (Figure 5). The urogenital folds surround the base of the cloaca, which differentiates into the posterior rectum and the anterior urogenital sinus (Figure 4), which is closed by a thin membrane (Ham and Veomett, 1980).

In males, testosterone secreted from the fetal testes results in masculinization of the external genitalia, while in the absence of testicular testosterone, female reproductive organs develop. For complete masculinization of external genital tissue to occur, the reduction of testosterone to $5\alpha$-dihydrotestosterone (DHT) by the enzyme $5\alpha$-reductase is required (Imperato-McGinley et al., 1979; Wilson et al., 1981; Brown and Migeon, 1984).

In females, the labioscrotal swellings differentiate into the labia majora. The urogenital folds form into the labia minora, which merge to form a hood over the clitoris, which develops from the genital tubercle (Figure 5). In males, the urogenital folds fuse over the opening of urogenital sinus from posterior to anterior forming the midline raphe. The genital tubercle elongates and forms the penis, which eventually encloses the urethra (Figure 6). The two genital swellings fuse with the genital tubercle and form the scrotum.

*Accessory reproductive organs in males.* Two essential secretions of the fetal testes occur after gonadal differentiation begins: (1) Müllerian-inhibiting substance, a glycoprotein, is secreted by the Sertoli cells and acts locally to suppress the development of the ipsilateral Müllerian duct; the effect of MIS is mediated via mesenchyme and does not involve the release of proteolytic enzymes from lysosomes (Donahoe et al., 1985; Josso, 1986); (2) testosterone is secreted by Leydig cells (Huhtaniemi, 1985) and mediates differentiation of the ipsilateral Wolffian duct; without exposure to testosterone during a restricted critical period, programmed death of Wolffian ducts occurs.

*Epididymis, ductus deferens, and ejaculatory duct.* In male embryos, the tubules associated with the cranial end of each mesonephric duct differentiate into the epididymis, which connects via the efferent ducts in the rete area of the testes with the seminiferous tubules (the embryonic seminiferous cords; Figure 3). The central segment of the Wolffian duct becomes the vas deferens. The seminal vesicle develops as a bud off of the lower portion of the Wolffian duct just before it joins the urogenital sinus (Figure 7). The duct below the seminal vesicle is referred to as the ejaculatory duct, which enters the urethra after passing through the utricular region of the prostate (Figure 8).

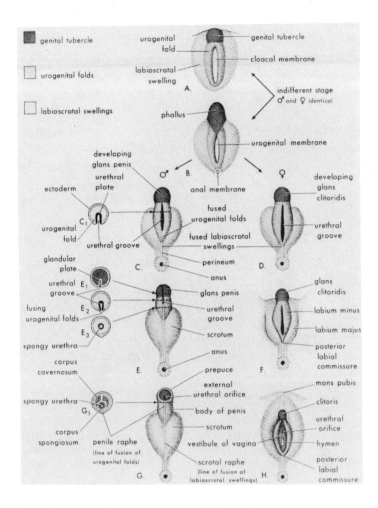

**FIGURE 5.** Diagrammatic representation of differentiation of external genitalia in human embryos. (A) Cloaca at 4 weeks gestation. Intestinal and genitourinary tracts are not yet separated. (B) Urogenital sinus (closed by a thin membrane) at 7 weeks. Male and female are indistinguishable at this stage. (C) and (D) Male and female at 9 weeks. Appearance remains similar except that the urogenital folds have begun to fuse in the male. Limited fusion of labioscrotal swellings in both sexes has increased the distance between the anus and urogenital sinus. (E) and (F) Male and female at 11 weeks. In the male, fusion of the genital folds to yield an elongated urethra is complete except near the end of the penis. A cleft has formed in the glans penis for the urethra. Labioscrotal swellings have fused, forming the scrotum. (G) and (H) Male and female at 12 weeks. Genital differentiation is essentially completed in both sexes. The male urethra extends to the tip of the penis. The prepuce (foreskin) is growing over the glans penis. A raphe (line of fusion) is clearly evident on both the scrotum and penis. In the female the urethra and vagina are fully separated. The genital tubercle has grown less rapidly than the surrounding tissue and has become the clitoris. the urogenital fold and labioscrotal swelling have become the labia minora (singular = labium minus) and the labia majora (singular = labium majus), respectively. (Figure from Moore, K.L. 1982, p. 282; text from Ham and Veomett, 1980, p. 626).

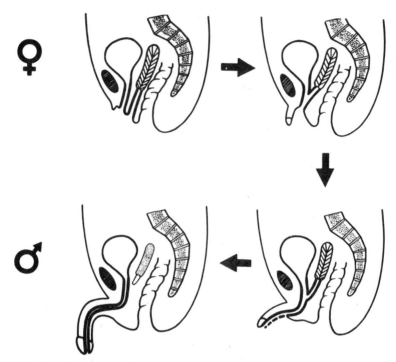

**FIGURE 6.** Diagram to illustrate the development of the normal male and female reproductive tract in man, and varying degrees of intersexuality. In the normal female (top left), the clitoris is vestigial and the urinary and genital ducts open separately. This basic pattern is established by the 16th week of gestation and cannot subsequently be altered. Masculinizing influences before the 16th week can produce enlargement of the clitoris and fusion of the urinary and genital ducts (top right), or an actual phallus with a penile urethra which may open at its base (bottom right). In the normal male (bottom left) the uterus has become vestigial. (From Overzier, 1963).

*Seminal vesicles.* Morphogenesis of the seminal vesicles has been extensively studied in the mouse. On Day 15 of fetal life seminal vesicle morphogenesis begins with dilation of the lower region of the Wolffian duct (Figure 7). After Day 17 of fetal life, buds growing into the mesenchyme are identifiable (Lung and Cunha, 1981). Differentiaiton of the seminal vesicles involves an inducing action of mesenchyme on epithelium, similar to findings in other accessory reproductive organs (Cunha et al., this volume). Lateral branching of ducts occurs during the first week after birth (Lung and Cunha, 1981) and, unlike the initial phase of differentiation, which is mediated by testosterone binding to androgen receptors, branching occurs as a result of 5$\alpha$-dihydrotestosterone binding to androgen receptors (Shima et al., 1990). In adult mice, seminal vesicle fluid influences sperm motility (Peitz, 1988) and removal of the seminal vesicles decreases fertility (Peitz and Olds-Clarke, 1986).

*Prostate.* The prostate develops from the embryonic urogenital sinus (Figure 7). The prostate is located just underneath the bladder and encloses the urethra (the

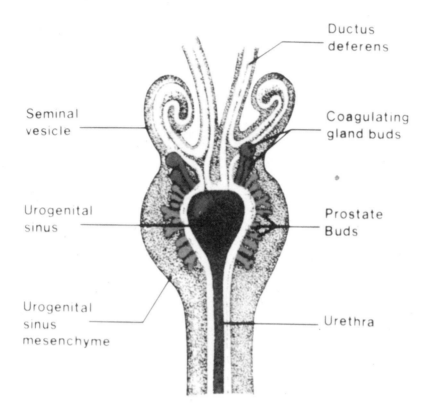

**FIGURE 7.** Ventral view of the reproductive tract of the 1-day-old mouse during growth of prostatic epithelial buds into the surrounding urogenital sinus mesenchyme. At this stage of development, the two large epithelial rudiments of the coagulating gland, which emanate from the cranial aspect of the urogenital sinus, are visible. The solid prostatic epithelial buds which are shown are destined to form the dorso-lateral prostate and are just beginning to branch. The bladder, which lies in front of the seminal vesicles and ductus deferens, has been removed for clarity (From Cunha, et al., 1987).

prostatic urethra) and the ejaculatory ducts (Figure 8; Figure 9). Sex steroids act via mesenchymal tissue to induce differentiation of the prostatic ducts; androgen binding in epithelial tissue is not required (Cunha et al., 1987). The ducts begin as solid mesenchymal-epithelial buds, which later branch extensively and canalize to form tubulo-alveolar glands (Cunha et al., this volume). While periurethral mesenchymal tissue is associated with the formation of prostatic buds, which originate from the urogenital sinus, subsequent ductal branching is associated with contact of the prostatic buds with mesenchymal tissue located in the dorsal and ventral regions of the urogenital sinus in rats (Timms and DiDio, 1990; Timms et al., 1992). In humans, the first lateral buds of the prostate are observed during the tenth week of gestation.

It is now accepted that glands in the prostate in adult men are best grouped into zones (peripheral, transition, periurethral and central; Figure 10) rather than

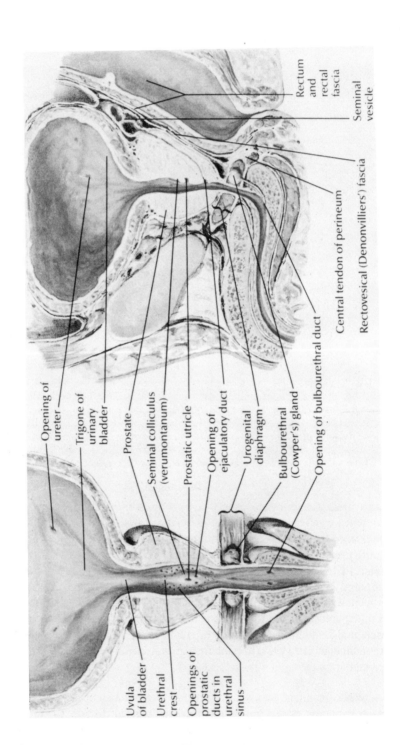

**FIGURE 8.** Drawing of a frontal (left) and mid-sagittal (right) view of the urogenital tract of the adult human male. (From Netter, 1989).

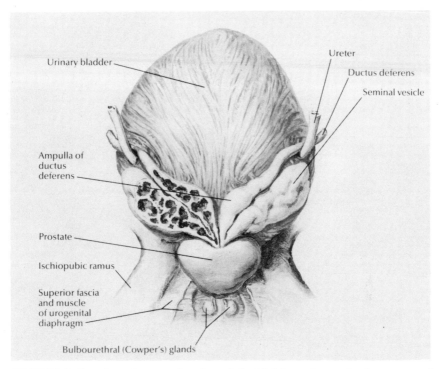

**FIGURE 9.** Drawing of a posterior view of the bladder and reproductive organs of the adult human male. (From Netter, 1989).

forming discrete lobes (Franks, 1954; McNeal, 1980; Blacklock, 1983; Aumuller, 1989). However, during fetal life in humans, the developing ducts of the prostate give the organ a lobular appearance (Shapiro, 1990). Lowsley (1912), who developed the idea of the human prostate having lobes, only examined tissue from fetuses and infants (Figure 11).

In the adult, each ejaculatory duct merges with the ipsilateral seminal vesicle duct (these are of Wolffian duct origin) and passes through the central zone as the common ejaculatory duct (Figure 9), each of which leads into the prostatic urethra next to an enlarged portion of the urethral crest, the verumontanum (also referred to as the colliculus seminalis); the ducts comprising the utricular prostate (McNeal's central zone) empty into the urethra at the verumontanum (Figure 8). The urethra passes posteriorly from the bladder to the verumontanum and then it bends and angles forward as it passes out of the anterior-caudal prostate through the external sphincter, which is striated muscle (Figure 10). The part of the urethra rostral to the verumontanum is surrounded by circular smooth muscle and is referred to as the preprostatic sphyncter (this functions to stop retrograde ejaculation into the bladder), which is continuous with the internal sphyncter above.

The urethra has gland openings throughout the prostate which form distinct sets of prostatic ducts extending from the prostatic urethra. Beginning in the cranial

Rostral

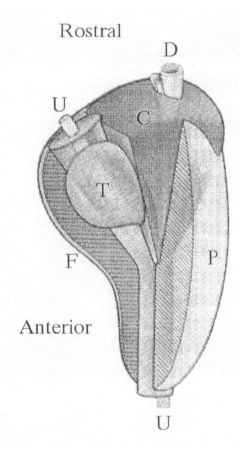

Anterior

**FIGURE 10.** Schematic diagram of the zones of the prostate in adult men. (D) ejaculatory duct (each duct enters the cranial prostate posterior and lateral to the urethra; see Figure 8); (U) urethra surrounded by preprostatic sphyncter muscles passes in a posterior direction to the verumontanum and then angles forward, after which it is surrounded by external sphyncter muscles, (T) transition zone, (P) peripheral zone - this is cut away to show the other zones, (C) central zone, (F) anterior fibromuscular stroma - this is cut away to show the other zones.

portion of the prostatic urethra in men, the periurethral glands open into the urethra above the verumontanum (because of the closing of the internal sphincter at ejaculation, these glands should not contribute to seminal fluid). The periurethral glands are very few in number as well as very short and straight. They comprise less than 1% of the prostate (Shapiro, 1990) and are contained within the preprostatic sphincter (referred to as the preprostatic segment) and the anterior fibromuscular stroma in the non-glandular region of the prostate (Figure 10). Second, the transition zone ducts extend out from a short urethral segment located just below the periurethral ducts and above the verumontanum; they comprise about 5% of the prostate. Third, the central zone (about 25% of the prostate) ducts open right at the verumontanum. The central zone is absent in dogs and cats; the seminal vesicles are also absent in these species. Fourth, the ducts leading to the peripheral zone, which forms the bulk (70%) of the prostate, extend out of the caudal prostatic urethra below the verumontanum (McNeal, 1980). Dogs and cats have homogenous prostate tissue similar to the peripheral zone in humans (McNeal, 1980, 1981; Aumuller, 1989).

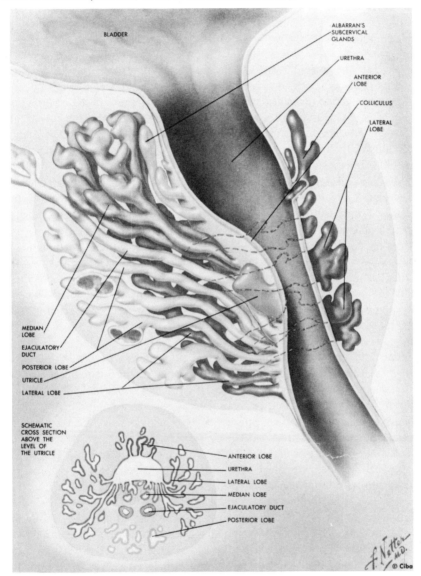

**FIGURE 11.** Drawing of the developing prostatic ducts (divided into lobes) in the newborn human male based on the findings of Lowsley (1912). (From Netter, 1954).

In mice, the coagulating glands develop from buds located on each side of the cranial portion of the urogenital sinus, just lateral to the opening of the Wolffian ducts (Figure 7; Lung and Cunha, 1981; Cunha et al., 1987). The coagulating gland of the rodent appears to be homologous to the craniodorsal lobe of the prostate in monkeys. The craniodorsal lobe of the prostate in the monkey secretes a substance that forms a coagulum when mixed with seminal vesicle fluid, which suggests a similarity of function with the coagulating gland in the rodent. The lateral tips of the dorsolateral lobe in the rat concentrate zinc, which is similar to the peripheral lobe in humans, also suggesting a homology (Blacklock, 1983).

The size of the utricular area of the prostate varies dramatically in men. Abnormal enlargement of this area of the prostate is implicated in fetal death, although this is rare (Zonadek and Zonadek, 1974). Because of the contribution of Müllerian tissue to this area of the prostate, it is possible that the size of this area of the prostate in men is related to differential exposure to estrogen (and/or MIS) during differentiation of the prostate (Zuckerman, 1936); another possibility is exposure to estrogenic chemicals in the environment (see below). This has clinical implications for men in that the transition and central zones of the prostate (which includes the utricular area) becomes hyperplastic in the majority (about 80%) of men who live beyond 70 years of age. Benign, hyperplastic enlargement of the prostate can result in occlusion of the urethra and is the most common (and expensive) disease associated with old age in humans (McNeal, 1978; Carter and Coffey, 1990). It is interesting that seminal vesicles and the central zone of the prostate are mostly resistant to the development of malignant carcinoma, which is restricted to the peripheral zone (70-80%) and transition zone (10-20%) of the prostate; 5-10% of cancers are in the central zone (Rotkin, 1983; Drago, 1989).

Administration of the synthetic estrogen, diethylstilbestrol (DES) to pregnant women resulted in marked hyperplasia and metaplasia of prostatic ducts near the verumontanum in the region of the utricular prostate (Lowsley's medial lobe and the central zone of the adult prostate; Driscoll and Taylor, 1980; Blacklock, 1983). Squamous metaplasia of prostatic and coagulating gland ductal epithelium in male mice and rats has also been reported after exposure to exogenous estrogen or estrogenic chemicals during early life (McLachlan et al., 1975; Arai et al., 1978), which is also characteristic of the effect of estrogen on rat prostatic cells in culture (Martikainen et al., 1987).

Estrogen given to adult, castrated guinea pigs resulted in atrophy of glands in the caudal prostate, while there was a continuation of secretion by glands in the rostral prostate, which have their origin near the utricular plate (Lipschutz et al., 1945). The finding that the degenerative changes induced by estrogen therapy for benign prostatic hyperplasia in old men are greater in the lower prostate than in the central zone, where ducts enter the urethra at and above the colliculus (similar to the finding in guinea pigs), provides evidence of differential sensitivity of regions of the prostate to estrogen (Blacklock, 1983). The estrogen sensitivity and Müllerian derivation of utricular area of the prostate (Glenister, 1962) suggests that the use of estrogen in the treatment of prostatic hyperplasia (to inhibit the brain-pituitary-gonadal axis) should be re-evaluated.

*Regression of Paramesonephric (Müllerian) ducts.* Müllerian inhibiting substance does not have an equivalent effect in males throughout the Müllerian duct system; sensitivity of Müllerian duct to MIS is greatest in the cranial portion of the duct and progressively decreases in the direction of the urogenital sinus (Josso, 1986). The lower part of the Müllerian duct becomes separated from the degenerating upper part of the duct and may persist in males, although this is highly variable (Zuckerman, 1936, 1938; Glenister, 1962). That this variability may be related to endogenous levels of estradiol in male fetuses (discussed further below) is suggested by the finding that treatment of pregnant females with diethylstilbestrol appears to interfere with the action of MIS on Müllerian duct regression in mice (McLachlan et al., 1975) and humans (Driscoll and Taylor, 1980).

The point at which the Müllerian ducts join the urogenital sinus is referred to as the vaginal plate in female embryos; this is a solid mass of cells separating the sac-like end of the Müllerian ducts (utricular region) from the urogenital sinus. In the male this tissue is more appropriately referred to as the utricular plate. This is an area where Wolffian, urogenital sinus and Müllerian epithelium all mingle, so it is embryologically very complex. This area gives rise to the prostatic utricle and primitive periurethral ducts, which extend cranially into the undifferentiated fibromuscular stroma. The periurethral glands in the female are homologous with this section of the prostate in the male (Blacklock, 1983). Below the utricular plate the epithelium is of urogenital sinus endodermal origin; the lower part of the definitive prostatic urethra and penile urethra differentiate from urogenital sinus below the utricular plate.

*Testicular androgen secretion.* The regulation of testosterone synthesis in fetal testes is still not completely understood in many species. In rats, testosterone content in the fetal testes dramatically increases between Day 15 and 18 of prenatal life, then remains constant for the remainder of intrauterine life (Warren et al., 1984). When the episodic pulsatile release of testosterone, which is characteristic of many adult male mammals, including men, begins is not known (Desjardins, 1981). Both LH in fetal serum and testicular LH receptors dramatically increase throughout the last third of pregnancy (Slob et al., 1980; Warren et al., 1984). There is LH-like activity in placental secretions as well as the fetal pituitary, but to date, there is no explanation for the onset and maintenance of testosterone secretion in male rat fetuses (e.g. Huhtaniemi et al., 1983; Habert and Picon, 1986; Habert et al., 1989). In humans, secretion of the placental glycoprotein, human chorionic gonadotropin (HCG), preceds secretion of testosterone by the fetal testes (Reyes et al., 1973; Rabinovici and Jaffe 1990). It has been recognized for some time that in humans, and many other mammals (excluding rabbits), anencephalic fetuses undergo normal sexual differentiation, which shows that a functional neuroendocrine system and/or pituitary is not required for the fetal testes to secrete testosterone (Zonadek and Zonadek, 1970; Jost, 1972, 1985).

*Accessory reproductive organs in females.* While the male gonads undergo marked changes immediately after invasion of the germ cells, the organization of the female gonad is delayed. The gonad in genetic females can only be recognized as a potential ovary by the continuing mitosis of the primordial germ cells and the failure to develop seminiferous cords. Later, condensation of the epithelial cells occurs as they surround the germ cells to form primordial follicles in the cortical (epithelial) region of the ovary, while the medullary cords regress. The follicular cells secrete an outer basement membrane, the membrana propria, and become the granulosa cells of the follicle. The germ cells stop mitotic activity and give rise to oogonia, which enter into the first meiotic division and then are arrested in the first meiotic prophase; MIS and estradiol (and possibly other substances) have been implicated in this process (Donahoe et al., 1985; Josso, 1986; Ueno et al., 1989). However, the role of MIS in the paracrine control of germ cells as well as other aspects of gonadal differentiation is still unresolved; MIS has also been suggested to play an active role in testicular differentiation (Vigier et al., 1989).

In females, the cranial portion of the Müllerian duct becomes the fallopian tube; the distal end of the fallopian tubes forms the ciliated fimbria. In some species (such as rodents, but not humans) a bursa encapsulates the fimbria and ovary such that when oocytes are shed from follicles at ovulation, the ova do not enter the peritoneal cavity proper. The caudal end of the Müllerian duct forms the uterus and upper part of the vagina. In the undifferentiated embryo, contact of the Müllerian duct with urogenital sinus induces the formation of the uterovaginal plate. The central cells of the plate break down to form the lumen of the upper vagina. The urogenital sinus differentiates into the lower one-half to two-thirds of the vagina. Wolffian ducts persist only in remnant form in females.

As will be discussed further below, during fetal life female fetuses have high circulating levels of testosterone relative to adulthood in many species (humans: Reyes et al., 1973, 1974; monkeys: Resko, 1975; mice: vom Saal, 1989a). However, due to the absence of the much higher levels of testosterone (both systemic and in the immediate vicinity of the testes) seen in males, the active processes of masculinization and defeminization do not occur. Differentiation of fetuses with XX genotype into females is thus generally assumed to not require gonadal hormones to induce tissues to differentiate in a feminine direction. However, there is evidence that some aspects of female development involve active processes which are influenced by ovarian secretions (Hendricks and Duffy, 1974; Pappas et al., 1978; Jansson and Frohman, 1987; Blizzard and Denef, 1973; Stenberg, 1975). For example, normal folliculogenesis (differentiation of oocytes and follicles) may require high levels of gonadotropins (of pituitary and/or placental origin) and estradiol (Reiter et al., 1972; Challoner, 1974, 1975; Angelova and Jordanov, 1986). Estradiol also acts to inhibit degeneration of

Müllerian ducts, while testosterone accelerates degeneration (Donahoe et al., 1985).

## Intrauterine Position

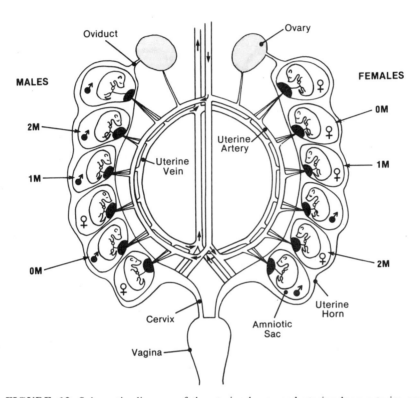

**FIGURE 12.** Schematic diagram of the uterine horns and uterine loop arteries and veins of a pregnant mouse at term. The intrauterine position of fetuses is determined at cesarean delivery. The labels 0M, 1M and 2M originally referred to the number of contiguous male fetuses. These labels are still used, even though fetuses are now classified based on proximity to both male and female fetuses; a 2M fetus is located between two male fetuses, a 1M fetus is located between a male and a female, and a 0M fetus is located between two female fetuses. Arrows within the uterine loop artery and vein indicate the direction of blood flow as revealed by injecting carbon dye into the maternal heart (for arterial flow) and into individual placentae (for venus flow; vom Saal and Dhar, 1992).

Naturally occurring variation in the levels of testosterone and estradiol in female mouse, rat and gerbil fetuses (due to being positioned *in utero* between male or between female fetuses) leads to marked differences in a wide range of reproductive traits: genital morphology, timing of puberty, length of estrous cycles, age at the cessation of fertility, aggressive and sexual behavior, and sexual attractiveness (Figure 12; Figure 13; vom Saal and Bronson, 1978, 1980; vom Saal, 1981, 1989a, 1989b; vom Saal and Moyer, 1985; vom Saal et al., 1990; Clark et al., 1991). These findings provide additional evidence that gonadal

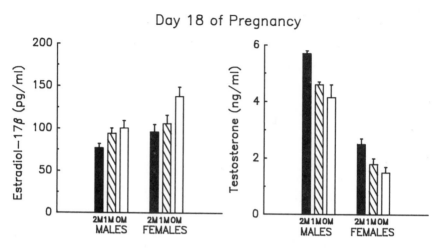

**FIGURE 13.** Serum concentrations of testosterone and estradiol-17β in mouse fetuses from different intrauterine positions on Day 18 of pregnancy (Day of mating = Day 0, parturition = Day 19). For both testosterone and estradiol, male vs. female, and within each sex, intrauterine position differences were statistically significant (From vom Saal, 1989a).

steroids have marked effects on the *normal* course of sexual differentiation in females. If variation in these traits is related to gonadal steroid levels in female rodents, then there is every reason to believe that a similar relationship occurs in other female mammals, such as humans, which also show marked individual variation in gonadal steroid levels during the fetal period of sexual differentiation (Reyes et al., 1973, 1974). This is a markedly different view of the normal process of sexual differentiation in female mammals than the view that endogenous gonadal steroids do not play an active role in the differentiation of the female phenotype. An important aspect of these findings is that variation inendogenous steroid concentrations within a "normal" range leads to marked variation in reproductive traits in female rodents without rendering any of the animals infertile (vom Saal and Bronson, 1978; vom Saal and Moyer, 1985; vom Saal et al., 1991).

*The freemartin syndrome in cattle.* The freemartin is an interesting condition which occurs most commonly in cattle, but may also occur less frequently in other domestic animals (Marcum, 1974). The freemartin describes a female calf born co-twin with a male. The two placentae form anastomoses with the result that the male and female fetus share a common blood supply, and virtually all freemartin females are sterile (Marcum, 1974); lower fertility has also been reported in the male co-twin in cattle (Dunn et al., 1979). Animals which produce litters appear to have evolved protective mechanisms against this possibility (vom Saal, 1989a). This phenomenon is unusual in that a freemartin may have one functional ovary while the other gonad may contain testicular tissue. Also, there is a variable degree of regression of Müllerian duct derivatives, development of Wolffian duct derivatives, and masculinization of the external genitalia, suggesting different degrees of action of androgen and MIS. Jost (1972) showed that injections of a variety of androgens into pregnant cattle did not result in the formation of ovotestes. This result was expected since, as described above, gonadal steroids do not mediate testicular differentiation. However, incubating sheep ovaries with MIS inhibited their capacity to synthesize estrogen (via inhibition of aromatase biosynthesis) and led to the formation of irregular seminiferous cord-like structures which secreted testosterone, which is characteristic of a freemartin's ovaries (Vigier et al., 1989). While the above finding is interesting, the etiology of the freemartin phenomenon is, as yet, not understood.

*Metabolism and Binding of Steroids in Target Cells*
In some tissues testosterone acts directly to regulate masculinization by binding to androgen receptors (for example, in the embryonic Wolffian ducts, which differentiate into the epididymides, vas deferens and seminal vesicles). In contrast, in other tissues intracellular steroid metabolizing enzymes alter the action of circulating testosterone. Intracellular enzymes may convert testosterone into an inactive metabolite or to another biologically active steroid, such as estradiol, which may then be secreted back into the circulation where it is available for entry into other target cells. Alternatively, intracellular enzymes may amplify the action of testosterone via conversion to a metabolite which has a greater biological activity in the cell than does testosterone. The same enzyme might serve each of the above functions in different cells.

*5α-reductase*. In organs which differentiate from Wolffian ducts, such as the seminal vesicles and epididymis, 5α-reductase is not required for normal differentiation, since human males with a genetic mutation resulting in a deficiency in 5α-reductase show normal Wolffian duct development (Wilson et al., 1981), and 5α-reductase is expressed after the initial period of sexual differentiation (Siiteri and Wilson, 1974). Thus, while intracellular formation of DHT is important for the functioning of these organs after differentiation, DHT is not involved in differentiation (Schultz and Wilson, 1974; Wilson et al., 1981; Schleicher et al., 1984). However, in mice, DHT is synthesized in seminal vesicles and epididymides during differentiation of these organs (Shima et al., 1990; Tsuji et al., 1991). This may explain why the female mouse differs from the human female in the response to elevated plasma levels of testosterone (or other synthetic androgenic compounds) during the fetal period of sexual differentiation. Exposure of female mouse fetuses to the synthetic androgen, testosterone propionate, (via administration to the mother) during the fetal period of sexual differentiation in mice results in differentiation of the seminal vesicles in females (vom Saal, 1979; 1989a). Testosterone levels during sexual differentiation in male mice are correlated with number of androgen receptors, 5α-reductase activity and weight of seminal vesicles in adulthood, which provides additional evidence for effects of circulating testosterone on seminal vesicle differentiation in mice (vom Saal et al., 1983; Keisler et al., 1991; Even and vom Saal, 1992; Nonneman et al., 1992).

Testosterone mediates differentiation of the embryonic urogenital sinus into the prostate and urethra (and associated glands) and masculinization of the external genitalia (penis and scrotum) after being metabolized by 5α-reductase to DHT; this also is observed in some areas of the brain (Negri-Cesi et al., 1986; Melcangi et al., 1988; Lephart et al., 1990). A deficiency in the capacity to synthesize 5α-reductase leads to a marked inhibition of masculinization of urogenital sinus tissue during the critical period of genital differentiation (Bardin and Catterall, 1981). The psycho-social consequences of the 5α-reductase-deficiency syndrome in humans is controversial (Imperato-McGinley et al., 1979; Baker, 1980; Ehrhardt and Meyer-Bahlburg, 1981). In skeletal muscle, testosterone acts to induce muscle growth (which is one reason why men are heavier than women) by binding to androgen receptors without first being metabolized to another steroid (Bardin and Catterall, 1981; Mooradian et al., 1987).

Of interest is the relationship between intracellular enzymes which amplify the action of steroids within target cells and the requirement that high concentrations of a steroid be available to the target tissue to regulate differentiation. As described above, in humans but not mice, testosterone acts within Wolffian duct structures, such as the seminal vesicles and epididymides, by binding to androgen receptors to regulate differentiation without the requirement of first being metabolized to the more potent androgen, DHT. As a result, higher intracellular concentrations of testosterone may be required to induce Wolffian duct differentiation than are required in tissues which can metabolize testosterone to DHT, such as in the urogenital sinus, since DHT has a higher binding affinity for the androgen receptor than does testosterone (Bardin and Catterall, 1981; Brown and Migeon, 1984). A higher concentration of testosterone within Wolffian ducts than would occur based on concentrations of testosterone present in blood might be accomplished via diffusion of testosterone from each testis to the ipsilateral Wolffian duct; diffusion of testosterone might occur within the mesonephric duct after it contacts the efferent ducts in the ipsilateral testis.

It appears that there is a requirement for higher concentrations of MIS and testosterone than are achieved via the systemic circulation to induce both the degeneration of the Müllerian ducts and stimulation of the Wolffian ducts. This hypothesis is supported by the persistence of the Müllerian duct and absence of the Wolffian duct ipsilateral (but not contralateral) to a congenitally absent or surgically removed testis in male fetuses (Short, 1972). Diffusion of MIS from the testis into the ipsilateral Müllerian duct may thus be required to achieve the high concentration of MIS needed for regression of these ducts during development in males. Since testosterone facilitates the action of MIS in Müllerian duct degeneration, also important may be the locally high concentrations of testosterone due to diffusion of testosterone from the ipsilateral testes. There is a cranial-caudal decrease in response of Müllerian duct to MIS, which is observed *in vitro* and thus reflects differential sensitivity of the duct to

MIS, not different concentrations of MIS and testosterone which reach the cranial and caudal portions of the duct (Josso, 1986).

*Sexual Differentiation of the Brain and Behavior*
It has been recognized for some time that testicular secretions have a profound influence on behavior (Medvei, 1982). It is accepted that testosterone (and its metabolites) initiate masculinization and defeminization of the brain and thus behavior in males. For example, administration of testosterone to pregnant guinea pigs caused the female offspring in adulthood to show male-like mounting behavior and inhibited sexual behaviors typical of females (Phoenix et al., 1959; Young et al., 1964). Over thirty years later, questions which remain to be answered include which behaviors are affected by testosterone vs. other steroids (i.e., estradiol, progesterone and glucocorticoids), neuropeptides, growth factors, etc. during sensitive periods in brain development, and which structures within the central nervous system interact to mediate specific behaviors. It is clear that the degree to which areas of the brain are interconnected (a single neuron can communicate directly with thousands of other neurons) means that complex social behaviors in mammals (such as any behavior relating to reproduction) are not mediated by a small number of neurons located together in one area of the brain (referred to as a nucleus of neurons).

Numerous studies have identified sexually dimorphic structural differences in the brain which are organized by steroid hormones. For example, in male rats, the volume of the sexually dimorphic nucleus of the preoptic area in the hypothalamus (SDN-POA) is greater in males than in females (Gorski et al., 1978; Jacobson and Gorski, 1981; Jacobson et al., 1985; Gorski, 1986). However, as with other sex differences in brain structure, no definitive functional correlate has, as yet, been determined for the sex difference in SDN-POA volume; there is conflicting evidence concerning the role of the SDN-POA on masculine sexual behavior (Arendash and Gorski, 1983; Commins and Yahr, 1984; de Jong et al., 1989; Baum et al., 1990). The importance of the discovery of numerous hormonally mediated sex differences in brain structure and physiology is that with time, the mechanisms underlying sex differences in behavior are likely to be clarified.

In rodents, exposure to testosterone during early life defeminizes both the neuroendocrine mechanisms regulating the cyclic release of LH and at least some aspects of female sexual behavior. If an adult male rat shows the capacity to respond to administration of exogenous estradiol by exhibiting a surge in LH, then this is taken as evidence that the normal process of defeminization did not occur (Gorski, 1979; Barraclough and Wise, 1982). There have been numerous attempts to relate the pattern of LH secretion in response to estrogen treatment with sexual orientation in adult men (Dorner et al. 1987). Yet, it was shown almost two decades ago that in primates, the capacity to release LH in response to an increase in estradiol (similar to the preovulatory LH surge in females) is normally present in adult males (Karsch et al., 1972; Norman and Spies, 1986).

This is also true in human males, and previous findings suggesting a link between the pattern of LH secretion in men (Dorner et al., 1976; Gladue et al., 1984) and sexual orientation have not been replicated (Hendricks et al., 1989). In fact, the link between sexual orientation and LH secretion may reflect the effects of viral infections (such as acquired immune deficiency syndrome-AIDS) prevalent in homosexual men on the functioning of the brain-pituitary-gonadal axis and thus the synthesis and release of LH and testosterone (Hendricks et al., 1989).

Beach (1979) pointed out the dangers associated with the misapplication of information obtained from animal studies to human psychosexual development. For example, there is no animal model for human homosexuality. While rats (and many other mammals) housed in same-sex groups may show mounting of each other, when given the option of engaging in sexual behavior with another rat of the same or opposite sex, it has never been reported that the member of the same sex was chosen. This has not stopped those promoting a political agenda regarding homosexuality from suggesting a link between developmental events and human homosexuality based on animal studies. Specifically, based on the finding in rats that a developmental event, stress during pregnancy, alters the pattern of testosterone secretion in male rat fetuses and also results in a reduction in sexual activity (not a change in sexual orientation) later in adult life (Ward and Weisz, 1980), maternal stress has been proposed to be the basis of human homosexuality (Dorner et al., 1987). In fact, the effects of maternal stress on morphology, physiology and behavior in rodents may not be mediated by stress-induced changes in gonadal steroids during fetal life (vom Saal et al., 1990). Findings from rodent studies provide important information about the relationship between developmental events and adult traits, but they are not relevant to a phenomenon (men and women with a homosexual orientation) which appears to be unique to humans.

*Ontogeny of steroid receptors in the brain.* The brain contains receptors for gonadal and adrenal steroids: estrogen, androgen, progestins, and glucocorticoids (McEwen et al., 1982). The development of specific receptors in target tissues allows steroids to exert effects on differentiation of the tissue, while the concentrations of receptors found in target tissues after differentiation are also modulated by their ligands during development (Tuohimaa and Niemi, 1972; Brown et al., 1988; Nonneman et al., 1992). Estrogen receptors in the brain are detectable by a number of different methods during both the fetal and neonatal period of sexual differentiation in rats and mice (Vito and Fox, 1982; Friedman et al., 1983). In contrast, brain androgen receptor concentrations are quite low in both rats and mice until after birth (Attardi and Ohno, 1976; Vito et al., 1979; Vito and Fox, 1982). Although several target organs (including brain regions) express receptors for different steroids, whether these receptors are localized in the same or different cells is, as yet, unclear (Jung-Testas et al., 1981; Döhler et al., 1986). However, in some cell lines, such as the MCF-7 line, individual cells express a variety of steroid receptors (Horowitz et al., 1975).

The absence of known genetic defects of estrogen receptors and the enzyme which synthesizes estrogen, aromatase, supports the fundamental importance of estrogen for implantation (penetration of the blastocyst into the uterus in humans) and thus embryonic survival, as well as the development and differentiation of the CNS and other target tissues (Wilson et al., 1981). In contrast, a defect in the synthesis of androgen receptors in androgen target cells (a mutation located on the X chromosome; Meyer et al., 1975) is responsible for the syndrome of testicular feminization (Tfm; Attardi et al., 1976; Brown and Migeon, 1984). The Tfm syndrome has been identified in humans, mice and rats (Fox, 1975; Meaney et al., 1983). The testes of Tfm males secrete testosterone, but since androgen target cells lack androgen receptors, the Wolffian ducts degenerate and the external genitalia differentiate in the female direction. The external appearance is thus as a phenotypic female. However, since the testes secrete MIS, the internal genitalia of females are absent due to the absence of derivatives of the Müllerian ducts. Thus, Tfm males show a blind vaginal pouch which is characteristically shorter than that of normal females (the cranial portion of the vagina is of Müllerian origin). The testes in Tfm (as well as normal) males secrete some estradiol (Setchell and Brooks, 1988), and there is also some conversion of testosterone to estradiol in Sertoli cells (Bardin et al., 1988) and adipose tissue (Simpson et al., 1989), so in species such as mice and rats in which estradiol exerts a masculinizing and defeminizing influence within selected areas of the brain, such as defeminization of the capacity to surge LH in response to estradiol, these developmental events still occur.

*Aromatization of testosterone in the brain.* Androstenedione, testosterone and 16α-hydroxyandrostenedione are metabolized to estrone, estradiol and estriol, respectively, via a series of steps by the microsomal enzyme, aromatase (Figure 14; Gibb and Lavoie, 1980; Mendelson et al., 1990). Aromatization refers to the fact that the A ring of estradiol is an aromatic ring. It was recognized almost 30 years ago that defeminization of the preovulatory LH surge system in newborn rats was mediated, at least in part, by aromatization of testosterone to estradiol within brain cells (Harris and Levine, 1965; Gorski, 1979). This led to the aromatization hypothesis, which was expanded to include all aspects of sexual differentiation of the brain and behavior. This model proposed that testosterone exerted its effect on the developing brain after being aromatized to estradiol, and that binding of estradiol to estrogen receptors mediated masculinization and defeminization of neuroendocrine function and behavior (Naftolin et al., 1975).

Support for the aromatization hypothesis has been provided by studies in which intrahypothalamic implants of testosterone and estradiol have been demonstrated to be equally effective in eliciting masculinization and defeminization of sexual behavior (MacLusky and Naftolin, 1981; Toran-Allerand, 1984). Nonaromatizable androgens, such as DHT, appeared to be ineffective, at least in terms of some aspects of sexual behavior and neuroendocrine function. Both testosterone-induced and estradiol-induced masculinization and defeminization of sexual behavior and neuroendocrine function can be blocked by antiestrogens,

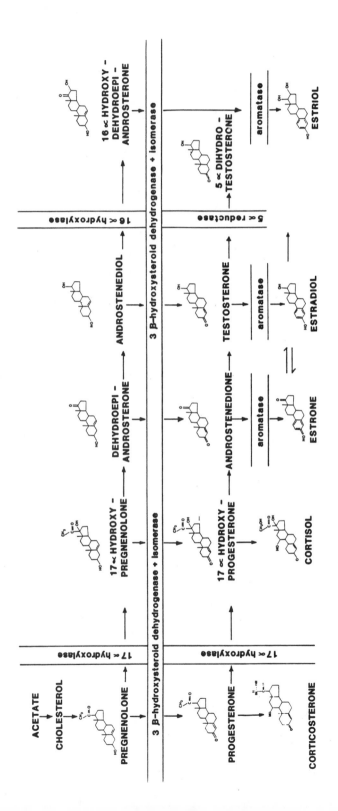

FIGURE 14. Diagram showing pathways for the synthesis of progesterone, glucocorticoids, androgen and estrogen. Enzymes are identified by parallel lines.

such as tamoxifen (Döhler et al., 1984b, 1986), and the masculinizing and de-feminizing effects of both endogenous and exogenous testosterone have been attenuated by aromatase inhibitors. For example, the inhibition of aromatase via treatment with ATD (1,4,6-androstatriene-3,17-dione) during sexual differentiation in male rats interferes with both defeminization (Clemens and Gladue, 1978; Davis et al., 1979) and masculinization (Gladue and Clemens, 1980) of sexual behavior. However, ATD also appears to interfere with the binding of androgen to androgen receptors, so, as with most pharmacological studies, one must use caution in interpreting results (Kaplan and McGinnis, 1989).

Given all of the above findings, it is clear that during sexual differentiation in rats, aromatization of testosterone to estradiol plays a role in the masculinization and defeminization of sexual behavior, masculinization of some brain structures (such as the SDN-POA; Döhler et al., 1984a, 1984b; Hines, this volume) and the defeminization of the neuroendocrine system regulating the preovulatory surge in LH (Yahr, 1988).

Aromatase activity is higher in the rat hypothalamus during perinatal life than in adulthood (George and Ojeda, 1982; Weisz et al., 1982). The activity of aromatase in the hypothalamus is also different in male and female rats during sexual differentiation (MacLusky et al., 1985; Tobet et al., 1985). There is evidence that both aromatase and $5\alpha$-reductase activity are modulated by circulating androgen during the fetal and neonatal period of sexual differentiation in rats (MacLusky and Naftolin, 1981; Wilson et al., 1981). Brain aromatase activity is also influenced by androgen levels during adult life (an activational effect), since castration results in a reduction in aromatase activity in the brain of adult male rats (Roselli et al., 1984; Paden and Roselli, 1987).

According to the aromatization model, high levels of both testosterone in the blood and aromatase activity in brain cells in the male rat during fetal and neonatal life are necessary for normal masculinization and defeminization of the brain (Paden and Roselli,1987; MacLusky et al., 1985). Normal female differentiation would occur when intracellular estrogen formation was low due to lower circulating testosterone levels and lower intracellular aromatase activity (MacLusky and Naftolin, 1981).

While the above information shows that the aromatization model explains some aspects of the regulation of the differentiation of sexual behavior by gonadal steroids, there are many aspects of the sexual differentiation of behavior which require the binding of androgen (testosterone or DHT) to androgen receptors (Döhler et al., 1986; Yahr, 1988). For example, the inhibition of androgen binding to androgen receptors (via treatment with the androgen receptor blocker, flutamide) around the time of birth interferes with both masculinization and defeminization of sexual behavior in male rats (Clemens et al., 1978; Gladue and Clemens, 1978). The defeminization of the neuroendocrine (LH surge) system in rats is influenced, at least partially, by binding of androgen to androgen receptors

(Gorski, 1986). Both the binding of androgen to androgen receptors and aromatization, with binding of estrogen to estrogen receptors, are involved in the differentiation of aggression during perinatal life and activation of aggression in adulthood in mice (Simon and Whalen, 1987). The available evidence is that only binding of androgen to androgen receptors mediates the differentiation of play behavior in rats (Meaney et al., 1983) as well as the sexually dimorphic spinal nucleus of the bulbocavernosus, a motor nucleus in the lumbar region of the spinal cord which innervates perineal striated muscles (Arnold and Breedlove, 1985).

In summary, the differentiation of sexual behaviors during early life, such as arousal, investigation, mounting, intromitting and ejaculation in males, and proceptive (initiating) and receptive (lordosis) behaviors in females is not regulated solely by one hormone acting on a single neural system for each behavior (Pfaff, 1980; Pfaff and Schwartz-Giblin, 1988; Sachs and Meisel, 1988). The above information is important in that it has often been suggested that aromatization of testosterone to estradiol mediates all aspects of brain sexual differentiation, while virtually all evidence supporting this model only relates to a few specific sexual behaviors. The wide array of behavioral differences, other than sexual behaviors, between males and females includes differences in infant play, aggression, learning, food intake and preference, activity level, exploratory activity, etc. While some of these sex differences reflect activational effects of the different gonadal hormones in the blood of adult males and females, many also are due to differences in brain function which were organized during early life. Sexual differentiation of the brain is thus an exceedingly complex process. It would be highly unlikely that a process as complicated as the differentiation of the neural areas which interact to mediate all of the above behaviors would be regulated by a single enzyme, aromatase, and a single type of steroid receptor for binding estradiol.

*Alphafetoprotein (AFP) and the aromatization model of sexual differentiation.* Estrogen (most importantly, estradiol) is present during development in the serum at very high concentrations, and, at least in some species (for example, humans, mice and cattle), estradiol is higher in blood and amniotic fluid in females than males during the prenatal period of brain sexual differentiaiton (Challis et al., 1974; Reyes et al., 1974; Robinson et al., 1977; Belisle and Tulchinsky, 1980; vom Saal and Bronson, 1980; vom Saal, 1989a). A critical part of the aromatization hypothesis thus required that virtually all circulating estrogen be inhibited from entering the brain and exerting masculinizing and defeminizing effects during sexual differentiation.

The plasma globulin, alphafetoprotein (AFP), is secreted into the blood in very high concentrations during embryonic development in vertebrates (Gitlin, 1975). AFP has been proposed to have major regulatory functions during development, independent of its capacity to bind estrogen (Gitlin, 1975; Ruoslahti and Seppala, 1979). AFP shows a high affinity for estrogen (but not testosterone) in rats and mice (Nunez et al., 1979; Keel and Abney, 1984), but this appears to be a property of AFP only in rats and mice and not in any other animal so far examined (Westphal, 1986). Similar to other steroid binding proteins, such as corticosteroid binding globulin (CBG), plasma concentrations of AFP are very high during the period of sexual differentiation in rats and mice (Figure 15; Germain et al., 1978; Ruoslahti and Seppala, 1979; Westphal, 1986; Montano et al., 1992). This finding led to the hypothesis that only male rats and mice would normally be masculinized and defeminized due to aromatization of testicular testosterone in the brain, since it was assumed (based on the high plasma concentrations of AFP) that too little estradiol was unbound (and thus biologically active) in the plasma of rats and mice to exert any physiological effect on developing tissues.

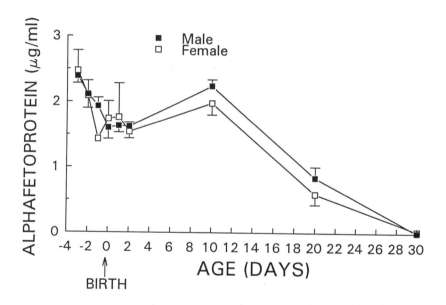

**FIGURE 15.** Concentrations of alphafetoprotein in male and female rats from 3 days prior to birth through 30 days after birth. Assays were conducted with the same serum pools used to measure testosterone and estradiol (see Figures 16 and 17) (Montano et al., 1992).

There have been numerous studies which have challenged the hypothesis that AFP acts to block passage of estrogen into brain cells during sexual differentiation. Internalization of AFP into mouse lymphoid tumor cells by receptor-mediated endocytosis has been reported (Naval et al., 1985). There is also considerable evidence (based on autoradiographic studies) that circulating AFP (presumably bound to estrogen) can enter selected cells in the brain in rats and mice (McEwen et al., 1975; Attardi and Rouslahti, 1976; Benno and Williams, 1978; Schachter and Toran-Allerand, 1982; Villacampa et al., 1984). Döhler (1986) has proposed that since deglycosylation of protein can facilitate entry into cells, AFP with the greatest degree of deglycosylation (which has the highest affinity for estrogen; Vallette et al., 1977) will preferentially enter target cells capable of internalizing AFP. In mice, mRNA for AFP is not present in brain areas in which AFP is localized within cells (AFP is synthesized mainly in the liver and yolk sac prior to birth and in the liver after birth; Schachter and Toran-Allerand, 1982). This finding suggested that AFP in brain cells had to be transported into the cells rather than synthesized within the cells, although subsequent studies have challenged this hypothesis (Poliard et al., 1988).

The presence of intraneuronal AFP in the CNS suggests that AFP may serve as a mediator of the transport of estrogen from the blood into brain cells. This possible source of intraneuronal estrogen may influence dendritic sprouting (Toran-Allerand, 1984). However, another possibility is that, within brain cells, AFP may serve as an alternate site for binding of estradiol, thus reducing the proportion of intracellular estradiol available to bind to nuclear receptors. Since AFP has been localized in brain cells in developing mice and rats (McEwen et al., 1975; Schachter and Toran-Allerand, 1982), one must also question whether AFP, itself, may play a role in neuronal development (Fox, 1987).

A finding from studies conducted by Pardridge and Mietus (1979) and McCall et al. (1981) is that fetal rat serum (with high concentrations of AFP) has a greater inhibitory effect on the passage of $^3$H-estradiol from the blood into brain tissue than does adult rat serum. However, in these experiments, $^3$H-steroids have only been injected into adult animals, not fetuses or neonates undergoing sexual differentiation. It was concluded that passage of estradiol into brain cells occurred purely by diffusion rather than as a result of active transport bound to AFP, since there was no evidence for saturation of active transport systems mediating passage of $^3$H-estradiol into brain as a result of increasing the concentration of unlabelled estradiol (McCall et al., 1981). Saturation of transport systems would be expected if the AFP-estradiol complex were being internalized by receptor-mediated endocytosis. The overwhelming evidence is that this conclusion is valid for adult animals, but these findings led to speculation that AFP was also not involved in transporting estradiol into neurons during the fetal/neonatal period of sexual differentiation. However, radiolabelled AFP ($^{125}$I-AFP) is internalized into the brain and other tissues of fetal and neonatal rats and mice, but internalization of $^{125}$-AFP into tissues does not occur after infancy (Villacampa et al., 1984; Laborda et al., 1989). These findings show that results from experiments concerning the active uptake of AFP associated with estradiol into tissues using adult animals are not relevant to models of sexual differentiation.

*Correlative and experimental evidence that circulating estradiol can enter cells and influence sexual differentiaiton.* A number of studies have suggested a correlation between the plasma concentration of estradiol during the fetal period of sexual differentiation and both adult sexual behavior and brain morphology in male rats and mice. Specifically, we measured both plasma testosterone and estradiol concentrations in male mice that developed between two other male fetuses *in utero* (2M males) and males that developed between two female fetuses (0M males) on Day 17 and 18 of fetal life (Figure 12). Overall, male fetuses had higher concentrations of testosterone than females, while females had higher concentrations of estradiol than males. Whereas 2M fetuses (male or female) had significantly higher plasma concentrations of testosterone, 0M fetuses had significantly higher plasma concentrations of estradiol relative to other fetuses of the same sex (Figure 13; vom Saal et al., 1983; vom Saal, 1989a). We have now demonstrated that this phenomenon, which is referred to as the intrauterine position phenomenon, is due to transport of steroids via diffusion from adjacent fetuses (Even et al., 1992; vom Saal and Dhar, 1992).

The importance of this naturally occurring source of individual differences in gonadal steroid concentrations during fetal life is that this phenomenon provides the only method for examining the relationship between the levels of endogenous hormones to which fetuses are exposed and postnatal traits. Because a 0M male fetus reliably has the highest plasma concentrations of estradiol and the lowest plasma concentrations of testosterone of any male fetus, we can deliver pups by cesarean section shortly before normal parturition, rear the pups with foster mothers, and study the consequences of differences in fetal hormone exposure during later life. Due to the fact that sexual differentiation occurs so early in development in single birth species with a long period of gestation, there is currently no method for assessing the levels of hormones in the blood of a fetus during sexual differentiation without killing the fetus, thus precluding examining the consequences of the very high degree of variability in gonadal steroid levels during fetal life in terms of postnatal traits. Since the available evidence in the mouse suggests that levels of gonadal steroids in amniotic fluid and blood are not always in equilibrium (unpublished observation), one cannot assume that amniotic fluid levels of hormones (determined by amniocentesis) will accurately reflect hormone concentrations in the fetal blood.

There are virtually identical findings from all experiments comparing 0M and 2M animals in rats and mice. Specifically, in rats, adult 0M males showed more mounts and intromissions, more ejaculations to satiety, and a larger volume of the sexually dimorphic nucleus of the preoptic area of the hypothalamus (SDN-POA) relative to 2M male siblings (vom Saal, Coquelin, Schoonmaker, Shryne, Jacobson and Gorski, unpublished observation). On Day 20 and 21 of fetal life, 0M male rat fetuses had significantly higher serum concentrations of estradiol than did 2M males (unpublished observation). Similarly, in mice, adult 0M males had higher rates of sexual behavior than 2M males, and 0M male fetuses had significantly higher serum levels of estradiol than 2M male fetuses (Figure 13; vom Saal et al., 1983; vom Saal, 1989a).

Adult 0M male mice were found to have a heavier prostate than 2M males, which was accounted for by a 3-fold higher number of androgen receptors in the prostate (per mg protein) of 0M than 2M males (Nonneman et al., 1992). The organization of androgen receptors in the mouse prostate is thus correlated with the levels of estradiol in the blood during fetal life. As discussed above, there is considerable evidence for estrogen responsiveness of prostate in rodents and other mammals (Tissel, 1971; Bashirelahi and Sidh, 1980; Mawhinney and Neubauer, 1979; Cunha et al, 1987). The induction by estrogen of epithelial metaplasia, as well as stimulation of fibromuscular tissue in the prostate, is presumably mediated directly via estrogen receptors (Cunha, 1986). Given the finding that stromal (mesenchyme) tissue regulates differentiation of the prostatic epithelium, and estrogen binding in rat ventral prostate is higher in stroma than epithelium (Jung-Testas et al., 1981), our findings suggest a regulatory role for endogenous estradiol in prostate differentiation. In particular, the concentration of estradiol in the blood during fetal life was positively correlated with the number of prostatic androgen receptors in adulthood.

One interesting aspect of the finding that there is a correlation between elevated estrogen levels during fetal life and enlarged prostates (which have elevated androgen-binding activity) in young adult 0M male mice is that in numerous studies involving exposure to very high doses of estrogens in male rats and mice during prenatal or neonatal life, inhibition of normal differentiation of the prostate has been observed. The prostate in these estrogen-treated males also shows little potential to subsequently respond to exogenous testosterone, indicating a down-regulation of androgen receptors. Both prenatal and neonatal treatment with a high dose of estrogen also markedly interferes with development of the seminal vesicles and testes, and thus reduces fertility (Kincl et al., 1963; Arai, 1970; McLachlan et al., 1975; Rajfer and Coffey, 1978, 1979; Vannier and Raynaud, 1980). However, these effects are not limited to administration of a high dose of estrogen to newborn rodents, since treatment with exogenous testosterone can have the same effect (Baranao et al., 1981). These findings from pharmacological studies show the dramatically different response which can occur when a developing fetus (or neonate) is exposed to physiological levels of an endogenous hormone vs. a very high dose of the hormone or a potent synthetic analog, such as diethylstilbestrol or other estrogenic xenobiotic (foreign chemical).

The findings from comparisons of 0M and 2M male rats and mice were initially quite surprising, since rates of sexual activity, volume of the SDN-POA, and prostate size (as well as androgen sensitivity) in adult males were negatively correlated with serum testosterone levels but positively correlated with serum estradiol levels during the fetal period of sexual differentiation. These correlational findings suggested that estradiol in male fetuses may have entered tissues in the brain and prostate of 0M males, thus elevating intracellular estradiol levels significantly above levels in the same cells in 2M males. The suggestion that this might have occurred led us to re-examine whether estradiol in the blood could enter brain cells in newborn rats. We also re-examined the literature concerning the aromatization of testosterone in the brain, since we had assumed that the higher plasma concentration of testosterone in 2M males should have meant that there was more testosterone to serve as a substrate for aromatization and that they should have shown the elevation in sexual activity and SDN-POA volume rather than 0M males.

The above findings have led to the hypothesis that, contrary to the prediction of the aromatization hypothesis, circulating estradiol might directly influence differentiation of selected target tissues due to passage of estradiol from the blood into cells, either by diffusion or by active transport while bound to AFP. We found (using Con A-sepharose to separate glycosylated and non-glycosylated proteins and centrifugal ultrafiltration dialysis to separate protein-bound and free steroids) that 89% of total circulating estradiol is bound to albumin, 10% is bound to AFP, and 1% is free (unbound to plasma proteins) in serum from 2-day old rats. Since AFP concentrations were between 1-2 mg/ml in these same fetuses (Figure 15), one would expect (based on the affinity of AFP for estradiol) that a greater proportion of estradiol would be bound to AFP. It thus appears that not all AFP measured by radioimmunoassay binds estradiol (Montano, 1991; Montano et al., 1992). Our findings are consistent with the observation that there are different forms of AFP which have markedly different degrees of glycosylation and binding affinities for estradiol; the form with the lowest glycosylation represents about 65% of AFP in fetal rat serum and shows high affinity binding to estradiol (Benassayag et al., 1975; Vallette et al., 1977). There may be marked changes during the perinatal period in the relative proportions of estrogen-binding and non-binding forms of AFP in the circulation, and further studies are needed to answer this question. A critical aspect of these findings is that fetuses have as much as 10 times higher circulating concentrations of total estradiol relative to average values observed during estrous cycles in adult female rats; except for the day of proestrus (right before ovulation), total circulating estradiol varies from 5-20 pg/ml serum in cycling rats (Smith et al., 1975).

Figure 16 and Figure 17 show the total, free, and protein bound (to both albumin and glycoproteins) serum concentrations of estradiol and testosterone in male and female rats from 3 days prior to delivery through 70 days after birth. Testosterone in serum collected from female rat fetuses is very high prior to parturition and then falls rapidly after birth (Montano, 1991). In rats and mice, most testosterone in the circulation of mothers and female fetuses is secreted by the placenta (Soares and Talamantes, 1982, 1983; Jackson and Albrecht, 1985), whereas in primates, the placenta secretes estrogen rather than androgen (Ryan, 1980). The extremely high free testosterone concentration in the blood of female fetuses may not have a masculinizing and defeminizing action on the brain in rats and mice due to the fact that androgen receptors in brain cells begin to increase dramatically beginning at birth (Vito and Fox, 1982), at exactly the time that the blood levels of testosterone in females drop dramatically associated with clearance from the blood of testosterone of placental origin; serum testosterone levels are significantly higher in male than female pups throughout the first week after birth (the neonatal period of sexual differentiation).

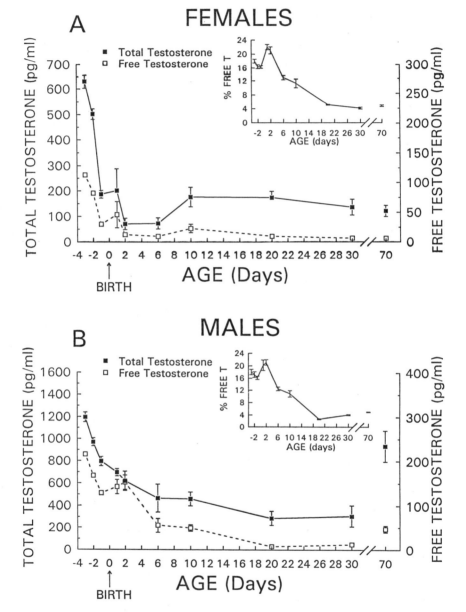

**FIGURE 16.** Total and free serum testosterone concentrations (mean ± SEM) throughout late fetal life, early postnatal development and young adulthood (Day 70) in the (A) female and (B) male rat (parturition = Day 0). From Day -3 (fetal life) to Day 10, serum was pooled across litters from animals of the same sex to achieve a volume of 0.5-1 ml; from Day 20 and Day 30 animals, serum was pooled from animals of the same sex from each litter. The free testosterone concentration in serum was calculated by multiplying percent free (measured by centrifugal ultrafiltration dialysis) x total testosterone (measured by RIA).

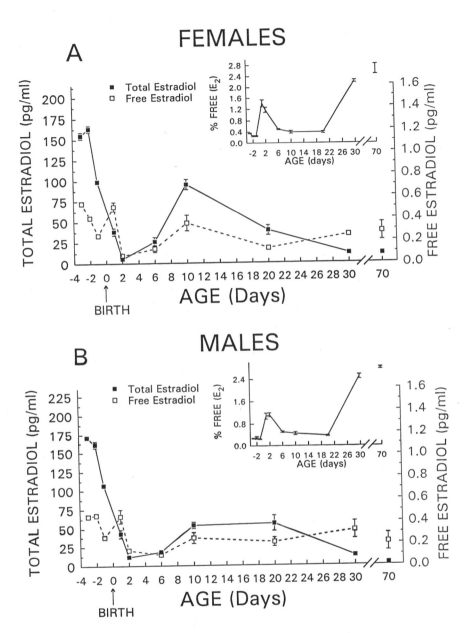

**FIGURE 17.** Total and free serum estradiol-17β concentrations (mean ± SEM) throughout late fetal life, early postnatal development and young adulthood (Day 70) in the (A) female and (B) male rat (parturition = Day 0). From Day -3 (fetal life) to Day 10, serum was pooled across litters from animals of the same sex to achieve a volume of 0.5-1 ml; from Day 20 and Day 30 animals, serum was pooled from animals of the same sex from each litter. The free estradiol concentration in serum was calculated by multiplying percent free (measured by centrifugal ultrafiltration dialysis) x total estradiol (measured by RIA).

Concentrations of total estradiol in serum drop from a high of between 160-170 pg/ml 2-3 days prior to birth to a low of 5 pg/ml at 48 hr after birth in female rats. The rise in estradiol at the end of the first week after birth in females is likely due to secretion from the adrenals (Weisz and Gunsalus, 1973; Meijs-Roelofs et al., 1973; Andrews and Ojeda, 1981). In mice, male fetuses typically have lower concentrations of estradiol 70-90 pg/ml than female fetuses (100-140 pg/ml serum) (vom Saal, 1989a). An interesting finding is that even though there was no sex difference in total circulating estradiol, 0M male rat fetuses had significantly higher serum concentrations of estradiol than did 2M male fetuses (unpublished observation).

A major problem in interpreting the literature relating to the role of AFP in protecting the developing brain from estrogen in the blood in rats and mice has been that different results concerning the binding of steroids in the developing brain have been reported with different techniques (MacLusky et al., 1979a, 1979b; Vito and Fox, 1982; Friedman et al., 1983; Brown et al., 1989). Occupancy of estrogen receptors was reported to be minimal in cell nuclei isolated from the brains of female rats aged 2-26 days (MacLusky et al., 1979a), presumably due to the presence of AFP. However, it is apparent from the data in Figure 17 that blood levels of estradiol are markedly lower by 48 hr after birth than during fetal life and the first 24 hr after birth, when many aspects of sexual differentiation occur. Also, in both rats and mice there appear to be a higher number of brain estrogen receptors prior to birth (Vito and Fox, 1982; Friedman et al., 1983) than had initially been reported (MacLusky et al., 1979b).

We re-examined the question concerning the capacity for circulating estradiol to enter brain cells and bind to estrogen receptors in newborn rats using a different technique than other investigators (MacLusky et al., 1979b; Brown et al., 1989). Rather than inject a bolus of radiolabelled estradiol ($^3$H-E$_2$), we implanted Silastic capsules containing $^3$H-E$_2$ into rat pups to achieve a stable, physiological concentration of $^3$H-E$_2$ in the blood (about 130 pg/ml, which is within the range observed during late fetal life and throughout most of the day of birth; Montano, 1991). We implanted rats 24 hr after birth and examined $^3$H-E$_2$ in brain cell nuclei at 48 hr after birth, when endogenous estradiol in the blood is at the lowest level (Figure 17). We found that $^3$H-E$_2$ passed from the blood into brain cells and was specifically bound to estrogen receptors (Montano et al., 1992). This finding thus shows that circulating estradiol can contribute to the intracellular pool of estradiol which is available to bind to estrogen receptors in brain cells during sexual differentiation. Since the free (biologically active) concentration of estradiol in serum in female fetuses is higher than in adult diestrous females, this finding suggests that sufficient estradiol can pass from blood into brain cells to influence sexual differentiation; this was predicted from correlational studies involving animals from different intrauterine positions. Other findings from this study suggested that estrogens were passing from the blood into brain cells by diffusion, not by active transport associated with internalization of AFP.

The results of other studies also are not consistent with the hypothesis that in the fetus, estrogen available within cells results solely from the intracellular aromatization of testosterone due to the inability of virtually all circulating estrogen to enter cells because they are bound to AFP. The apparent binding affinity of aromatase for testosterone has been reported to be around $0.3$-$0.4$ x $10^{-6}$ M (Reed and Ohno, 1976). Serum concentrations of testosterone during sexual differentiation in male and females rats are in the $10^{-8}$ M range (Figure 16; Weisz and Ward, 1980). These findings suggest that *in vivo*, saturation of aromatase by testosterone is unlikely to occur. An estimate based on *in vitro* studies is that the percent conversion of testosterone to estradiol is less than 0.1% (George and Ojeda, 1982). In homogenates of hypothalamus from adult rats, the conversion of testosterone to estrogen is less than 1% (Roselli et al., 1985). The low percent conversion of testosterone to estradiol in brain cells could explain why the 40% higher concentration of plasma testosterone in 2M than 0M male mouse fetuses (Figure 13) does not lead to an enhancement of differentiation of tissues with estrogen receptors, while the approximately 30% higher concentration of plasma estradiol in 0M than 2M male fetuses contributes enough supplemental estradiol within brain (and prostate) cells to markedly influence differentiation.

Studies involving injection of a high dose of estradiol into neonatal rats have shown that testosterone-derived estradiol binds to approximately 50% of estrogen receptors in the brain that are bound by saturating doses of estradiol (Krey et al., 1980). However, in studies in which both androgen and estrogen receptor occupancy were measured after administration of physiological doses of radiolabelled testosterone ($^3$H-T), binding was primarily to androgen receptors (Krey et al., 1979).

There also appears to be an independence of expression of aromatase and estrogen receptors. Certain brain areas that contain very high levels of estrogen receptors in neonates (e.g., hypothalamus: Vito and Fox, 1982; cerebral cortex: Sheridan, 1979) exhibit low levels of aromatase activity (George and Ojeda, 1982). However, immunohistochemical localization of the aromatase enzyme, which would allow for a more detailed anatomical localization, has not been examined using a highly specific antibody. Other studies have indicated that hypothalamic aromatase activity in rats is regulated, at least in part, by androgen binding to androgen receptors during both prenatal and adult life (Roselli et al., 1984; Paden and Roselli, 1987). The induction of aromatase in the hypothalamic-preoptic area appears to require binding of androgen to androgen receptors, and the inductive effects of testosterone on aromatase were blocked by concomitant administration of an androgen-receptor antagonist (Roselli and Resko, 1984).

The implications of the above findings for the model that virtually all estrogen binding to estrogen receptors in developing rat brain derives from intracellular aromatization of androgen have not been addressed. There may be some brain cells which contain estrogen receptors but not aromatase, and in these cells, circulating estrogen would have to be the source of intracellular estrogen which binds to estrogen receptors. It is also possible that in neurons which contain aromatase and androgen receptors, but not estrogen receptors, aromatase serves to inactivate testosterone (Sar and Stumpf, 1977). Alternatively, the estrogen formed by aromatization in these brain cells may pass back into the systemic circulation and would be available for uptake into other cells with estrogen receptors. Since AFP was presumed to block the uptake of plasma estrogens into brain cells, this hypothesis has not been considered in rodents, although this occurs in birds (Schlinger and Arnold, 1991).

Many of the models concerning sexual differentiaiton are based primarily on studies which have used rats and mice. While general principles concerning the phenomena of masculinization and defeminization appear to be similar among mammals, many specific aspects of these phenomena differ markedly between species, and this has led to considerable confusion. For example, a major problem with the aromatization hypothesis is that in no mammal other than rats and mice does AFP bind estrogen (Westphal, 1986). While there are other plasma globulins which bind gonadal steroids in other mammals, none of these plasma proteins specifically binds estrogen and not testosterone, and a mechanism for selectively inhibiting estradiol from entering cells (a central tenet of the aromatization hypothesis) thus does not exist. For example, many mammals have a sex steroid binding globulin that binds both estradiol and testosterone, but human sex steroid binding globulin has a higher affinity for testosterone than for estradiol (Pardridge, 1981, 1986). The available evidence is that rodents do not have a sex steroid binding globulin (Corvol and Bardin, 1973; Renoir et al., 1980), and the data in Figure 16 show that the concentrations of free testosterone are extremely high during the perinatal period of sexual differentiation in rats; all testosterone which is not free is bound to albumin, since there is no binding of testosterone to androgen binding protein in fetal-neonatal rat serum (Danzo and Eller, 1985; Montano, 1991). Thus, the concept that females are not masculinized and defeminized by estradiol, due to the presence of plasma binding proteins that selectively sequester estradiol in the blood, does not explain why estrogen does not act to masculinize and defeminize female mammals other than rats and mice (Baum et al., 1990).

The effects of steroids on target tissues during pregnancy (and for a period of time after birth in both mothers and fetuses) is greatly complicated by the dramatic increase in plasma steroid-binding proteins that occurs during pregnancy (Siiteri et al., 1982). Speculation concerning why such dramatic changes in binding protein concentrations are seen during pregnancy has focused on clearance rate, since most protein-bound steroids are cleared from the circulation relatively slowly in comparison to free steroids (Schroeder and Henning, 1989).

High concentrations of steroid-binding plasma proteins provide a pool for replenishing free hormone and reduce the magnitude of oscillations in plasma steroid concentrations due to transient changes in secretion.

Again, we found that the free concentration of estradiol in female fetuses is higher than the free concentration in adult females, at which time estradiol clearly enters cells and regulates cell function. Also, most circulating estradiol in 2-day-old female rats is bound to albumin (not AFP), and albumin-bound steroids may pass out of capillaries in some tissues (see below). In addition, even the fraction of estradiol bound to AFP may be selectively transported into some target tissues (Toran-Allerand, 1984). Thus, the hypothesis that AFP serves as a barrier to the movement of virtually all estradiol into cells appears to be incorrect.

Studies to investigate the paradoxical finding that estradiol is involved in masculinization, yet is present in higher concentrations in the plasma of female than male fetuses, should focus on the dynamic relationship between plasma concentrations of testosterone, estradiol and blood binding proteins vs. the capacity for tissues to metabolize and bind testosterone and estradiol throughout the period of sexual differentiation. Thus, various tissues become sensitive to the effects of steroids at different stages in development, and a change in the concentrations of a particular steroid in plasma at one time in development will only have an effect on differentiation of tissues which have already begun the process of synthesizing enzymes and receptors which allow a response to the steroid. For example, the testes of neonatal rats do not respond to estradiol and also do not show evidence of estrogen receptors until after the early neonatal period (Huhtaniemi, 1985).

The one certainty concerning the hormonal regulation of sexual differentiation is that testosterone secreted from the testes during early fetal life in males initiates this complex process. We do not yet understand the subsequent events which result in all of the different aspects of sexual differentiation. However, there appears to be an interaction between androgen and estrogen, as well as other hormones and "factors" involved in regulating the differentiation of tissues, during early life which is far more complex than current models would suggest.

*Binding of Steroids to Albumin and Glycoproteins in Plasma*
Most published information concerning concentrations of circulating steroids in pregnant females and fetuses, as well as in animals after birth, involves mea-surement of only the total amount of steroid present in the blood. In these stud-ies steroids are extracted from blood using techniques which do not allow one to discriminate between the fraction of steroid that is bound to plasma proteins vs. the fraction that is free. Thus, while there is some information concerning total estradiol and testosterone present in blood, and less information concerning the *in vitro* dialyzable fraction of free estradiol and testosterone in blood, there are few studies which have investigated the fraction of either steroid that is biologi-

cally active *in vivo* at various stages in an animal's life. The biologically active fraction of circulating steroid is the fraction of steroid that can pass from capillaries into cells and is available to bind to intracellular receptors. There are findings which suggest that the biologically active fraction of estradiol in blood may be different from the *in vitro* dialyzable fraction, which is determined using *in vitro* dialysis techniques (vom Saal, 1983b; Toran-Allerand, 1984; Pardridge, 1986).

Even though the concentration of total steroid measured by radioimmunoassay may be very high in fetuses and pregnant females relative to values observed in nonpregnant adult animals, it is generally assumed that only a small (free) fraction of the total steroid that is assayed is biologically active. For example, it has often been assumed that because of the high concentrations of sex steroid binding globulin during fetal development in humans, cellular uptake of estradiol and testosterone, and the eventual occupation of estrogen and androgen receptors in target tissues, is less than in adulthood due to the low proportion of free (unbound) steroid. The results of our study concerning the free serum concentration of estradiol in developing rats showed that during late fetal life and on the day of birth, the free concentration of estradiol in the blood was higher than levels observed in adult diestrous females (Figure 17). This finding (in conjunction with our finding of circulating $^{3}$H-estradiol uptake into brain cells in neonatal rats) argues strongly that the free circulating concentration of estradiol is within a range which is biologically active during sexual differentiation in rats.

Several factors have been proposed to influence concentrations of steroids within tissues. These include the rate of secretion of the steroid into plasma, concentration of albumin and specific plasma binding proteins, plasma flow rate, and the rate constant for dissociation of the steroid-protein complex (Ekins et al., 1982; Mendel, 1989). There are differences in the influx of steroids into various tissues which have been related to configuration of the capillary beds and the capillary transit time through a tissue (this is the time required for a substance to pass from the afferent to efferent vessels through capillaries). When capillary transit times are slow, as in liver (Pardridge and Mietus, 1979) or uterus (Laufer et al., 1983), steroids may dissociate from binding globulins (such as corticosteroid binding globulin) as well as from albumin during transit through the tissue. A variable fraction of steroid (including some globulin-bound in addition to albumin-bound steroid) may thus pass into the tissue. Recent evidence suggests that neither the albumin or globulin bound fraction of cortisol accounts for the passage of cortisol into liver (Mendel et al., 1988), while the opposite may hold for progesterone (Mendel, 1989). The controversy concerning whether other steroids, such as estradiol or testosterone, bound to plasma albumin or specific globulins dissociate during transit through capillaries and enter tissues in target organs such as the brain remains to be resolved. It is possible that different results will be found for each steroid in each tissue, so general conclusions concerning the transport of steroids into tissues are not warranted at this time. However, it appears that the unidirectional uptake of hormones by some tissues can exceed the free hormone fraction due to the rapid dissociation of steroids from albumin relative to the blood transit time through capillaries (Pardridge, 1986).

Plasma proteins leave capillaries and return to the circulation via the lymphatic ducts (Sandberg et al., 1960). Slow movement of plasma proteins in the extracellular space also influences equilibrium of steroid between plasma and intracellular binding sites for steroids. The net availability of steroid to bind to intracellular receptors is thus determined by multiple equilibrium relationships (Tait and Burstein, 1964). Further complicating the picture is the observation that vascular permeability to protein is variable and under hormonal control (Peterson and Spaziani, 1969). Given the complexity of the problem, it is not surprising that there are conflicting views (based on studies of the transport of different steroids into different tissues) concerning the exact model which best describes the passage of steroids from capillaries into tissues (Ekins et al., 1982; Tait, 1982; Pardridge, 1986; Mendel, 1989; Ekins, 1990).

The question of the bioavailability of albumin-bound steroid is often raised, primarily because of the weak binding involved. Since albumin is present in the blood in very high concentrations, it plays an important role in influencing the capacity for steroids to enter cells. Results from some studies are consistent with the uptake of albumin by fetal tissues, including the brain (Laborda et al., 1989). There may be a marked difference in the capacity for albumin to pass through capillaries into tissues during development and in adulthood. For example, the transfer of albumin from blood to cerebrospinal fluid in the immature animal is considerably greater than in the adult in the chicken (Moro et al., 1984) and in the rat (Hulsebosch and Fabian, 1989). This finding does not appear to be due to immaturity of tight junctions in the choroid plexus; tight junctions may be by-passed by a transcellular route which is present only at immature stages of choroid plexus development (Mollgard and Saunders, 1977). Direct cellular uptake of albumin (with or without a weakly bound steroid) from cerebrospinal fluid or from blood can also occur by receptor-mediated transcytosis and/or endocytosis (Pardridge, 1986).

The results of most studies have been interpreted within the model that steroids must first dissociate from plasma steroid-binding proteins prior to entering cells (the free hormone hypothesis). Thus, plasma steroid-binding globulins are presumed to only serve as a passive reservoir for replenishing free $\alpha$-hormone, which is rapidly cleared. However, as discussed above, an alternative hypothesis is that globulin-bound steroid (such as estradiol bound to AFP) can enter cells via receptor-mediated endocytosis; for example, this has been identified as the mechanism by which lipoproteins are internalized into cells (Brown and Goldstein, 1986). The protein-internalization hypothesis predicts that plasma binding proteins serve an important regulatory function in determining the proportion of a circulating steroid which will enter selected target tissues (those with membrane receptors for the protein; Rosner and Hochberg, 1976). Once inside a target cell, the steroid would presumably dissociate from the plasma protein and become available for binding to specific intracellular receptors, due to the lower binding affinity of plasma proteins for steroids relative to intracellular receptors (Toran-Allerand, 1984). For example, the identification of membrane receptors for corticosteroid binding globulin in pituitary corticotroph cells suggests that internalization of the corticosteroid binding globulin-corticosteroid complex may occur (Perrot-Applanat et al., 1984; Kuhn et al., 1986). Evidence exists that in pituitary corticotrophs, corticosteroids bound to CBG are biologically active (Rosner and Hochberg, 1976).

Siiteri et al., (1982) suggested that binding proteins may play a role in creating an intracellular pool of bound steroid which is protected from metabolism but is in equilibrium with the pool of steroid bound to intracellular receptors. This may explain the discrepancy between the amount of a steroid, such as estradiol, that is present in serum vs. that required to saturate intracellular receptors. Sakly and Koch (1983) also proposed that binding proteins internalized by target cells may modulate the cellular response to steroids by competing with receptors. For example, the testes in neonatal rats contain AFP, which has led to the suggestion that intracellular AFP may serve to bind, and thus render biologically inactive, intracellular estradiol (Huhtaniemi, 1985).

### Effects of Estrogenic Xenobiotics on Fetal Development
While the information covered in this chapter is relevant for understanding the mechanisms of sexual differentiation, it is also of considerable importance for understanding the potential effects that man-made substances might have on developing organisms; this also holds for naturally occuring estrogenic substances produced by plants and fungi, such as the mycotoxin, zearealonone (Kuiper-Goodman, 1991). Synthetic estrogen-like molecules, such as diethyl-stilbestrol, some lower chlorinated PCB's, DDT (particularly o,p'-DDT) and other ingredients in pesticides have the capacity to bind to and activate intracellular estrogen receptors (Korach et al., 1987; Gray, this volume; Soto et al., this volume).

Steroid binding proteins present in the blood may serve to bind (and possibly sequester from some tissues) much (but not all) of the estradiol present in blood during differentiation of the reproductive tract, brain, and other estrogen target tissues. However, while the best studied synthetic estrogen, diethylstilbestrol, has a slightly higher affinity than estradiol for estrogen receptors (Soto, et al., this volume), it shows only very weak binding to plasma glycoproteins (alphafetoprotein in rats and sex steroid binding globulin in humans; Sheehan and Young, 1979). If this were also true for other estrogenic xenobiotics, any barrier function that plasma glycoproteins might serve in terms of restricting the entry of plasma estradiol into cells would not be effective for estrogenic xenobiotics.

Estrogenic xenobiotics can have devastating effects on development, although these effects might not become apparent until individuals reach adulthood or even old age (Takasugi and Bern, 1988). A tragic example is the high incidence of infertility and tumors seen in the offspring of animals and women treated with diethylstilbestrol during pregnancy (McLachlan et al., 1975; Arai et al., 1978; Barber, 1986; Takasugi and Bern, 1988). The timing of exposure to the xenobiotic in relation to the onset of synthesis of estrogen receptors in target tissues, the binding affinity of the xenobiotic to both estrogen receptors and other blood and intracellular proteins, and the presence of enzymes which can metabolize the xenobiotic are all factors which will determine the effects of a particular dose of a xenobiotic on a developing fetus and newborn.

## ACKNOWLEDGEMENTS

We thank Drs. Gerald R. Cunha and Thomas O. Fox for reviewing this chapter. Support was provided by NSF grant DCB-9004806.

## REFERENCES

Allan, F.D. (1960). *Essentials of Human Embryology*. Oxford University Press, New York.

Andrews, W. and Ojeda, S. (1981). A quantitative analysis of the maturation of steroid negative feedbacks controlling gonadotropin release in the female rat: The infantile-juvenile periods, transition from an androgenic to a predominantly estrogenic control. *Endocrinol.* **108**, 1313-1320.

Angelova, P. and Jordanov, J. (1986). Meiosis-inducing and meiosis-preventing effects of sex steroid hormones on hamster fetal ovaries in organ culture. *Arch. d'Anat. Micro.* **75**, 149-159.

Arai, Y. (1970). Nature of metaplasia in rat coagulating glands induced by neonatal treatment with estrogen. *Endocrinol.* **86**, 918-920.

Arai, Y., Chen, C.Y., and Nishizuka, Y. (1978). Cancer development in male reproductive tract in rats given diethylstilbestrol at neonatal age. *Gann.* **69**, 861-862.

Arendash, G. and Gorski, R. (1983). Effects of discrete lesions of the sexually dimorphic nucleus of the preoptic area or other medial preoptic regions on the sexual behavior of male rats. *Brain Res. Bull.* **10**, 147-154.

Arnold, A. (1980). Sexual differences in the brain. *Amer. Scientist* **68**, 165-173.

Arnold, A. and Breedlove, M. (1985). Organizational and activational effects of sex steroids on brain and behavior: A re-analysis. *Horm. Behav.* **19**, 469-498.

Attardi, B. and Ohno, S. (1976). Androgen and estrogen receptors in the developing mouse brain. *Endocrinol.* **99**, 1279-1290.

Attardi, B. and Rouslahti, E. (1976). Foetoneonatal estradiol-binding protein in mouse brain cytosol is alpha-foetoprotein. *Nature* **263**, 658-687.

Attardi, B., Geller, L.N., and Ohno, S. (1976). Androgen and estrogen receptor in brain cytosol from male, female, and testicular feminized (tfm) mice. *Endocrinol.* **98**, 864-874.

Aumuller, G. (1989). Morphologic and regulatory aspects of prostatic function. *Anat Embryol.* **179**, 519-531.

Baker, S. (1980). Psychosexual differentiation in the human. *Biol. Reprod.* **22**, 61-72.

Baker, T.G. (1972). Oogenesis and ovulation. In *Germ Cells and Fertilization*, ed. C.R. Austin and R.V. Short. Cambridge Univ. Press, Cambridge, pp. 14-45.

Balinsky, B.I. (1975). *An Introduction to Embryology*. W. B. Saunders Co., Philadelphia.

Baranao, J., Chemes, H., Tesone, M., Chauzzi, V., Scacchi, P.., Calvo, J., Faugon, M., Moguilevsky, J. Charreau, E., and Calandra, R. (1981). Effects of androgen treatment of the neonate on rat testis and sex accessory organs. *Biol. Reprod.* **25**, 851-858.

Barber, H. (1986). An update on DES in the field of reproduction. *Int. J. Fertil.* **31**, 130-134.

Bardin, C.W. and Catterall, J.F. (1981). Testosterone: A major determinant of extragenital sexual dimorphism. *Science* **211**, 1285-1294.

Bardin, C.W., Cheng, C.Y., Musto, N.A., and Gunsalus, G.L. (1988). The Sertoli cell. In *Physiology of Reproduction*, ed. E. Knobil and J. Neill. Raven Press, New York, 933-974.

Barraclough, C.A. and Leathem, J. (1954). Infertility induced in mice by a single injection of testosterone propionate. *Proc. Soc. Exp. Biol. Med.* **85**, 673-674.

Barraclough, C.A. and Wise, P.M. (1982). The role of catecholamines in the regulation of pituitary luteinizing hormone and follicle stimulating hormone secretion. *Endocrine Rev.*, **3**, 91-119.

Bashirelahi, N. and Sidh, S.M. (1980). Estrogen receptors in male genital organs. *Advances in Sex Hormone Research*, **4**, 1-26.

Bassett, S.G. and Pete, G.J. (1987). Utilization of circulating androstenedione and testosterone for estradiol production during gestation in the rat. *Biol. Reprod.* **37**, 606-611.

Baum, M.J. (1979). Differentiation of coital behavior in mammals: A comprehensive analysis. *Neurosci. Biobehav. Rev.* **3**, 265-284.

Baum, M.J., Carroll, R., Cherry, J., and Tobet, S. (1990) Steroidal control of behavioral, neuroendocrine and brain sexual differentiation: Studies in a carnivore, the ferret. *J. Neuroendocrinol.* **2**, 401-418.

Beach, F.A. (1945). Bisexual mating behavior in the male rat. Effects of castration and hormone administration. *Physiol. Zool.* **18**, 390-402.

Beach, F.A. (1975). Hormonal modification of sexually dimorphic behavior. *Psychoneroendocrinol.* **1**, 3-23.

Beach, F.A. (1979). Animal models for human sexuality. In *Sex, Hormones and Behaviour*. Ciba Foundation Symposium 62, Excerpta Medica, New York, pp. 113-132.

Becak, W. (1983). Evolution and differentiation of sex chromosomes in lower vertebrates. In *Mechanisms of Gonadal Differentiation in Vertebrates*. Springer-Verlag, Berlin, pp. 3-12.

Belisle, S. and Tulchinsky, D. (1980). Amniotic fluid hormones. In *Maternal-Fetal Endocrinology*, ed. D. Tulchinsky and K.J. Ryan. Saunders, Philadelphia, pp. 169-195.

Benassayag, C., Vallette, G., Cittanova, N., Nunez, E. and Jayle, M. (1975). Isolation of two forms of rat alpha-fetoprotein and comparison of their binding parameters with estradiol-17$\beta$. *Biochem. Biophys. Acta* **412**, 295-305.

Benno, R. and Williams, T. (1978). Evidence for intracellular localization of alpha-fetoprotein in the developing rat brain. *Brain Res.* **142**, 182-186.

Bianchi, N.O. (1991). Sex determination in mammals: How many genes are involved? *Biol. Reprod.* **44**, 393-397.

Blacklock, N.J. (1983). The development and morphology of the prostate. In *The Endocrinology of Prostate Tumours*, ed. R. Ghanadian. MTP Press, Lancaster, England, pp. 1-13.

Blizzard, D. and Denef, C. (1973). Neonatal androgen effects on open-field activity and sexual behavior in the female rat: the modifying enfluence of ovarian secretions during development. *Physiol. Behav.* **11**, 65-69.

Borum, K. (1966). Oogenesis in the mouse. A study of the origin of the mature ova. *Exp. Cell. Res.*, **45**, 39-47.

Brawer J.R., Naftolin, F., Martin, J., and Sonnenschein, C. (1978). Effects of a single injection of estradiol valerate on the hypothalamic arcuate nucleus and on the reproductive function in female rat. *Endocrinol.* **103**, 501-512.

Brown, M. and Goldstein, J. (1986). A receptor-mediated pathway for cholesterol homeostasis. *Science* **232**, 34-47.

Brown, T.R. and Migeon, C.J. (1984). Androgen receptors in normal and abnormal male sexual differentiation. In *Steroid Hormone Resistance*, ed. G. Chrousos, D. Loriaux, and M. Lipsett. Plenum Press, New York, pp. 227-255.

Brown, T., Hochberg, R., Zielinski, J., and MacLusky, N. (1988). Regional sex differences in cell nuclear estrogen-binding capacity in the rat hypothalamus and preoptic area. *Endocrinol.* **123**,1761-1770.

Brown, T.J., MacLusky, N.J., Toran-Allerand, C.D., Zielinski, J.E., and Hochbert, R.B. (1989). Characterization of 11ß-methoxy-16 alpha-[$^{125}$I]iodoestradiol binding: Neuronal localization of estrogen-binding sites in the developing rat brain. *Endocrinol.* **124**, 2074-2088.

Bull, J.J. (1980). Sex determination in reptiles. *Quart. Rev. Biol.* **55**, 3-21.

Bull, J.J. (1983). *Evolution of Sex Determining Mechanisms.* Benjamin Cummings Pub., Menlo Park, CA.

Burns, R.K. (1961). Role of hormones in the differentiation of sex. In *Sex and Internal Secretions*, ed. W. Young. Williams and Wilkins, Baltimore, pp. 76-158.

Byskov, A. and Hoyer, P. (1988). Embryology of Mammalian gonads and ducts. In *The Physiology of Reproduction*, ed. E. Knobil et al. Raven Press, Ltd., New York, pp 265-302.

Carter, J.B. and Coffey, D.S. (1990). The prostate: An increasing medical problem. *The Prostate* **16**, 39-48.

Challoner, S. (1974). Studies of oogenesis and follicular development in the golden hamster. 1. A quantitative study of meiotic prophase *in vitro. J. Anat.*, **117**, 373-383.

Challoner, S. (1975). Studies of oogenesis and follicular development in the golden hamster. 3. Initiation of follicular growth *in vitro. J. Anat.*, **119**,157-162.

Challis, J., Kim, C., Naftolin, F. Judd, H., Yen, S., and Benirschke, K. (1974). The concentrations of androgens, oestrogens, progesterone and luteinizing hormone in the serum of foetal calves throughout the course of gestation. *J. Endocrinol.* **60**, 107-115.

Chang, C.Y. and Witschi, E. (1956). Genetic control and hormonal reversal of sex differentiation in Xenopus. *Proc. Soc. Exp. Biol. Med.* **93**,140-144.

Clark, M., Crews, D., and Galef, B. (1991). Sex-steroid levels of pregnant and fetal Mongolian gerbils. *Physiol. Behav.* **49**, 239-243.

Clemens, L. and Gladue, B. (1978). Feminine sexual behavior in rats enhanced by prenatal inhibition of androgen aromatization. *Horm. Behav.* **11**, 190-201.

Clemens, L., Gladue, B., and Coniglio, L. (1978). Prenatal endogenous androgenic influences on masculine sexual behavior and genital morphology in male and female rats. *Horm. Behav.* **10**, 40-53.

Colby, H.D. (1980). Regulation of hepatic drug and steroid metabolism by androgens and estrogens. In *Advances in Sex Hormone Research*, Vol. 4. ed. J. Thomas and R. Singhal, Urban and Schwarzenberg, Baltimore. pp. 27-71.

Commins, D. and Yahr, P. (1984). Lesions of the sexually dimorphic area disrupt mating and marking in male gerbils. *Brain Res. Bull.* **13**, 185-193.

Cook, H.J., Fantes, J., and Green, D. (1983). Structure and evolution of the human Y chromosome DNA. *Differentiation* 23 (Suppl.), S48-S55.

Corvol, P. and Bardin, C. (1973). Species distribution of testosterone-binding globulin. *Biol. Reprod.* **8**, 277-282.

Cunha, G. (1986). Development of the male reproductive tract. In *Urologic Endocrinology*, ed. J. Rajfer. Saunders, Philadelphia, pp. 6-35.

Cunha, G.R., Boutin, E.L., Turner, T., and Donjacour, A.A. (1992). Role of mesenchyme in the development of the urogenital tract. In *Chemically Induced Alterations in Sexual Development: The Wildlife/Human Connection.* ed. T. Colborn, Elsevier Applied Science, pp. 85-105.

Cunha, G., Donjacour, A., Cooke, P., Mee, S., Bigsby, R., Higgins, S., and Sugimura, Y. (1987). The endocrinology and developmental biology of the prostate. *Endocr. Rev.* **8**, 338-362.

Danzo, B. and Eller, B. (1985). The ontogeny of biologically active androgen-binding protein in rat plasma, testis and epididymis. *Endocrinol.* **117**, 1380-1388.

Davis, P.G., Chaptal, C.V., and McEwen, B.S. (1979). Independence of the differentiation of masculine and feminine sexual behavior in rats. *Horm. Behav.* **12**,12-19.

de Jong, F., Louwerse, A., Ooms, M., Evers, P. Endert, E. and van de Pol, N. (1989). Lesions of the SDN-POA inhibit sexual behavior of male Wistar rats. *Brain Res. Bull.* **23**, 483-492.

De Moor, P., Verhoeven, G., and Heyns, W. (1973). Permanent effects of foetal and neonatal T secretion on steroid metabolism and binding. *Differentiation,* **1**, 241-253.

Desjardins, C. (1981). Endocrine signaling and male reproduction. *Biol. Reprod.* **24**, 1-21.

Diczfalusy, E. (1968). Steroid metabolism in the feto-placental unit. In *The Feto-placental Unit,* ed. A. Pecile and C. Finzi. Excerpta Medica, Amsterdam, pp 65.

Döhler, K. (1986). The special case of hormonal imprinting, the neonatal influence of sex. *Experientia* **42**, 759-769.

Döhler, K.D., Hancke, J.L., Srivastava, S.S., Shryne, J.E., and Gorski, R.A. (1984a). Participation of estrogens in female sexual differentiation of the brain: neuroanatomical, neuroendocrine and behavioral evidence. *Prog. Brain Res.* **61**, 97-115

Döhler, K.D., Srivastava, S.S., Shryne, J.E., Jarzab, B., Sipos, A., and Gorski, R.A. (1984b). Differentiation of the sexually dimorphic nucleus in the preoptic area of the rat brain is inhibited by postnatal treatment with estrogen antagonist. *Neuroendocrinol.* **38**, 297-301.

Döhler, K., Coquelin, A., Davis, F., Hines, M., Shryne, J., and Gorski, R. (1986). Aromatization of testicular androgens in physiological concentrations does not defeminize sexual brain function. In *Monogr. Neural Sci. Vol 12. Systemic Hormones, Neurotransmitters and Brain Developement,* ed. G. Dorner, S. McCann and L. Martini. Karger, Basel, pp. 28-35.

Donahoe, P.K., Hutson, J.M., MacLaughlin, D.T., and Budzik, G.P. (1985). Steroid interactions with Mullerian inhibiting substance. In *The Endocrine Physiology of Pregnancy and the Peripartal Period.* Serono Symposia Pub., Vol 21, Raven Press, New York, pp. 101-116.

Dorner, G., Docke, F., Goyz, F., Rohde, W., Stahl, F., and Tonjes, R. (1987). Sexual differentiation of gonadotropin secretion, sexual orientation and gender role behavior. *Steroid Biochem.* **27**,1081-1987.

Dorner, G., Rohde, W., Seidel, K., Haas, W., and Schott, G. (1976). On the evocability of a positive oestrogen feedback action on LH secretion in transexual men and women. *Endokrinologie* **67**, 20-25.

Drago, J.R. (1989). The role of new modalities in the early detection and diagnosis of prostate cancer. *CA-A Cancer Journal for Clinicians* **39**, 326-336.

Driscoll, S. and Taylor, S. (1980). Effects of prenatal maternal estrogen on the male urogenital system. *J. Am. Coll. Obstet. Gynecol.* **56**, 537-542.

Dullaart, J., Kent, J., and Ryle, M. (1975). Serum gonadotrophin concentrations in infantile female mice. *J. Reprod. Fertil.* **43**,189-192.

Dunn, H., McEntee, K., Hall, C., Johnson, R., and Stone, W. (1979). Cytogenetic and reproductive studies of bulls born co-twin with freemartins. *J. Reprod. Fertil.* **57**, 21-30.

Ehrhardt, A.A., and Meyer-Bahlburg. F.L. (1981). Effect of prenatal sex hormones on gender-related behavior. *Science* **211**, 1312-1318.

Einarsson, K., Gustafsson, J., and Stanbag, A. (1973). Neonatal imprinting of liver microsomal hydroxulation and reduction of steroids. *J. Biol. Chem.* **248**, 4987-4997.

Ekins, R. (1990). Measurement of free hormones in blood. *Endocr. Rev.* **11**, 5-46.

Ekins, R., Edwards, P., and Newman, B. (1982), The role of binding proteins in hormone delivery. In *Free Hormones in Blood*, ed. A. Albertini and R. Ekins. Elsevier. Amsterdam, pp. 3-43.

Even, M. and vom Saal, F. (1992). Seminal vesicle and preputial gland response to steroids in adult male mice is influenced by prior intrauterine position. *Physiol. Behav.* **51**, 11-16.

Even, M.D., Dhar, M., and vom Saal, F.S. (1992). Transport of steroids between fetuses via amniotic fluid mediates the intrauterine position phenomenon in rats. *J. Reprod. Fertil*, in press.

Feder, H.H. and Goy, R.W. (1983). Effects of neonatal estrogen treatment of female guinea pigs on mounting behavior in adulthood. *Horm. Behav.* **17**, 284-291.

Ford, J.J. and D'Occhio, M.J. (1989). Differentiation of sexual behavior in cattle, sheep and swine. *J. Anim. Sci.* **67**, 1816-1823.

Ford, J.J., Chrinsenson, R.K., and Maurer, R.R. (1980), Serum testosterone concentrations in embryonic and fetal pigs during sexual differentiation. *Biol. Reprod.* **23**, 583-587.

Fox, T.O. (1975). Androgen and estrogen binding macromolecules in developing mouse brain: biochemical and genetic evidence. *Proc. Nat. Acad. Sci.* (USA) **72**, 4303-4307.

Fox, T.O. (1987). AFP in sexual differentiation of mouse and rat brain. In *Biological Activities of Alpha-fetoprotein*. Vol. 1. ed. G. Mizejewski and H. Jacobson. CRC Press, Boca Raton, pp. 181-189.

Franks, L.M. (1954). Benign nodular hyperplasia of the prostate: a review. *Ann. Roy. Coll. Surg. Engl.* **14**, 92-106.

Fredga, K. (1983). Aberrant sex chromosome mechanisms in mammals. *Differentiation*, 23 (Suppl.), S23-S30.

Friedman, W.J., McEwen, B.S., Toran-Allerand, C.D., and Gerlach, J.L. (1983). Perinatal development of hypothalamic and cortical estrogen receptors in mouse brain: methodological aspects. *Dev. Brain Res.* **11**, 19-27.

George, F.W. and Ojeda, S.R. (1982). Changes in aromatase activity in the rat brain during embryonic, neonatal, and infant development. *Endocrinol.* **111**, 522-529.

George, F. and Wilson, J. (1987). Conversion of androgen to estrogen by the human fetal ovary. *J. Clin. Endocrinol. Metab.* **47**, 550-555.

George, F.W., Simpson, E.R., Milewich, L., and Wilson J.D. (1979). Studies on the regulation of the onset of steroid hormone biosynthesis in fetal gonads. *Endocrinol.* **105**, 1100-1106.

Germain, B., Campbell, P., and Anderson, J. (1978). Role of serum estrogen-binding protein in the control of tissue estradiol levels during postnatal development in the female rat. *Endocrinol.* **103**, 1401-1410.

Gibb, W. and Lavoie, J. (1980). Substrate specificity of the placental microsomal aromatase. *Steroids* **36**, 507-519.

Gibori, G., and Sridaran, R. (1981). Sites of androgen and estradiol production in the second half of pregnancy in the rat. *Biol. Reprod.*, **24**, 249-256.

Gitlin, D. (1975). Normal biology of alpha-fetoprotein. *Ann. N.Y. Acad. Sci.* **259**, 7-16.

Gladue, B. and Clemens, L. (1978). Androgenic influences on feminine sexual behavior in male and female rats: defeminization blocked by prenatal antiandrogen treatment. *Endocrinol.* **103**, 1702-1709.

Gladue, B. and Clemens, L. (1980). Masculinization diminished by disruption of prenatal estrogen biosynthesis in male rats. *Physiol. Behav.* **25**, 589-593.

Gladue, B., Green, R., and Hellman, R. (1984). Neuroendocrine response to estrogen and sexual orientation. *Science* **225**, 1496-1499.

Glenister, T.W. (1962). The development of the utricle and of the so-called "middle" or "median" lobe of the human prostate. *J. Anat. (Lond)* **96**, 443-455.

Gosden, R.G., Laing, S.C., Felicio, L.S., Nelson, J.F., and Finch, C.E. (1983). Imminent oocyte exhaustion and reduced follicular recruitment mark the transition to acyclicity in aging C57BL/6J mice. *Biol. Reprod.* **28**, 255-260.

Goldman, B.D., Grazia,Y.R., Kamberi, I.A., and Porter, J.C. (1971). Serum gonadotropin concentrations in intact and castrated neonatal rats. *Endocrinol.*, **88**, 771-776.

Goodfellow, P. (1983). Expression of the 12E7 antigen is controlled independently by genes on the human X and Y chromosomes. *Differentiation*, **23**(Suppl.), S35-S39.

Gorski, R. (1979). The neuroendocrinology of reproduction: An overview. *Biol. Reprod.* **20**, 111-127.

Gorski, R. (1986). Sexual differentiation of the brain: A model for drug-induced alterations of the reproductive system. *Environ. Health Perspectives.* **70**, 163-175.

Gorski, R., Gordon, J., Shryne, J., and Southam, A. (1978). Evidence for a morphological sex difference within the medial preoptic area of the rat brain. *Brain Res.* **148**, 333-346.

Gower, D.B. and Cooke, G.M. (1983). Regulation of steroid-transforming enzymes by endogenous steroids. *J. Steroid Biochem.* **19**, 1527-1556.

Gray, L.E. (1992). Compound-induced alterations of sexual differentiation: A review of effects in humans and rodents. In *Chemically Induced Alterations in Sexual Development: The Wildlife/Human Connection.* eds. T. Colborn and C. Clement, Princeton Scientific Publishing Co., pp. 203-230.

Gubbay, J., Collignon, J., Koopman, P., Capel, B., Economou, A., Münsterberg, A., Vivian, N., Goodfellow, P., and Lovell-Badge, R. (1990). A gene mapping to the sex-determining region of the mouse Y chromosome is a member of a novel family of embryonically expressed genes. *Nature* **346**, 245-250

Gupta, C. (1988). Activation of phospholipases during masculine differentiation of embryonic genitalia. *Proc. Soc. Exp. Biol. Med.* **188**, 489-494.

Habert R, and Picon, R. (1986). Relationships between plasma progesterone levels and testicular testosterone production in the rat fetus: Effects of maternal ovariectomy. *J. Endocrinol.* **108**, 361-367

Habert, R., Veniard, B., Brignaschi, P., Gangnerau, M.N., and Picon, R. (1989). Absence of development of late steroidogenic lesions in rat testis during the end of the fetal life. *Arch. Androl.*, **22**, 41-48

Hall, P.F. (1988). Testicular steroid synthesis: Organization and regulation. In *The Physiology of Reproduction.* ed. E. Knobil et al., Raven Press, Ltd., New York, pp. 975-998.

Ham, R. and Veomett, M. (1980). *Mechanisms of Development.* Mosby, St. Louis.

Harlow, H.F., Joslyn, W.P., Senke, M.G., and Dopp, A. (1966). Behavioral aspects of reproduction in primates. *J. Anim. Sci.* **25**, 49-67.

Harrington, R.W. (1961). Oviparous hermaphroditic fish with internal self fertilization. *Science* **134**, 1749-1750.

Harris, G.W. (1964). Sex hormones: Brain development and brain function. *Endocrinol.* **75**, 627-651.

Harris, G.W. and Jacobson, D. (1952). Functional grafts of the anterior pituitary gland. *Proc. Roy. Soc., Series B.* **139**, 263-276.

Harris, G.W. and Levine, S. (1965). Sexual differentiation of the brain and its experimental control. *J. Physiol.* **181**, 379-400.

Hendricks, S.E. and Duffy, J.A. (1974). Ovarian influences on the development of sexual behavior in neonatally androgenized rats. *Develop. Psychobiol.* **7**, 297-303.

Hendricks, S.E., Graber, B., and Rodriguez-Sierra, J.F. (1989). Neuroendocrine responses to exogenous estrogen: No differences between heterosexual and homosexual men. *Psychoneuroendocrinol.* **14**, 177-185.

Hines, M. (1992). Surrounded by estrogens? Considerations for neurobehavioral development in human beings. In *Chemically Induced Alterations in Sexual Development: The Wildlife/Human Connection.* eds. T. Colborn and C. Clement, Princeton Scientific Publishing Co., pp. 261-281.

Hines, M. and Green, R. (1991). Human hormonal and neural correlates of sex-typed behaviors. *Rev. Psychiat.* **10**, 536-555.

Hodgkin, J. (1990). Sex determination compared in Drosophila and xenorabditis. *Nature* **344**, 721-728.

Horowitz, K., Costlow, M., and McGuire, W. (1975). MCF-7: a human cancer cell line with estrogen, androgen, progesterone and glucocortocoid receptors. *Steroids* **26**, 785-795

Huhtaniemi, I.T. (1985). Functional and regulatory differences between the fetal and adult populations of rat Leydig cells. In *The Endocrine Physiology of Pregnancy and the Peripartal Period*, ed. R.B. Jaffe and S. Dell'Acqua. Serono Symposia Pub., Vol 21. Raven Press, New York, pp. 65-85.

Huhtaniemi, I.T., Warren, D.W., Apter, D., and Catt, K.J. (1983). Absence of gonadotropin-induced desensitization of testosterone production in the neonatal rat testis. *Mol. Cell Endocrinol.* **32**, 81-89

Hulsebosch, C. and Fabian, R. (1989). Penetration of IgGs into the neuroaxis of the neonatal rat. *Neurosci. Let.* **98**, 13-18.

Imperato-McGinley, J., Peterson, R., Gautier, T., and Sturla, E. (1979). Androgens and the evolution of male-gender identity among male pseudohermaphrodites with 5α-reductase defiency. *New Engl. J. Med.* **300**, 1233-1237.

Jackson, J.A. and Albrecht, E.D. (1985). The development of placental androstenedione and testosterone production and their utilization by the ovary for aromatization to estrogen during rat pregnancy. *Biol. Reprod.* 33, 451-457.

Jacobson, C.D., Davis, F.C., and Gorski, R.A. (1985). Formation of sexually dimorphic nucleus of the preoptic area: Neuronal growth, migration and changes in cell number. *Dev. Brain. Res.* **21**, 7-18.

Jacobson, C.D. and Gorski, R.A. (1981). Neurogenesis of the sexually dimorphic nucleus of the preoptic area in the rat. *J. Comp. Neurol.* **196**, 519-529.

Jansson, J.O. and Frohman, L.A. (1987). Inhibitory effect of the ovaries on neonatal androgen imprinting of growth hormone secretion in female rats. *Endocrinol.* **121**, 1417-1423.

Janzen. F.J. and Paukstis, G.L. (1991). Environmental sex determination in reptiles: Ecology, evolution, and experimental design. *Quart. Rev. Biol.* **66**, 149-179.

Jesionowska, H., Karelus, K., and Nelson, J.F. (1990). Effects of chronic exposure to estradiol on ovarian cyclicity in C56BL/6J mice: Potentiation at low doses and only partial suppression at high doses. *Biol. Reprod.* **43**, 312-317

Josso, N. (1986). AntiMüllerian hormone: New perspectives for a sexist molecule. *Endocr. Rev.* **7**, 421-433

Jost, A. (1972). A new look at the mechanisms controlling sex differentiation in mammals. *Johns Hopkins Med. J.* **130**, 38-53.

Jost, A. (1985). Sexual organogenesis. In *Handbook of Behavioral Neurobiology*, ed. N. Adler, D. Pfaff and R. Goy. Plenum Press, New York, pp. 3-20.

Jung-Testas, Groyer, M-T, Bruner-Lorand, J., Hechter, O., Baulieu, E-E, and Robel, P. (1981). Androgen and estrogen receptors in rat ventral prostate epithelium and stroma. *Endocrinol.* **109**, 1287-1289.

Kaplan, M. and McGinnis, M. (1989). Effects of ATD on male sexual behavior and androgen receptor binding: A reexamination of the aromatization hypothesis. *Horm. Behav.* **23**, 10-26.

Karsch, F., Dierschke, D., and Knobil, E. (1972). Sexual differentiation of pituitary function: Apparent difference between primates and rodents. *Science* **179**, 484-486.

Keel, B. and Abney, T. (1984). The kinetics of estrogen binding to rat α-fetoprotein. *Experientia* **40**, 503-505.

Keisler, L., vom Saal, F., Keisler, D., and Walker, S. (1991). Hormonal manipulation of the prenatal environment alters reproductive morphology and increases longevity in autoimmune NZB/W mice. *Biol. Reprod.* **44**, 707-716.

Kincl, F., Pi, A., and Lasso, L. (1963). Effects of estradiol benzoate treatment in the newborn male rat. *Endocrinol.* **72**, 966-968.

Koopman, P., Gubbay, J., Vivian, N., Goodfellow, P., and Lovell-Badge, R. (1991). Male development of chromosomally female mice transgenic for Sry. *Nature* **351**, 117-121.

Korach, K.S., Sarver, P., Chae, K., McLachlan, J.A., and McKinney J.D. (1987). Estrogen receptor-binding activity of polychlorinated hydroxybiphenyls Conformationally restricted structural probes. *Mol. Pharmacol.* **33**, 120-126.

Krey, L., Lieburg, I., Roy, E., and McEwen, B. (1979). Oestradiol plus receptor complexes in the brain and anterior pituitary gland: quantitation and neuroendocrine significance. *J. Steroid. Biochem.* **11**, 279-284.

Krey, L., Kamel, F., and McEwen, B. (1980). Parameters of neuroendocrine aromatization and estrogen receptor occupation in the male rat. *Brain Res.* **193**, 277-283.

Kuhn, R., Green, A., Raymoure, W., and Siiteri, P. (1986). Immunocytochemical localization of corticosteroid-binding globulin in rat tissues. *J. Endocrinol.* **108**, 31-36.

Kuiper-Goodman, T. (1991). Risk assessment to humans of mycotoxins in animal-derived food products. *Vet. Hum. Toxicol.* **33**, 325-333.

Laborda, J., Naval, J., Calvo, M., Lampreave, F., and Uriel, J. (1989). Alpha-fetoprotein and albumin uptake by mouse tissues during development. *Biol. Neonate* **56**, 332-341.

Langman, J. (1975). *Medical Embryology*, 3rd ed. The Williams and Wilkins Co., Baltimore.

Laufer, L.R., Gambone, J.C., Chaudhuri, G., Pardridge, W.M., and Judd, H.L. (1983). The effect of membrane permeability and binding by human serum proteins on sex steroid influx into the uterus. *J. Clin. Endo. Metab.* **56**, 1282-1287.

Lee, F., Torp-Pedersen, S.T., and Siders, D.B. (1989). The role of transrectal ultrasound in the early detection of prostate cancer. *CA-A cancer Journal for Clinicians* **39**, 337-360.

Lephart, E.D., Andersson, S., and Simpson, E.R. (1990). Expression of Neural 5 alpha-reductase activity during prenatal development in the rat. *Endocrinology* **127**, 1121-1128.

LeVay, S. (1991). A difference in hypothalamic structure between heterosexual and homosexual men. *Science* **253**, 1034-1037.

Lipschutz, A., Yanine, D., Schwartz, J., Beuzzone, S. Acuna, J., and Silberman, S. (1945). Induction and prevention of fibromyoepithelioma of utricular bed in male guinea-pigs. *Cancer Res.* **5**, 515-523.

Lowsley, O.S. (1912). The development of the human prostate gland with reference to the development of other structures at the neck of the urinary bladder. *Am. J. Anat.* **13**, 299-349.

Lung., B. and Cunha, G. (1981). Development of seminal vesicles and coagulating glands in neonatal mice. I. the morphogenetic effects of various hormonal conditions. *Anat. Rec.* **199**, 73-88.

Lyon, M. (1970). Genetic activity of sex chromosomes in somatic cells of mammals. *Phil. Trans. Royal Soc. Lond.* (B) **259**, 41.

MacLusky, N., Chaptal, C. and McEwen, B. (1979a). The development of estrogen receptor systems in the rat brain and pituitary: Postnatal development. *Brain Res.* **178**, 143-160.

MacLusky, N., Lieberburg, I., and McEwen, B. (1979b). The development of estrogen receptor systems in the rat brain: Perinatal development. *Brain Res.* **178**, 129-142.

MacLusky, N. and Naftolin, F. (1981). Sexual differentiation of the central nervous system. *Science* **211**, 1294-1303.

MacLusky, N., Philip, A., Hurlburt, C., and Naftolin, F. (1985). Estrogen formation in the developing rat brain: Sex differences in aromatase activity during early postnatal life. *Psychoneuroendocrinol.* **10**, 355-361.

Marcum, J.B. (1974). The freemartin syndrome. *Anim. Breed. Abst.* **42**, 228-242.

Martikainen, P., Makela, S., Santti, R., Harkonen, P., and Souminen, J. (1987). Interaction of male and female sex hormones in cultured rat prostate. *Prostate* **11**, 291-303.

Mawhinney, M. and Neubauer, B. (1979). Actions of estrogen in the male. *Inves. Urol.* **16**, 409-420.

Mazur, M. and Younglai, E. (1986). Role of the pituitary in controlling oogenesis in the rabbit. *Biol. Reprod.* **35**, 191-197.

McCall, A., Han, S., Millington, W., and Baum, M. (1981). Non-saturable transport of [$^3$H]estradiol across the blood-brain barrier in female rats is reduced by neonatal serum. *J. Reprod. Fertil.* **61**, 103-108.

McEwen, B.S., Biegon, A., Davis, P.G., Krey, L.C., Luine, V.N., McGinnis, M.Y., Paden, C.M., Parsons, B., and Rainbow, T.C. (1982). Steroid hormones: humoral signals which alter brain cell properties and function. *Recent Prog. Horm. Res.* **38**, 41-92.

McEwen, B.S., Plapinger, L., Chaptal, C., Gerlach, J., and Wallach, G. (1975). Role of fetoneonatal estrogen binding protein in the association of estrogen with neonatal brain cell nuclear receptor. *Brain Res.* **96**, 400-406.

McKelvie, P. Jaubert, F., and Nezelof, C. (1987). Is true hermaphroditism a primary germ cell disorder? *Pediatric Path.* **7**, 31-41.

McLachlan, J., Newbold, R., and Bullock, B. (1975). Reproductive tract lesions in male mice exposed prenatally to diethylstibestrol. *Science* **190**, 991-992.

McLaren, A. (1991). Development of the mammalian gonad: The fate of the supporting cell lineage. *BioEssays* **13**, 151-156.

McNeal, J.E. (1978). Origin and evolution of benign prostatic enlargement. *Inves. Urol.* **15**, 340-345.

McNeal, J. E. (1980). The anatomic heterogeneity of the prostate. In *Models of Prostate Cancer*. ed. D. Coffey, D. Merchant and G. Murphy. Liss, New York, pp. 149-160.

McNeal, J.E. (1981). The zonal anatomy of the prostate. *Prostate* **2**, 35-49.

Meaney, M.J., Stewart, J., Poulin, P., and McEwen, B.S. (1983). Sexual differentiation of social play in rat pups is mediated by neonatal androgen-receptor system. *Neuroendocrinol.* **37**, 85-90.

Medvei, V.C. (1982). *A History of Endocrinology*. MTP Press, Lancaster, Pa.

Meijs-Roelofs, H.A., Uilenbroek, J.J., de Jong, F.H., and Welschen, R. (1973). Plasma estradiol-17-beta and its relationship to serum follicle-stimulating hormone in immature female rats. *J. Endocrinol.* **59**, 295-304.

Melcangi, R., Celotti, F., Ballabio, M., Poletti, A., Castano, P., and Martini, L. (1988). Testosterone 5-alpha-reductase activity in the rat brain is highly concentrated in white matter structures and in purified myelin sheaths of axons. *J. Steroid Biochem.* **31**, 173-179,

Mendel, C. (1989). The free hormone hypothesis: A phlogically based mathematical model. *Endocr. Rev.* **10**, 232-274.

Mendel, C., Cavalieri, R., and Weisiger, R. (1988). Uptake of thyroxine by the perfused rat liver: Implications for the free hormone hypothesis. *Am. J. Physiol.* **255**, E110-E119.

Mendelson, C.R., Means, G.D., Mahendroo, M.S., Corbin, C.J., Steinkampf, M.P., Graham-Lorence, S., and Simpson, E.R. (1990). Use of molecular probes to study regulation of aromatase cytochrome P-450. *Biol. Reprod.* **42**, 1-10.

Meyer, W.J., Migeon, B.R., and Migeon, C.J. (1975). Locus on human X chromosome for dihydrotestosterone receptor and androgen insensitivity. *Proc. Nat. Acad. Sci.* **72**, 1469-1472.

Miller, W.L. (1990). Editorial: Immunoassays for human Mullerian inhibitory factor (MIF): New insight into the physiology of MIF. *J. Clin. Endocr. Metab.* **70**, 8-10.

Mittwoch, U. (1973). Genetics of Sex Differentiation. *Academic Press*, New York.

Mittwoch, U., Delhanty, J., and Beck, F. (1969). Growth of differentiating testes and ovaries. *Nature* **224**, 1323-1325.

Mollgard, K. and Saunders, M.R. (1977). A possible transepithelial pathway via endoplasmic reticulum in foetal sheep choroid plexus. *Proc. Roy. Soc. Lond. B* **199**, 321-326.

Montano, M.M. (1991). *In vitro* and *in vivo* studies of free, AFP-bound and albumin-bound estradiol in blood: Evidence for uptake and binding in rat brain during sexual differentiation. Ph.D. thesis, University of Missouri-Columbia.

Montano, M.M., Wang, M-H., Even, M.D., and vom Saal, F.S. (1991). Serum corticosterone in fetal mice: Sex differences, circadian changes, and effect of maternal stress. *Physiol. Behav.* **50**, 323-329.

Montano, M.M., Welshons, W.V., Keel, B., and vom Saal, F.S. (1992). Estradiol passes from blood into brain cells and binds to estrogen receptors in newborn female rats. Paper presented at the 25th meeting of the Society for the Study of Reproduction, Raleigh, N.C., July 12-15.

Mooradian, A.D., Morley, J.E., and Korenman, S.G. (1987). Biological actions of androgens. *Endocr. Rev.* **8**, 1-28.

Moore, K.L. (1982). *The Developing Human: Clinically Oriented Embryology.* W.B. Saunders, Philadelphis.

Moro, R., Fielitz, W., Esteves, A., Grunberg, J., and Uriel. (1984). *In vivo* uptake of heterologous alphafetoprotein and serum albumin by ependymal cells of developing chick embryos. *Int. J. Dev. Neurosci.* **2**, 143-148.

Naftolin, F., Ryan, K.J., Davies, I.J., Reddy, V.V., Flores, F., Petro, Z., Kuhn, M., White, R.J., Takoaka, Y., and Wolin, L. (1975). The formation of estrogens by central neuroendocrine tissues. *Rec. Prog. Horm. Res.* **31**, 295-315.

Naval, J., Villacampa, M., Goguel, A., and Uriel, J. (1985). Cell-type-specific receptors for alpha-fetoprotein in a mouse T-lymphoma cell line. *Proc. Natl. Acad. Sci.* (USA) **82**, 3301-3305.

Negri-Cesi, P., Celotti, F., and Martini, L. (1986). Androgen metabolism in the brain: Role in sexual differentiation and in the control of gonadotropin secretion. *Monogr. Neural. Sci.* **12**, 7-16.

Netter, F.H. (1954). *The CIBA collection of medical illustrations. Reproductive System Vol. II.* CIBA-GEIGY Corp., Summit, N.J.

Netter, F.H. (1989). *Atlas of Human Anatomy.* CIBA-GEIGY Corp., West Caldwell, N.J.

Nonneman, D.J., Ganjam, V.K., Welshons, W.V., and vom Saal, F.S. (1992). Intrauterine position effects on steroid metabolism and steroid receptors of reproductive organs in male mice. *Biol. Reprod*, in press.

Nordeen, E. and Yahr, P. (1983). A regional analysis of estrogen binding to hypothalamic cell nuclei in relation to masculinization and defeminization. *J. Neurosci*. **3**, 933-941.

Norman, R.L. and Spies, H.G. (1986). Cyclic ovarian function in a male macaque: additional evidence for a lack of sexual differentiation in the physiological mechanisms that regulate the cyclic release of gonadotropins in primates. *Endocrinol*. **118**, 2608-2610.

Nunez, E.A., Benassayag, C., Savu, L., Vallette, G., and DeLorne, J. (1979). Oestrogen binding function of alpha-fetoprotein. *J. Steroid. Biochem*. **11**, 237-243.

Ohno, S. (1967). *Sex Chromosomes and Sex-Linked Genes*. Springer Verlag, Berlin.

Overzier, C. (1963). *Intersexuality*. Academic Press, New York.

Paden, C.M. and Roselli, C.E. (1987). Modulation of aromatase activity by testosterone in transplants of fetal rat hypothalamic-preoptic area. *Dev. Brain Res*. **33**, 127-133.

Page, D.C., Mosher, R., Simpson, E.M., Fisher, E.M.C., Mardon, G., Pollak, J., McGillivray, B., de la Chapelle, A., and Brown, L.G. (1987). The sex-determining region of the human Y chromosome encodes a finger protein. *Cell* **51**, 1091-1104.

Painter, T. (1923). Studies in mammalian spermatogenesis. II. The spermatogenesis of man. *J. Exp. Zool*. **37**, 291-335.

Palmer, M.S., Sinclair, A.H., Berta, P., Ellis, N.A., Goodfellow, P.N., Abbas, N.E., and Fellous, M. (1989). Genetic evidence that ZYF is not the testis-determining factor. *Nature* **342**, 937-939.

Pappas, C.T., Diamond, M.C., and Johnson, R.E. (1978). Effects of ovariectomy and differential experience on rat cerebral cortical morphology. *Brain. Res.* **154**, 53-60.

Pardridge, W.M. (1981). Transport of protein-bound hormones into tissues *in vivo*. *Endocrine Rev*. **2**, 103-123.

Pardridge, W.M. (1986). Receptor-mediated peptide transport through the blood-brain barrier. *Endocr. Rev*. **7**, 314-330.

Pardridge, W.M. and Mietus, L.J. (1979). Transport of protein-bound steroid hormones into liver *in vivo*. *Am. J. Physiol*. **237**, E367-E372.

Peitz, B. (1988). Effects of seminal vesicle fluid components on sperm motility in the house mouse. *J. Reprod. Fertil*. **83**, 169-176.

Peitz, B. and Olds-Clarke, P. (1986). Effects of seminal vesicle removal on fertility and uterine sperm motility in the house mouse. *Biol. Reprod*. **35**, 608-617.

Pelliniemi, L.J. and Dym, M. (1980). The fetal gonad and sexual differentiation. In *Maternal-Fetal Endocrinology*, ed. D. Tulchinsky and K.J. Ryan. Saunders, Philadelphia, pp. 252-280.

Pelliniemi, L.J. and Niemi, M. (1969). Fine structure of the human foetal testis. I. The interstitial tissue. *Z. Zellforsch*. **99**, 507-522.

Perrot-Applanat, M., Racadot, O., and Milgrom, E. (1984). Specific localization of plasma corticosteroid binding globulin immunoreactivity in pituitary corticotrophs. *Endocrinol*. **115**, 559-569.

Peterson, R.P. and Spaziani, E. (1969). Cyclohexamide and cortisol inhibition of estradiol stimulated uterine uptake and distribution of homologous serum albumin and alpha globulin in the rat. *Endocrinol*. **85**, 932-940.

Pfaff, D. (1980). *Estrogens and Brain Function*. Springer-Verlag, New York.

Pfaff, D. and Schwartz-Giblin, S. (1988). Cellular mechanisms of female reproductive behaviors. In *Physiology of Reproduction*, ed. E. Knobil and J. Neill. Raven Press, New York, pp. 1487-1568.

Pfeiffer, C.A. (1936). Sexual differences of the hypophyses and their determination by the gonads. *Am. J. Anat.* **58**, 195-225.

Phoenix, C.H., Goy, R.W., Geral,l A.A., and Young, W.C. (1959). Organizing action of prenatally administered testosterone propionate on the tissue mediating mating behavior in the female guinea pig. *Endocrinol* **65**, 369-382.

Poliard, A., Feldman, G., and Bernuau, D. (1988). Alpha-fetoprotein and albumin gene transcripts are detected in distince cell populations of the brain and kidney of the developing rat. *Differentiat.* **39**, 59-65.

Rabinovici, J. and Jaffe, R. (1990). Development and regulation of growth and differentiated function in human and subhuman primate fetal gonads. *Endocr. Rev.* **11**, 532-557.

Rajfer, J. and Coffey, D. (1978). Sex steroid imprinting of the immature prostate long-term effects. *Inves. Urol.* **16**, 186-190.

Rajfer, J. and Coffey, D. (1979). Effects of neonatal steroids on male sex tissues. *Inves. Urol.* **17**, 3-8.

Real, L. (1980). On uncertainty and the law of diminishing returns in evolution and behavior. In *Limits to Action*, ed. J. Staddon. Academic Press, New York, pp 37.

Reed, K. and Ohno, S. (1976). Kinetic properties of human placental aromatase. *J. Biol. Chem.* **251**, 1625-1631.

Reiter, E.O., Goldenberg, R.L., Vaitukaitis, J.L., and Ross, G.T. (1972). A role for endogenous estrogen in normal ovarian development in the neonatal rat. *Endocrinol.*, **91**, 1537-1539.

Renoir, J., Mercier-Bodard, C., and Balieu, E. (1980). Hormonal and immunological aspects of the phylogeny of sex steroid binding plasma protein. *Proc. Natl. Acad. Sci.* (USA) **77**, 4578-4582.

Resko, J.A. (1975). Fetal hormones and their effect on the differentiation of the central nervous system in primates. *Fed. Proc.* **34**, 1650-1655.

Resko, J.A., Ploem, J.G., and Stadelman, H.L. (1975). Estrogens in fetal and maternal plasma of the rhesus monkey. *Endocrinol.* **97**, 425-430.

Reyes, F., Boroditsky, R., Winter, J., and Faiman, C. (1974). Studies on human sexual development. II. Fetal and maternal serum gonadotropin and sex steroid concentrations. *J. Clin. Endocrinol. Metab.* **38**, 612-617.

Reyes, F., Winter, J., and Faiman, C. (1973). Studies on human sexual development. I. Fetal gonadal and adrenal sex steroids. *J. Clin. Endocrinol. Metab.* **37**, 74-78.

Richardson, S.J., Senikas, Z., and Nelson, J.F. (1987). Follicular depletion during the menopausal transition: evidence for accelerated loss and ultimate exhaustion. *J. Clin. Endocrinol. Metab.* **65**, 1231-1237.

Robinson, J., Judd, H., Young, P., Jones, O., and Yen, S. (1977). Amniotic fluid androgens and estrogens in midgestation. *J. Clin. Endocrinol. Metab.* **45**, 755-761.

Rories, C. and Spelsberg, T.C. (1989). Ovarian steroid action on gene expression: Mechanisms and models. *Annual Rev. Physiol.* **51**, 653-681.

Roselli, C.E. and Resko, J.A. (1984). Androgens regulate brain aromatase activity in adult male rats through a receptor mechanism. *Endocrinol.* **114**, 2183-2189.

Roselli, C.E., Ellinwood, W.E., and Resko, J.A. (1984). Regulation of brain aromatase activity in rats. *Endocrinol.* **114**, 192-200.

Roselli, C.E., Horton, L.E., and Resko, J.A. (1985). Distribution and regulation of aromatase activity in the rat hypothalamus. *Endocrinol.* **117**, 2471-2477.

Rosner, W. and Hochberg, R. (1976). Corticosteroid binding globulin in the rat: isolation and studies of its influence on cortisol action *in vivo*. *Endocrinol.* **91**, 626-632.

Rotkin, I.D. (1983). Origins, distribution, and risk of benign prostatic hypertrophy. In *Benign Prostatic Hypertrophy*, ed. F. Hinman. Springer-Verlag, New York, pp. 10-21.

Ruoslahti, E. and Seppala, M. (1979). alpha-fetoprotein in cancer and fetal development. *Adv. Cancer Res.* **29**, 275-346.

Ryan, K.J. (1980). Placental synthesis of steroid hormones. In *Maternal-Fetal Endocrinology*, ed. D. Tulchinsky and K.J. Ryan. Saunders, Philadelphia, pp. 3-16.

Sachs, B. and Meisel, R. (1988). The physiology of male sexual behavior. In *Physiology of Reproduction*, ed. E. Knobil and J. Neill. Raven Press, New York, pp. 1393-1485.

Sakly, M. and Koch, B. (1983). Ontogenitical variation of transcortin modulates glucocorticoid receptor function and corticotrophic activity in the pituitary gland. *Horm. Metab. Res.* **15**, 92-96.

Sandberg, A.A., Slaunwhite, W.R., and Carter, A.C. (1960). Transcortin: a corticosteroid-binding protein of plasma. III. The effects of various steroids. *J. Clin. Invest.* **39**: 1914-1926.

Sar, M. and Stumpf, W.E. (1977). Distribution of androgen target cells in rat forebrain and pituitary after [$^3$H]-dihydrotestosterone administration. *J. Steroid Biochem.* **8**, 1131-1135.

Schachter, B.S. and Toran-Allerand, C.D. (1982). Intraneuronal alpha-fetoprotein and albumin are not synthesized locally in the developing brain. *Dev. Brain Res.* **5**, 93-98.

Schlegel, R., Farias, E., Russo, N., Moore, J., and Gardner, L. (1967). Structural changes in the fetal gonads and gonaducts during maturation of an enzyme, steroid 3b-ol-dehydrogenase, in the gonads adrenal cortex and placenta of fetal rats. *Endocrinol.* **81**, 565-572.

Schleicher, G., Drews, U., Stumpf, W.E., and Sar, M. (1984). Differential distribution of dihydrotestosterone and estradiol binding sites in the epididymis of the mouse: an autoradiographic study. *Histochem.* **81**, 139-147.

Schellhas, H.F. (1974). Malignant potential of dysgenetic gonad. *Obstet. Gynecol.* **44**, 455-462.

Schlinger, B.S. and Arnold, A.P. (1991). Brain is the major site of estrogen synthesis in a male songbird. *Proc. Nat. Acad. Sci.* **88**, 4191-4194.

Schroeder, R.J. and Henning, S.J. (1989). Roles of plasma clearance and corticosteroid-binding globulin in the developmental increase in circulating corticosterone in infant rats. *Endocrinol.* **124**, 2612-2618.

Schultz, M.F. and Wilson, J.D. (1974). Virilization of the Wolffian duct in the rat fetus by various androgens. *Endocrinol.* **94**, 979-986.

Setchell, B.P. and Brooks, D.E. (1988). Anatomy, vasculature, innervation, and fluids of the male reproductive tract. In *Physiology of Reproduction*, ed. E. Knobil and J. Neill. Raven Press, New York, pp. 753-836.

Shapiro, B., Goldman, A., Steinbeck, H., and Neumann, F. (1976). Is feminine differentiation of the brain hormonally determined? *Experientia* **32**, 650-651.

Shapiro, E. (1990). Embryological development of the prostate. *Urol. Clin. N. Amer.* **17**, 487-493.

Sheehan, D.M. and Young, M. (1979). Diethylstilbestrol and estradiol binding to serum albumin and pregnancy plasma of rat and human. *Endocrinol.* **104**, 1442-1446.

Sheridan, P. (1979). Estrogen binding in the neonatal cortex. *Brain Res.* **178**, 201-206.

Shima, H., Tsuji, M., Young, P., and Cunha, G. (1990). Postnatal growth of mouse seminal vesicle is dependent on 5$\alpha$-dihydrotestosterone. *Endocrinol.* **127**, 3222-3233.

Short, R.V. (1972). Sex determination and differentiation. In *Reproduction in Mammals: 2. Embryonic and Fetal Development*, ed. C.R. Austin and R.V. Short. Cambridge University Press, London, pp. 43-71.

Siiteri, P.K. and Wilson, J.D. (1974). Testosterone formation and metabolism during male sexual differentiation in the human embryo. *J. Clin. Endocrinol. Metab.* **38**, 113-125.

Siiteri, P.K., Murai, J.T., Hammond, G.L., Nisker, J.A., Raymoure, W.J., and Kuhn, R.W. (1982). The serum transport of steroid hormones. *Rec. Prog. Horm. Res.* **38**, 457-510.

Simon, N.G., and Whalen, R.E. (1987). Sexual differentiation of androgen-sensitive and estrogen-sensitive regulatory systems for aggressive behavior. *Horm. Behav.* **21**, 493-500.

Simpson, E.R., Merrill, J.C., Hollub, A.J., Graham-Lorence, S., and Mendelson, C.R. (1989). Regulation of estrogen biosynthesis by human adipose cells. *Endocr. Rev.* **10**, 136-148.

Sinclair, A.H., Berta, P., Palmer, M.S., Hawkins, J.R., Griffins, B.L., Smith, M.J., Foster, J.W., Fridchauf, A.-M., Lovell-Badge, R., and Goodfellow, P. (1990). A gene from the human sex-determining region encodes a protein with homology to a conserved DNA-binding motif. *Nature* **346**, 240-244.

Slob, A.K., Oom, M.P., and Vreeburg, T.M. (1980). Prenatal and early postnatal sex differences in plasma and gonadal testosterone and plasma luteinizing hormone in female and male rats. *J. Endocrinol.* **87**, 81-87

Smith, M., Freeman, M., and Neill, J. (1975). The control of progesterone secretion during the estrous cycle and early pseudopregnancy in the rat: prolactin, gonadotropin and steroid levels associated with rescue of the corpus luteum of pseudopregnancy. *Endocrinol.* **96**, 219-226.

Soares, M.J., and Talamantes, F. (1982). Gestational effects on placental and serum androgen, progesterone and prolactin-like activity in the mouse. *J. Endocrinol.* **95**, 29-36.

Soares, M.J., and Talamantes, F. (1983). Mid-pregnancy elevation of serum androstenedione levels in the C3H/HeN mouse: placental origin. *Endocrinol.* **113**, 1408-1412.

Sodersten, P., Pettersson, A., and Eneroth, P. (1983). Pulse administration of estradiol-17β cancels sex differences in behavioral estrogen sensitivity. *Endocrinol.* **112**, 1883-1885.

Sopelak, V.M. and Butcher, R.L. (1982). Contribution of the ovary versus hypothalamus-pituitary to termination of estrous cycles in aging rats using ovarian transplants. *Biol. Reprod.* **27**, 29-37.

Soto, A., Lin, T., Justicia, H., Silvia, R., and Sonnenschein, C. (1992) An "in culture" bioassay to assess the estrogenicity of xenobiotics (E-SCREEN). In *Chemically Induced Alterations in Sexual Development: The Wildlife/Human Connection*. eds. T. Colborn and C. Clement, Princeton Scientific Publishing Co., pp. 295-309.

Speed, R.M. and Chandley, A.C. (1983). Meiosis in the foetal mouse ovary. II Oocyte development and age-related aneuploidy. Does a production line exist? *Chromosoma* **88**, 184-189.

Sridaran, R., and Gibori, G. (1987). Placental-ovarian relationship in the control of testosterone secretion in the rat. *Placenta* **8**, 327-333.

Stenberg, A. (1975). On the modulating effects of ovaries on neonatal androgen programming of rat liver enzymes. *Acta Endocrinol.* (Copenh) **78**, 294-301.

Stiff, M., Bronson, F., and Stetson, M. (1974). Plasma gonadotropins in prenatal and prepubertal female mice: Disorganization of pubertal cycles in the absence of a male. *Endocrinol.* **94**, 492-496.

Tait, J. (1982). The biological availability of free and protein bound steroid. In *Free Hormones in Blood*, ed. A. Albertini and R. Ekins. Elsevier, Amsterdam, pp. 65-70.

Tait, J.F. and Burstein, S. (1964). *In vivo* studies of steroid dynamics in man. In *The Hormones*, ed. G. Pincus, K.V. Thimann, and E.D. Astwood. Academic Press, New York, pp. 441-557.

Takasugi, N. and Bern, H.A. (1988). Introduction: Abnormal genital tract delopment in mammals following early exposure to sex hormones. In *Toxicity of Hormones in Perinatal Life*, ed. J. Mori and H. Nagasawa. CRC Press, Boca Raton, pp. 1-7.

Tapanainen, J., Kellokumpu-Lehtinen, P., Pelliniemi, L.J., and Huhtaniemi, I.T. (1981). Age-related changes in endogenous steroids of human fetal testes during early and midpregnancy. *J. Clin. Endocrinol. Metab.* **52**, 98-102.

Tapanainen, J., Kuopio, T., Pelliniemi, L.J., and Huhtaniemi, I.T. (1984). Rat testicular endogenous steroids and number of Leydig cells between the fetal period and sexual maturity. *Biol. Reprod.* **31**, 1027-1035.

Terada, N., Kuroda, H., Namiki, M., Kitamura, Y., and Matsumoto, K. (1984). Augmentation of aromatase activity by FSH in ovaries of fetal and neonatal mice in organ culture. *J. Steroid. Biochem.* **20**, 741-745.

Timms, B. and DiDio, L.J.A. (1990). The effect of intrauterine position on the occurrance of female prostatic bud development. *Anat. Rec.* **226**, 1048.

Timms, B., Larson, B., Lee, C., Newbauer, B., Goode, R., Seiz, J., and Aumuller, G. (1992). Lobe specific secretory protein production in heterotypic recombinants from rat urogenital sinus and adult prostate epithelium. *Anat. Rec.*, in press.

Tissel, L-E. (1971). The growth of the ventral prostate, the dorsolateral prostate, the coagulating glands and the seminal vesicles in castrated adrenalectomized rats injected with E2 and/or cortisone. *Acta Endocrinol.* **86**, 485-501.

Tobet, S., Baum, M., Tang, H., Shim, J., and Canik, J. (1985). Aromatase activity in the perinatal rat forebrain: Effects of age, sex and intrauterine position. *Develop. Brain Res.* **23**, 171-178.

Toran-Allerand, C.D. (1984). On the genesis of sex differences of the central nervous system: morphogenetic consequences of steroidal exposure and possible role of alpha-fetoprotein. *Prog. Brain Res.* **61**, 63-98.

Tsuji, M., Shima, H., and Cunha, G.R. (1991). *In vitro* androgen-induced growth and morphogenesis of the Wolffian duct within urogenital ridge. *Endocrinol.* **128**, 1805-1811.

Tulchinsky, D., Hobel, C.J., Yeager, E., and Marshall, J.R. (1972). Plasma estradiol, estriol, estradiol, progesterone and 17-hydroxyprogesterone in human pregnancy. I. Normal pregnancy. *Am. J. Obstet. Gynecol.* **112**, 1095-1100.

Tuohimaa, P. and Niemi, M. (1972). *In vitro* uptake of tritiated sex steroids by the hypothalamus of adult male rats treated neonatally with an antiandrogen (cyproterone). *Acta Endocrinol.* (Copen) **71**, 45-54.

Ueno, S., Takahashi, M., Manganaro, T., Ragin, R., and Donahoe, P. (1989). Cellular localization of Mullerian inhibiting substance in the developing rat ovary. *Endocrinol.* **124**, 1000-1006.

Vallette, G., Benassayag, C., Belanger, C., Nunez, EA., and Jayle, MF. (1977). Rat iso-alpha-fetoprotein: purification and interaction with estradiol-17-beta. *Steroids* **29**, 277-289.

van Niekirk, W. (1974). *True Hermaphroditism*. Harper and Row, New York.

Vannier, B and Raynaud, J. (1980). Long-term effects of prenatal oestrogen treatment on genital morphology and reproductive function in the rat. *J. Reprod. Fertil.* **59**, 43-49.

Vigier, B., Forest, M., Eychenne, B., Bazard, J., Garrigou, O. Robel, P., and Josso, N. (1989). Anti-Mullerian hormone produces endocrine sex reversal of fetal ovaries. *Dev. Biol.* **86**, 3684-3688.

Villacampa, M., Lampreave, F., Calvo, M., Naval, J., Pineiro, A., and Uriel, J. (1984). Incorporation of radiolabelled alphafetoprotein in the brain and other tissues of the developing rat. *Dev. Brain Res.* **12**, 77-82.

Vito, C. and Fox, T. (1982). Androgen and estrogen receptors in embryonic and neonatal rat brain. *Dev. Brain Res.* **2**, 97-110.

Vito, C.C., Wieland, S.J., and Fox, T.O. (1979). Androgen receptor exists thoughout the "critical period" of brain sexual differentiation. *Nature* **282**, 308-310.

vom Saal, F. (1979). Prenatal exposure to androgen influences morphology and aggressive behavior of male and female mice. *Horm. Behav.* **12**, 1-11.

vom Saal, F. (1981). Variation in phenotype due to random intrauterine positioning of male and female fetuses in rodents. *J. Reprod. Fertil.* **62**, 633-650.

vom Saal, F. (1983a). Models of early hormonal effects on intrasex aggression in mice. In *Hormones and Aggressive Behavior*, ed. B. Svare. Plenum, New York, pp. 197-222.

vom Saal, F. (1983b). The interaction of circulating estrogens and androgens in regulating mammalian sexual differentiation. In *Hormones and Behavior in Higher Vertebrates*, ed. J. Balthazart, E. Prove and R. Giles. Springer Verlag, Berlin, pp. 159-177.

vom Saal, F. (1984). The intrauterine position phenomenon: Effects on physiology, aggressive behavior and population dynamics in house mice. In *Prog. Clin. Biol. Res.*, Vol. 169, Biological Perspectives on Aggression, ed. K. Flannelly, R. Blanchard and D. Blanchard. Liss, New York, pp. 135-179.

vom Saal F., (1989a). Sexual differentiation in litter bearing mammals: influence of sex of adjacent fetuses *in utero. J. Anim. Sci.* **67**, 1824-40.

vom Saal, F. (1989b). The production of and sensitivity to cues that delay puberty and prolong subsequent oestrous cycles in female mice are influenced by prior intrauterine position. *J. Reprod. Fertil.* **86**, 457-471.

vom Saal, F., and Bronson, F. (1978). *In utero* proximity of female mouse fetuses to males: Effect on reproductive performance during later life. *Biol. Reprod.* **19**, 842-853.

vom Saal, F. and Bronson, F. (1980). Sexual characteristics of adult female mice are correlated with their blood testosterone levels during prenatal development. *Science* **208**, 597-599.

vom Saal, F.S. and Dhar, M. D. (1992). Blood flow in the uterine loop artery and loop vein is bi-driectional in the mouse: Implications for intrauterine transport of steroids. *Physiol. Behav.*, in press.

vom Saal, F. and Finch, C. (1988). Reproductive senescence: Phenomena and mechanisms in mammals and selected vertebrates. In *Physiology of Reproduction*, ed. E. Knobil and J. Neill. Raven Press, New York, pp. 2351-2413.

vom Saal, F. and Moyer, C. (1985). Prenatal effects on reproductive capacity during aging in female mice. *Biol. Reprod.* **32**, 1116-1126.

vom Saal, F.S., Even, M.D., and Quadagno, D.M., (1991). Effects of maternal stress on puberty, fertility and aggressive behavior of female mice from different intrauterine positions. *Physiol. Behav.* **49**, 1073-1078

vom Saal, F., Grant, W., McMullen, C., and Laves, K. (1983). High fetal estrogen titers correlate with enhanced adult sexual performance and decreased aggression in male mice. *Science* **220**,1306-1309.

vom Saal, F., Quadagno, D., Even, M., Keisler, L., Keisler, D., and Khan, S. (1990). Paradoxical effects of maternal stress on fetal steroids and postnatal reproductive traits in female mice from different intrauterine positions. *Biol. Reprod.* **43**, 751-761.

Ward, I. and Weisz, J. (1980). Maternal stress alters plasma testosterone in fetal males. *Science* **207**, 328-329.

Warren, D., Haltmeyer, G., and Eik-Nes, K. (1973). Testosterone in the fetal rat testis. *Biol. Reprod.* **8**, 560-565.

Warren, D.W., Huhtaniemi, T., Tapanainen, J., Dufau, M.L., and Catt, K.J. (1984). Ontogeny of gonadotropin receptors in the fetal and neonatal rat testis. *Endocrinol.* **114**, 470-476

Weisz, J. and Gunsalus, O. (1973). Estrogen levels in immature female rats: true or spurious-ovarian or adrenal? *Endocrinol.* **93**, 1057-1065.

Weisz, J. and Ward, I. (1980). Plasma testosterone and progesterone titers in pregnant rats, their male and female fetuses, and neonatal offspring. *Endocrinol.* **106**, 306-316.

Weisz, J., Brown, B.L., and Ward, I.L. (1982). Maternal stress decreases steroid aromatase activity in the brain of male and female rat fetuses. *Neuroendocrinol.* **35**, 374-379.

Weniger, J.P. (1989). Aromatase activity in fetal rat gonads. *J. Reprod. Fertil.* **87**, 355-357.

Westphal, U. (1986). *Steroid-protein Interactions.* II. Springer Verlag, Berlin.

Wilson, J., George, F., and Griffin, J. (1981). The hormonal control of sexual development. *Science* **211**, 1278-1284.

Witschi, E. (1959). Age of sex determining mechanisms in vertebrates. *Science* **130**, 372-375.

Witschi, E. (1967). Biochemistry of sex differentiation in vertebrate embryos. In *The Biochemistry of Animal Development. Vol II*, ed. R. Weber. Academic Press, New York. pp. 193.

Yahr, P. (1988). Sexual differentiation of behavior in the context of developmental psychobiology. In *Handbook of Behavioral Neurobiology, Vol 9*, ed. E. Blass. Plenum, New York, pp. 197-243.

Young, W.C., Goy, R.W., and Phoenix, C.H. (1964). Hormones and sexual behavior. *Science* **143**, 212-218.

Zuckerman, S. (1936). The endocrine control of the prostate. *Proc. Roy. Soc. Med.* **29**, 1557-1568.

Zuckerman, S. (1938). Effects of prolonged estrogen stimulation on the prostate. *J. Anat. (Lond)* **72**, 264-276.

Zuckerman, S. and Baker, T.G. (1977). The development of the ovary and the process of oogenesis. In *The Ovary, Vol I -General Aspects*, ed. S. Zuckerman and B.J. Weir. Academic Press, New York, pp. 42-68.

Zonadek, L.H. and Zonadek, T. (1970). The human prostate in anencephaly. Acta. *Endocrinol.* **64**, 548-556.

Zonadek, L.H. and Zonadek, T. (1974). The prostatic utricle in the fetus and infant. *Urol. Int.* **29**, 458-465.

# ROLE OF MESENCHYME IN THE DEVELOPMENT OF THE UROGENITAL TRACT

**Gerald R. Cunha**
Anatomy Department and Reproductive Endocrinology Center,
University of California San Francisco, California

**Eugenie L. Boutin**
Anatomy Department and Reproductive Endocrinology Center,
University of California San Francisco, California

**Tim Turner**
Anatomy Department and Reproductive Endocrinology Center,
University of California San Francisco, California

**Annemarie A. Donjacour**
Anatomy Department and Reproductive Endocrinology Center,
University of California San Francisco, California

## INTRODUCTION

All vertebrate embryos exhibit an ambisexual phase of sex differentiation before overt sex differentiation takes place. During this period the gonads are morphologically undifferentiated, and the developing internal genitalia are represented by the Mullerian and Wolffian ducts, mesonephric tubules, and the urogenital sinus. These structures constitute the rudiments of both the male and female genital tracts. In females the gonads differentiate into ovaries, the mesonephric tubules and the Wolffian ducts regress (due to the absence of androgens), and the Mullerian ducts persist and give rise to the oviduct, uterus, cervix and upper vagina (Forsberg, 1978; Koff, 1933; O'Rahilly, 1973). The lower vagina, urethra and bladder are derived from the urogenital sinus in females. During masculine development the undifferentiated gonads differentiate into testes, and the Leydig cells of the testes produce testosterone (Jirasek, 1967; Winter et al., 1981). This hormone prevents the programmed cell death of the mesonephric tubules and Wolffian ducts and stimulates the mesonephric tubules to differentiate into the efferent ducts (Wilson et al., 1981a). Once survival of the Wolffian ducts is ensured, further stimulation by androgens elicits regional development of the Wolffian ducts into the epididymis, ductus deferens, and seminal vesicles (SV). Androgens also elicit the development of the prostate and bulbourethral glands from the urogenital sinus (UGS) as well as evoking masculine development of the urethra and external genitalia. However, metabolic conversion of testosterone to dihydrotestosterone by the enzyme 5α-reductase is a critical step in the differentiation of these UGS-derived organ rudiments and the

1. Corresponding Author: Gerald R. Cunha, Anatomy Department and Reproductive Endocrinology Center, University of California, San Francisco, California, USA 94143.

2. This chapter supported by NIH grants DK32157, HD17491, CA05388, HD21919, CA49996, and HD11979.

developing external genitalia (Wilson et al., 1981b). A second hormone, Mullerian Inhibiting Substance (MIS), is produced by Sertoli cells of the fetal testes and triggers the destruction of the Mullerian duct in males (Donahoe et al., 1982; Josso et al., 1977). While the role of endogenous estrogens and estrogen receptors is unclear during normal fetal and neonatal sex development of the genital tract, it is evident that exogenous estrogens (and androgens) have teratogenic effects in both male and female fetuses (Arai et al., 1983; Bern and Talamantes, 1981; Burns, 1961; Forsberg and Kalland, 1981; McLachlan, 1981b; Takasugi, 1976).

*Mesenchyme as an Inducer of Epithelial Development*
All glandular accessory sexual organs in males and females are composed of an epithelial parenchyma embedded in a fibromuscular stroma. The development of all such organs occurs via mesenchymal-epithelial interactions. Indeed, the effects of steroidal and nonsteroidal sex hormones on morphogenesis and differentiation of male and female accessory sexual structures are mediated via mesenchymal-epithelial interactions. For example, embryonic epithelia of male urogenital gland rudiments grown *in vitro* by themselves fail to undergo morphogenesis and remain undifferentiated (Cunha, 1976a). Likewise, mesenchyme grown by itself *in vitro* or *in vivo* remains undifferentiated and fails to form complex structures (Cunha, 1972; Cunha, 1976b). If, however, epithelium and mesenchyme of an organ rudiment are isolated, directly recombined homotypically and grown in association (i.e., homotypic tissue recombinant), the epithelium undergoes its normal morphogenesis and differentiation (Cunha et al., 1980; 1983a), and the mesenchyme differentiates into fibromuscular elements which are essential for normal organ function (Cunha et al., 1989). Such homotypic tissue recombinants, if grown under *in vivo* conditions as grafts to appropriate hosts, will ultimately achieve functional activity (Cunha, 1972; 1976b; Cunha et al., 1983c; 1991; Donjacour et al., 1988; Higgins et al., 1989a; 1989b; Takeda et al., 1990).

Investigation of heterotypic tissue recombinants, in which mesenchyme from one organ rudiment is grown in association with epithelium from another, has shown that mesenchyme induces and specifies patterns of epithelial morphogenesis, regulates epithelial proliferation, promotes epithelial cytodifferentiation, and induces and specifies epithelial functional or biochemical activity (Cunha et al., 1983b). Recent progress in the analysis of the developing seminal vesicle (SV) emphasizes the important interplay between mesenchyme and epithelium in the development of an androgen-dependent gland. In the developing SV we have recently shown that seminal vesicle mesenchyme (SVM) can *instructively* induce SV development in epithelia of the following structures: embryonic Wolffian duct (Higgins et al., 1989b), adult epididymis (Turner et al., 1989), adult ductus deferens and adult ureter (Cunha et al., 1991). (An instructive induction is one in which the normal prospective developmental fate of the epithelium is reprogrammed by the mesenchyme.) In all of these inductions the epithelia were induced to change their original phenotype and to express the SV phenotype morphologically and functionally (Figure. 1). In recent studies in which SVM was combined with either wild-type or Tfm (testicular feminization) ureter epithelium (URE), the URE was induced to change from a multilayered transitional urothelium to a simple columnar epithelium exhibiting the highly folded morphology characteristic of the SV (Cunha and Young, 1991a; Cunha et al., 1991). In SVM + *wild-type* URE tissue recombinants these morphological changes in epithelial differentiation culminated in the expression of epithelial androgen receptors and the complete spectrum of SV secretory proteins (Cunha et al., 1991). However, in SVM + *Tfm* URE recombinants, the androgen-insensitive Tfm epithelium is incapable of expressing functional androgen receptors, and SV secretory proteins were absent even though the SVM had induced SV morphology (Cunha and Young, 1991). Thus, certain "androgenic" effects (epithelial morphogenesis, proliferation, and change in epithelial cytodifferentiation) are elicited via paracrine influences from androgen-receptor-positive SV mesenchyme in Tfm epithelium. By contrast, the expression of androgen-dependent secretory proteins appears to be dependent upon intra-epithelial androgen receptors and, thus, cannot be expressed in Tfm URE (Cunha et al., 1991).

The importance of mesenchyme as an inducer of epithelial development is also applicable to the female genital tract in so far as similar observations have been made in tissue recombinants composed of uterine and vaginal epithelium and mesenchyme. Again, both uterine and vaginal mesenchyme have the ability to instructively induce changes in epithelial morphogenesis, cytodifferentiation, and functional or biochemical activities (Boutin et al., 1991; Cooke et al., 1987; Cooke et al., 1986; Cunha, 1976b). Mesenchyme-induced changes in functional cytodifferentiation have not been examined in depth in uterine or vaginal inductions, but in tissue recombinants composed of vaginal mesenchyme + uterine epithelium, the epithelium is induced to undergo vaginal cytodifferentiation and to express a novel set of cytokeratins characteristic of vaginal differentiation (Bigsby and Cunha, unpublished). The induced epithelium cycles from a mucified to a cornified state through the estrous cycle, which is one of the functional hallmarks of vaginal epithelium. Associated with these mesenchyme-induced changes in epithelial differentiation is an alteration at the biochemical level in the expression of a cell surface heparan sulfate proteoglycan (syndecan) characterized by Bernfield's group (Jalkanen et al., 1985; Rapraeger et al., 1985). Both the cellular location and the molecular weight (MW) of the syndecan molecule are different in uterine and vaginal epithelia (Boutin et al., 1991; Hayashi et al., 1988; Sanderson and Bernfield, 1988) even though syndecan has the same 69 kD protein core in all tissues. The number and size of the heparan sulfate and chondroitin sulfate glycosaminoglycan side chains vary in different tissues which appears to account for the variation in syndecan's molecular weight (Sanderson and Bernfield, 1988). Syndecan in uterine epithelium of an adult mouse has an average MW of 110 kD and is localized by the rat monoclonal 281-2 to the basolateral borders of the simple columnar epithelial cells (Boutin et al., 1991). This pattern of expression is altered in

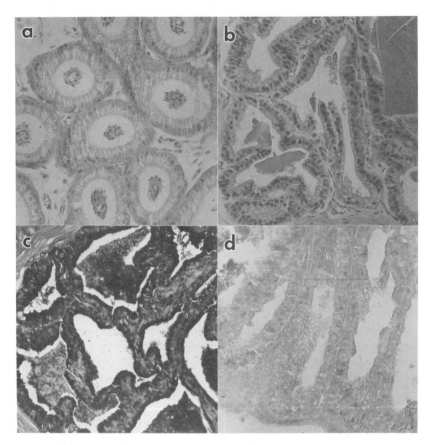

**FIGURE 1.** Histological sections of (a) adult mouse epididymis compared with (b) a tissue recombinant composed of neonatal rat seminal vesicle mesenchyme (SVM) plus epithelium of the adult mouse epididymis (EPE) at the end of 1 month of growth in a male nude mouse host. Note that the rat SVM has induced the mouse EPE to express the complex morphological pattern characteristic of the seminal vesicle. Immunocytochemical staining of a rat SVM + adult mouse EPE recombinant reveals the expression of mouse (c) but not rat (d) seminal vesicle secretory proteins. *250*x.

neonatal uterine epithelium that has been recombined with rat vaginal stroma and allowed to develop *in vivo* as a transplant for 5 weeks. Under these conditions vaginal epithelial cytodifferentiation is induced, and syndecan staining changes dramatically as well. Cells of the basal and intermediate layers of the stratified epithelium are surrounded by intense syndecan staining. In addition, syndecan immunoprecipitated by monoclonal antibody 281-2 has a smaller average MW of 92 kD (Boutin et al., 1991). This is the same pattern of syndecan expression detected in adult mouse vaginal epithelium (Boutin et al., 1991; Hayashi et al., 1988; Sanderson and Bernfield, 1988). Hence, in this heterotypic recombinant the vaginal stroma induced the uterine epithelium to alter both the synthesis and the localization of syndecan such that its pattern of expression correlated with the induced vaginal epithelial phenotype. Reciprocal changes are elicited when uterine mesenchyme induces uterine differentiation in vaginal epithelium (Boutin et al., 1991).

*Mesenchyme as a Mediator of Androgenic and Estrogenic Effects upon Epithelium*

For years it has been tacitly assumed that effects of androgens on target epithelial cells result from binding of hormone to receptors within the responding epithelial cells themselves. The following observations support this concept: (a) Androgen receptors are detectable biochemically in prostatic extracts as well as in prostatic epithelial and stromal cells by autoradiography or immunocytochemistry (Cooke et al., 1991a; Husmann et al., 1991; Jung-Testas et al., 1981; Krieg et al., 1981; Lahtonen et al., 1983; Prins et al., 1991; Shannon and Cunha, 1984; Stumpf and Sar, 1976; Tilley et al., 1985). (b) Androgens elicit prostatic growth and specifically stimulate prostatic epithelial proliferation in the intact prostate (Bruchovsky et al., 1975; Coffey, 1974; Evans and Chandler, 1987; Tuohimaa, 1980; Tuohimaa and Niemi, 1974). Thus, androgen-induced prostatic epithelial proliferation has been thought to result from the receptor-mediated action of androgens on prostatic epithelial cells themselves mediated by the epithelial androgen receptor. This quite reasonable conclusion is based solely on the correlation between androgen-induced epithelial proliferation and epithelial androgen receptors, but does not by any means establish a causal relationship. An alternate mechanism by which androgens might elicit epithelial proliferation in the prostate or other target organs is based on the idea that androgens act upon cells of the mesenchyme or stroma which then elaborate regulatory substances controlling epithelial proliferation (Cunha et al., 1980; 1983c; 1987). This idea has been derived in part from investigation of mesenchymal-epithelial interactions between normal and androgen-insensitive Tfm tissues. Tfm mice are insensitive to androgens due to a defect in the androgen receptor (Attardi and Ohno, 1974; Bardin et al., 1973; He et al., 1991; Ohno, 1979; Wilson et al., 1981a, b; 1984). Nonetheless, in tissue recombinants composed of normal urogenital sinus mesenchyme (UGM) + Tfm bladder epithelium (BLE) androgen-induced prostatic development occurred in the Tfm epithelial cells (Cunha and Chung, 1981; Cunha and Lung, 1978; Lasnitzki and Mizuno, 1980; Shannon and Cunha, 1984; Sugimura et al., 1986). In fact, when all four possible tissue recombinants between Tfm and wild-type tissues are analyzed (Figure 2), the androgen-receptor status of the epithelium did not affect the results as both wild-type and Tfm epithelia developed into prostate in association with normal wild-type UGM. In contrast, prostatic differentiation did not occur in tissue recombinants constructed with Tfm mesenchyme (Cunha et al., 1980; Cunha and Lung, 1978; Lasnitzki and Mizuno, 1980) even when wild-type epithelium was used. Prostatic development in tissue recombinants composed of wild-type UGM + Tfm BLE and seminal vesicle development in tissue recombinants composed of wild-type SVM + Tfm URE involved three major processes: ductal morphogenesis, epithelial growth, and secretory cytodifferentiation. All of these processes were induced by androgens, but were expressed in androgen-insensitive Tfm epithelia which lack functional androgen receptors (Cunha and Young, 1991a; Shannon

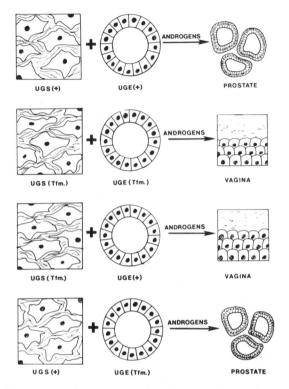

**FIGURE 2.** A summary of tissue recombination experiments between urogenital sinus mesenchyme and epithelium from Tfm and wild-type embryos. A positive androgenic response (prostatic morphogenesis) occurs when wild-type mesenchyme is grown in association with either wild-type or Tfm epithelium. Conversely, vagina-like differentiation occurs when either wild-type or Tfm epitheliam are grown in association with Tfm mesenchyme. (From Cunha et al., 1980 with permission.)

and Cunha, 1984; Sugimura et al., 1986; Takeda et al., 1985). These observations in conjunction with similar experiments in the embryonic mouse mammary gland (Drews and Drews, 1977; Kratochwil and Schwartz, 1976) suggest that the mesenchyme is the actual target and mediator of androgenic effects upon the epithelium. This idea is supported by the observation that in the normal wild-type male genital tract and mammary gland mesenchymal cells possess androgen receptors during fetal periods while associated epithelial cells, in most cases, lack androgen receptors (Cooke et al., 1991a; Husmann et al., 1991; Shannon and Cunha, 1983; Takeda et al., 1985; Wasner et al., 1983). Indeed, epithelial androgen receptors in normal androgen sensitive animals are not detectable until quite late in the organogenesis of the male genital tract and in many organs are not expressed until after birth (Cooke et al., 1991a; Husmann et al., 1991).

In the female genital tract estrogen-induced effects on epithelial differentiation and proliferation may also be mediated, in part, by stromal factors. This idea is supported by a number of findings. Even though estrogen receptors (ER) are undetectable in uterine epithelium of the early neonatal mouse, exogenous estrogen increases the rate of epithelial proliferation, thus, implicating an indirect mechanism of estrogen action mediated by estrogen-receptor-positive mesenchymal cells (Bigsby et al., 1990; Bigsby and Cunha, 1986; Cunha et al., 1982; Taguchi et al., 1988; Yamashita et al., 1989). In addition, a direct proliferative effect of estrogen has never been demonstrated in primary cultures of mammary, uterine, or vaginal epithelial cells (Casimiri et al., 1980; Flaxman et al., 1973; Iguchi et al., 1985b; Imagawa et al., 1982; Kirk et al., 1978; Liszezak et al., 1977; Nandi et al., 1984; Tomooka et al., 1986; Uchima et al., 1987), while in mixed cultures of epithelial and stromal cells estrogen may stimulate epithelial proliferation (Haslam, 1986; Inaba et al., 1988; McGrath, 1983). Furthermore, vaginal and uterine epithelial cells that fail to respond to estrogen *in vitro* (Iguchi et al., 1983; 1985a; Uchima et al., 1987) exhibit an estrogen-induced mitogenic response when recombined with their respective stromas and grown as grafts beneath the renal capsule of the appropriate host (Cooke et al., 1986). Evidence of indirect estrogenic action has also been proposed from studies on the primate oviduct and uterus in that epithelial cells of the regenerating monkey uterus lack ER at a time when estrogen induces epithelial DNA synthesis (McClellan et al., 1990). Although a specific mesenchymal factor has not yet emerged as the mediator of androgenic or estrogenic responses within epithelium, a number of growth factors must be considered as paracrine mediators of mesenchymal effects on epithelium: epidermal growth factor, (EGF), insulin-like growth factor-I, transforming growth factor-B and -α, basic fibroblast growth factor (b-FGF) and keratinocyte growth factor (KGF) (Alarid et al., 1991; Di Augustine et al., 1988; Dickson and Lippman, 1987; Finch et al., 1989; Mukku and Stancel, 1985a; 1985b; Murphy et al., 1987; Snedeker et al., 1991). EGF receptors have also been reported in the uterus, and they have been shown to be estrogen-regulated (Mukku and Stancel, 1985a; 1985b).

Experimental tissue recombination studies provide additional support for a paracrine role of stroma in estrogen-induced epithelial proliferation. To test the idea that stroma plays a paracrine role in epithelial growth or is causally involved in estrogenic response in estrogen-target epithelia, tissue recombinants constructed with epithelium and mesenchyme of the vagina (estrogen target) and urinary bladder (nontarget) were analyzed (Cunha and Young, 1991b). Urinary bladder epithelium (BLE) is not an estrogen target epithelium since it lacks estrogen receptors (Schulze and Barrack, 1987), and its proliferation is not affected by estrogens. Moreover, BLE normally has an extremely low proliferative activity (Hicks, 1975). These features of BLE have facilitated an examination of paracrine growth effects of stroma on estrogen-regulated epithelial differentiation and proliferation. For this purpose, the four possible tissue recombinants were prepared with vaginal and bladder tissues. The experimental protocol and results for this experiment are given in Figure 3. As reported in earlier studies (Cooke et al., 1986; 1987; Cunha, 1976b; Cunha et al., 1977), in homotypic vaginal tissue recombinants (VS + VE) the epithelium continued to express the vaginal phenotype in both oil- and estradiol-treated

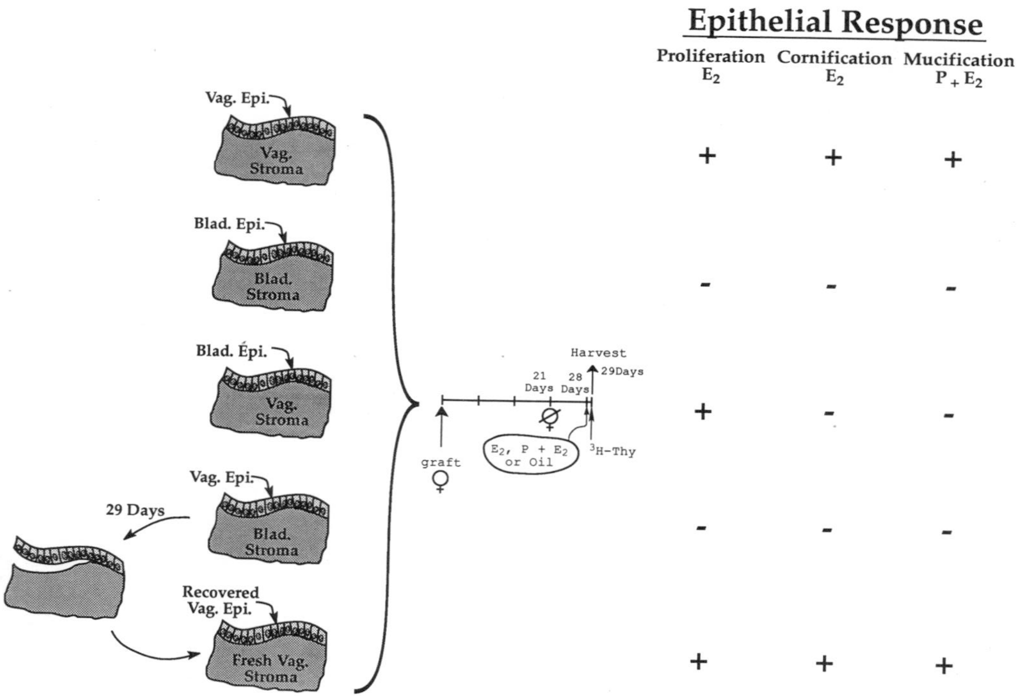

**FIGURE 3.** Experimental protocol and summary of results of tissue recombinant experiments using vaginal and urinary bladder tissues. Vaginal epithelium and stroma (Vag. Epi. and Vag. Stroma, respectively) and bladder epithelium and stroma (Blad. Epi. and Blad. stroma, respectively) from 3-day-old mice were combined as indicated and the tissue recombinants grafted underneath the renal capsule of normal female hosts, which after 21 days were ovariectomized. Seven days later the hosts were injected with estradiol ($E_2$), progesterone (P) plus $E_2$ or with oil and sacrificed 24 hours later. Two hours before harvest the hosts were injected with $^3$H-thymidine ($^3$H-Thy.) As a variation, tissue recombinants of Blad. Stroma plus Vag. Epi. were grown for 29 days (in intact females which were ovariectomized at 21 days), and the Vag. Epi. was recovered, combined with fresh Vag. Stroma and then tested as above for hormonal response. In all cases hormonal response was found to be in an all (+) or none (-) event.

hosts. This was displayed as cyclic production of cornified and mucified layers during the initial 3 weeks of growth in intact, cycling female hosts. This continued cycling implies that progesterone as well as estrogen was affecting the VS+VE tissue recombinant. Subsequent ovariectomy and oil treatment of the hosts resulted in typical epithelial atrophy, while treatment with estradiol elicited epithelial proliferation and cornification in VS+VE recombinants. However, the vaginal epithelium remained atrophic irrespective of the hormonal status of the host when grown in association with bladder stroma, that is, the epithelium of BLS+VE tissue recombinants failed to show evidence of cycling between the cornified and mucified states and failed to proliferate in response to estrogen. This suggests that normal cytodifferentiation and hormonal responsiveness of vaginal epithelium requires a specific stromal environment provided by the estrogen-receptor-positive vaginal stroma, but not the estrogen-receptor-negative bladder stroma.

In reciprocal tissue recombinants of vaginal stroma plus bladder epithelium (VS+BLE), the BLE continued to express its normal urothelial phenotype. This was manifested by the continued presence of large "umbrella" cells apically and the absence of cycling of epithelial differentiation between the cornified and mucified states. However, when BLE was grown in association with VS, proliferation of the BLE became estrogen-dependent. These observations implicate the stroma as an important factor in estrogen-induced epithelial proliferation and hormonal regulation of epithelial differentiation. Of the four possible tissue recombinations between epithelium and stroma of the vagina and bladder, estrogenic stimulation of epithelial proliferation was observed in only those tissue recombinants in which an estrogen-receptor-positive (Cunha et al., 1982; Stumpf and Sar, 1976) vaginal stroma was utilized (VS+VE and VS+BLE) (Figure 4).

In addition, it should be stressed that vaginal epithelium grown in association with bladder stroma failed to cornify in response to estrogen even though the host's vaginal epithelium and the epithelium of VS+VE tissue recombinants cornified in response to estradiol. Thus, estrogen was without effects on VE when grown in association with bladder stroma (BLS + VE) while full estrogenic response was observed only when VE was grown in association with VS. Significantly, normal vaginal epithelial differentiation (cornification and mucification) and hormonal responsiveness (both to estrogen and progesterone) could be completely reestablished (Figs. 3-4) by recovering the unresponsive mouse VE from BLS+VE recombinants and reassociating it with fresh vaginal stroma from a neonatal rat to generate a secondary (2°) rVS + mVE recombinant which was grown *in vivo* in a second host for an additional month prior to analysis of hormonal response (Cunha and Young, 1991c).

In an analogous model, cultured uterine and vaginal epithelium, which were shown to be unresponsive to estrogen *in vitro* (Iguchi et al., 1983; 1985b), can re-express normal estrogen responsiveness when reassociated with their

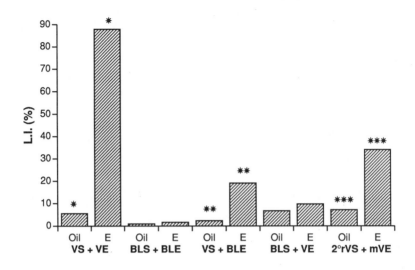

**FIGURE 4.** Relative epithelial labelling index with $^3$H-Thymidine of tissue recombinants composed of vaginal and bladder epithelium and stroma. Homotypic vaginal and bladder recombinants (VS+VE and BLS+BLE) and heterotypic recombinants (VS+BLE and BLS+VE) were prepared with mouse tissues. Secondary (2°) rVS + mVE are tissue recombinants in which the epithelium from mouse BLS + mouse VE recombinants was isolated after 1 month and recombined with fresh rat VS according to the protocol in Figure 3. E = estradiol-treated. Note that in VS+VE and VS+BLE recombinants epithelial labelling index is estrogen responsive while in BLS+BLE and BLS+VE epithelial labelling index is not estrogen responsive. The estrogenic responsiveness of VE in BLS+VE recombinants is re-established in 2° rVS + mVE recombinants which were grown for 1 month *in vivo* prior to analysis of hormonal response. Differences in epithelial labelling index are statistically significant (*, **, *** = .05). Multiple comparisons were made using the Anova analyses of variance, and significance was established using Scheffe's test. Abbreviations: m = mouse; r = rat; 2° = secondary; all other abbreviations as per text.

homotypic stromas (Cooke et al., 1986). Thus, the failure of VE to respond to estrogen and progesterone when grown on BLS was not due to irrevocable damage to the epithelium, but instead may be due to a failure of the estrogen-receptor-negative bladder stroma to provide the appropriate permissive environment or to maintain the appropriate state of epithelial differentiation required for response to estrogen (cornification and proliferation) and progesterone (mucification). These results demonstrate that the responsiveness of vaginal epithelium to estrogen and progesterone is critically dependent upon the stromal environment, and are consistent with the idea that estrogenic effects on vaginal epithelial proliferation are elicited via paracrine influences from vaginal stroma. Estrogenic and progestational effects could certainly occur via paracrine mechanisms since vaginal stromal cells are known to have both estrogen and progesterone receptors (Cunha et al., 1982; Stumpf and Sar, 1976). Alternately, the vaginal stroma may promote a state of vaginal epithelial differentiation which is crucial (permissive) for responsiveness to estrogen and progesterone. In this regard, vaginal stroma from neonatal and adult mice is known to be a specific inducer of the vaginal epithelial differentiation (Cunha, 1976b; Cooke et al., 1986; 1987; Boutin et al., 1991).

*Paracrine Factors in Urogenital Development; Use of the Neonatal Mouse Seminal Vesicle as a Model System*
The androgen-dependent neonatal mouse seminal vesicle (SV) rudiment is a particularly versatile model to investigate paracrine factors in urogenital development because its development can be regulated *in vitro* in a completely physiological manner by adding or deleting androgens from serum-free medium. This makes possible comparisons between developing and developmentally quiescent SVs (Shima et al., 1990). Recent findings demonstrate that this model provides unique opportunities for investigating androgenic effects in terms of morphogenetic cell-cell interactions, androgen metabolism, androgen receptors, and growth factors.

The neonatal mouse seminal vesicle (SV) develops from the lower Wolffian duct (WD) under the inductive influence of SVM (Cunha, 1976a; Higgins et al., 1989a). Mesenchyme of the fetal prostate (urogenital sinus mesenchyme, UGM) can also induce SV differentiation when associated with Wolffian duct-derived epithelium (Cunha, 1972). In fact, both SVM and UGM can function as prostatic inductors (Cunha, 1972; Donjacour and Cunha, In preparation). This suggests that SVM and UGM share common inductive activities. Postnatal growth and branching morphogenesis of the SV is dependent upon dihydrotestosterone (DHT) produced from testosterone (T) by $5\alpha$-reductase (Shima et al., 1990). Neonatal mouse SVs grown in a chemically defined serum-free medium (containing EGF, BSA, insulin, transferrin, cholera toxin and either T or DHT) undergo branching morphogenesis, growth and express epithelial androgen receptors (AR) which are undetectable prior to culture (Shima et al., 1990). Dose-response studies have shown that DHT is about 10 times more effective in eliciting SV branching morphogenesis than T (Shima et al., 1990), and more recently deletion experiments have shown that only insulin, transferrin and androgen are required to promote SV morphogenesis *in vitro* (Shima and Cunha, unpublished). Transferrin is absolutely required, but appears to function solely as a carrier of iron, since a lipophilic iron chelator, ferric pyridoxal isonicotinoyl hydrazone (Landschulz et al., 1984) can replace transferrin (Shima and Cunha, unpublished). When added to a basal medium (containing transferrin, BSA, EGF and cholera toxin), insulin stimulates mesenchymal cell proliferation in a dose-dependent manner without affecting SV epithelial morphogenesis or growth. Testosterone in the absence of insulin (basal medium plus transferrin BSA, EGF, and cholera toxin) has a modest effect on epithelial growth and branching morphogenesis and a modest effect on mesenchymal growth, but when both T and insulin are added together epithelial growth and branching morphogenesis are markedly stimulated as is mesenchymal growth (Tsuji et al., 1991b). Thus, in SV organ cultures insulin is an essential permissive agent required to express maximal response to T. Insulin is known to have a spectrum of metabolic effects and to stimulate growth and proliferation of a variety of cells *in vitro* (Hill and Milner, 1985; Straus, 1984). It can act through its own high affinity receptor (Barnes and Sato, 1980; Straus, 1984), as well as through low affinity binding to the IGF-I receptor (De Pablo et al., 1990; Rechler et al., 1976; Rechler et al., 1977; Straus, 1984). Receptors for insulin or IGF-I have not been described for the developing or adult SV even though a variety of developing tissues are responsive to insulin (De Pablo et al., 1990; Persson, 1980); insulin receptors have been reported for the closely related ventral prostate (Carmena et al., 1986) which responds proliferatively to insulin (Buchanan and Riches, 1986; McKeehan et al., 1984). Insulin has been detected in the embryonic rat and mouse pancreas as early as day 11 of gestation (Clark and Rutter, 1972; De Pablo et al., 1990; Kakita et al., 1983) and plasma insulin levels are appreciable (about 50% of adult levels) in the neonatal rat (Bonner-Weir et al., 1981). While it is unclear at this time whether insulin is acting on the developing SV through the IGF-I receptor or through a high affinity insulin receptor, it is known that insulin is not acting on the developing SV by increasing conversion of T to DHT (Tsuji et al., 1991a). However, the possibility remains that insulin could be involved in the initial expression of SV epithelial androgen receptors (AR) since plasma insulin levels increase during the neonatal period (Bonner-Weir et al., 1981) when epithelial AR are making their initial appearance (Cooke et al., 1991a; Husmann et al., 1991). A relationship between AR and insulin is also suggested by the report that prostatic cytosolic AR levels are diminished in diabetic rats (Ho, 1991). In any case, the responsiveness of the developing mouse SV to insulin *in vitro* (Shima et al., 1990) is consistent with a role of insulin as a metabolic and growth regulator in development.

Preliminary studies have recently implicated keratinocyte growth factor (KGF) in the development of the SV in so far as a neutralizing antibody to KGF provided by Dr. Stuart Aaronson inhibits androgen-dependent development of the SV grown *in vitro* under serum-free conditions (Alarid and Cuhna, in preparation). Thus, the actions of androgens are likely to be mediated in part by the actions of known growth factors, some of which may function as paracrine mediators between the interacting epithelium and mesenchyme of the developing genital tract.

*Relevance of Epithelial-Mesenchymal Interactions to Chemically Induced Alterations in Sexual Development*

Chemical toxicants introduced into the environment are known to influence the developing endocrine system. This leads to profound developmental consequences because of the crucial role of hormones in the organogenesis of the urogenital system and other hormone target organs. As a general rule the developing organism is extremely sensitive to estrogenic xenobiotic agents which have been shown to adversely affect the endocrine system at virtually all points of regulation (Bern and Talamantes, 1981; Herbst and Bern, 1981; McLachlan, 1981a; 1985; Mori and Nagasawa, 1988). Neuroendocrine development is perturbed morphologically and functionally (Bookstaff et al., 1990a; 1990b; Whitten and Naftolin, 1991). The gonads are likewise affected resulting in gonadal tumors in fish (Down et al., 1990), gonadal feminization in male gull embryos (Fry and Toone, 1981) and reductions in testosterone biosynthesis in mammals (Kleeman et al., 1990; Subramanian et al., 1987). The net result is impaired reproduction (Kubiak et al., 1989; Mably et al., 1991; Whitten and Naftolin, 1991). Abnormalities associated with exposure to hormonally active xenobiotics are observed within hormone target organs of male and female genital tracts and are due to disruption of endocrine function at the systemic level as well as from direct action of the toxicants on developing hormone target organs. To fully understand the etiology of genital tract lesions elicited by xenobiotic agents will require an understanding of the normal developmental mechanisms (e.g., hormone-receptor interactions and epithelial-mesenchymal interactions), and how these noxious agents perturb the complex process of sex differentiation. Suitable *in vitro* models will be essential since many of the uncontrolled systemic variables can be eliminated through use of organ culture and *in vitro* analysis of epithelial-mesenchymal interactions.

In this regard organ cultures of the neonatal mouse SV and bulbourethral gland (BUG) are ideal for detecting substances that may act as reproductive toxicants by virtue of interfering with the early critical steps in the organogenesis of the male reproductive tract particularly those substances that are teratogenic by virtue of their estrogenic, androgenic or antiandrogenic activity. The BUG is known to have mesenchymal estrogen receptors. While the role of estrogen and estrogen receptors is unclear in the developing BUG, its development is inhibited by estradiol or methoxychlor and thus, the BUG may be a good model for investigating the teratogenic effect of estrogenic substances in the male (Cooke and Eroschenko, 1990). Since the developing SV also has estrogen receptors (Cooke et al., 1991b) and is adversely affected by exogenous estrogens *in vivo* (Chung and MacFadden, 1980; Higgins et al., 1981), it too may be useful for examining the potential teratogenicity of estrogenic substances in the developing male genital tract. Parameters which are amenable to analysis in cultures of SVs or BUGs inlcude epithelial and mesenchymal growth, epithelial branching morphogenesis, expression of epithelial androgen receptors, or, in the case of the SV, secretory proteins. Growth factors certainly play a role in organogenesis of the genital tract and have been implicated as the mediators of steroidal sex hormones (Alarid et al., 1991; Bossert et al., 1990; Di Augustine et al., 1988; Dickson and Lippman, 1987; Mukku and Stancel, 1985a; 1985b; Murphy et al., 1987; Snedeker et al., 1991; Tsuji et al., 1991a). The neonatal mouse SV culture system may also be useful for identifying xenobiotic agents that perturb the action of growth factors or epithelial-mesenchymal interactions. Since proper morphogenesis and function of the SV is important for optimal fertility (Curry and Atherton, 1990), the developing mouse SV (and BUG) provides a versatile economical mammalian model to study the effects of environmental toxicants that adversely affect development of the reproductive tract.

# REFERENCES

Alarid, E.T., Cunha, G.R., Young, P., and Nicoll, C.S. (1991). Evidence for a possible organ- and sex-specific role of bFGF in the development of the fetal mammalian reproductive tract. *Endocrinology*, **129**, 2148-2154.

Arai, Y., Mori, T., Suzuki, Y., and Bern, H. (1983). Long-term effects of perinatal exposure to sex steroids and diethylstilbestrol on the reproductive system of male mammals. *Int. Rev. Cytology*, **84**, 235-268.

Attardi, B. and Ohno, S. (1974). Cytosol androgen receptor from kidneys of normal and testicular feminized (Tfm). mice. *Cell*, **2**, 205-12.

Bardin, C.W., Bullock, L.P., Sherins, R.J., Mowszowicz, I., and Blackburn, W.R. (1973). Androgen metabolism and mechanism of action in male pseudohermaphroditism: A study of testicular feminization. *Recent Prog. Horm. Res.*, **29**, 65-109.

Barnes, D. and Sato, G. (1980). Methods for growth of cultured cells in serum-free medium. *Analytical Biochemistry*, **102**, 255-270.

Bern, H.A. and Talamantes, F.J. (1981). Neonatal mouse models and their relation to disease in the human female. In *Developmental Effects of Diethylstilbestrol (DES). in Pregnancy*, ed. A. Herbst and H. A. Bern. Thieme Stratton Inc., New York, pp. 129-147.

Bigsby, R.M. and Cunha, G.R. (1986). Estrogen stimulation of deoxyribonucleic acid synthesis in uterine epithelial cells which lack estrogen receptors. *Endocrinology.*, **119**, 390-396.

Bigsby, R.M., Aixin, L., Luo, K., and Cunha, G.R. (1990). Strain differences in the ontogeny of estrogen receptors in murine uterine epithelium. *Endocrinology*, **126**, 2592-2596.

Bonner-Weir, S., Trent, D.F., Honey, R.N., and Weir, G.C. (1981). Responses of neonatal rat islets to streptozotocin. *Diabetes*, **30**, 64-69.

Bookstaff, R.C., Kamel, F., Moore, R.W., Bjerke, D.L., and Peterson, R.E. (1990a). Altered regulation of pituitary gondotropin-releasing hormone (GnRH). receptor number and pituitary responsiveness to GnRH in 2,3,7,8-tetrachlorobenzo-p-dioxin-treated male rats. *Toxicology and Applied Pharmacology*, **105**, 78-92.

Bookstaff, R.C., Moore, R.W., and Peterson, R.E. (1990b). 2,3,7,8-tetrachlorodibenzo-p-dioxin increases the potency of androgens and estrogens as feedback inhibitors of luteinizing hormone secretion in male rats. *Toxicology and Applied Pharmacology*, **104**, 212-224.

Bossert, N.L., Nelson, K.G., Ross, K.A., Takahashi, T., and McLachlan, J.A. (1990). Epidermal growth factor binding and receptor distribution in the mouse reproductive tract during development. *Develop. Biol.*, **142**, 75-85.

Boutin, E.L., Sanderson, R.D., Bernfield, M., and Cunha, G.R. (1991). Epithelial-mesenchymal interactions in uterus and vagina influence the expression of syndecan, a cell surface proteoglycan. *Develop. Biol.*, **148**, 63-74.

Bruchovsky, N., Lesser, B., van Doorn, E.V., and Craven, S. (1975). Hormonal effects on cell proliferation in rat prostate. *Vitam. Horm.*, **33**, 61-102.

Buchanan, L.J. and Riches, A.C. (1986). Proliferative responses of rat ventral prostate: Effects of variations in organ culture media and methodology. *Prostate*, **8**, 63-74.

Burns, R.K. (1961). Role of hormones in the differentiation of sex. In *Sex and Internal Secretions*, ed. W. C. Young. Williams and Wilkins, Baltimore, pp. 76-158.

Carmena, M.J., Fernandez-Moreno, M.D., and Prieto, J.C. (1986). Characterization of insulin receptors in isolated epithelial cells of rat ventral prostate: Effect of fasting. *Cell Biochem Function*, **4**, 19-24.

Casimiri, V., Rath, N.C., Parvez, H., and Psychoyos, A. (1980). Effect of sex steroids on rat endometrial epithelium and stroma cultured separately. *J. Steroid Biochem.*, **12**, 293-298.

Chung, L.W. and MacFadden, D.K. (1980). Sex steroids imprinting and prostatic growth. *Investigative Urol.*, **17**, 337-342.

Clark, W.R. and Rutter, W.J. (1972). Synthesis and accumulation of insulin in the fetal rat pancreas. *Develop. Biol.*, **29**, 468-481.

Coffey, D.S. (1974). The effects of androgens on DNA and RNA synthesis in sex accessory tissue. In *Male Accessory Sex Organs: Structure and Function*, ed. D. Brandes. Academic Press, New York, pp. 307-328.

Cooke, P.S. and Eroschenko, V.P. (1990). Inhibitory effects of technical grade methoxychlor on development of neonatal male mouse reproductive organs. *Biol Reproduction*, **42**, 585-596.

Cooke, P.S., Uchima, F.-D.A., Fujii, D.K., Bern, H.A., and Cunha, G.R. (1986). Restoration of normal morphology and estrogen responsiveness in cultured vaginal and uterine epithelia transplanted with stroma. *Proc. Nat'l. Acad. Sci. USA*, **83**, 2109-2113.

Cooke, P.S., Fujii, D.K., and Cunha, G.R. (1987). Vaginal and uterine stroma maintain their inductive properties following primary culture. *In Vitro Cell. Dev. Biol.*, **23**, 159-166.

Cooke, P.S., Young, P., and Cunha, G.R. (1991a). Androgen receptor expression in developing male reproductive organs. *Endocrinology*, **128**, 2867-2873.

Cooke, P.S., Young, P., Hess, R.A., and Cunha, G.R. (1991b). Estrogen receptor expression in developing epididymis, efferent ductules and other male reproductive organs. *Endocrinology*, **128**, 2874-2879.

Cunha, G.R. (1972). Epithelio-mesenchymal interactions in primordial gland structures which become responsive to androgenic stimulation. *Anat. Rec.*, **172**, 179-196.

Cunha, G.R. (1976a). Epithelial-stromal interactions in development of the urogenital tract. *Int. Rev. Cytol.*, **47**, 137-194.

Cunha, G.R. (1976b). Stromal induction and specification of morphogenesis and cytodifferentiation of the epithelia of the Mullerian ducts and urogenital sinus during development of the uterus and vagina in mice. *J. Exp. Zool.*, **196**, 361-370.

Cunha, G.R. and Chung, L.W.K. (1981). Stromal-epithelial interactions: I. Induction of prostatic phenotype in urothelium of testicular feminized (Tfm/y). mice. *J. Steroid Biochem.*, **14**, 1317-1321.

Cunha, G.R. and Lung, B. (1978). The possible influences of temporal factors in androgenic responsiveness of urogenital tissue recombinants from wild-type and androgen-insensitive (Tfm). mice. *J. Exp. Zool.*, **205**, 181-194.

Cunha, G.R. and Young, P. (1991). Inability of Tfm (testicular feminization). epithelial cells to express androgen-dependent seminal vesicle secretory proteins in chimeric tissue recombinants. *Endocrinology*, **128**, 3293-3298.

Cunha, G.R. and Young, P. (1992). Role of stroma in estrogen-induced epithelial proliferation. *Epithelial Cell Biol.*, **1**, 18-31.

Cunha, G.R., Lung, B. and Kato, K. (1977). Role of the epithelial-stromal interaction during the development and expression of ovary-independent vaginal hyperplasia. *Develop. Biol.*, **56**, 52-67.

Cunha, G.R., Chung, L.W.K., Shannon, J.M., and Reese, B.A. (1980). Stromal-epithelial interactions in sex differentiation. *Biol. Reprod.*, **22**, 19-43.

Cunha, G.R., Shannon, J.M., Vanderslice, K.D., Sekkingstad, M., and Robboy, S.J. (1982). Autoradiographic analysis of nuclear estrogen binding sites during postnatal development of the genital tract of female mice. *J. Steroid Biochem.*, **17**, 281-286.

Cunha, G.R., Shannon, J.M., Taguchi, O., Fujii, H., and Chung, L.W.K. (1983a). Epithelial-mesenchymal interactions in hormone-induced development. In *Epithelial-Mesenchymal Interactions in Development*, ed. R. H. Sawyer and J. F. Fallon. Praeger Scientific Press, New York, pp. 51-74.

Cunha, G.R., Fujii, H., Neubauer, B.L., Shannon, J.M., Sawyer, L.M., and Reese, B.A. (1983b). Epithelial-mesenchymal interactions in prostatic development. I. Morphological observations of prostatic induction by urogenital sinus mesenchyme in epithelium of the adult rodent urinary bladder. *J. Cell Biol.*, **96**, 1662-1670.

Cunha, G.R., Chung, L.W.K., Shannon, J.M., Taguchi, O., and Fujii, H. (1983c). Hormone-induced morphogenesis and growth: Role of mesenchymal-epithelial interactions. *Recent Prog. Horm. Res.*, **39**, 559-598.

Cunha, G.R., Donjacour, A.A., Cooke, P.S., Mee, S., Bigsby, R.M., Higgins, S.J. and Sugimura, Y. (1987). The endocrinology and developmental biology of the prostate. *Endocrine Rev.*, **8**, 338-363.

Cunha, G.R., Young, P., and Brody, J.R. (1989). Role of uterine epithelium in the development of myometrial smooth muscle cells. *Biol. of Reprod.*, **40**, 861-871.

Cunha, G.R., Young, P., Higgins, S.J., and Cooke, P.S. (1991). Neonatal seminal vesicle mesenchyme induces a new morphological and functional phenotype in the epithelia of adult ureter and ductus deferens. *Development*, **111**, 145-158.

Curry, P.T. and Atherton, R.W. (1990). Seminal vesicles: development, secretory products, and fertility. *Archives of Andrology*, **25**, 107-113.

De Pablo, F., Scott, L.A., and Roth, J. (1990). Insulin and insulin-like growth factor I in early development: peptides, receptors and biological events. *Endocrine Rev.* **11**, 558-577.

Di Augustine, R.P., Petrusz, P., Bell, G.I., Brown, C.F., Korach, K.S., McLachlan, J.A., and Teng, C.T. (1988). Influence of estrogens on mouse uterine epidermal growth factor precursor protein and messenger ribonucleic acid. *Endocrinology*, **122**, 2355-2363.

Dickson, R.B. and Lippman, M.E. (1987). Estrogenic regulation of growth and polypeptide growth factor secretion in human breast carcinoma. *Endocr Rev*, **8**, 29-43.

Donahoe, P.K., Budzik, G., Trelstad, R., Mudgett-Hunter, M., Fuller, A.F.J., Hutson, J., Ikawa, H., Hayashi, A., and MacLaughlin, D. (1982). Mullerian Inhibiting Substance: An update. *Rec. Prog. Horm. Res.*, **38**, 279-330.

Donjacour, A.A., Cunha, G.R., and Higgins, S.F. (1988). Detection of specific prostatic proteins in an epithelium that lacks androgen receptors. *Endocrinol. Suppl.*, **122**, 502.

Down, N.E., Peter, R.E., and Leatherland, J.F. (1990). Seasonal changes in serum gonadotropin, testosterone, 11-ketotestosterone, and estradiol-17b levels and their relation to tumor burden in gonadal tumor-bearing carp x goldfish hybrids in the Great Lakes. *General and Comparative Endocrinology,* **77**, 192-201.

Drews, U. and Drews, U. (1977). Regression of mouse mammary gland anlagen in recombinants of Tfm and wild-type tissues: Testosterone acts via the mesenchyme. *Cell*, **10**, 401-404.

Evans, G.S. and Chandler, J.A. (1987). Cell proliferation studies in rat prostate. I. The proliferative role of basal and secretory epithelial cells during normal growth. *Prostate*, **10**, 163-178.

Finch, P.W., Rubin, J.S., Miki, T., Ron, D., and Aaronson, S.A. (1989). Human KGF is FGF-related with properties of a paracrine effector of epithelial cell growth. *Science*, **245** 752-755.

Flaxman, B.A., Chopra, D.P., and Newman, D. (1973). Growth of mouse vaginal epithelial cells *in vitro. In Vitro*, **9**, 194-201.

Forsberg, J.G. (1978). Development of the human vaginal epithelium. In *The Human Vagina*, ed. E. S. E. Hafez and T. N. Evans. Elsevier, No. Holland, New York, pp. 3-20.

Forsberg, J.-G. and Kalland, T. (1981). Neonatal estrogen treatment and epithelial abnormalities in the cervicovaginal epithelium of adult mice. *Cancer Res*, **41**, 721-734.

Fry, D.M. and Toone, C.K. (1981). DDT-induced feminization of gull embryos. *Science*, **213**, 922-924.

Haslam, S.Z. (1986). Mammary fibroblast influence on normal mouse mammary epithelial cell responses to estrogen *in vitro*. *Cancer Res.*, **45**, 310-316.

Hayashi, K., Hayashi, M., Boutin, E., Cunha, G.R., Bernfield, M., and Trelstad, R.L. (1988). Hormonal modification of epithelial differentiation and expression of cell surface heparan sulfate proteoglycan in the mouse vaginal epithelium: An immunohistochemical and electron microscopic study. *Lab. Invest.*, **58**, 68-76.

He, W.W., Kumar, M.V., and Tindall, D.J. (1991). A frameshift mutation in the androgen receptor gene causes complete androgen insensitivity in the testicular-feminized mouse. *Nucleic Acids Res.*, **19**, 2373-2378.

Herbst, A. and Bern, H., (1981). *Developmental effects of DES in pregnancy*. Thieme Stratton, New York, 1981.

Hicks, R.M. (1975). The mammalian urinary bladder: An accommodating organ. *Biol. Rev.*, **50**, 215-246.

Higgins, S.J., Brooks, D.E., Fuller, F.M., Jackson, P.J., and Smith, S.E. (1981). Functional development of sex accessory organs of the male rat: Use of oestradiol benzoate to identify the neonatal period as critical for development of normal protein-synthetic and secretory capabilities. *Biochem. J.*, **194**, 895-905.

Higgins, S.J., Young, P., Brody, J.R., and Cunha, G.R. (1989a). Induction of functional cytodifferentiation in the epithelium of tissue recombinants. I. Homotypic seminal vesicle recombinants. *Development*, **106**, 219-234.

Higgins, S.J., Young, P., and Cunha, G.R. (1989b). Induction of functional cytodifferentiation in the epithelium of tissue recombinants. II. Instructive induction of Wolffian duct epithelia by neonatal seminal vesicle mesenchyme. *Development*, **106**, 235-250.

Hill, D.J. and Milner, R.D.G. (1985). Insulin as a growth factor. *Pedriatric Research*, **19** 879-886.

Ho, S.M. (1991). Prostatic androgen receptor and plasma testosterone levels in streptozotocin-induced diabetic rats. *J. Steroid Biochem. Mol. Biol.*, **38**, 67-72.

Husmann, D.A., McPhaul, M., and Wilson, J.D. (1991). Androgen receptor expression in the developing rat prostate is not altered by castration, flutamide, or suppression of the adrenal axis. *Endocrinology*, **128**, 1902-1906.

Iguchi, T., Uchima, F.D.A., Ostrander, P.L., and Bern, H.A. (1983). Growth of normal mouse vaginal epithelial cells in and on collagen gels. *Proc. Natl. Acad. Sci. USA*, **80**, 3743-3747.

Iguchi, T., Ostrander, P.L., Mills, K.T., and Bern, H.A. (1985a). Induction of abnormal epithelial changes by estrogen in neonatal mouse vaginal transplants. *Cancer Res*, **45**, 5688-5693.

Iguchi, T., Uchima, F.-D.A., Ostrander, P.L., Hamamoto, S.T., and Bern, H.A. (1985b). Proliferation of normal mouse uterine luminal epithelial cells in serum-free collagen gel culture. *Proc. Jpn. Acad.*, **61**, 292-295.

Imagawa, W., Tomooka, Y., and Nandi, S. (1982). Serum-free growth of normal and tumor mouse mammary epithelial cells in primary culture. *Proc. Natl. Acad. Sci. USA*, **79**, 4074-4077.

Inaba, T., Wiest, W.G., Strickler, R.C., and Mori, J. (1988). Augmentation of the response of mouse uterine epithelial cells to estradiol by uterine stroma. *Endocrinology.*, **123**, 1253-1258.

Jalkanen, M., Nguyen, H., Rapraeger, A., Kurn, N., and Bernfield, M. (1985). Heparan sulfate proteoglycans from mouse mammary epithelial cells: Localization on the cell surface with a monoclonal antibody. *J. Cell Biol.*, **101**, 976-984.

Jirasek, J.E. (1967). The relationship between the structure of the testis and differentiation of the external genitalia and phenotype in man. *Ciba Symp.*, **16**, 3-29.

Josso, N., Picard, J.Y., and Tran, D. (1977). The anti-Mullerian hormone. *Rec. Prog. Hormone Res.*, **33**, 117-160.

Jung-Testas, I., Groyer, M.T., Bruner-Lorand, J., Hechter, O., Baulieu, E.-E., and Robel, P. (1981). Androgen and estrogen receptors in rat ventral prostate epithelium and stroma. *Endocrinology.*, **109**, 1287-1289.

Kakita, K., Giddings, S.J., Rotwein, P.S., and Permutt, M.A. (1983). Insulin gene expression in the developing rat pancreas. *Diabetes*, **32**, 691-696.

Kirk, D., King, R.J.B., Heyes, J., Peachy, L., Hirsch, P.J., and Taylor, R.W.T. (1978). Normal human endometrium in cell culture. *In Vitro*, **14**, 651-662.

Kleeman, J.M., Moore, R.W., and Peterson, R.E. (1990). Inhibition of testicular steroidogenesis in 2,3,7,8-tetrachlorodibenzo-p-dioxin-treated rats: Evidence that the key leision occurs prior to or during pregnenolone formation. *Toxicology and Applied Pharmacology*, **106**, 112-125.

Koff, A.K. (1933). Development of the vagina in the human fetus. *Contrib. Embryol. Carnegie Inst. Wash.*, **24**, 59-90.

Kratochwil, K. and Schwartz, P. (1976). Tissue interaction in androgen response of embryonic mammary rudiment of mouse: Identification of target tissue of testosterone. *Proc. Natl. Acad. Sci. USA*, **73**, 4041-4044.

Krieg, M., Klotzl, G., Kaufmann, J., and Voigt, K.D. (1981). Stroma of human benign prostatic hyperplasia: preferential tissue for androgen metabolism and oestrogen binding. *Acta Endocrinol.*, **96**, 422-432.

Kubiak, T.J., Harris, H.J., Smith, L.M., Schwartz, T.R., Stalling, D.L., Trick, J.A., Sileo, L., Docherty, D.E., and Erdman, T.C. (1989). Microcontaminants and reproductive impairment of the Forster's tern on Green Bay, Lake Michigan— 1983. *Arch. Environ. Contam. Toxicol.*, **18**, 706-727.

Lahtonen, R., Bolton, N.J., Kontturri, M., and Vihko, R. (1983). Nuclear androgen receptors in the epithelium and stroma of human benign prostatic hypertrophic glands. *Prostate*, **4**, 129-139.

Landschulz, W., Thesleff, I., and Ekblom, P. (1984). A lipophilic iron chelator can replace transferrin as a stimulator of cell proliferation and differentiation. *J. Cell Biol.*, **98**, 596-601.

Lasnitzki, I. and Mizuno, T. (1980). Prostatic induction: interaction of epithelium and mesenchyme from normal wild-type mice and androgen-insensitive mice with testicular feminization. *J. Endocrinol.*, **85**, 423-428.

Liszezak, T.M., Richardson, G.S., MacLaughlin, D.T., and Kornblith, P.L. (1977). Ultrastructure of human endometrial epithelium in monolayer culture with and without steroid hormones. *In Vitro*, **3**, 344-356.

Mably, T.A., Moore, R.W., Bjerke, D.L., and Peterson, R.E. (1991). The male reproductive system is highly sensitive to *in utero* and lactational TCDD exposure. *Banbury Report*, **35**, 1.

McClellan, M.C., Rankin, S., West, N.B., and Brenner, R.M. (1990). Estrogen receptors, progesterone receptors and DNA synthesis in the macaque endometrium during the luteal-follicular transition. *J. Steroid Biochem. Molec. Biol.*, **37**, 631-641.

McGrath, C.M. (1983). Augmentation of response of normal mammary epithelial cells to estradiol by mammary stroma. *Cancer Res.*, **43**, 1355-1360.

McKeehan, W.L., Adams, P.S., and Rosser, M.P. (1984). Direct mitogenic effects of insulin, epidermal growth factor, glucocorticoid, cholera toxin, unknown pituitary factors and possibly prolactin, but not androgen, on normal rat prostate epithelial cells in serum-free, primary cell culture. *Cancer Res.*, **44**, 1998-2010.

McLachlan, J.A. (1981a). *Estrogens in the Environment.* Elsevier/North Holland, New York.

McLachlan, J.A. (1981b). Rodent models for perinatal exposure to diethylstilbestrol and their relation to human disease in the male. In *Developmental Effects of Diethylstilbestrol (DES). in pregnancy*, ed. H. A and H. Bern. Thieme Stratton, New York, pp. 147-158.

McLachlan, J.A. (1985). *Estrogens in the Environment II: Influences on Development.* Elsevier, New York.

Mori, T. and Nagasawa, H. (1988). *Toxicity of Hormones in Perinatal Life.* CRC Press, Inc., Boca Raton, Florida.

Mukku, V.R. and Stancel, G.M. (1985a). Receptors for epidermal growth factor in the rat uterus. *Endocrinology*, **117**, 149-154.

Mukku, V.R. and Stancel, G.M. (1985b). Regulation of epidermal growth factor receptor by estrogen. *J. Biol. Chem.*, **260**, 9820-9824.

Murphy, L.J., Murphy, L.C., and Friesen, H.G. (1987). A role for the insulin-like growth factors as estromedins in the rat uterus.. *Trans. Assoc. Am. Physicians*, **100**, 204-214.

Nandi, S., Imagawa, W., Tomooka, Y., McGrath, M.F., and Edery, M. (1984). Collagen gel culture system and analysis of estrogen effects on mammary carcinogenesis. *Arch. Toxicol.*, **55**, 91-96.

O'Rahilly, R. (1973). The embryology and anatomy of the uterus. In *The Uterus*, ed. H. J. Norris, A. T. Hertig and M. R. Abell. Williams and Wilkins Co., Baltimore, pp. 17-39.

Ohno, S. (1979). *Major Sex Determining Genes.* Springer-Verlag, New York.

Persson, B. (1980). Insulin as a growth factor in the fetus. In *The Biology of Normal Human Growth*, ed. M. Ritzen, K. Hall, A. Zettereberg, A. Aperia, A. Larson and R. Zetterstrom. Raven Press, New York, pp. 213-221.

Prins, G., Birch, L. and Greene, G. (1991). Androgen receptor localization in different cell types of the adult rat prostate. *Endocrinology*, **129**, 3187-3199.

Rapraeger, A., Jalkanen, M., Endo, E., Koda, J., and Bernfield, M. (1985). The cell surface proteoglycan from mouse mammary epithelial cells bears chondroitin sulfate and heparan sulfate glycosaminoglycans. *J. Chem. Biol.*, **260**, 11046-11052.

Rechler, M.M., Podskalny, J.M., and Nissley, S.P. (1976). Interaction of multiplication-stimulating activity with chick embryo fibroblasts demonstrates a growth receptor. *Nature*, **259**, 134-136.

Rechler, M.M., Posskalny, J.M., and Nissley, S.P. (1977). Characterization of the binding of multiplication-stimulating activity to a receptor for growth polypeptides in chick embryo fibroblasts. *J. Biol. Chem.*, **252**, 3898-3910.

Sanderson, R. and Bernfield, M. (1988). Molecular polymorphism of a cell surface proteoglycan: Distinct structures on simple and stratified epithelia. *Proc. Nat'l. Acad. Sci. USA*, **85**, 9562-9566.

Schulze, H. and Barrack, E.R. (1987). Immunocytochemical localization of estrogen receptors in the normal male and female canine urinary tract and prostate. *Endocrinology*, **121**, 1773-1783.

Shannon, J.M. and Cunha, G.R. (1983). Autoradiographic localization of androgen binding in the developing mouse prostate. *Prostate*, **4**, 367-373.

Shannon, J.M. and Cunha, G.R. (1984). Characterization of androgen binding and deoxyribonucleic acid synthesis in prostate-like structures induced in testicular feminized (Tfm/Y). mice. *Biol. Reprod.,* **31** 175-183.

Shima, H., Tsuji, M., Young, P.F., and Cunha, G.R. (1990). Postnatal growth of mouse seminal vesicle is dependent on 5a-dihydrotestosterone. *Endocrinology,* **127,** 3222-3233.

Snedeker, S.M., Brown, C.F., and DiAugustine, R.P. (1991). Expression and functional properties of transforming growth factor a and epidermal growth factor during mouse mammary gland ductal morphogenesis. *Proc. Natl. Acad. Sci. USA,* **88,** 276-280.

Straus, D.S. (1984). Growth stimulatory actions of insulin *in vitro* and *in vivo. Endocrine Rev.,* **5,** 356-369.

Stumpf, W. and Sar, M. (1976). Autoradiographic localization of estrogen, androgen, progestin, and glucocorticosteroid in "target tissues" and "non-target tissues". In *Receptors and Mechanism of Action of Steroid Hormones,* ed. J. Pasqualini. Marcel Dekker Inc., New York, pp. 41-84.

Subramanian, A.N., Tanabe, S., Tatsukawa, R., Saito, S., and Miyazaki, N. (1987). Reduction in the testosterone levels by PCBs and DDE in Dall's porpoises of Northwestern North Pacific. *Marine Pollution Bulletin,* **18,** 643-646.

Sugimura, Y., Cunha, G.R., and Bigsby, R.M. (1986). Androgenic induction of deoxyribonucleic acid synthesis in prostatic glands induced in the urothelium of testicular feminized (Tfm/y). mice. *Prostate,* **9,** 217-225.

Taguchi, O., Bigsby, R.M., and Cunha, G.R. (1988). Estrogen responsiveness and the estrogen receptor during development of the murine female reproductive tract. *Growth, Differentiation and Develop.,* **30,** 301-313.

Takasugi, N. (1976). Cytological basis for permanent vaginal changes in mice treated neonatally with steroid hormones. *Int. Rev. Cytol.,* **44,** 193-224.

Takeda, H., Mizuno, T., and Lasnitzki, I. (1985). Autoradiographic studies of androgen-binding sites in the rat urogenital sinus and postnatal prostate. *J. Endocrinol.,* **104,** 87-92.

Takeda, H., Suematsu, N., and Mizuno, T. (1990). Transcription of prostatic steroid binding protein (PSBP). gene is induced by epithelial-mesenchymal interaction. *Development,* **110,** 273-282.

Tilley, W.D., Horsfall, D.J., McGee, M.A., Henderson, D.W., and Marshall, V.R. (1985). Distribution of oestrogen and androgen receptors between the stroma and epithelium of the guinea-pig prostate. *J. Steroid Biochem.,* **22,** 713-719.

Tomooka, Y., DiAugustine, R.P., and McLachlan, J.A. (1986). Proliferation of mouse uterine epithelial cells *in vitro. Endocrinology.,* **118,** 1011-1018.

Tsuji, M., Shima, H., and Cunha, G.R. (1991a). Morphogenetic and proliferative effects of testosterone and insulin on the neonatal mouse seminal vesicle *in vitro. Endocrinology,* **129,** 2289-2297.

Tsuji, M., Shima, H., and Cunha, G.R. (1991b). Morphogenetic and proliferative effects of testosterone and insulin on the neonatal mouse seminal vesicle *in vitro. Endocrinology,* **129,** 2289-2297.

Tuohimaa, P. (1980). Control of cell proliferation in male accessory sex glands. In *Male Accessory Sex Glands,* ed. E. Spring-Mills and E.S.E. Hafez. Elsevier/North Holland, New York, pp. 131-153.

Tuohimaa, P. and Niemi, M. (1974). Cell renewal and mitogenic activity of testosterone in male sex accessory glands. In *Male Accessory Sex Organs: Structure and Function in Mammals,* ed. D. Brandes. Academic Press, pp. 329-343.

Turner, T., Young, P., and Cunha, G.R. (1989). Seminal vesicle induction of adult mouse epididymal epithelium by newborn mouse and rat seminal vesicle mesenchyme. *J. Cell Biol.* (Abstract), **109,** 69a.

Uchima, F.D.A., Edery, M., Iguchi, T., Larson, L., and Bern, H.A. (1987). Growth of mouse vaginal epithelial cells in culture: Functional integrity of the estrogen receptor system and failure of estrogen to induce proliferation. *Cancer Ltrs.*, **35**, 227-235.

Wasner, G., Hennermann, I., and Kratochwil, K. (1983). Ontogeny of mesenchymal androgen receptors in the embryonic mouse mammary gland. *Endocrinology*, **113**, 1771-1780.

Whitten, P.L. and Naftolin, F. (1991). Xenoestrogens and neuroendocrine development. In *Prenatal Exposure to Environmental Toxicants: Developmental Consequences*, ed. H. L. Needleman and D. Bellinger. Johns Hopkins University Press.

Wilson, J., George, F., and Griffin, J. (1981a). The hormonal control of sexual development. *Science*, **211**, 1278-1284.

Wilson, J.D., Griffin, J.E., Leshin, M., and George, F.W. (1981b). Role of gonadal hormones in development of the sexual phenotypes. *Human Genetics*, **58**, 78-84.

Wilson, J.D., Griffin, J.E., George, F.W., and Leshin, M. (1984). Recent studies on the endocrine control of male phenotypic development. In *Sexual Differentiation: Basic and Clinical Aspects*, ed. M. Serio, M. Zanisi, M. Motta, and L. Martini. Raven Press, New York, pp. 223-232.

Winter, J.S.D., Faiman, C., and Reyes, F. (1981). Sexual endocrinology of fetal and perinatal life. In *Mechanisms of Sex Differentiation in Animals and Man*, ed. C. R. Austin and R. G. Edwards. Academic Press, New York, pp. 205-254.

Yamashita, S., Newbold, R.R., McLachlan, J.A., and Korach, K.S. (1989). Developmental pattern of estorgen receptor expression in female mouse genital tracts. *Endocrinology*, **125**, 2888-2896.

# ENVIRONMENTAL ESTROGENS: ORPHAN RECEPTORS AND GENETIC IMPRINTING

### John A. McLachlan, Retha R. Newbold, Christina T. Teng, and Kenneth S. Korach

Laboratory of Reproductive and Developmental Toxicology, National Institute of Environmental Health Sciences, Research Triangle Park, North Carolina

*Many chemicals in the environment function like female sex hormones-- estrogens. This functional signal apparently is mediated by a member of the nuclear hormone receptor gene family. This gene family and the chemicals it recognizes seem to be growing; family members for which no known ligand exists are called orphan receptors. One consequence of exposure to estrogens early in development is the feminization of the male reproductive system which occurs at both the gross structural and genetic levels. This imprinting of genes has implications for reproductive health which are only now being considered.*

Humans and other animals live in an increasingly complex environment. While our external chemical milieu has changed dramatically in the last half century, many millions of years were required for living organisms to evolve strategies to deal with their internal environment. There are many ways to interpret environmental signals; one is through receptors which respond to cues from both the internal and external environment. Receptors are molecules with specific and high affinity binding for effector molecules (ligands); this binding results in a functional change. A class of receptor molecules which interact with specific parts of the genome is called the nuclear hormone receptors (Parker, 1991). These molecules comprise a super gene family that recognize such important biomolecules as steroid hormones (including the female sex hormones, estrogen, and progesterone; the male sex hormone, androgen; the adrenal hormones, glucocorticoid and mineralocorticoid), thyroid hormone (thyroxine), vitamins (Vitamin D), and retinoic acid. The hormone-receptor complex binds to specific regulatory regions of DNA in the cell nucleus and apparently alters expression of key target genes; in fact, regulation of gene expression is the hallmark of hormone action and leads predictably to functional alterations in cells, tissues and organs. Thus, an understanding of receptor binding and action lies at the basis for understanding a key element in interpreting signals from our internal environment.

The nuclear receptor gene family has two unique features which may provide a crucial link in understanding how signals from our external environment are also

[1]Corresponding author: Dr. John A. McLachlan, Laboratory of Reproductive and Developmental Toxicology, National Institute of Environmental Health Sciences, P. O. Box 12233, Research Triangle Park, North Carolina 27709.

interpreted. One feature is that there are apparently members of this family for which there are no known ligands—hence the term "orphan receptors" (O'Malley, 1990). As more orphan receptors are found and their natural ligands are discovered, the picture of cell regulation and differentiation by steroid hormones, vitamins, and retinoids will change. A case in point was the discovery of a natural ligand, 9-cis retinoic acid, for an orphan member of the retinoid subfamily of receptors, opening new pathways for understanding effector ligands involved in hormone action (Heyman et al., 1992).

An additional feature of this gene family involves their association with foreign chemicals. This occurs in at least two primary ways: (1) receptors for which there are no known endogenous ligands which recognize exogenous chemicals or (2) receptors of known function which bind and respond to foreign chemicals of diverse structures. In the first case, a recently discovered member of the nuclear receptor family apparently recognizes a class of foreign chemicals called peroxisome proliferators which includes industrial plasticizers, herbicides, and hypolipidemic agents (Issemann and Green, 1990). Similarly, a receptor (although from another gene family) exists for the ubiquitous xenobiotic, dioxin or TCDD (Lucier, In Press).

The second case, that of foreign chemicals interacting with known receptors, is exemplified by the many xenobiotics which interact with the estrogen receptor. These compounds elicit many of the same cellular and physiological effects of the natural female sex hormone, estradiol. In fact, this may be considered a kind of hormone mimicry in which compounds which are not made in an organism can stimulate specific responses associated with compounds that are made. Thus, foreign chemicals, which are not known to be hormones, will interact with the estrogen receptor and, when given to gonadectomized animals, mimic estrogen-like physiological effects, including development, growth and functional stimulation of the vagina, cervix, uterus, and mammary gland. There are numerous compounds with estrogenic effects (Fig. 1); these have been described elsewhere (McLachlan, 1985; and McLachlan et al., 1987).

Estrogenic xenobiotics may be natural constituents of our environment such as those found in plants (phytoestrogens such as coumestrol) or the product of fungi (mycotoxin estrogens-zearalenone); both plant estrogens and mycotoxin estrogens are variable parts of our diet. Other estrogenic xenobiotics are synthetic compounds; these include diethylstilbestrol (DES) which was used therapeutically in pregnant women as well as given to livestock and poultry as a growth promoter for many years. A class of synthetic estrogenic xenobiotics which are widespread environmentally are the chlorinated hydrocarbons; DDT and DDE are the best known examples. More recently, we have demonstrated that another group of ubiquitous chlorinated hydrocarbons, the polychlorinated biphenyls (PCBs), are also weakly estrogenic (Korach et al., 1988).

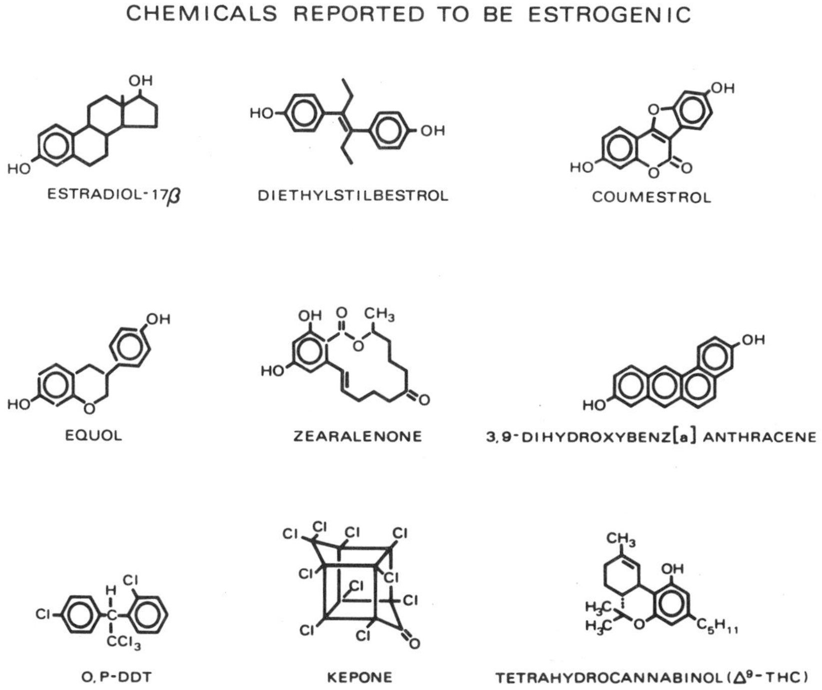

CHEMICALS REPORTED TO BE ESTROGENIC

**FIGURE 1.** Environmental estrogens. The structures of selected chemicals for which estrogenic activity has been described is very diverse. The specific references for these chemicals is given in McLachlan et al., 1987.

Although the hormonal activity of numerous foreign chemicals is clearly demonstrated, the adverse effect of these compounds on health is less clear. Certainly, it has been shown that environmental estrogens contained in plants can adversely effect reproduction in wild animals and livestock which eat them (Hughes, 1988). In the case of humans, contamination of food with DES has been associated with precocious puberty in young boys and girls (New, 1985); in fact, a reported outbreak of precocious breast development among young girls in Puerto Rico in the 1980s raised the possibility of environmental estrogen exposures, but the extent and etiology of the outbreak were never determined.

These reports, however, highlight the fact that estrogenic effects may be most significant in younger individuals. In fact, work in experimental animals suggests that developmental exposures to estrogens have irreversible and deleterious effects. [The long-term sequalae following treatment with DES during fetal or neonatal life in humans or experimental animals has been extensively reviewed (Mori and Nagasawa, 1988) and is well summarized in the present volume by Bern et al., Chapter 2.] While there are many changes induced by exogenous estrogens in early life, a hallmark of such exposures in mice following prenatal treatment is failure of testicular descent and retention of the female genital tract in a genetic male (McLachlan et al., 1975; Newbold et al., 1987; Newbold and McLachlan, 1988).

Early in sexual development the mammalian fetus exists as a pseudohermaphrodite with gonads genetically determined to become an ovary or testes and the rudiments for both the male and female genital tract coexisting. During normal sexual differentiation of a genetic male, the male reproductive system (Wolffian duct) persists and develops while the female system (Müllerian duct) regresses; later in development, the testes, which are intra-abdominal in the fetus, descend into the scrotum. Administration of DES to a pregnant mouse during this critical period of sexual development blocks much of the process and retains a fetal-like condition—intra-abdominal testes and the retention of both male and female genital systems—an adult pseudohermaphrodite (Fig. 2).

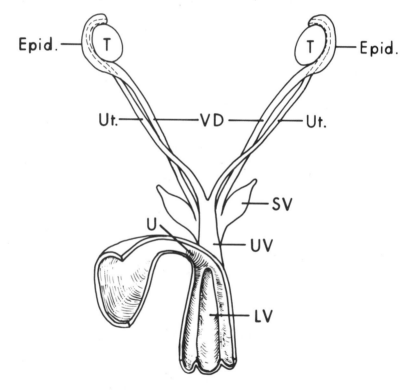

**FIGURE 2.** Feminization of the male reproductive system associated with developmental estrogenization. A schematic representation of the adult reproductive tract in a genetic male mouse exposed prenatally to diethylstilbestrol (DES). In addition to the male reproductive system including undescended testes (T), epididymus (Epid.), vas deferens (VD), seminal vesicle (SV), and urethra (U), the mouse also exhibits a coexisting female reproductive system including uterus (Ut.), upper vagina (UV), and lower vagina (LV). Summarized from data in Newbold et al., 1987.

So, certainly at the structural level, prenatal exposure to exogenous estrogens alters sexual development in a predictable way leading in the male to undescended testes and the retention of the Müllerian or fetal female duct system. The question arises then, whether aspects of estrogen-associated feminization of the male genital system occurs at a more subtle level. In other words, can female genes be imprinted in the male reproductive system such that they may be functionally active later in life?

To this end we have identified a major estrogen-inducible secretory protein from the mouse uterus (Teng et al., 1986; Pentecost and Teng, 1987; Teng et al., 1989). This protein, lactoferrin, is found in low amounts in the male mouse reproductive system (primarily the dorsolateral lobes of the prostate) but is absent from the seminal vesicle (an organ derived entirely from the Wolffian or fetal male duct). However, when an adult male mouse, which was exposed prenatally to DES, is gonadectomized and treated secondarily with estrogens, its seminal vesicle expresses lactoferrin messenger RNA and protein with the same intensity as the uterus of an estrogen-treated female (Pentecost et al., 1988; Newbold et al., 1989). Further evidence for feminization at the gene level is the expression of the estrogen receptor in the seminal vesicle of developmentally estrogenized mice, but not controls (Newbold et al., 1989). These, and other data, suggest molecular pseudohermaphroditism associated with develop mental imprinting by estrogen of female genes in the male reproductive system. The functional significance of this hormonally associated genetic imprinting is not clear as yet, although it has been reported that male offspring of mice treated prenatally with DES have reduced sperm count and increased epididymal cysts, undescended testes, and infertility (Newbold and McLachlan, 1988).

Therefore, chemicals in the environment with estrogenic activity may have long lasting effects on sexual development both prominent and subtle. These effects are apparently mediated through intracellular receptors, the ontogeny of which is just beginning to be studied. Only by a mechanistic understanding of the role of estrogen in the normal and abnormal development of the genital system will strategies for a healthy reproductive life be assured.

## REFERENCES

Heyman, R.A., Mangelsdorf, D.J., Dyck, J.A., Stein, R.B., Eichele, G., Evans, R.M., and Thaller, C.T. (1992). 9-*Cis* retinoic acid is a high affinity ligand for the retinoid X receptor. *Cell*, **68**, 396-406.

Hughes, C.L., Jr. (1988). Phytochemical mimicry of reproductive hormones and modulation of herbivore fertility by phytoestrogens. *Environ. Health. Perspect.*, **78**, 171-174.

Issemann, I. and Green, S. (1990). Activation of a member of the steroid hormone receptor superfamily by peroxisome proliferators. *Nature*, **347**, 645-649.

Korach, K.S., Sarver, P., Chae, K., McLachlan, J.A., and McKinney, J.D. (1988). Estrogen receptor binding activity of polychlorinated hydroxybiphenyls: conformationally restricted structural probes. *Mol. Pharm.*, **33**, 120-126.

Lucier, G.W. (In Press). Receptor-mediated carcinogenesis. In *Approaches to Classifying Carcinogens According to Mechanims of Action,* ed. H. Vainiv. International Agency for Research on Cancer, IARC Scientific Publications.

McLachlan, J.A. (ed.) (1985). *Estrogens in the Environment II: Influences on Development.* Elsevier North Holland, New York.

McLachlan, J.A, Newbold, R., and Bullock, B. (1975). Reproductive tract lesions in male mice exposed prenatally to diethylstilbestrol. *Science,* **190,** 991-992.

McLachlan, J.A., Newbold, R.R., Korach, K.S., and Hogan, M. (1987). Risk assessment considerations for reproductive and developmental toxicity of oestrogenic xenobiotics. In *Human Risk Assessment: The Roles of Animal Selection and Extrapolation,* ed. M.V. Roloff and A.W. Wilson. Taylor and Francis, Ltd, London, pp. 187-193.

Mori, T. and Nagasawa, H. (eds.) (1988). *Toxicity of Hormones in Perinatal Life.* CRC Press, Inc., Boca Raton, Florida.

New, M.I. (1985). Premature thelarche and estrogen intoxication. In *Estrogens in the Environment II: Influences on Development,* ed. J.A. McLachlan. Elsevier North Holland, New York, pp. 349-357.

Newbold, R.R. and McLachlan, J.A. (1988). Neoplastic and non-neoplastic lesions in male reproductive organs following perinatal exposure to hormones and related substances. In *Toxicity of Hormones in Perinatal Life,* eds. T. Mori and H. Nagasawa. CRC Press, Inc., Boca Raton, Florida, pp. 89-109.

Newbold, R.R., Bullock, B.C., and McLachlan, J.A. (1987). Müllerian remnants of male mice exposed prenatally to diethylstilbestrol. *Teratogen. Carcinogen. Mutagen.,* **7,** 377-389.

Newbold, R.R., Pentecost, B.T., Yamashita, S., Lum, K., Miller, J.V., Nelson, P., Blair, J., Kong, H., Teng, C., and McLachlan, J.A. (1989). Female gene expression in the seminal vesicle of mice after prenatal exposure to diethylstilbestrol. *Endocrinology,* **124,** 2568-2576.

O'Malley, B. (1990). The steroid receptor superfamily: more excitement predicted for the future. *Mol. Endo.,* **4,** 363-369.

Parker, M.G. (ed.) (1991). *Nuclear Hormone Receptors,* Academic Press, London.

Pentecost, B.T. and Teng, C.T. (1987). Lactoferrin is the major estrogen inducible protein of mouse uterus secretions. *J. Biol. Chem.,* **262,** 10134-10139.

Pentecost, B.T., Newbold, R.R., Teng, C.T., and McLachlan, J.A. (1988). Prenatal exposure of male mice to diethylstilbestrol alters the expression of the lactotransferrin gene in seminal vesicles. *Mol. Endo.,* **2,** 1243-1248.

Teng, C.T., Walker, M.P., Bhattacharyya, S.N., Klapper, D.G., DiAugustine, R.P., and McLachlan, J.A. (1986). Purification and properties of an oestrogen-stimulated mouse uterine glycoprotein (approx. 70kDa). *Biochem. J.,* **240,** 413-422.

Teng, C.T., Pentecost, B.T., Chen, Y.H., Newbold, R.R., Eddy, E.M., and McLachlan, J.A. (1989). Lactotransferrin gene expression in the mouse uterus and mammary gland. *Endocrinology,* **124,** 992-999.

# EFFECTS OF KRAFT MILL EFFLUENT ON THE SEXUALITY OF FISHES: AN ENVIRONMENTAL EARLY WARNING?

**William P. Davis**
Environmental Research Laboratory, Gulf Breeze Florida

**Stephen A. Bortone**
Biology Department, University of West Florida, Pensacola, Florida

## INTRODUCTION

In this report we describe arrhenoidy (i.e., masculinization) in females of the fish family Poeciliidae sampled from streams receiving kraft mill effluent (KME) and among fish experimentally exposed to microbially degraded phytosterols. The masculinization response involves development of male secondary sex morphological characters, including modification of the anal fin into a gonopodium-like structure, often concomitant with male fish behavior, including mating attempts.

Initial discovery of arrhenoid female mosquitofish, *Gambusia affinis*, was made during a field survey of Elevenmile Creek (Fig. 1, Escambia Co., Florida) investigating the distributional boundaries of the eastern *G. holbrooki* and western *G. affinis*, mosquitofish.

The investigators were startled to observe well developed modification of the anal fin, resembling a gonopodium, (i.e., Fig. 4, male intermittent or copulatory organ) on pregnant, female mosquitofish. Additional investigation established that masculinization among these fish occurred only downstream from the discharge of KME; none were collected upstream or in tributary streams (Howell et al., 1980). Discussing this "environmentally induced sex inversion," Reinboth (1980) stated: "...phenotypical expression of sex depends on a vulnerable chain of events the links of which remain in total obscurity to us." Subsequently, KME-induced acquisition of male secondary sex characteristics in female poeciliid fishes has been reported both for laboratory and *in situ* exposures (Bortone and Drysdale, 1981; Drysdale, 1981, 1984; Rosa-Molinar and Williams, 1984; Bortone et al., 1989; Davis, 1989; Drysdale and Bortone, 1989).

Induction of precocious sexual maturity in salmonid fishes is reported by Funk and Donaldson (1972) resulting from induction by gonadotropins. McLeay et al. (1987) review the diverse reports of pulp and paper mill effluent toxicities, and a number of authors (e.g., McLeay and Brown, 1974; Anokas et al., 1976; Roald, 1977; McLeay and Brown, 1979; McLeay et al., 1979; Oikari et al., 1982, 1983, 1984, 1985, 1988; Myllyvirta et al., 1989; Lehtinen et al., 1990) have reported biochemical, physiological, metabolic, and behavioral types of toxicity associated with KME effluents.

---

1. Corresponding Author: W. P. Davis, Environmental Research Laboratory, Gulf Breeze, FL 32561.

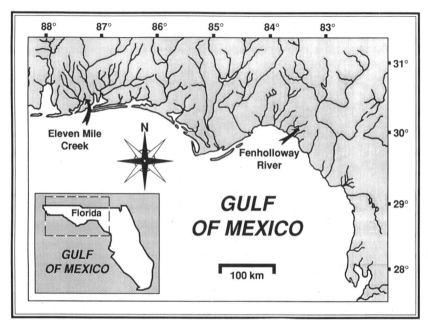

**FIGURE 1.** Enlargement of west Florida indicating the two sites where KME induces masculinization of female poeciliid fishes: Elevenmile Creek, Escambia Co. and Fenholloway River, Taylor Co., Florida.

Environmental investigators have reported reduced numbers of species, indications of physiological stress, biochemical responses, behavioral changes, and reproductive inhibition in fishes surviving in KME, which Owens (1991) summarized in his review of pulp and paper effluent, aquatic environment hazard assessment. Most reported investigations have been conducted in regions at higher latitudes and no others have described similar masculinization effects among fishes exposed to KME.

Sex change in fishes has been inferred in some reports without the corroborating evidence of gonad histology. We use masculinization or arrhenoidy in this report to represent changes of secondary sex characteristics (Bortone et al., 1989; Drysdale and Bortone, 1989). Additionally, we focus on species which have not demonstrated delayed maturation, for example, that occurs in species of mollies, *Poecilia* (Farr and Travis, 1989; Trexler and Travis, 1990a,b). Masculinization should not be conceptually confused with "sex reversal" or adaptive ambisexuality (Reinboth, 1988). Sex determination among fishes is diverse and most previous research has focused on the adaptive aspects of sex changes among fishes. Sex determination has been genetically described as a polygenic process in fishes (Winge, 1934; Kosswig, 1964). However, Kallman (1984) emphasizes that this idea should be more adequately tested and provides a thorough and clear elaboration of sex determination in poeciliid fishes. The two mosquitofish species (*G. holbrooki* and *G. affinis*) in our observations apparently have different sex determination chromosome systems (Angus, 1989).

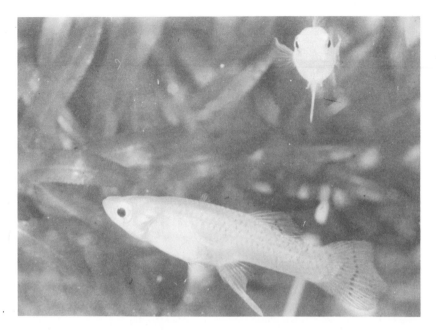

**FIGURE 2.** Lateral and head-on views of masculinized *Gambusia holbrooki* as indicated by gonopodial development of the anal fin. These mosquitofish, about 26-30 mm total length, were captured in the Fenholloway River.

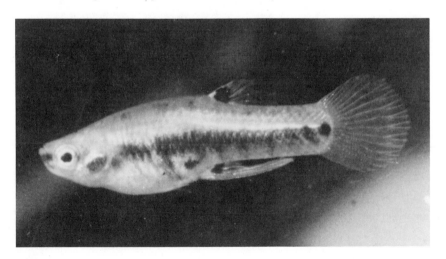

**FIGURE 3.** A highly masculinized female *Heterandria formosa*, about 20-25 mm length, which retains the female pigment spot on the base of the anal fin transformed into a gonopodium.

Masculinization is observed in the female anal fin (Figs. 2, 3, 5, 6) by increased numbers of segments and consequent elongation of the third through fifth fin rays (Turner, 1941a,b; 1942a,b; Howell and Denton, 1989). Experimentally,

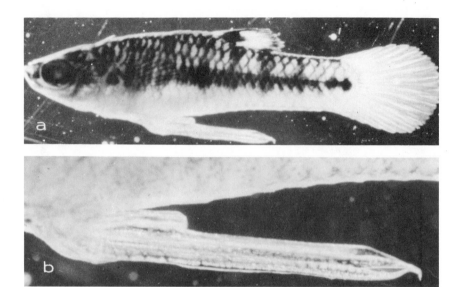

**FIGURE 4.** a) Normal male *Heterandria formosa*, least killifish, about 10 mm length. b) Enlarged view of the gonopodium, normally the male intromittent organ which lacks any pigmentation.

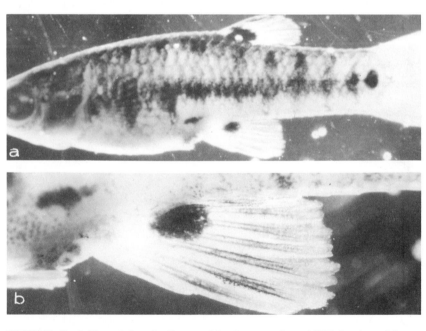

**FIGURE 5.** a) Normal female *Heterandria formosa*, least killifish, about 26 mm length. b) Enlarged view of the unmodified female anal fin with the typical pigment spot which characterizes this sex.

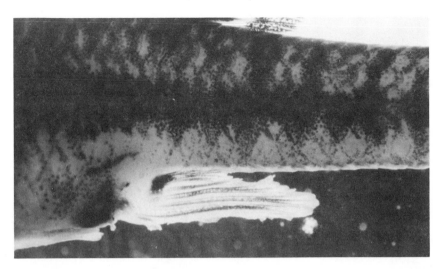

**FIGURE 6.** An enlarged view of an anal fin of a female *Heterandria formosa* which has begun to elongate into a gonopodium from a fish captured in the Fenholloway River.

masculinization of female mosquitofish has been induced using methyltestosterone (Turner, 1941a; 1942a,b; 1960; Okada and Yamashita, 1944), androstenedione, androstanol and spironolactone (Hunsinger and Howell, 1991). These examples from the literature have reinforced the generally accepted notion that poeciliid masculinization observed in wild populations has been induced by androgens associated with KME. Conner et al. (1978) reported that phytosterols in tall (pine) oil may be microbially converted to C-19 steroids. Tall oil, a by-product of kraft pulping, is composed of 20-25% resin acids, 46-48% fatty acids and 25-35% phytosterols (Casey, 1980). The 800,000 tons of tall oil produced in the U.S. during 1974 could potentially produce 20,000 tons (U.S.) of phytosterols (Conner et al., 1978).

## EXPERIMENTAL AND *IN-SITU* COMPARISONS

We have experimentally exposed *G. affinis*, mosquitofish (Fig. 2) and *Heterandria formosa* least killifish to KME effluent stream water in both outdoor pools and laboratory aquaria. In the stream-side pool experiments, fish from non-KME sites were exposed to KME stream water and subsampled to observe temporal effects of KME exposure. Several morphological variables were measured including preanal length, anal-fin length, dorsal-fin height, pelvic-fin length, interorbital width, eye diameter and body depth, each divided by standard length, were used to establish group assignment (Bortone et al., 1989). KME exposed groups were compared with fish from a non-KME site (source of exposed fish) and highly masculinized fish from another KME field site (Fig. 1, Fenholloway River). After three or more weeks of exposure, KME treated female *G. affinis* constituted a group statistically intermediate between nonmasculinized and masculinized reference samples. Comparable results with laboratory exposures of new-born *G. affinis* to KME were reported by Drysdale (1984) and

Drysdale and Bortone (1989). Masculinization of female *H. formosa* in the pool KME exposure was not statistically discernable; (two escaped fish, later recovered from the KME stream did become masculinized).

Laboratory exposures to microbially treated phytosterol were conducted with *G. affinis* and *H. formosa*. The exposure technique described by Denton et al., (1985) and Howell and Denton (1989) utilized a mixture of the phytosterols sitosterol and stigmastanol in perforated dialysis bags or packets with cultures of the bacterium, *Mycobacterium smegmatis*. We performed test exposures in various sized containers (100 ml bowls, 2 and 6 litre jars) comparing different numbers of fish to establish an appropriate test design. In our tests the masculinization responses of *H. formosa* to this "androgen generator" packet were equivalent to, or more pronounced than, the responses of *G. affinis*.

Use of *H. formosa* for laboratory exposure has distinct experimental advantages: (1) this poeciliid species is typically docile with minimal aggression among individuals; (2) the anal fin of female is marked with a dark pigment spot which remains as an indicator of genetic sex during and after masculinization (Figs. 3, 5, 6). The first advantage is important since behavioral changes during masculinization can induce increased levels of aggression and potential damage to body and fins. The degree of masculinization response we observed ranged from virtually no anal fin modification to well developed gonopodial growth during the same exposure periods. Despite differences in the fin transformation responses between containers, fish (n = 8-12) within a specific exposure container consistently became masculinized to the same degree. These variable degrees of masculinization response probably reflect different amounts of androgenic steroid produced or released by each of these androgen generator packets.

The degree of masculinization may sometime prove to be a useful indicator in field samples as well. During periods of drought when streams receiving KME are intensely stained, captured poeciliids are smaller, less abundant and often exhibit the greatest gonopodial development among females, typically more developed than fish exposed in laboratory experiments. In these circumstances, it is difficult to determine whether certain individual *G. affinis* are genetically male or arrhenoid females. In contrast, *H. formosa* females, regardless of the degree of gonopodial fin modification, retain characteristic snout to dorsal fin proportion and the melanin pigment spot on anal fin base (Figs. 3, 5, 6).

These preliminary results demonstrate the sensitivity of the response of these fish to exposure variables. The masculinization responses observed in laboratory exposures are related specifically to microbially degraded phytosterol components per se. KME-effluents additionally contain a plethora of other pulp mill byproducts, halogenated organics including dioxins and furans, which may also induce other endogenic responses.

Although laboratory experiments induce masculinized morphology closely resembling the arrhenoid female poeciliids exposed to KME effluent, there have been no chemical identifications of specific androgenic steroidal compounds present in KME. Furthermore, how the masculinization response may vary and interact with various environmental factors including the seasonal levels of phytosterol precursors in the processed trees (Casey, 1980) as well as environmental parameters such as dissolved oxygen, temperature, microbial activity, and other chemical components in KME, all remain to be investigated.

Effects of KME masculinizing agents on aquatic species, other than poeciliid fishes, has scarcely been assessed. However, Caruso et al. (1988) reported the occurrence of precocious secondary male sex characters (eye enlargement and gonadal development) in juvenile American eels, *Anguilla rostrata*. The features described are inconsistent with the size and time of normal sexual maturation (Facey and Helfman, 1985; Helfman et al., 1987). The affected eels were also collected from Elevenmile Creek, where arrhenoid mosquitofish were first discovered.

## HOW FAR MASCULINIZATION?

Turner and Steeves (1989) used the steroid, 11-ketotestosterone, to induce spermatogenesis in the otherwise all-female species, *Poecilia formosa*. Riehl (1991) described anal fin morphology and hermaphroditic gonad in a single individual least killifish, *H. formosa*. He stated that it was the first reported example of masculinization for this species (but see Bortone and Drysdale, 1981) and presented no data regarding the environmental circumstances which produced the arrhenoid fish. Rasotto and Zulian (1989) reported 158 of 264 (60%) female *G. affinis* from a thermal spring in northern Italy were masculinized. One masculinized fish in their study exhibited a hermaphroditic condition with degenerating vitellogenic oocytes and many cysts of spermatids and spermatozoa. They did not provide evidence of potential effects of any environmental factors in their report, but effluent from pharmaceutical manufacture may have been present (Marconato, A., 1990, pers. comm.). Masculinized *G. affinis* captured from Elevenmile Creek, as well as both *G. holbrooki* and *H. formosa* that were sampled from Fenholloway River, in central north Florida have included a few hermaphroditic individuals (Drysdale and Bortone, pers. obs.).

Both field and laboratory studies represent ephemeral observations of the masculinization response. Field captured poeciliids are removed from the conditions which induced masculinization when observed in aquaria. Data presently available do not reflect continuous life history observations, thus timing of modification steps and the terminal stage(s) of the masculinization process are not known. Information is lacking on the concomitant fate of masculinized poeciliid populations or the other species subjected to continued exposures to KME androgens. Potentially, the observed masculinization may represent stages of intersexuality in a progression toward hermaphroditism or sex reversal. Our field collections and observations revealed very few hermaphroditic states among the KME exposed fish. However, KME-exposed fish in nature may not survive sustained exposure to high levels of the androgen. We have noticed that highly masculinized females from the field, maintained in aquaria, generally have higher mortality than non-masculinized cohorts. Additionally, we have observed only a few large specimens (e.g. >25 mm SL (standard length)) among the masculinized poeciliids in the more concentrated KME effluents (e.g. Fenholloway River). In contrast, in situations where KME received aerobic waste treatment, *G. affinis* often exhibit masculinization at more moderate levels and achieve considerably larger sizes (>30 mm SL). However, it is not apparent whether the larger fish become masculinized during later life history stages or if lower concentrations of KME stimulated growth (e.g. Sandstrom et al., 1988).

The "degree" of masculinization, as judged by modifications of anal fin and behavioral elements, does not continue in fish after removal from KME streams in the field while maintained in aquaria without androgen treatment. However, one of us (WPD) was initially skeptical regarding the published statement: "When three pregnant, masculinized females were placed into an aquarium with three normal, control females, the masculinized females exhibited only behavioral patterns of typical males, i.e., chasing the control females with gonopodial swinging and thrusting, in vain attempts at fertilization" (Howell et al., 1980). During our observations of masculinized *G. affinis* from Elevenmile Creek (1986-1990) no modified behavioral patterns were detected in behavioral experiments conducted after two months removal from KME exposure (Bortone et al., 1989). However, during periods when female *G. affinis* were directly exposed to microbially treated phytosterol products and in the process of masculinization, they did exhibit the male behavior reported by Howell et al., (1980) and Larkin (1986). Furthermore, we have observed individual arrhenoid females which, judging by loss of body weight, were nearing the end of their life span which exhibited elements of male courting behavior to other females in aquaria free of androgenic treatment. The question of how the presence of androgens interacts, or continues to influence or modify physiological, behavioral and morphological states remains unresolved.

Masculinized females placed in laboratory aquaria have reproduced, typically birthing nonarrhenoid offspring. Hunsinger et al., (1988) and our observations confirm that *G. affinis* and *H. formosa* may produce viable offspring in aquaria (at least in the early stages of masculinization) while free of KME/androgen exposure.

In a study rarely cited, Okada and Yamashita (1944) described results of subcutaneously implanted crystals of methyl-dihydro-testosterone in pregnant *G. affinis*. Young born on the fourth day after treatment showed no effects, while those born on the fifth day were characterized by body curvature and "longer than normal" anal fins. Offspring due for later birth were not parturated and perished in the female's body. Examination of the unborn embryos revealed conspicuous body curvature, and increased segmentation with elongation of anal fin rays and noticeable thickening of the third anal ray by the tenth day after implantation.

Another parental fish whose embryos had not attained the developmental stage prior to parturition did not manifest the same embryonic relationship(s) between development and sensitivity to the implanted steroid.

## ECOLOGICAL SIGNIFICANCE OF POLLUTION INDUCED SEX ALTERATION

From our collecting experience, the Fenholloway River represents a worst-case scenario, with poeciliid fishes virtually the only species present during times of drought and intensely stained concentrated KME. In a geographic region with moderately high aquatic species biodiversity (Swift et al., 1986), the Fenholloway River is distinctly impoverished in fish species downstream from the KME entry point. Downstream, each entering tributary stream, spring or peripheral pool is rich in fish species, and the female poeciliids in these adjacent habitats show no indication of masculinized anal fin. In the confluences of spring fed tributaries, where startling plumes of clear water curl into the dark KME stain, fish collected represent mixtures of masculinized and unaffected poeciliid fish. Collections from a few meters up these tributary spring "runs" never included masculinized females.

Similar cases of local restriction of masculinized female fish to the KME per se, have also been observed in small tributaries along Elevenmile Creek. Although territorial behavior has been suggested, this phenomenon has been observed immediately after receded floods, when it would be assumed that fishes and specific territorial stations should be "scrambled" or transported or modified. Perhaps there is suggestion here of an "attractive nuisance" phenomenon involved with the androgenic factor. Gordon et al. (1978) report attraction of salmonids to KME stained waters, but with the implication of "cover" rather than biochemical. Observation of this curious phenomenon would not be possible, were it not for the distinctive tag provided by masculinized anal fin of female poeciliids.

The combination of various studies and our observations of the "highly" masculinized females from KME effluents, lead us to strongly suspect that reproductive function becomes impaired, if not entirely lost, after continued KME exposure. As already noted, few highly masculinized females occurred in field samples; such fish are essential to make the needed observations and assessments. Studies which have addressed the question of response to continuing KME exposure (Sandstrom et al., 1988; Munkittrick et al., 1991) have not discerned androgenic effects, but have noted male gonadal recrudescence and abnormal or atricial oocytes in females. We suspect that the long term effects of KME androgens would include reduced embryo viability and modification or, perhaps, neutering of female reproductive function.

Until another method of detection is developed, other than measurements of body proportions, one is faced with the tautology that masculinization response is morphological change per se. Poeciliids, due to their small size, are difficult subjects to obtain sufficient blood or plasma samples for most currently used biochemical analytical techniques. Yet, due to their ecological habits, these fishes have numerous advantages as both environmental sentinels and laboratory research subjects. One can only speculate that it may be possible that in response to continued androgen exposure, or perhaps as a function of ontogenetic development, affected fish proceed through a complete series of intersexual steps, eventually becoming hermaphroditic; then, if they should survive, they may become functionally male. The complex biochemical environment of KME exposure may continue to confound attempts to predict the ultimate fate of exposed fishes. For example, Asahina et al., (1989) report experimental evidence that different androgenic compounds produce different levels or degrees of morphological response in medaka fish, and the responses differ between medaka and a goby species.

Certain poeciliid species express latent maturing males, possibly as a genetic or adaptive trait, (Travis et al., 1989; Trexler and Travis, 1990a,b) so that time-series observations and samples must be carefully made. If the polygenic sex determination theory is correct, there could exist multiple, genetically based, and variable responses to exposure to endogenically active substances.

Masculinization of poeciliid fish has been treated mostly as a scientific curiosity or research specialization. Potential importance as bioindication of endogenic effects of exposure to xenobiotic substances has received scant attention. It was pointed out during this conference that the poeciliid fish observations represent a unique case of masculinization of vertebrate species populations in the field. Generally, it is believed that androgenic steroids are aromatized to induce estrogenic effects (Wester et al., 1986). Few studies elucidate the potentially disruptive effects of hormones or endocrine mimicking substances upon natural vertebrate populations in the field. Among invertebrates, e.g. the snail American oyster drill (*Urospinax cinerea*), there are data indicating decline in populations where females were masculinized (termed imposex) by environmental exposures to tributyltin (Gibbs et al., 1991).

Poeciliids, especially with the world-wide distribution of *Gambusia affinis* (Krumholtz, 1948), offer an important opportunity as aquatic indicator species, a sentinel to alert attention to potential effects upon other vertebrate species in the same environments.

We submit that the early maturation of the American eel (Caruso et al., 1988) represents a model of ontogenetic dysfunction by developmental acceleration or premature maturation (i.e., normal timing or sequence of life history stages is irreversibly disrupted). Normally, male eels mature just prior to migration to open sea. It is highly improbable that presumably juvenile eels with precocious testicular development could successfully complete the migration to the Sargasso Sea to spawn (Facey and Helfman, 1985; Helfman et al., 1987).

Although no surveys have been reported, arrhenoid poeciliids have not been reported or recognized widely over the warmer latitudes. The unique commonality of Elevenmile Creek and Fenholloway River include industrial use of virtually the entire flow (25 and 50 mgd respectively) for KME discharge. Discovery and observation of the masculinization phenomenon was facilitated by easy access to the effluent. Most pulp mills discharge to larger waterways. This practice dilutes and potentially obscures effects described herein. Larger bodies of water will potentially have different ecological circumstances influencing microbial exposures and pathways to potentially sensitive species. Such features may be crucial in the production and availability of KME androgen precursors. It is essential to illuminate these processes and increase understanding in order to evaluate and choose potential strategies for mitigation.

## SUMMARY

Masculinization, or arrhenoidy, has been reported among livebearing poeciliid fishes living in streams receiving effluent from kraft pulp mills. The principal characteristic indicating adrogenic effects of the effluent is elongation of the female anal fin into a gonopodium, which serves to transfer and insert sperm from functional male poeciliid fish. Apparent duplication of the environmentally masculinized females may be accomplished in the laboratory after exposure to various steroids. Specific phytosteroids, microbially transformed, simulate the morphological and behavioral effects observed in fishes captured from kraft mill effluent. However, specific substances in effluents remain unidentified.

Masculinization of poeciliid females appears to be permanent, the degree of response graded to concentration and/or duration and, therefore, may affect a number of life history elements that influence longevity and fitness. Exposure during early stages of the life history appears to produce the most severe responses, potentially including hermaphroditism.

The apparent graded masculinization response to presence or concentration of the androgenic factor presents a potential assessment technique to monitor effectiveness of stream water quality and treatment processes.

## ACKNOWLEDGEMENTS

Field sampling and pool exposures in KME effluent streams was a task with few pleasures, but made possible by the able assistance of a number of co-workers. We especially wish to acknowledge the dedication of Roxanna Hinzman, as well as the frequent assistance from R. A. Davis, M. R. Davis, and M. Wilson. We appreciate the effort of all those unnamed who also have contributed to this investigation.

Contribution No. 772, Environmental Research Laboratory, Gulf Breeze, Florida 32561 U.S.A. The information in this document has been funded wholly by the

U.S. Environmental Protection Agency, and has been subjected to the Agency's peer and administrative review. Mention of commercial products or trade names does not constitute the Agency's endorsement or recommendation for use.

## REFERENCES

Ahokas, J.T., Karta, N.T., Oikari, A., and Soivio, A. (1976). Mixed function monooxygenase of fish as an indicator of pollution of aquatic environment by industrial effluent. *Bull. Environ. Contam. Toxicol.*, **16**(3), 270-274.

Angus, R.A. (1989). A genetic overview of poeciliid fishes. In *Ecology and Evolution of Livebearing Fishes*, ed. G.K. Meffe and F.F. Snelson, Jr. Prentice Hall, Englewood Cliffs, New Jersey, pp. 51-68.

Asahina, K.A., Urabe, T., Sakai, T., Hirose, H., and Hibiya, T. (1989). Effects of various androgens on the formation processes on the anal fin rays in the female medaka *Oryzias latipes*. *Nippon Suisan Gakkaisi,* **55**(10), 1871.

Bortone, S.A. and Drysdale, D.T. (1981). Additional evidence for environmentally induced intersexuality in poeciliid fishes. *Bull. Assoc. Southeast Biol.*, **28**, 67.

Bortone, S.A., Davis, W.P., and Bundrick, C.M. (1989). Morphological and behavioral characters in mosquitofish as potential bioindication of exposure to kraft mill effluent. *Bull. Environ. Contam. Toxicol.*, **43**, 370-377.

Caruso, J.H., Suttkus, R.D., and Gunning, G.E. (1988). Abnormal expression of secondary sex characters in a population of *Anguilla rostrata* (Pisces: Anguillidae) from a dark colored Florida stream. *Copeia*, **4**, 1077-1079.

Casey, J.P. (1980). *Pulp and Paper, Chemistry and Chemical Technology, Third Edition, Volume 1*, ed. J.P. Casey. John Wiley and Sons, New York, 820 pp.

Conner, A.H., Nagaoka, M., Rowe, J.W., and Perlman, D. (1978). Microbial conversion of tall oil sterols to C-19 steroids. *Applied and Environ. Microbiol.*, **32**(2), 310-311.

Davis, W.P. (1989). Review of the androgenic effects on poeciliid and other fishes living in streams receiving kraft mill effluents. *EPA/600/X-89/184.*

Denton, T.E., Howell, W.M., Allison, J.J., McCollum, J., and Marks, B. (1985). Masculinization of female mosquitofish by exposure to plant sterols and *Mycobacterium smegmatis*. *Bull. Environ. Contam. Toxicol.*, **35**, 627-632.

Drysdale, D.T. (1981). Histological examination of intersexual mosquitofish, *Gambusia affinis* (Pices: Poeciliidae). *Bull. Assoc. Southeast. Biol.*, **28**, 67.

Drysdale, D.T. (1984). Intersexuality in the mosquitofish, *Gambusia affinis*. Unpubl. MS thesis, University of West Florida, Pensacola, Florida, pp. 55.

Drysdale, D.T. and Bortone, S.A. (1989). Laboratory induction of intersexuality in the mosquitofish, *Gambusia affinis,* using paper mill effluent. *Bull. Environ. Contam. Toxicol.*, **43**, 611-617.

Facey, D.E. and Helfman, G.S. (1985). Reproductive migrations of American eels. *Proc. Ann. Conf. SEAFWA*, pp. 132-138.

Farr, J.A. and Travis, J. (1989). The effect of ontogenic experience on variation in growth, maturation, and sexual behavior in the sailfin molly, *Poecilia latipinna*, (Pisces: Poeciliidae). *Environ. Biol. Fishes*, **26**, 39-49.

Gibbs, P.E., Spencer, B.E., and Pascoe, P.L. (1991). The American oyster drill, *Urosalpinx cinerea* (Gastropoda): evidence of decline in an imposex-affected population (R. Blackwater. Essex). *J. Mar. Biol. Ass. U.K.*, **71**, 827-838.

Gordon, M.R. and McLeay, D.J. (1978). Avoidance reactions of salmonids to pulp mill effluents. *CPAR Rep. 688 Environ. Prot. Serv.*, Ottawa, Ontario, Canada.

Helfman, G.S., Facey, D.E., Hales, Jr., L.S., and Bozeman, E.L. (1987). Reproductive ecology of the American eel. *Am. Fish. Soc. Symp.*, **1**, 42-56.

Howell, W.M., Black, D.A., and Bortone, S.A. (1980). Abnormal expression of secondary sex characters in a population of mosquitofish, *Gambusia affinis holbrooki*: evidence for environmentally induced masculinization. *Copeia*, **4**, 676-681.

Howell, W.M. and Denton, T.E. (1989). Gonopodial morphogenesis in female mosquitofish, *Gambusia affinis affinis* masculinized by exposure to degradation products from plant sterols. *Environ. Biol. Fish.*, **24**, 43-51.

Hunsinger, R.N., Byram, B.R., and Howell, W.M. (1988). Unchanged gonadal morphology of mosquitofish masculinized by exposure to degraded plant sterols. *J. Fish. Res. Board Can.*, **32**, 795-796.

Hunsinger, R.H. and Howell, W.M. (1991). Treatment of fish with hormones: solubilization and direct administration of steroids into aquaria water using acetone as a carrier solvent. *Bull. Environ. Contam. Toxicol.*, **47**, 272-277.

Kallman, K.D. (1984). A new look at sex determination in poeciliid fishes. In *Evolutionary Genetics of Fishes*, ed. B.J. Turner. Plenum Publ. Co., New York, pp. 95-171.

Kosswig, C. (1964). Polygenic sex determination. *Experientia*, **20**, 190-199.

Krumholz, L.A. (1948). Reproduction in the western mosquitofish, *Gambusia affinis affinis* (Baird and Girard), and its use in mosquito control. *Ecol. Monogr.*, **18**(1), 1-43.

Larkin, M.J. (1986). The effects of induced masculinization on reproductive and aggressive behaviors of female mosquitofish, *Gambusia affinis affinis*: evidence for environmentally induced masculinization. Unpubl. MS thesis, Samford University, Birmingham, Alabama.

Lehtinen, K.J., Kierkegaard, A., Jakobsson, E., and Wandell, A. (1990). Physiological effects in fish exposed to effluents from mills with six different bleaching processes. *Ecotoxicol. Environ. Safety*, **19**, 33-46.

McLeay, D.J. and Brown, D.A. (1974). Growth stimulation and biochemical changes in juvenile coho salmon (*Oncorhynchus kisutch*) exposed to bleached kraft mill effluent for 200 days. *J. Fish. Res. Bd. Can.*, **31**, 1043-1049.

McLeay, D.J., Walden, C.C., and Munro, J.R. (1979). Influence of dilution water on the toxicity of kraft pulp mill effluent, including mechanisms of effect. *Water Res.*, **13**, 151.

McLeay, D.J. and Brown, D.A. (1979). Stress and chronic effects of treated and untreated bleached kraft mill effluent on the biochemistry and stamina of juvenile coho salmon (*Oncorhynchus kisutch*). *J. Fish. Res. Bd. Can.*, **36**(9), 1049-1059.

McLeay, D.J. and Associates Ltd. (1987). Aquatic toxicology of pulp and paper mill effluent: a review. *Rep. EPS* 4/PF/1, Environment Canada, Ottawa, Canada, 191 pp.

Munkittrick, K.R., Portt, C., Van Der Kraak, G.C., Smith, I., and Rokosh, D.A. (1991). Impact of bleached kraft mill effluent on population characteristics, liver MFO activity and serum steroid levels of a Lake Superior white sucker (*Catastomus commersoni*) population. *Can. J. Fish. Aquat. Sci.*, **48**, 1-10.

Myllyvirta, T. and Vuorinen, P.J. (1989). Effects of bleached kraft mill effluent (BKME) on the schooling behavior of vendace (*Coregonus albula* L.). *Bull. Environ. Contam. Toxicol.*, **42**, 262-269.

Oikari, A., Lonn, B.E., Castren, M., Nakari, T., Snickars-Nikinmaa, B., Bister, H., and Virtanen, E. (1983). Toxicological effects of dehydroabietic acid (DHAA) on the trout, *Salmo gairdneri* Richardson, in fresh water. *Water Res.*, **17**, 81-89.

Oikari, A., Anas, E., Kruzynsky, G., and Holmbom, B. (1984). Free and conjugated resin acids in the bile of rainbow trout, *Salmo gairdneri*. *Bull. Environ. Contam. Toxicol.*, **33**, 233-240.

Oikari, A., Holbom, B., Anas, E., Miilunpalo, M., Kruzynski G., and Castren, M. (1985). Ecotoxicological aspects of pulp and paper mill effluents discharged to an inland water system: distribution in water, and toxicant residues and physiological effects in caged fish (*Salmo gairdneri*). *Aquatic Toxicol.*, **6**, 219-239.

Oikari, A., Lindstrom-Seppa, P., and Kukkonen, J. (1988). Subchronic metabolic effects and toxicity of a simulated pulp mill effluent on juvenile lake trout, *Salmo trutta* m. *lacustris. Ecotoxicol. Environ. Safety*, **16**, 202-218.

Oikari, A.O.J. and Nakari, T. (1982). Kraft pulp mill effluent components cause liver dysfunction in trout. *Bull. Environ. Contam. Toxicol.*, **28**, 266-270.

Okada, Y.K. and Yamashita, H. (1944). Experimental investigation of the sexual characters of poeciliid fish. *J. Fac. Sci. Imp. Univ. Tokyo Instit. Zool.*, **6**, 589-633.

Owens, J.W. (1991). The hazard assessment of pulp and paper effluents in the aquatic environment: a review. *Environ. Toxicol. Chem.*, **10**, 1511-1540.

Reinboth, R. (1980). Can sex inversion be environmentally induced? *Biol. Reprod.*, **22**, 49-59.

Reinboth, R. (1988). Physiological problems of teleost ambisexuality. *Environ. Biol. Fishes*, **22**(4), 249-259.

Riehl, R. (1991). Masculinization in a hermaphroditic female of the mosquitofish *Heterandria formosa. Japan J. Ichthyol.*, **37**(4), 374-379.

Roald, S.O. (1977). Effects of sublethal concentrations of lignosulfates on growth, intestinal flora and some digestive enzymes of rainbow trout. *Aquaculture*, **12**, 327.

Rosa-Molinar, E. and Williams, C.S. (1984). Notes on fecundity of an arrhenoid population of mosquitofish, *Gambusia affinis holbrooki. Northeast. Gulf Science*, **7**(1), 121-125.

Rasotto, M.B. and Zulian, E. (1989). Abnormal hermaphroditism in *Gambusia affinis holbrooki* from a thermal spring of north-eastern Italy. *J. Fish Biol.*, **35**, 593-595.

Sandstrom, O., Neuman, E., and Karas, P. (1988). Effects of a bleached pulp mill effluent on growth and gonad function in Baltic coastal fish. *Wat. Sci. Tech.*, **20**(2), 119-129.

Swift, C.C., Gilbert, C.R., Bortone, S.A., Burgess, G.H., and Yerger, R.W. (1986). Zoogeography of the freshwater fishes of the southeastern United States: Savannah River to Lake Pontchartrain. In *The Zoogeography of North American Freshwater Fishes,* ed. C.H. Hocutt and E.O. Wiley. John Wiley and Sons Inc., New York, pp. 213-265.

Travis, J., Farr, J.A., McManus, M., and Trexler, J. (1989). Environmental effects on adult growth patterns in the male sailfin molly, *Poecilia latipinna* (Poeciliidae). *Environ. Biol. Fishes*, **26**, 119-127.

Trexler, J. and Travis, J. (1990a). Phenotypic plasticity in the sailfin molly, *Poecilia latipinna* (Pisces: Poeciliidae) I. Field experiments. *Evol.*, **44**(1), 143-156.

Trexler, J. and Travis, J. (1990b). Phenotypic plasticity in the sailfin molly, *Poecilia latipinna* (Pisces: Poeciliidae) II. Laboratory experiment. *Evol.*, **44**(1), 157-167.

Turner, B. J. and Steeves III, H. R. (1989). Induction of spermatogenesis in an all-female fish species by treatment with an exogenous androgen. In *Evolution and Ecology of Unisexual Vertebrates,* ed. R.M. Dawley and J.P. Bogart. New York State Mus. Bull. 466, pp. 113-122.

Turner, C.L. (1941a). Gonopodial characteristics produced in the anal fins of females of *Gambusia affinis affinis* by treatment with ethynyl testosterone. *Biol. Bull.*, **80**, 371-383.

Turner, C.L. (1941b). Morphogenesis of the gonopodium in *Gambusia affinis affinis. J. Morphol.*, **69**(1), 161-185.

Turner, C.L. (1942a). A quantitative study of the effects of different concentrations of ethynyl testosterone and methyl testosterone in the production of gonopodia in females of *Gambusia affinis. Phys. Zool.*, **15**, 263-280.

Turner, C.L. (1942b). Morphogenesis of the gonopodia suspensorium in *Gambusia affinis* and the induction of male suspensorial characters in the female by androgenic hormones. *J. Exp. Zool.*, **91**, 167-193.

Turner, C.L. (1960). The effects of steroid hormones on the development of some secondary sexual characters in cyprinodont fishes. *Trans. Amer. Microscop. Soc.*, **79**, 320-333.

Wester, P.W., Canton, J.H., and Bisschop, A. (1985). Histopathological study of *Poecilia reticulata* after long-term B-hexachlorocyclohexane exposure. *Aquat. Toxicol.*, **6**, 271-296.

Winge, O. (1934). The experimental alteration of sex chromosomes into autosomes and vice versa, as illustrated by *Lebistes. C. R. Trav. Lab. Carlsberg Ser. Physiol.*, **21**, 1-49.

# ENDOCRINE AND REPRODUCTIVE FUNCTION IN GREAT LAKES SALMON

**John F. Leatherland**
Institute of Ichthyology, Department of Zoology, University of Guelph
Guelph, Ontario, Canada

*Since the early 1970s, epizootics of disease in fish, particularly epizootics of tumors, have been used as indicators of the "health" of the ecosystems in the Great Lakes. The justification for such an approach was based on contemporary evidence that demonstrates a chemical etiology for most known animal tumors. Consequently, clustering of neoplastic lesions in populations of fish in a particular locale might provide a means of identifying "hot spot" sources of waterborne carcinogens. Such an approach has advantages over reliance on chemical screening, since it does not require* a priori *knowledge of the chemistry of the biologically active factor(s).*

*Pacific salmon (genus* Oncorhynchus*) have been introduced into the Great Lakes since the early 1960s. These salmon have been studied with regard to their value as "sentinel" organisms. This paper reviews the data available in which these species have been used in the exploration of the presence of environmental factors that adversely affect endocrine (specifically thyroid) function, reproductive success or developmental processes.*

*All Great Lakes salmon suffer an epizootic of thyroid hyperplasia that appears to have an environmental etiology other than that of iodide deficiency. Indirect evidence is indicative of the presence of goitrogens in the Great Lakes. In order to determine whether such goitrogens are accumulated in the adult salmon, Great Lakes salmon diets were fed to fish (coho salmon and rainbow trout) and rodents (rats and mice). The recipient fish did not develop thyroid lesions, suggesting that the putative factor(s) effecting thyroid enlargement in the wild salmon is not bioaccumulated in their body tissues. However, the salmon-fed rodents did exhibit thyroid lesions, which may be associated with the halogenated aromatic hydrocarbon mix that was present in the Great Lakes salmon.*

*Some of the Pacific salmon stocks in the Great Lake exhibit a variety of reproductive problems. The paper reviews what is known of these conditions, and discusses the evidence for and against an environmental etiology.*

1. Corresponding Author: John Leatherland, Institute of Ichthyology, Department of Zoology, University of Guelph, Guelph, Ontario N1G 2W1, Canada.

# INTRODUCTION

*Great Lakes Salmon*

The Great Lakes ecosystems are intensely managed systems that contain a diverse array of intentionally or accidentally introduced aquatic species. Many of the dominant native fishes extant at the turn of the century have either disappeared entirely (e.g., Atlantic salmon, *Salmo salar* in Lake Ontario), or are greatly reduced in biomass (e.g., lake whitefish, *Coregonus clupeaformis* and lake charr (trout) *Salvelinus namaycush*). A prime example of the great altering of the Great Lakes systems is the composition of the salmonid populations or stocks in the various lakes.

The salmon species that presently form a significant component of the salmonid fish communities in the Great Lakes are Pacific Ocean salmon (*Oncorhynchus*), species that were introduced into the lakes from Oregon and British Columbia populations periodically since the late nineteenth century. Several thousand coho salmon (*Oncorhynchus kisutch*) fry were introduced into Lake Erie and its tributary rivers by Great Lakes States and Provinces between 1873 and 1878, and again in 1933, but there were no reports of survivors, and the program was considered a failure (Scott and Crossman, 1973). It was not until the 1960s that further plantings of Pacific salmon were attempted as part of the Great Lakes restoration program. Sockeye salmon, and their landlocked form, kokanee salmon (*Oncorhynchus nerka*), pink salmon (*Oncorhynchus gorbuscha*), chinook salmon (*Oncorhynchus tshawytscha*) and coho salmon have all been introduced into different lakes at various times.

Some of these species (e.g., pink salmon) were introduced in one lake, spread to all of the Great Lakes and became self-reproducing, whereas others (e.g., sockeye salmon), failed to gain a substantial foothold in the Great Lakes. From a management perspective, the annual stocking programs for coho and chinook salmon have been successful in the sense that they provide the basis of a 2.5 billion dollar sportsfishing industry in the Great Lakes region. However, from an ecological perspective, the deliberate introduction, on a massive scale, of exotic species into the largest body of freshwater in the world has to be viewed with some concern. The coho and chinook programs were designed so that natural spawning activity was discouraged since the species would compete for spawning areas in streams used by other commercially important salmonid species; to minimize competition for spawning areas the post-smolts were usually released into rivers that had physical barriers to prevent the returning adults migrating away from the lakes, or in rivers in which hatcheries were built to ensure that all potomadromous sexually mature adults could be prevented from moving upstream. Gametes were taken from the returning adults each year, and the fish were raised through the parr stage and allowed to undergo smoltification in the hatchery. Smolts were introduced into the "natal" river annually, either in the fall or spring, from where they migrated into the lake to feed, grow and become sexually mature. The new generation of sexually mature adults returned to their "natal" rivers and were harvested for gamete collection and the to complete the cycle.

These programs are still based on this principle of annual release of smolts, although in most lakes, some individuals have established spawning runs in other than the "natal" streams, and have established themselves, sometimes at the cost of other desired species (e.g., brown trout, *Salmo trutta*) that use the same streams and rivers for spawning.

*Great Lakes Salmon as "Sentinel" Systems*
Although the oncorhynchid salmon species are not native to the Great Lakes, some species have certain biological characteristics that lend themselves to biomonitoring of environmental toxicants. This concept of using aquatic organisms as "sentinel" systems has been proposed on several occasions (Sonstegard, 1976; Sonstegard and Leatherland, 1979, 1984). The Pacific salmon are predatory fish that roam through large areas of a particular lake during the lacustrine period of their life history, and large numbers return to their "natal" river as sexually mature animals of known age, at a predictable time of the year. They feed on lake invertebrates and vertebrates of appropriate size, and in their final year (coho salmon) or two years (chinook salmon) of their life cycle, they are predominantly piscivorous, and one of the top predators in the aquatic food web. This position on the food chain ensures that they are exposed to a wide range of existing xenobiotics, many of which are "biomagnified" up the food chain. Thus, the total tissue burden of xenobiotics in Great Lakes Pacific salmon represents a relative measure of the presence of these compounds in a particular lake ecosystem. For example, inter-lake comparisons of the levels of the xenobiotics that are accumulated by Great Lakes salmon provide a measure of the relative contamination among the lake ecosystems, and annual measurement of the xenobiotic burdens have been used as a measure of the temporal changes in toxicant levels within the Great Lakes.

Because of the "biomagnification" characteristics of food chains, identification of potentially toxic agents is more likely to occur by analysis of tissue burdens of xenobiotics, than by analysis of lake water samples. An example of this biomagnification is the comparison of the levels of polychlorinated biphenyls (PCBs) in Lake Ontario coho salmon and Lake Ontario water based on levels found in the 1970s. Two to three hundred grams of salmon (the equivalent of a single meal) would have contained the same amount of PCB as several million liters of lake water.

In addition to their value as biomonitors of toxicant levels in the food chain, salmon (and fish generally) are ideal subjects for the biomonitoring of waterborne environmental toxicants. Unlike terrestrial vertebrates that are exposed to water-borne contaminants via drinking water (or via the skin in the case of aquatic amphibians), fish are exposed to the aquatic environment for their entire lives, including the early sensitive stages of ontogeny, and their blood is brought into close contact with the ambient medium across the large surface area of the gill epithelium, thus providing the opportunity for diffusion into the blood of low molecular weight toxicants. As these compounds are removed from the circulation and accumulated in tissue, a diffusion gradient between the environment and the tissue is maintained.

Studies of the comparative physiology of salmon taken from different Great Lakes have also been used as a means of assessing the toxicological effects of contaminants on aspects of growth, energy partitioning, reproduction, ionoregulation, and early ontogeny. In addition, by feeding salmon to laboratory animals (fish or rodents), it has been possible to assess the toxicity of the accumulated xenobiotic mixtures as they are transferred along the food chain, and thus, to explore the hazards to human health of consuming Great Lakes salmon.

Although the salmon are valuable marker organisms for this type of study, there are factors that have to be taken into consideration when analysing the information gained. Firstly, there are differences in the origin of the various stocks of salmon in the Great Lakes. The resulting genetic differences, which can be significant, may explain some of the physiological differences that are found. To some extent, this is alleviated by the fact that similar genetic stocks were introduced into several lakes (e.g., coho salmon of a similar stock are to be found in Lakes Michigan, Ontario, Superior and Erie). Further, in Lake Ontario, there are two distinct genetic stocks originating from Oregon (via Lake Michigan) and British Columbia stocks, respectively. Secondly, each of the Great Lakes is a unique ecosystem (and very different from that of the Pacific Northwest), with respect to latitude, water temperature and depth, forage base, and biomass. Any or all of these parameters can have pronounced epigenetic effects on the biology and life history of fish. Thirdly, the xenobiotic mixture in salmon in different lakes is lake-specific, and the toxicity is not related in a simple manner to total xenobiotic burdens. Consequently, although these salmon "sentinel" systems have considerable value, particularly in the early identification of a concern, there is no valid "control" group, and the results of studies have to be evaluated with care, and interpreted conservatively.

An additional concern, and one that was justifiably emphasized by one of the reviewers of this paper, is that a distinction is made between relationals that "parallel" one another, and those that have a bona fide "cause-effect" relationship. This fact warrants emphasis. The following review of endocrine and reproductive indicators in Great Lakes salmon must be read with the caveat that, with few exceptions, studies of the type described here do not offer direct evidence of cause-effect relationships, and postulations of such links are speculative.

*Sensitive Versus Insensitive Species as Indicator Species*
Our first interest in the Great Lakes salmon was initiated by the descriptions of epizootics of thyroid lesions (see below for references). Not all species of Great Lakes teleost fish, nor even all species of Great Lakes salmonid fish exhibit

thyroid lesions. Thus, if, as we believe, such lesions have an environmental etiology, it is reasonable to conclude that the exotic salmon species are more sensitive to the putative toxicant than the native species. Similarly, not all stocks of teleost fish in the Great Lakes, native or exotic, suffer the kind of reproductive problems that characterize lake charr and some salmon stocks (see below). In fact, some exotic stocks of salmon have been remarkably successful in establishing themselves as self-reproducing populations (e.g., Lake Michigan coho salmon), although this was not the intent of the supposedly controlled introduction of these species into the lakes. Since this is the case, it begs the question as to whether we should rely on observations of "sensitive" species, that can often indicate cause for concern, or of the majority of species that are apparently less sensitive. The latter would suggest that the concerns are over-rated.

Historically, biological markers or "sentinel" species were chosen because of their sensitivity to a specific situation. The miner's canary is an example. Given the somewhat primitive levels of understanding of the physiological processes in teleosts, and the incomplete knowledge of the sites of possible intervention of xenobiotics in these processes, it is reasonable to take the responses of the sensitive species as indicators of potential problems.

For the most part, the responses that we monitored are gross pathological events, such as lesions or major decreases in reproductive success. Our ability to monitor subtle changes in the health of fish species in the wild (or even of captive domesticated species) is limited, and we cannot assume that the absence of overt pathological signs in certain species or stocks represents an "all clear" signal for a given ecosystem, particularly when apparently unaffected species share the same lake systems as affected fish.

When taken in isolation, one might wish to dismiss the evidence of endocrine and reproductive problems of wild Great Lakes fish, particularly of the exotic species, as an aberration. However, the similarities and parallels that are found between the sensitive fish species and other forms of wildlife, such as the fish-eating birds and mammals in the Great Lakes region, provide strong (albeit indirect) evidence of a common and omnipresent etiology. If one adds to that the remarkable parallels between endocrine and reproductive problems of wildlife and human populations in the region (see other papers in this issue, and below), one has little choice but to take the evidence into consideration.

## ENDOCRINE AND REPRODUCTIVE DYSFUNCTION IN GREAT LAKES SALMON

Epizootics of thyroid hyperplasia and hypertrophy (affecting 100% of the population) have been reported in pink, coho and chinook salmon taken from every one of the Great Lakes. Drongowski et al. (1975) indicated lower fertility of Great Lakes salmon compared with Pacific Northwest populations. Some stocks of Great Lakes coho salmon have extremely low fertility and high prevalence of embryo mortality associated with low plasma steroid hormone levels. These dysfunctional conditions form the basis of this section of the paper.

*Thyroid Hyperplasia and Hypertrophy (Goitres or Tumours)*
Reports of thyroid enlargement of salmonid fish held in certain trout farms in the Great Lakes region were published in the early part of this century by Marine and Lehnhart and Gaylord and Marsh (see Leatherland et al., 1992 for review of the literature). Subsequent reports of thyroid enlargement in Great Lakes salmonids appeared in the literature from the early 1950s by Robertson and Chaney (1952) on Lake Michigan steelhead trout (*Oncorhynchus mykiss*), Black and Simpson (1974) on Lake Erie coho salmon, and Drongowski et al. (1975) on steelhead trout and coho salmon in Lake Michigan. In all three papers, the authors proposed that the thyroid lesions represented endemic iodide-deficiency tumours, a diagnosis that was based on the generally accepted fact that iodide content of water in the Great Lakes region is low.

Subsequent papers from my laboratory and that of my colleague, Dr. R. A. Sonstegard, confirmed the presence of thyroid hyperplasia in coho salmon collected from Lakes Erie, Ontario, Michigan and Superior. We also described the histopathology of the lesions at a light and electron microscope level, related the prevalence and the size of the lesions to the animal's ability to secrete the thyroid hormones, thyroxine ($T_4$) and triiodothyronine ($T_3$), and expanded the studies to include chinook and pink salmon from some of the Great Lakes (Sonstegard and Leatherland, 1976; Moccia et al., 1977, 1978, 1981; Leatherland and Sonstegard, 1980a, 1981a, b, 1984, 1987; Leatherland et al., 1978, 1992; Noltie et al., 1988).

Our studies have shown that from the early 1970s, when we began the series of investigations, up to the present, every sexually mature Great Lakes salmon that we examined had an enlarged thyroid (relative to comparable species at comparable developmental stages, sampled from the Pacific Northwest).

The prevalence of the *grossly visible* thyroid lesions of the Lake Ontario coho salmon stock has tended to decline in the last two decades; in the 1970s, the prevalence was 20-30%, but is currently less than 1%. However, there have been no marked changes in the prevalences of gross thyroid lesions in the Lake Erie stocks in the last 18 years; prevalences of 80-90% in these stocks are considered "normal". The lowered values in the Lake Ontario stock was coincident with the introduction of different genetic stocks of coho salmon by the Ontario Ministry of Natural Resources since the early 1970s. However, despite some changes in gross lesions, it has to be emphasized that, in our experience, the *prevalence of thyroid hyperplasia has been consistently 100%* for the last 18 years, regardless of salmon species, lake of origin, or gender.

Normal thyroid tissue of salmon is in the form of scattered follicles around the ventral aorta in the midline of the lower jaw. In Great Lakes salmon, thyroid tissue is present from the tip of the jaw to the tip of the heart, and extends laterally from the midline to invade the bases of the gill arches. Histological analysis is required to diagnose the thyroid lesions in some salmon, but in many specimens, the lesions are readily evident by gross examination of the base of the gill arches. In these instances, thyroid tissue invades major blood vessels, and the gill arches are eroded as a result of the proliferative process. Estimates of the relative enlargement of the thyroid tissue of Great Lakes salmon compared with the Pacific Ocean stocks are difficult because, unlike the thyroid of tetrapods which have a discrete encapsulated thyroid gland, the thyroid tissue in salmonids is diffuse and thus cannot be dissected and weighed. Using serial sections of lower jaw tissue of Great Lakes and Pacific Ocean stocks, we estimate that the degree of enlargement of thyroid tissue ranges from $1 \times 10^3$, for the smallest histological lesion, to $1 \times 10^{12}$ for the gross lesions.

Samples of thyroid tissue were taken from adult coho salmon during the 1991 spawning migration to assess the thyroid hormone reserve of animals from the two lakes. For this assessment I used immunostaining of the tissue with monoclonal $T_4$ antibody; for reference I examined the thyroid of hatchery reared rainbow trout and pink salmon. As expected, immunostained $T_4$ was located in the thyroid follicle lumina of the references specimens and of the Lake Ontario coho salmon. In the latter the colloid was much-reduced in quantity. There was no evidence of $T_4$ immunostaining in the thyroid tissue of the Lake Erie salmon, even in the small areas of colloid that remained. The results suggest that both stocks have limited reserves of $T_4$, but there is clearly a marked difference in the ability of the stocks in the two lakes to synthesize $T_4$ at this stage in their life cycle (unpublished data).

The overall results of our studies, and those of other researchers over the years, led us to question whether the iodide-deficiency theory could explain the observations of thyroid enlargement of the Great Lakes salmon species. Of particular interest were reports from various laboratories of thyroid lesions in marine species that clearly had access to abundant iodide (see Leatherland et al., 1992, for review), suggesting that iodide deficiency was not the only possible factor. Details of the arguments against an iodide-deficiency condition in Great Lakes salmon have been published previously (Leatherland and Sonstegard, 1984). Briefly, they can be summarized as follows: a. flesh iodide levels of Great Lakes salmon do not support an iodide-deficiency argument, b. the species' position in the food web as top predators ensures an adequate iodide supply that together with the enterohepatic cycling of iodide, meets their low iodide requirement, c. gender differences are not evident, despite the fact that the ovary (which represents 25-30% of body weight) competes with the thyroid for available iodide, and females, therefore, have a substantially higher iodide need than males, d. Great Lakes salmon *can* secrete thyroid hormones, sometimes at extremely high levels, an ability that belies the argument that they have insufficient iodide with which to produce iodotyrosines and iodothyronines.

Seasonal and inter-lake studies strongly suggested an etiology based on an environmental biologically-active agent. Since halogenated aromatic hydrocarbons are present at high levels in the tissues of some Great Lakes salmon stocks, and are known to have "anti-thyroid" effects in mammals (Bastomsky, 1977a, b; McKinney et al., 1985a, b), the major components (polychlorinated biphenyls, PCBs) were suspect etiological factors for the thyroid lesions. However, we were unable to find any indication of thyroid enlargement in either rainbow trout (*Oncorhynchus mykiss*) (Leatherland and Sonstegard, 1979, 1980b) or coho salmon that had been fed PCB-contaminated diets (Leatherland and Sonstegard, 1978). Moreover, in the Great Lakes salmon themselves, there was no evidence of a correlation between tissue organochlorine content and degree of thyroid enlargement. Furthermore, in "fish-to-fish" feeding trials in which Great Lakes salmon were fed to immature hatchery-reared rainbow trout or coho salmon, there was no evidence of thyroid enlargement in the recipient fish in response to the organochlorine burden of the salmon (Leatherland and Sonstegard, 1982).

To date, we have no evidence of a direct link between the organochlorine burden of Great Lakes salmon and the epizootics of thyroid hyperplasia and hypertrophy in these species. In view of the known actions of some of these molecules on the thyroid hormone economy of mammals, this finding is significant. Several possible explanations can be offered. First, the total body burdens, which represent accumulations of the xenobiotics in lipid-rich tissues, may not reflect the blood levels of biologically active toxicants. The accumulation of the xenobiotics by these tissues represents a form of detoxification. Second, there is evidence of selective metabolism of some halogenated aromatic hydrocarbon molecules by salmonid fish; it could be argued that the biologically active congeners are either metabolized or stored, thus reducing their biological impact. Third, there is increasing evidence of biological effects of organochlorine metabolites that are present in the forage base of Great Lakes ecosystems. These metabolites were not measured in the samples taken from wild fish, nor were they a component of the PCB-contaminated diets that we used to evaluate organochlorine effects on salmonid thyroid function. However, if these metabolites are involved in the process, it would appear that they are not bioaccumulated by the Great Lakes salmon, since "fish-to-fish" feeding trials failed to induce thyroid lesions in juvenile coho salmon and rainbow trout that were fed diets containing Great Lakes coho salmon (see below). A fourth possibility centres around the differences in thyroid hormone economy of salmonids and mammals. McKinney et al. (1985a, b, c) propose that thyroid hormone binding proteins are likely candidates as receptors for halogenated aromatic hydrocarbons. Such binding would have profound effects on the overall thyroid hormone economy of the animal, since the serum free/bound ratios of the thyroid hormones would be changed, as would the availability of $T_4$ for the production of $T_3$ by peripheral monodeiodination of $T_4$; as a consequence, there would be major shifts in the overall balance between the hypothalamus, pituitary gland and thyroid gland. Thus, the "anti-thyroid" effects of these compounds in mammals might be linked to perturbations in the normal partitioning of thyroid hormones within the different compartments, and the subsequent changes in the secretory dynamics of the thyroid hormones rather than to direct effects on the thyroid gland per se. These responses to altered availability of binding sites for thyroid hormones would be far more marked in mammals in which the free:bound ratios of $T_4$ and $T_3$ are low, than in salmonid fish in which the thyroid hormone binding is much lower. Consequently, the potential impact of interactions of the xenobiotic halogenated aromatic hydrocarbon molecules with blood proteins may have less significance in fish.

In addition to consideration of possible impact of halogenated compounds, other factors warrant consideration. For example, there is good correlation between the size of the thyroid lesions in coho salmon from the different Great Lakes and the degree of eutrophication of the lake of origin of the salmon (see above for references). The demonstration by Gaitán and co-workers that some products of bacterial metabolism cause goitres in human populations (see Gaitán, 1973; Gaitán et al., 1980 for reviews) led us to consider whether similar factors are etiological agents in the epizootics of thyroid lesions in Great Lakes salmon. If these factors are involved, we must postulate that they are omnipresent but at different concentrations in the different regions of the Great Lakes basin. There is preliminary support for this hypothesis from recent testing of samples of Lake Erie water using a bioassay based on porcine thyroid slices cultured *in vitro* (E. Gaitán, J. F. Leatherland and R. A. Sonstegard, unpublished data); Lake Erie water samples, collected in mid-summer, impaired the synthesis of iodinated organic tyrosine compounds. Clearly, considerably more work is needed to test this hypothesis. Equally clear is the potential importance of such studies to human medicine. Dr. William Beierwaltes' reports in the Washington City Medical Society Bulletin documenting the prevalence of endemic goitre in the U.S.A., and specifically in the State of Michigan, "*that cannot be attributed to iodine deficiency*" emphasizes the potential extent of the problem in the Great Lakes region (Beierwaltes, 1987a, b).

*Disorders of the Reproductive System*
Since the early part of this century, some native salmonid stocks have exhibited low or little reproductive success. The most cited example is the lake charr (trout) which exhibits a high mortality of the early ontogenic stages. In addition, life history studies indicate a low recruitment of adults into the breeding population (E.C./D.F.O./H.W.C., 1991). There is considerable evidence to suggest that the species is extremely sensitive to halogenated aromatic hydrocarbon contaminants, and the studies by Mac and co-workers (see Mac and Schwartz, 1992, for review) provide convincing evidence in support of a xenobiotic etiology for the high mortality of the early ontogenic stages. The problems appear to be related in large part to maternally transferred PCB congeners (Mac and Schwartz, 1992). It is interesting to note that this embryo mortality continues to occur, despite the major reduction in overall levels of halogenated aromatic hydrocarbon contaminants in many species of Great Lakes fish in the last two decades. The lake charr studies clearly indicate that these "lower" levels are still adversely affecting

developmental processes of sensitive species, presumably because of the bioconcentration of maternal xenobiotics in the egg yolk. It is less clear whether the poor recruitment into the breeding population of the survivors is similarly related to the presence of contaminants, or the result of other changes in the lake ecosystems.

Anecdotal accounts of impaired reproductive function of introduced species have also been reported. For example, Drongowski et al. (1975) commented on the lower "fertility" of Lake Michigan salmon eggs relative to the Oregon stocks; the authors correlated this to the hypothyroidism (presumed to be an iodide-deficiency) of the Great Lakes stocks. However, it is not clear whether this general assumption of a lower egg fertility is valid because of the genetic variability between the extant Great Lakes and Pacific Northwest stocks. There is, however, convincing evidence of a marked reproductive problem in the Fairview, Pennsylvania Lake Erie stock of coho salmon. Survival to hatch of this stock between 1980 and 1990 has ranged from a high of 48% (1981) to a low of <5% (1990). The problem appears to reside in the quality of eggs, and is possibly associated with a breakdown in the mechanisms that initiate ovulation, since "over-ripe" eggs are commonly found still attached to the ovarian membranes of these females (Flett et al., 1992). Other factors that are associated with this infertility syndrome of the Lake Erie stock include lower plasma levels of gonadotropin and gonadal steroid hormones of males (testosterone and ll-ketotestosterone) and females (testosterone, $17\alpha$, $20\beta$ dihydro-4-pregnen-3-one) (Leatherland et al., 1982; Morrison et al., 1985a; Flett et al., 1992), low egg thyroid hormone content (Leatherland et al., 1989), high prevalence of embryo deformities (Morrison et al., 1985b), poor expression of secondary sexual characteristics of the males (Leatherland et al., 1982; Morrison et al., 1985a), and high prevalence of precocious sexual maturation of the males (Morrison et al., 1985a).

It is not clear whether the pathological changes reported in these stocks are related to one another, or whether they are independent events. It is possible that the apparently impaired ability of the Pennsylvania stock to secrete gonadal steroid hormones is a factor in the low egg quality, and ovulatory problems of these fish. There is also a marked inverse relationship between fertilization rates of the eggs taken from individual females, and embryo deformity rates (Flett et al., 1992), but whether these factors are specifically related has yet to be determined.

Since egg thyroid hormone levels are derived from maternal hormone sources, it is likely that the lowered egg thyroid hormone content is linked directly to the severe hypothyroidism of the Lake Erie coho salmon stock. However, the low egg hormone content of the Fairview coho salmon stock does not appear to be a factor in the low fertility of this stock. Fertility rates of a self-reproducing Lake Erie coho salmon stock (Fishers Creek stock) were >80%, despite the fact that egg thyroid hormone contents of this stock were also low. It might be argued that the differences in egg $T_3$ content between the Fairview and Fishers Creek stock might account for the lower fertility of the Fairview salmon. However, elevation of egg $T_3$ content by administering the hormone to the pre-ovulatory females, had no effect on fertility (Leatherland and Sonstegard, 1987; Leatherland et al., 1989; Flett et al., 1992).

Gender dimorphism in salmon is a heritable characteristic, and the hatchery management practices used to harvest gametes provides no mechanism for the selection of these characteristics by the usual mate-selection methods. Consequently, in hatchery managed stocks, the expression of the secondary sexual characteristics of the "kype" (growth of the upper and lower jaw permitting the teeth to be exteriorized for fighting conspecifics), and red colouration of the flanks of adult (but not precocious) males (Fleming and Gross, 1989) tends to be diminished. In the Lake Erie Fairview stock, the loss of secondary sexual characteristics can be explained in part by this shift in the gene pool of the stock, but the change is much more marked than other examples of "managed" stocks in the Great Lakes or Pacific Northwest regions. Whether there is an endocrine basis for the loss of gender characteristics remains to be determined, and requires a better understanding of the physiological processes involved in the control of the expression of secondary sexual characteristics by salmon.

The physiological control of precocious sexual maturation of male salmon, "grilse" in Atlantic salmon, and "jacks" in Pacific salmon, is still controversial, and is based on studies of Atlantic salmon. These studies suggest that rapid growth during critical ontogenic stages leads to the physiological "decision" being made so that the fish mature sexually at the time of smoltification (in Atlantic salmon) or one or two years after smoltification, depending on the species (in Pacific salmon) (e.g., Metcalfe et al., 1988). Thus, high prevalences of precocious sexual maturation of male salmon may be a developmental problem resulting from inappropriate hatchery-management. However, this explanation does not fully explain the extremely high prevalences of precocious sexual maturation of the Fairview Lake Erie coho salmon stock (>90% in some years), since hatchery management practices of the Pennsylvania Fisheries Commission are similar to those of comparable agencies in New York State, Michigan and Ontario. Further work is needed in this poorly-understood field before the phenomenon can be adequately explained.

## EFFECTS OF CONSUMPTION OF GREAT LAKES SALMON ON THE ENDOCRINE SYSTEM OF SALMONID FISH OR RODENTS

Although the consumption of Great Lakes coho salmon diets (100% ground fish diets, supplemented with essential fatty acids, vitamins and minerals) by immature salmonid fish resulted in significant increases in the tissue levels of organochlorine compounds, and liver enlargement in the recipient fish, there was no evidence of thyroid hyperplasia or changes in plasma thyroid hormone levels in these fish (Leatherland and Sonstegard, 1982).

In the late 1970s my colleague, Dr. R.A. Sonstegard and I attempted to determine the effects of feeding Great Lakes coho salmon to rodents with a view to evaluating the possible hazards of consumption of Great Lakes salmon by human beings. We were specifically interested in determining if such diets effect changes in thyroid physiology, and if so, whether these changes could be correlated with the organochlorine content of the salmon. In our preliminary experiments we employed 100% salmon diets (supplemented with essential fatty acids, minerals and vitamins), and in the later studies we used a 30% fish diet (+ mineral and vitamin supplements) mixed with rat chow. The rodents were fed the experimental diets for 30 to 180 days. Table 1 summarizes the responses of rats that were fed diets containing Great Lakes salmon (30% by weight) for 80 days. Rats fed the Lake Ontario salmon diet exhibited hepatomegaly as indicated by the increased hepatosomatic index. In addition, all groups that were fed Great Lakes salmon diets had elevated levels of hepatic mixed function oxidase activity. Increases in the activity of these enzyme systems are usually interpreted to indicate an increase in hepatic detoxification activity. In the groups fed Lake Ontario or Lake Michigan salmon there was thyroid enlargement and plasma $T_4$ concentration was lowered; the changes in thyroid function in the different rat treatment groups were correlated with dietary organochlorine content (Sonstegard and Leatherland, 1979; Leatherland and Sonstegard, 1980c; R.A. Sonstegard, S. Safe and J.F. Leatherland, unpublished data). Reduced thyroid capability was also found in mice fed Lake Ontario salmon diets (Cleland et al., 1988). Similar studies by Villeneuve and co-workers were essentially similar to our studies in the demonstration of anti-thyroid effects of Great Lakes salmon consumption by rats (Villeneuve et al., 1981; Chu et al., 1984), and recent studies by Daly and co-workers have shown profound neurobiological effects of such salmon diets on rodents (Daly et al., 1989).

The apparent discrepancies between the results of the "fish-to-fish" and "fish-to-rodent" studies have been discussed earlier in the report. A better interpretation of these findings depends on advances in our understanding of the chemical nature of the toxicants, and of the metabolic pathways of degradation and storage of these toxicants. Equally important is a more comprehensive understanding of the manner in which these compounds exert their biological effects.

The absence of a response in the "fish-to-fish" studies does not necessarily "prove" that there are no toxicants in the Great Lakes fish, but may indicate that the experimental subjects were not fed during critical ontogenic stages, that there is efficient metabolism of such toxicants by the recipient fish, or the effective removal of the toxicants from the blood compartment. Equally, the suspect goitrogen may be readily metabolized and thus not accumulated; this does not preclude the possibility that it has an effective biological action whilst it is present in the circulation.

The results of the "fish-to-rodent" studies appear to be easier to interpret. The degree of the "anti-thyroid" response by rodents to the Great Lakes salmon diets

TABLE 1.    Hepatosomatic index (HSI), and N-demethylase activity (ND), B[a]P hydroxylase activity (BPH), and cytochrome P-450 content (CP) in male rats fed diets of coho salmon from either the Pacific Ocean, or one of Lakes Ontario, Erie or Michigan, or rat chow for 80 days[1]

| Diet/source of salmon | HSI[2] | ND[3] | BPH[4] | CP[5] |
|---|---|---|---|---|
| Rat chow | 3.3±0.2 | 2.5±0.5 | 2.9±0.4 | 4.1±0.7 |
| Pacific Ocean | 3.3±0.2 | 3.3±0.6 | 3.7±0.7 | 4.1±0.2 |
| Lake Ontario | 4.2±0.3* | 5.1±0.2** | 14.1±0.4** | 9.1±0.1** |
| Lake Erie | 3.8±0.1 | 4.4±0.5* | 5.0±0.6* | 5.2±0.3** |
| Lake Michigan | 4.0±0.3 | 6.2±0.4** | 12.5±1.2** | 7.5±0.6** |

[1]Salmon were collected from the 1978 spawning run, and 30% diets were used;
[2]expressed as % body weight;
[3]nmol HCHO formed per mg protein per min;
[4]expressed as nmol B[a]P metabolized per mg protein per 10 min;
[5]expressed as nmol per 10 mg protein. All data are shown as mean±SEM (n=4).
*, ** significantly different (p<0.05 and 0.01, respectively) from the Pacific Ocean salmon-fed group.
[Sonstegard, R.A., Safe, S. and Leatherland, J.F., unpublished data].

appears to be related to the level of organochlorine content of the salmon. Moreover, the thyroid response resembled that seen in PCB-treated rats (Bastomsky, 1977a, b). Thus, it is possible that the organochlorine body burden of the salmon is the etiological factor; however, cause-effect relationships have yet to be established. It may be that the etiological agents are chemicals present in levels that parallel the levels of the halogenated aromatic hydrocarbon compounds, but are chemically unrelated.

## CONCLUSIONS

The epizootic of thyroid hyperplasia in Great Lakes oncorhynchid salmon (prevalence of 100%), that cannot be explained on the basis of an iodide-deficient etiology, provides the most convincing evidence of a biologically active environmental factor affecting the function of the endocrine system in Great Lakes fish. Low lake iodide content *may* be a contributory factor in the thyroid hyperplasia, but there is no convincing experimental or epizootiological evidence to support such an hypothesis. Most evidence points toward the omnipresence of a goitrogen(s) in the Great Lakes. The nature of the putative goitrogen has yet to be determined, but there is currently no experimental evidence of it being bioaccumulated and laterally transferred from fish to fish along a food chain. This may suggest a water-borne factor, but short half-life tissue-associated xenobiotics cannot be excluded as possible agents.

Thyroid enlargement was found in rodents fed Great Lakes salmon diets, thus providing evidence of environmental anti-thyroid substances in the Great Lakes food chain. However, it is not yet clear as to whether the putative goitrogens effecting thyroid enlargement in the salmon is the same as that affecting the thyroid hormone economy of rodents that were fed these salmon.

The status of some native salmonid species in the Great Lakes, such as the lake charr (trout), provides continuing evidence, of developmental problems that are probably related to environmental toxicants. These problems continue to exist despite the decline in level of bioaccumulated xenobiotics in Great Lakes species during the last two decades. These toxicants appear to affect the survival of early ontogenic stages, and the recruitment of adults into the breeding population. This may also be true for some introduced salmon species. There is convincing evidence of a dysfunctional reproductive syndrome in at least one Great Lakes salmon stock, the Fairview Lake Erie stock; the etiology remains to be fully elucidated.

Two other putative reproductive/developmental problems have been identified in some Great Lakes salmon stocks, namely the loss of expression of secondary sexual characteristics (particularly of males), and the high prevalence of precocious sexual maturation of males. However, the physiological basis of precocious sexual maturation is too poorly understood for its significance as an indicator of environmental problems to be established at this time. Similarly, without a fuller understanding of the processes that determine the expression of sexual dimorphism, it is not possible to explain the phenomenon in Great Lakes salmon on the basis of environmental factors; however, the extent of the loss of dimorphism in some stocks does not appear to be explicable on the basis of genetic drift alone.

There is a fundamental need for additional studies of the basic physiological processes of salmonids and other Great Lakes species of teleosts. A rudimentary understanding of the "normal" reproductive and developmental processes of these species is absolutely essential if we propose to use dysfunctional reproductive/developmental states of these species as environmental indicators.

## ACKNOWLEDGEMENTS

I wish to acknowledge with heartfelt thanks the contributions made through the years by my Students, Postdoctoral Fellows and Colleagues. They are, in alphabetical order: Mr. S. Barrett, Dr. G. Cleland, Dr. P. Copeland, Dr. E.M. Donaldson, Dr. N.E. Down, Mr. P.A. Flett, Dr. M.V.H. Holdrinet, Mrs. L.

Lin, Dr. D. Noltie, Mr. R. Moccia, Mr. P.A. Morrison, Dr. K.R. Munkittrick, Dr. R.A. Sonstegard, Dr. J. Sumpter, and Dr. G. Van Der Kraak.

## REFERENCES

Bastomsky, C.H. (1977a). Goiters in rats fed polychlorinated biphenyls. *J. Physiol. Pharmacol.*, **55**, 288-292.

Bastomsky, C.H. (1977b). Enhanced thyroxine metabolism and high uptake goiters in rats after a single does of 2,3,7,8-tetrachlorodibenzo-*p*-dioxin. *Endocrinology*, **101**, 292-296.

Beierwaltes, W.H. (1987a). The most common thyroid disease in the State of Michigan is endemic goiter not due to iodine deficiency. *Washington City Med. Soc. Bull.* September 1987: 3-10.

Beierwaltes, W.H. (1987b). The diagnosis and treatment of endemic goiter, the most common thyroid disease in the United States: a challenge to physicians. *Washington City Med. Soc. Bull.* October 1987: 2-10.

Black, J.J. and Simpson, C.L. (1974). Thyroid enlargement in Lake Erie coho salmon. *J. Natl. Cancer Inst.*, **53**, 725-729.

Chu, I., Villeneuve, D.C., Valli, V.E., Ritter, L., Norstrom, R. J., Ryan, J.J., and Becking, G.C. (1984). Toxicological response and its reversibility in rats fed Lake Ontario or Pacific coho salmon for 13 weeks. *J. Env. Sci. Health*, **B19**,713-731.

Cleland, G., Leatherland, J.F., and Sonstegard, R.A. (1988). Toxic effects in CS7B1/6 and DBA/2 mice following consumption of halogenated aromatic hydrocarbon contaminated Great Lakes coho salmon (*Oncorhynchus kisutch Walbaum*). *Envir. Health Perspect.*, **75**, 153-157.

Daly, H.B., Hertzler, D.R., and Sargent, D.M. (1989). Ingestion of environmentally contaminated Lake Ontario salmon by laboratory rats increases avoidance of unpredictable aversive nonreward and mild electric shock. *Behav. Neurosci.*, **6**, 1356-1365.

Drongowski, R.A., Wood, J.S., and Bouck, G.R. (1975). Thyroid activity in coho salmon from Oregon and Lake Michigan. *Trans. Am. Fish. Soc.*, **2**, 349-352.

E.C./D.F.O./H.W.C. (1991). Toxic chemicals in the Great Lakes and associated effects. Joint Report of Environment Canada, the Department of Fisheries and Oceans and Health and Welfare Canada, Ottawa, Canada.

Fleming, I.A. and Gross, M.R. (1989). Evolution of adult female life history and morphology in a Pacific salmon (coho: *Oncorhynchus kisutch*). *Evolution*, **43**, 141-157.

Flett, P.A., Munkittrick, K.R., Van Der Kraak, G., and Leatherland, J.F. (1992). Reproductive problems in Lake Erie coho salmon. In *Proceedings of the 4th International Symposium on the Reproductive Physiology of Fish*, eds. A.P. Scott, J.P. Sumpter, D.E. Kime, and M.S. Rolfe. Fish Symp 91, Sheffield, pp. 151-153.

Gaitán, E. (1973). Water-borne goitrogens and their role in the etiology of endemic goiter. *World Rev. Nutr. Dietetics*, **17**, 53-90.

Gaitán, E., Medina, P., DeRouen, T.A. and Zia, M.S. (1980). Goitre prevalence and bacterial contamination of water supplies. *J. Clin. Endocrinol. Met.*, **51**, 957-961.

Leatherland, J.F. and Sonstegard, R.A. (1978). Lowering of serum thyroxine and triiodothyronine levels in yearling coho salmon, *Oncorhynchus kisutch*, by dietary Mirex and PCBs. *J. Fish. Res. Bd. Can.*, **35**, 1285-1289.

Leatherland, J.F. and Sonstegard, R.A. (1979). Effects of dietary Mirex and PCB (Aroclor 1254) on thyroid activity and lipid reserves in rainbow trout, *Salmo gairdneri. J. Fish Dis.,* **2**, 43-48.

Leatherland, J.F. and Sonstegard, R.A. (1980a). Seasonal changes in thyroid hyperplasia, serum thyroid hormone and lipid concentrations, and pituitary gland structure in Lake Ontario coho salmon (*Oncorhynchus kisutch*) and a comparison with coho salmon from Lakes Michigan and Erie. *J. Fish Biol.,* **16**, 539-562.

Leatherland, J.F. and Sonstegard, R.A. (1980b). Effect of dietary polychlorinated biphenyls (PCBs) or Mirex in combination with food deprivation and testosterone administration on serum thyroid hormone concentration and bioaccumulation of organochlorines in rainbow trout (*Salmo gairdneri*). *J. Fish Dis.,* **3**, 115-124.

Leatherland, J.F. and Sonstegard, R.A. (1980c). Structure of the thyroid and adrenal glands in rats fed diets of Great Lakes coho salmon. *Envir. Res.,* **23**, 77-86.

Leatherland, J.F. and Sonstegard, R.A. (1981a). Thyroid dysfunction in Great Lakes coho salmon, *Oncorhynchus kisutch* (Walbaum): Seasonal and interlake differences in serum $T_3$ uptake and serum total and free $T_4$ and $T_3$ levels. *J. Fish Dis.,* **4**, 413-423.

Leatherland, J.F. and Sonstegard, R.A. (1981b). Thyroid function, pituitary structure and serum lipids in Great Lakes coho salmon, *Oncorhynchus kisutch* Walbaum, 'jacks' compared with sexually immature spring salmon. *J. Fish Biol.,* **18**, 643-654.

Leatherland, J.F. and Sonstegard, R.A. (1982). Bioaccumulation of organochlorines by yearling coho salmon (*Oncorhynchus kisutch* Walbaum) fed diets containing Great Lakes coho salmon, and the pathophysiological responses of the recipients. *Comp. Biochem. Physiol.,* **72**C, 91-99.

Leatherland, J.F. and Sonstegard, R.A. (1984). Pathobiological responses of feral teleosts to environmental stressors: Interlake studies of the physiology of Great Lakes salmon. In *Contaminant Effects on Fisheries,* eds. V. W. Cairns, P. V. Hodson, and J.O. Nriagu. John Wiley and Sons, Toronto, pp. 115-149.

Leatherland, J.F. and Sonstegard, R.A. (1987). Comparative fecundity and egg survival in two stocks of goitred coho salmon (*Oncorhynchus kisutch* Walbaum) from Lake Erie. *Can. J. Zool.,* **65**, 2780-2785.

Leatherland, J.F., Moccia, R.D., and Sonstegard, R.A. (1978). Ultrastructure of the thyroid gland in goitered coho salmon (*Oncorhynchus kisutch*). *Cancer Res.,* **38**, 149-158.

Leatherland, J.F., Copeland, P., Sumpter, J.P., and Sonstegard, R.A. (1982). Hormonal control of gonadal maturation and development of secondary sexual characteristics in coho salmon, *Oncorhynchus kisutch,* from Lakes Ontario, Erie and Michigan. *Gen. Comp. Endocrinol.,* **48**, 196-204.

Leatherland, J.F., Lin, L., Down, N.E., and Donaldson, E.M. (1989). Thyroid hormone content of eggs and early developmental stages of three stocks of goitred salmon (*Oncorhynchus kisutch*) from the Great Lakes of North America, and a comparison with a stock from British Columbia. *Can. J. Fish. Aquat. Sci.,* **46**, 2146-2152.

Leatherland, J.F., Down, N.E., Falkmer, S., and Sonstegard, R.A. (1992). Endocrine and reproductive system. In *Pathobiology of Spontaneous and Induced Neoplasms in Fishes: Comparative Characterization, Nomenclature and Literature,* (eds.), C. Dawe and J. Harshbarger. Academic Press, New York (in press).

Mac, M.J. and Schwartz, T.R. (1992). Investigations into the effects of PCB congeners on reproduction in lake trout from the Great Lakes. Jackpine Warbler. Special Issue on Cause-Effect Linkages II Symposium. Traverse City Michigan, September 1991 (in press).

# EPIDEMIOLOGICAL AND PATHOBIOLOGICAL EVIDENCE OF CONTAMINANT-INDUCED ALTERATIONS IN SEXUAL DEVELOPMENT IN FREE-LIVING WILDLIFE

**Glen A. Fox**
Wildlife Toxicology Division, Canadian Wildlife Service
National Wildlife Research Centre, Environment Canada, Hull, Quebec, Canada

## INTRODUCTION

We live in a chemically contaminated world and the situation in North America is not an exception. Our coastal ocean waters, the Laurentian Great Lakes and many of our rivers are polluted with a wide variety of toxic chemicals. These marine and freshwater ecosystems are of great biological and ecological significance and support diverse faunas. For example, the Great Lakes represent 20% of our planet's fresh surface water. The rich resources of our marine coastlines and the Great Lakes have attracted large segments of North America's human population and associated industries to their shores.

In three of the many contaminated ecosystems that have been identified in North America - the coast of southern California, Puget Sound, and the Laurentian Great Lakes - various wildlife populations have been the subject of extensive descriptive epidemiological and pathobiological investigations. Several cases of contaminant-related effects on wildlife health have been documented in these areas. In this manuscript I will review three cases related to alterations in sexual development: evidence of feminization and altered sex ratios in fish-eating birds; pseudohermaphroditism in snails; and abnormal reproductive physiology in fish and birds exposed to pulp and paper mill effluents.

## SUPERNORMAL CLUTCHES, FEMALE-FEMALE PAIRING AND HISTOLOGICAL EVIDENCE OF CONTAMINANT-INDUCED ALTERATIONS IN THE SEX RATIO OF FISH-EATING BIRDS

The number of eggs a female bird lays in a clutch and the mating strategy typical of that species have evolved as a result of various ecological pressures. Gulls (Laridae) and terns (Sternidae) are generally long-lived, monogamous species which usually lay 2 or 3 eggs, the number and size of eggs diminishing when food is scarce. Therefore, when over 10% of nests of Western Gulls (*Larus occidentalis*) in colonies on the Channel Islands off the coast of southern California were observed to contain 5 or 6 eggs in the late 1960s and early 1970s (Schreiber, 1970; Harper, 1971; Hunt and Hunt, 1973), biologists recognized that this was an abnormal phenomenon. Further epidemiological investigations and experimentation have shown that these supernormal clutches are the product

1. Corresponding Author: Glen A. Fox, Wildlife Toxicology Division, Canadian Wildlife Service, National Wildlife Research Centre, Environment Canada, Hull, Quebec, K1A 0H3, Canada.

of multiple females engaging in a shared breeding attempt (Hunt and Hunt, 1977). These cooperative female-female pairings and polygynous associations (Shugart and Southern, 1977; Shugart, 1980) in this and other gull species are behavioral responses to a female-biased operational sex ratio, resulting either from range expansion and colonization or high differential male mortality and/or embryonic feminization as a result of local environmental factors (Fox and Boersma, 1983; Fry et al., 1987).

A comprehensive review of data in published and unpublished field studies and museum collections has shown that supernormal clutches are a very rare and recent (post-1950) phenomenon in Western Gulls, the Great Lakes population of Herring Gulls, and Caspian Terns (*Sterna caspia*) nesting in U.S. waters (Conover, 1984). In Western Gulls, there has also been a recent marked skew in the adult sex ratio towards females, and a similar trend exists for Herring Gulls (Conover and Hunt, 1984). The breeding population of Western Gulls on Santa Barbara Island was severely impacted by organochlorine pollutants, particularly DDT, in the decade prior to the period of highest incidence of female-female pairing, and the breeding population of the colony declined from 3000 birds in 1972 to 850 in 1978 (Sowls et al., 1980).

Total DDT (tDDT) as measured in the myctophid fish *Stenbrachius leucopsarus* increased in the ocean off southern California between 1949 and 1970 (MacGregor, 1974). This has been confirmed with dated sediments from the southern California Bight (Hom et al., 1974). Sand crabs (*Emerita analoga*) collected in 1970-1971 near the White's Point outfall of the Los Angeles County sewer system contained over 45 times as much tDDT as crabs collected near major agricultural drainage areas (Burnett, 1971). Sediments near the outfall probably contain over 100 metric tons of tDDT. The major source of this insecticide was the wastes discharged into the Los Angeles County sewer system by the Montrose Chemical Corporation—an estimated 2 million kg of tDDT were released between 1949 and 1970 (MacGregor, 1974). This effluent was rich in o,p'-DDT, the most estrogenic isomer.

Herring Gulls nesting in the Great Lakes, particularly Lakes Ontario and Michigan have had a high incidence of supernormal clutches and female-female pairing (Shugart, 1980; Fox, in prep.). Gulls in these colonies have also suffered from embryonic and chick mortality, edema, growth retardation and deformities (Gilbertson and Fox, 1977; Gilbertson et al., 1991) and altered nest defense and incubation behavior (Fox et al., 1978), resulting in severely reduced reproductive success. These effects were associated with high levels of a number of organochlorine contaminants in the 1960s and early 1970s; reproductive success has increased concomitant with declining contaminant levels in the late 1970s and 1980s (Mineau et al., 1984; Peakall and Fox, 1987).

Although Caspian Terns nesting in the United States have also been heavily contaminated with organochlorines, their reproductive success was not markedly affected in the 1970s (Snedon and Weseloh, in prep.). However, poor reproductive success and evidence of developmental toxicity have been observed in several U.S. colonies in the 1980s (Gilbertson et al., 1991). Long-term studies of marked populations in the Great Lakes suggest that although U.S. colonies are maintaining their size, this is only accomplished by extensive recruitment from less contaminated Canadian colonies, and that the mortality rate is higher for birds originating in U.S. colonies than in Canadian colonies (Ludwig, 1979; L'Arrivee and Blokpoel, 1988). There is a consistent pattern among these species populations; the incidence of supernormal clutches and polygynous associations coincide with organochlorine contamination, both spatially and temporally. In contrast, supernormal clutches and female-female pairing have not been observed in stable breeding colonies of Western and Herring Gulls in less polluted areas.

In Lake Ontario Herring Gulls, supernormal clutches were most prevalent in 1977 (70 per 1000), declining rapidly over the next four years to 10 per 1000. Since Herring Gulls do not breed until they are at least 3 or 4 years of age, the peak incidence occurred during the period in which cohorts hatching in the late 1960s and early 1970s would be expected to be recruiting into the colonies. Gull embryos have been shown to be quite sensitive to the teratogenic effects of estrogenic substances (Boss, 1943; Boss and Witschi, 1947). Organochlorine contaminants such as DDT, methoxychlor, and mirex and/or their metabolites are known to be estrogenic in birds (Fry and Toone, 1981; Eroschenko and Palmiter, 1980) and Peterson et al. (chapter 10) have shown that perinatal exposure of male rats to 2,3,7,8-tetrachlorodibenzo-*p*-dioxin (TCDD) results in marked feminization at the anatomical, physiological and behavioral levels. There is histological and anatomical evidence that *in ovo* concentrations of o,p'-DDT (2 and 5 ppm and higher) and p,p'-DDE (20 and 100 ppm) induce feminization in male gull embryos (Fry and Toone, 1981; Fry et al., 1987). Fry (pers. comm.) also examined 17 formalin-preserved near-term embryos and newly hatched chicks I collected from Lake Ontario colonies in 1975 and 1976. Five (71%) of the seven males were significantly feminized (primordial germ cells present in testes), and in two cases the gonads were visibly abnormal. Five of 9 (56%) females had significant-sized right oviducts and three had enlarged left mesonephros which Fry suggested "could indicate the influence of exogenous estrogenic substances". DDE, mirex and TCDD residues in Herring Gull eggs apparently peaked in Lake Ontario in 1972 (72 ppm DDE, 11.4 ppm mirex, 2347 ppt TCDD) and in or before 1971 in Lake Michigan (90 ppm DDE, 1.2 ppm mirex, 249 ppt TCDD) and declined by 50-75% by 1976. It is therefore probable that many male embryos were feminized during the period of peak contamination in Lakes Ontario and Michigan. If the majority of males in these numerically weak cohorts were feminized and incapable of reproduction, then the operational sex ratio in colonies in these Lakes in the late 1970s would be markedly skewed towards females.

Very few eggs in supernormal clutches of Herring Gulls (Shugart et al., 1988) and Western Gulls (Schreiber, 1970; Hunt and Hunt, 1977), are fertile, although female-female pairs provide excellent parental care (Hunt and Hunt, 1977; Fitch, unpubl.). Hence, the adaptive significance of this reproductive strategy is not immediately apparent (Shugart et al., 1988).

Both new recruits and widows have been shown to form female-female pairs, and many of these pairs persist for more than one breeding season (Hunt and Hunt, 1977; Shugart et al., 1988). There are no significant hormonal or behavioral differences between females paired with females and those paired with males (Wingfield et al., 1982; Hunt et al., 1984). However, embryonic feminization of males may result in suppression of sexual behavior and self-exclusion from the breeding colony. The large numbers of nonbreeding Herring Gulls we flushed from breeding colonies in Lake Ontario in the 1970s have not been observed in the 1980s since reproductive success has returned to normal. Although I have never observed significant adult mortality in Lake Ontario colonies in the 1970s or 1980s, it did occur regularly on Lake Michigan colonies and, based on size, most of the dead individuals appeared to be males (J.A. Keith, J.P. Ludwig, and G. Shugart, pers. comm.).

Whether the underlying skewed operational sex ratio is due to self-exclusion of feminized males, markedly increased differential mortality or both, the occurrence of supernormal clutches, female-female pairs and polygynous associations in Western and Herring Gulls represents yet another documented example of contaminant-induced effects at the population level.

## PSEUDOHERMAPHRODITISM OR 'IMPOSEX' IN GASTROPOD MOLLUSCS

A syndrome characterized by the superimposition of male characters on females has recently been identified in a number of marine gastropod (snail) species. Smith (1971, 1980) conducted a very extensive study of the mud snail, *Nassarius obsoletus*, an estuarine, dioecious (sexes distinct) neogastropod, on the Connecticut shoreline of Long Island Sound. He reported female snails possessing one or more of the following male secondary sex characteristics; (i) penises with a penal duct, (ii) vas deferens, or (iii) convoluted gonadal oviducts. Smith coined the term 'imposex' for this syndrome. The condition was environmentally induced rather than genetically controlled (Smith, 1980), and was associated with marinas (Smith, 1981a). Smith (1981 b,c) tested a wide variety of substances associated with marina activities, including paints, disinfectant, detergent, leaded gasoline and exhaust emissions; only tributyltin (TBT) compounds or paints containing them induced imposex in mud snails. These biocidal paints were first introduced in the late 1960s to prevent the settlement and growth of aquatic organisms on boats and fish cages.

Extensive field and laboratory studies have shown that very low concentrations of TBT have the same effect on the dogwhelk *Nucella lapillus*, another neogastropod and a dominant carnivore in intertidal rocky shore communities on both sides of the North Atlantic (Bryan et al., 1986, 1987; Gibbs and Bryan, 1986). The sexes of dogwhelks are separate and development is direct, taking place over a period of 3-4 months within a durable egg capsule attached to a low-tidal rock surface. The juveniles hatch as miniature adults. Pseudohermaphroditism (imposex) in dogwhelks was first described by Blaber (1970) in the population residing in Plymouth Sound in 1969-70. More recent studies of the same population and many others around southwest England have shown that both the incidence and the intensity of this condition are now quite marked, and many populations are in decline, particularly those close to centers of boating and shipping activities (Bryan et al., 1986). The severity of the symptoms vary but the female develops a penis and vas deferens and, in the most extreme cases, the latter may occlude the oviduct, resulting in sterility and, in some cases, death (Gibbs and Bryan, 1986). Imposex is nonreversible. The most affected populations suffer from reproductive failure and high female mortality, and are characterized therefore by relatively small numbers of juveniles and adult females. The condition can eventually lead to the local extinction of the species (Bryan et al., 1986).

Tank experiments and *in situ* transfer experiments have shown that imposex in *N. lapillus* is initiated at remarkably low tin concentrations—less than 1 ng/L of TBT-derived (hexane extractable) tin (Bryan et al., 1986). Sterilization of some females occurs at localities averaging around 1-2 ng/L of TBT tin and is total in areas averaging about 6-8 ng/L with a concomitant reduction in recruitment to zero. At extremely high concentrations of TBT, masculinization of females also occurs in the ovary (Gibbs et al., 1988), leading to complete sex reversal. TBT appears to interfere directly or indirectly with endocrine control of sex determination by inducing a morphogenic factor within the pedal ganglia. Despite the lack of recruitment, populations continue to exist for many years because of the longevity of the species. Imposex appears to increase female mortality and thus populations near extinction are usually composed predominantly, if not solely, of males.

In view of the high toxicity of TBT, Britain banned the use of TBT-containing anti-fouling paints on small boats and aquaculture cages under the Food and Environment Protection Act in July 1987. After comparing data collected for dogwhelk populations on the Northumbrian coast in 1986 and 1989, Evans et al. (1991) report a marked recovery within these populations since the introduction of this partial ban. The severity of imposex is reduced, recruitment of juveniles has improved and there is evidence of much better survivorship of females.

To date, imposex has also been detected in dogwhelks in the Pacific Ocean at sites as distant as Auke Bay, Alaska (Short et al., 1989), Puget Sound (Saavedra Alvarez and Ellis, 1990), the Strait of Juan de Fuca and Georgia Strait on the British Columbia coast (Bright and Ellis, 1990), and was widespread in New Zealand coastal waters in 1988 but was not detected at some of the same sites in 1970-71 (Smith and McVeagh, 1991). Imposex is also prevalent in coastal waters of Singapore, Malaysia and Indonesia in southeast Asia (Ellis and Pattisina, 1990). These data suggest that this is now a global environmental problem, and to date at least 45 species of gastropod have been affected. Of concern are the findings of Moore and Stevenson (1991) who recently documented intersexuality in harpticoid copepods of several species along the Scottish coastline, suggesting that other phyla may be affected. The highest incidence was in the vicinity of a major sewage discharge where 93% of the specimens examined of the dominant crustacean zooplankton species exhibited intersexuality.

## ABNORMAL REPRODUCTIVE PHYSIOLOGY IN FISH AND BIRDS EXPOSED TO PULP AND PAPER EFFLUENTS

Society's demand for bleached, white paper has resulted in the conversion of much of the world's forests into fiber and the release of large quantities of by-product chemicals into rivers, lakes and coastal waters as complex pulp mill effluent. A number of reports describe the abnormal expression of modified secondary sexual characteristics in populations of the sexually dimorphic mosquito fish, *Gambusia affinis* and *G. holbrookii*, in streams receiving paper mill effluents in the southeastern United States (Howell et al., 1980; Rosa-Molinar and Williams, 1984; Bortone et al., 1989; Davis and Bortone, chapter 6). Masculinized fish were found as far as 4 miles downstream, but not upstream, of two pulp mill effluent discharge sites. Females were strongly masculinized showing both the presence of a fully developed gonadopodium, the intromittent organ, and sexual behavior characteristic of the male of this species. It was concluded that some chemical or combination of chemicals associated with pulp mill effluent was exerting a strong androgenic effect on females in these populations of fish.

Microbial degradation of plant sterols such as sitosterols and stigmastanol, abundant in the resin fraction of coniferous trees used in the pulping industry, was suspected as the source of androgenic steroids responsible for altering the secondary sexual characteristics of these fish (Davis and Bartone, herein). Mosquito fish experimentally exposed to plant sterols, particularly B-sitosterol and stigmastanol, in the presence of *Mycobacterium* developed gonadopodial characteristics in 6 days (Denton et al., 1985). These characteristics did not regress when the transformed fish were removed to an environment free of plant sterols. These and other (Drysdale and Bortone, 1989) simple laboratory experiments demonstrate that such a cause-effect hypothesis is reasonable.

When compared to fish from three other areas of Lake Superior, White Sucker (*Catostomis commersoni*) collected from Jackfish Bay, a site receiving primary-treated kraft mill effluent exhibited an increased age to maturity, smaller gonads, lower fecundity with age, an absence of secondary sex characteristics in males, and lack of an increase in egg size with increasing female age. These findings were accompanied by marked induction of hepatic mixed-function oxidase (AHH) activity, decreases in serum levels of estradiol and testosterone and dysfunction of normal hypothalamic hormonal control at multiple sites in the pituitary-gonadal axis (Munkittrick et al., 1991). The lowered growth rate and decreased energetic commitment to reproduction suggest that there is a decreased conversion of energy into somatic or reproductive tissue. Similarly, in their studies of the physiology of Perch (*Perca fluviatilis*) inhabiting a site on the coast of the Gulf of Bothnia whose waters receive effluent from a kraft pulp mill, Andersson et al. (1988) found marked induction of hepatic mixed-function oxidase activity (EROD), abnormalities in carbohydrate metabolism and that gonad size was smaller in both male and female fish caught near the mill outlet compared with control fish. These effects showed a graded response along the pollution gradient 2-8 km from the mill.

Some bird populations also appear to be affected by the kraft mill in Jackfish Bay. Most of the eggs in the 35 nests in the Herring Gull colony in the Bay failed to hatch in 1991 and no young were successfully raised. Our biochemical studies of adults and 28-day old chicks from a colony in an adjacent bay revealed marked induction of hepatic mixed-function oxidase (EROD)—much higher than that in another Lake Superior site not near any pulp mills. However, chemical analyses did not reveal any significant differences in levels of TCDD and other persistent organochlorine contaminants between these colonies. In contrast, studies of Great Blue Heron (*Ardea herodias*) chicks from nesting colonies along the Fraser River estuary in British Columbia's Georgia Strait have shown elevated hepatic mixed-function oxidase (EROD) levels (Bellward et al., 1990), subcutaneous edema, growth retardation (Hart et al., 1991), and morphometric and histological changes in their brains (Henshel et al., 1992) which correlated with 2,3,7,8-TCDD levels in paired eggs from these nests. At peak contamination, the most contaminated colony failed to produce any young (Elliott et al., 1989). The Georgia Strait receives wastes from the greatest concentration of forest product industries in Canada; the TCDD contamination in fish-eating wildlife in the area is associated with these industries (Elliott et al., 1989). Some of these effects are consistent with TCDD-induced toxicity, however experimental evidence suggests that some may result from chronic exposure to other, as yet unidentified, substances such as steroids derived from plant sterols.

## CONCLUSIONS

Supernormal clutches in gulls, the distinctive tag provided by the masculinized anal fin of poeciliid fishes, and the development of a penis by female snails have provided ecoepidemiologists with conspicuous flags signalling otherwise subtle alterations in sexual development. Wildlife studies suggest that the underlying manifestations of toxicity have severely affected the reproduction of some populations of these organisms and that affected populations can be geographically widespread. It is time to ask "what effects have these and other chemicals had on human populations?" and, more important, "what can be done to detect, control and eliminate environmental chemicals capable of altering sexual development?"

The gull data suggest that feminization was widespread in the most contaminated populations during the period of peak contamination and that males either died or were feminized and chose not to attempt to breed. Although a large proportion of some regional populations was affected at the time, the developmental abnormality associated with this functional deficit was detected accidentally, and no dysfunctional adults were ever identified. It was the occurrence of nests containing twice the normal number of eggs, which proved to be the result of female-female pairing, that alerted investigators to a problem. Later studies showed a change in sex ratio and suggested a probable connection between the structural developmental abnormality in the testes of the embryo/newborn and functional deficits in these males when they reached breeding age. In contrast, the masculinizing effects of pulp mill effluent on mosquito fish and of TBT on molluscs are grossly manifested at very low concentrations and, with time, functional deficits associated with these anatomical abnormalities are reflected in the demography of the population. The abnormalities responsible for the reproductive dysfunction in egg-laying fish such as the White Sucker and Perch associated with exposure to pulp mill effluent are only detected when the structure and physiology of local fish populations are studied in detail.

Peterson et al. (chapter 10) have shown that perinatal exposure of male rats to 2,3,7,8-TCDD decreased their androgenic status from the fetal stage into adulthood, decreased the mass of their testes and epididymis, and decreased their daily sperm production thus delaying testicular development and permanently inhibiting spermatogenesis, resulting in a reduction in male fertility. Such exposure also demasculinized and feminized their sexual behavior and increased their pituitary and/or hypothalamic responsiveness to ovarian steroids in adulthood, indicating that regulation of LH secretion was permanently feminized. These effects apparently result from alterations in sexual differentiation of the central nervous system. Some of these or similar effects have been observed in contaminant-exposed fish and fish-eating birds. Since the sources of contaminants involved vary greatly, we must conclude that chronic exposure or exposure at a critical stage in development to a variety of environmental contaminants can alter sexual development and/or functions.

Although structural and biochemical abnormalities may occur during embryonic development, the critical functional deficit is only manifested at sexual maturity. Current premarket chemical testing requirements and other regulations do not provide sufficient information about effects on reproduction to allow regulators to prevent the widespread release of such man-made chemicals as DDT, TBT, TCDD, PCBs, etc. and the occurrence of such subtle reproductive effects as reported herein. Widespread use of such persistent products, which also have the ability to bioaccumulate, results in numerous point sources that eventually amalgamate to become a global problem.

Effluents vary from manufacturer to manufacturer, mill to mill, etc., depending upon the feedstock and exact process used. Effluents also interact with a host of site-specific factors, both physical and biological, resulting in the release of a complex and potentially greatly modified discharge containing numerous, little-studied compounds. Although most components of pulp and paper effluents are not known to be persistent or bioaccumulative, they are released continuously in vast quantities. The pulp mill near Jackfish Bay releases >70,000 L of effluent per minute and, as is frequently the case, is only one of several mills on the shoreline! Such inputs are thus a source of chronic toxic contamination. The biologically significant contamination of San Francisco Bay by DDT from the Montrose Chemical Corporation and of the world's largest freshwater lake by pulp mill effluent clearly illustrate that the industrial engineering philosophy that "the solution to pollution is dilution" is totally unacceptable.

Policy decisions affecting ecosystem and public health may have to be made on the basis of observational evidence alone. In prevention, it is necessary to identify an exposure without necessarily identifying the ultimate cause of the disease. According to Lilienfeld and Lilienfeld (1980), a causal relationship would be recognized to exist "whenever evidence indicates that the factors form part of the complex of circumstances that increases the probability of the occurrence of the disease and that a diminution of one or more of these factors decreases the frequency of that disease".

The weight of ecoepidemiological evidence suggests that the relationships are real, probably causal, and biologically or ecologically significant enough to warrant the attention of those engaged in the protection of health and the environment. We should be willing to initiate preventative or remedial action and to risk that the findings we accept as true may turn out to be untrue--rather than learn that we were not protective enough of human health and planet Earth, the only place in the universe known to sustain life. Wildlife will continue to be the sentinels and sensors whose responses will critically monitor our decisions and actions.

## REFERENCES

Andersson, T., Forlin, L., Hardig, I., and Larsson, A. (1988). Physiological disturbances in fish living in coastal water polluted with bleached kraft mill effluents. *Can. J. Fish. Aquat. Sci.*, **45**, 1525-1536.

Bellward, G.D., Nortstom, R.J., Whitehead, P.E., Elliott, J.E., Bandiera, S.M., Dworschak, C., Chang, T., Forbes, S., Cedario, B., Hart, L.E., and Cheng, K.M. (1990). Comparison of polychlorinated dibenzodioxin levels with hepatic mixed-function oxidase induction in Great Blue Herons. *J. Toxicol. Environ. Health*, **30**, 33-52.

Blaber, S.J.M. (1970). The occurrence of a penis-like outgrowth behind the right tentacle in spent females of *Nucella lapillus* (L). *Proc. Malacol. Soc. Lond.*, **39**, 231-233.

Bortone, S.A., Davis, W.B., and Bundrick, C.M. (1989). Morphological and behavioral characters in mosquito fish as potential bioindication of exposure to kraft mill effluent. *Bull. Environ. Contam. Toxicol.*, **43**, 370-377.

Boss, W.R. (1943). Hormonal determination of adult characters and sex behavior in Herring Gulls (*Larus argentatus*). *J. Exp. Zool.*, **94**, 181-209.

Boss, W.R. and Witschi, E. (1947). The permanent effects of early stilbesterol injections on the sex organs of the Herring Gull (*Larus argentatus*). *J. Exp. Biol.*, **105**, 61-77.

Bright, D.A. and Ellis, D.V. (1990). A comparative survey of imposex in the northeast Pacific gastropods (Prosobranchia) related to tributyltin contamination, and choice of a suitable indicator. *Can. J. Zool.*, **68**, 1915-1924.

Bryan, G.W., Gibbs P.E., Hummerstone, L.G., and Burt, G.R. (1986). The decline of the gastropod *Nucella lapillus* around south-west England:Evidence for the effect of tributyltin from antifouling paints. *J. Mar. Biol. Ass. U.K.*, **66**, 611-640.

Bryan, G.W., Gibbs, P.E., Burt, G.R., and Hummerstone, L.G. (1987). Effects of tributyltin (TBT) accumulation on adult dog-whelks, *Nucella lapillus*: long-term field and laboratory experiments. *J. Mar. Biol. Ass. U.K.*, 67, 524-544.

Burnett, R. (1971). DDT residues: Distribution of concentrations in Emerita analoga (Stimpson) along coastal California. *Science*, **174**, 606-608.

Conover, R.M. (1984). Occurrence of supernormal clutches in Laridae. *Wilson Bull.*, **96**, 249-267.

Conover, R.M. and Hunt, G.L. (1984). Female-female pairing and sex ratios in gulls: A historical perspective. *Wilson Bull.*, **96**, 619-625.

Denton, T.E., Howell, W.M., Allison, J.J., McCollum, J., and Marks, B. (1985). Masculinization of female mosquito fish by exposure to plant sterols and *Mycobacterium smegmatis*. *Bull. Environ. Contam. Toxicol.*, **35**, 627-632.

Drysdale, D.T. and Bortone, S.A. (1989). Laboratory induction of intersexuality in the mosquito fish, *Gambusia affinis*, using paper mill effluent. *Bull. Environ. Contam. Toxicol.*, **43**, 611-617.

Elliott, J.E., Butler, R.W., Norstrom, R.J., and Whitehead, P.E. (1989). Environmental contaminants and reproductive success of Great Blue Herons *Ardea herodias* in British Columbia, 1986-87. *Environ. Pollut.*, **59**, 91-114.

Ellis, D.V.and Pattisina, L.A.(1990). Widespread neogastropod imposex: a biological indicator of global TBT contamination. *Mar. Pollut. Bull.*, **21**, 248-253.

Evans, S.M., Hutton, A., Kendall, M.A., and Samosir, A.M. (1991). Recovery in populations of dogwhelks *Nucella lapillus* (L) suffering from imposex. *Mar. Pollut. Bull.*, **22**, 409-413.

Eroschenko, V.P. and Palmiter, R.D. (1980). Estrogenicity of kepone in birds and mammals. In *Estrogens in the Environment*, ed. J.A. McLachlan. Elsevier/ North-Holland, New York, pp. 305-325.

Fox, G.A. and Boersma, D. (1983). Characteristics of supernormal ring-billed gull clutches and their attending adults. *Wilson Bull.*, **95**, 522-559.

Fox, G.A., Gilman, A.P., Peakall, D.B., and Anderka, F.W. (1978). Behavioral abnormalities of nesting Lake Ontario Herring Gulls. *J. Wildlife Manage.*, **43**, 477-483.

Fry, D.M. and Toone, C.K. (1981). DDT-induced feminization of gull embryos. *Science*, 213, 922-924.

Fry, D.M., Toone, C.K., Speich, S.M., and Peard, R.J. (1987). Sex ratio skew and breeding patterns of gulls: demographic and toxicological considerations. *Stud. Avian Biol.*, **10**, 26-43.

Gibbs, P.E.and Bryan, G.W. (1986). Reproductive failure in populations of the dog-whelk, *Nucella lapillus*, caused by imposex induced by tributyltin from antifouling paints. *J. Mar. Biol. Ass. U.K.*, 66, 767-777.

Gibbs, P.E., Pascoe, P.L., and Burt, G.R. (1988). Sex change in the female dog-whelk, *Nucella lapillus*, induced by triorganotin from antifouling paints. *J. Mar. Biol. Ass. U.K.*, **68**, 715-731.

Gilbertson, M. and Fox, G.A. (1977). Pollutant-associated embryonic mortality of Great Lakes Herring Gulls. *Environ. Pollut.*, **12**, 211-216.

Gilbertson, M., Kubiak, T., Ludwig, J., and Fox, G. (1991). Great Lakes embryo mortality, edema, and deformities syndrome (GLEMEDS) in colonial fish-eating birds: Similarity to chick edema disease. *J. Toxicol. Environ. Health*, **33**, 455-520.

Harper, C.A. (1971). Breeding biology of a small colony of Western Gulls (*Larus occidentalis wymani*) in California. *Condor*, **73**, 337-341.

Hart, L.E., Cheng, K.M., Whitehead, P.E., Shah, R.M., Lewis, R.J., Ruschkowski, S.R., Blair, R.W., Bennett, D.C., Bandiera, S.M., Norstrom, R.J., and Bellward, G.D. (1991). Dioxin contamination and growth and development in Great Blue Heron embryos. *J. Toxicol. Environ. Health*, **32**: 331-344.

Henshel, D.S., Cheng, K.M., Norstrom, R., Whitehead, P., and Steeves, J.D. (1992). Morphometric and histological changes in brains of Great Blue Heron hatchlings exposed to PCDDs: Preliminary analyses. In *Environmental Toxicology and Risk Assessment: Aquatic, Plant, Terrestrial, 1st. Symposium, ASTM STP 1179*, ed. W.G. Landis, J. Hughes, and M. Lewis. American Society for Testing and Materials, Philadelphia, (in press).

Hom,W., Risebrough, R.W., Soutar, A., and Young, D.R. (1974). Deposition of DDE and polychlorinated biphenyls in dated sediments of the Santa Barbara Basin. *Science*, **184**, 1197-1199.

Howell, W.M., Black, D.A., and Bortone, S.A. (1980). Abnormal expressions of secondary sex characters in a population of mosquito fish, *Gambusia affinis holbrookii*: Evidence for environmentally-induced masculinization. *Copeia*, **4**, 676-681.

Hunt, G.L. and Hunt, M.W. (1973). Clutch size, hatching success, and eggshell thinning in Western Gulls. *Condor*, **75**, 483-486.

Hunt, G.L. and Hunt, M.W. (1977). Female-female pairing in Western Gulls (*Larus occidentalis*) in southern California. *Science*, **196**, 1466-1467.

Hunt, G.L., Newman, A.L., Warner, M.H., Wingfield, J.C., and Kaiwi, J. (1984). Comparative behavior of male-female and female-female pairs among Western Gulls prior to egg laying. *Condor*, **86**, 157-162.

L'Arrivee, L. and Blokpoel, H. (1988). Seasonal distribution and site fidelity in Great Lakes Caspian terns. *Colonial Waterbirds*, **11**, 202-214.

Lilienfeld, A.M. and Lilienfeld, D.E. (1980). *Foundations of Epidemiology*, 2nd Ed. Oxford University Press, New York.

Ludwig, J.P. (1979). Present status of the Caspian Tern population of the Great Lakes. *Mich. Academician*, **12**, 69-77.

MacGregor, J.S. (1974). Changes in the amount and proportions of DDT and its metabolites, DDE and DDD, in the marine environment off southern California, 1949-72. *Fishery Bull.*, **72**, 275-293.

Mineau, P., Fox, G.A., Norstrom, R.J., Weseloh, D.V., Hallet, D.J., and Ellenton, J.A. (1984). Using the Herring Gull to monitor levels and effects of organochlorine contamination in the Canadian Great Lakes. In *Toxic Contamination in the Great Lakes*, ed. J.O. Nriagu and M.S. Simmons.Wiley and Sons, New York, pp. 425-452.

Moore, C.G.and Stevenson, J.M. (1991). The occurrence of intersexuality in harpticoid copepods and its relationship with pollution. *Mar. Pollut. Bull.*, **22**, 72-74.

Munkittrick, K.R., Port, C.B., Van Der Kraak, G.J., Smith, I.R., and Rokosh, D.A. (1991). Impact of bleached kraft mill effluent on population characteristics, liver MFO activity, and serum steroid levels of a Lake Superior white sucker (*Catostomus commersoni*) population. *Can. J. Fish. Aquat. Sci.*, **48**, 1371-1380.

Peakall, D.B. and Fox, G.A. (1987). Toxicological investigations of pollutant-related effects in Great Lakes gulls. *Environ. Health Persp.*, **71**, 187-193.

Rosa-Molinar, E. and Williams, C.S. (1984). Notes on fecundity of an arrhenoid population of mosquito fish *Gambusia affinis holbrookii*. *Northeast Gulf Sci.*, **7**, 121-125.

Saavedra Alvarez, M.M. and Ellis, D.V. (1990). Widespread neogastropod imposex in the Northeast Pacific: Implications for TBT contamination surveys. *Mar. Pollut. Bull.*, **21**, 244-247.

Schreiber, R.W. (1970). Breeding biology of Western Gulls (*Larus occidentalis*) on San Nicolas Island, California, 1968. *Condor*, **72**, 133-140.

Short, J.W., Rice, S.D., Brodersen, C.C., and Stickle, W.B. (1989). Occurrence of tri-N-butyltin caused imposex in the North Pacific marine snail *Nucella lima* in Auke Bay, Alaska. *Mar. Biol.*, **102**, 291-297.

Shugart, G.W. (1980). Frequency and distribution of polygyny in Great Lakes Herring Gulls in 1978. *Condor*, **82**, 426-429.

Shugart, G.W. and Southern, W.E. (1977). Close nesting; a result of polygyny in Herring Gulls. *Bird-Banding*, **48**, 276-277.

Shugart, G.W., Fitch, M.A., and Fox, G.A. (1988). Female pairing: A reproductive strategy for Herring Gulls? *Condor*, **90**, 933-935.

Smith, B.S. (1971). Sexuality in the American mud snail, *Nassarius obsoletus* Say. *Proc. Malacol. Soc. Lond.*, **39**, 377-378.

Smith, B.S. (1980). The estuarine mud snail, *Nassarius obsoletus* abnormalities in the reproductive system. *J. Moll. Stud.*, **46**, 247-256.

Smith, B.S. (1981a). Reproductive anomalies in stenoglossan snails related to pollution from marinas. *J.Appl.Toxicol.*, **1**, 15-21.

Smith, B.S. (1981b). Male characteristics on female mud snails caused by antifouling bottom paints. *J. Appl. Toxicol.*, **1**, 22-25.

Smith, B.S. (1981c). Tributyltin compounds induce male characteristics on mud snails, *Nassarius obsoletus = Ilyanassa obsoleta. J. Appl. Toxicol.*, **1**, 141-144.

Smith, P.J. and McVeagh, M. (1991). Widespread organotin pollution  in New Zealand coastal waters as indicated by imposex in dogwhelks. *Mar. Pollut. Bull.*, **22**, 409-413.

Sowls, A.L., Degange, A.R., Nelson, J.W., and Lester, G.S. (1980). *Catalog of California Seabird Colonies*. Coastal Ecosystems Project, Fish and Wildlife Service, U.S. Department of the  Interior, Washington D.C. p.371.

Wingfield, J.C., Newman, A.L., Hunt, G.L., and Farner, D.S. (1982). Endocrine aspects of female-female pairing in the Western Gull (*Larus occidentalis wymani*). *Anim. Behav.*, **30**, 9-22.

# XENOBIOTIC INDUCED HORMONAL AND ASSOCIATED DEVELOPMENTAL DISORDERS IN MARINE ORGANISMS AND RELATED EFFECTS IN HUMANS; AN OVERVIEW

**Peter J.H. Reijnders**
Research Institute for Nature Management, Dept. Estuarine Ecology,
Den Burg, The Netherlands

**Sophie M.J.M. Brasseur**
Research Institute for Nature Management, Dept. Estuarine Ecology,
Den Burg, The Netherlands

*This review discusses the noxious effects on marine organisms of contaminants that disrupt physiological processes controlled by the endocrine system. It outlines the impacts of several groups of contaminants—heavy metals, chlorinated hydrocarbons, and polyaromatic hydrocarbons—on both the endocrine system and early phases in the reproductive cycles of different marine organisms. A series of respective case studies are reviewed ending in an evaluation of the wildlife/human connection.*

*Xenobiotic effects are observed throughout all trophic levels in the marine system, ranging from zooplankton to top predators such as seals. Impacts can occur at the level of steroid biosynthesis, biotransformation, gametogenesis, oogenesis, and spermatogenesis. This chapter reviews the associations between xenobiotics and corresponding mechanisms in light of the limited information available. The complex, multiple role of cytochrome P-450 in controlling toxicity of chemicals and the balance of steroids will be extensively elaborated.*

*A suite of disturbances in the early phase of reproductive cycles has been associated with xenobiotics and postulated to be linked to hormonal imbalance from the lower to the higher trophic levels in the marine ecosystem. Several classes of effects are described, such as: lowered egg production, retarded maturation of oocytes, decreased ovarian growth, lowered vitellogenesis, retarded follicle development, follicle phagocytosis, pseudohermaphroditism, implantation failure and pathological disorders in the genital tract.*

*Epidemiological studies on interference of xenobiotics within the reproductive system of humans are sporadic and scarcely reveal conclusive results. Within the toxicological investigations on this*

1. Corresponding Author: Peter Reijnders, Research Institute for Nature Management, Dept. Estuarine, Ecology, P.O. Box 167, 1790 AD Den Burg, The Netherlands.

*subject the effects attributed to polychlorinated biphenyls (PCBs), poly-chlorinated dibenzodioxins (PCDDs) and polychlorinated dibenzofurans (PCDFs) are the most manifest. Some effects of these contaminants on embryonic development, follicular maturation, and sperm function are described.*

*Considered from a global viewpoint, in particular, PCB concentrations in ecosystems will continue to rise in the future. The increasing concern about the potential hazards for marine systems, as well as other wildlife and humans, is documented.*

## INTRODUCTION

Xenobiotic effects on early phases in the reproductive cycle of organisms are observed in almost every component of the global marine ecosystem. For some compounds the endocrine and developmental toxicological properties are studied in detail. However, in most cases the modes of action have not been elucidated, partly because of the complexity of the endocrine system but certainly also due to the fact that mixtures of various contaminants are involved.

Toxicity proceeds through interference by compounds or their metabolites in the control of physiological processes. Many physiological processes are coordinated by hormones. The purpose of this chapter is to summarize the xenobiotic induced alteration of endocrine functioning as expressed by hormonal imbalance and associated developmental disorders in marine organisms.

Three different classes of case studies will be considered; (1) studies where a clear relation between biosynthesis of hormones and effects are described, (2) studies which describe an impact via biotransformation of steroids and (3) studies where developmental disorders are observed but no clear relation to hormonal imbalance could be established. For each class, case studies representing different trophic levels will be provided in successive order where information is available. This review will therefore not be exhaustive.

The toxicological implications of human exposure to a limited number of xenobiotics is also discussed. Finally the long term global effects of a group of persistent environmental contaminants (the PCBs) on the marine ecosystem will be outlined.

## BIOSYNTHESIS

Chemical pollutants have been shown to act as environmental inhibitors of gonadal activity. Short term cadmium exposure of sea stars, *Asteria rubens*, affected steroid synthesis and tissue levels of progesterone and testosterone (Voogt et al., 1987). It was found in the same animal that both cadmium and PCBs significantly reduced levels of progesterone and testosterone in the pyloric caeca of males and females (den Besten, 1991). No effect of cadmium was found in the gonads and PCB exposure resulted in an increase of testosterone in testes and ovaries. The latter effect may be explained by the different forms of PCB-induced synthesis or conversion activities in steroid metabolism. This will be elaborated in the next section on biotransformation. Although the exact impact of progesterone and testosterone in sea stars is still unknown, it has been suggested that changes in their levels represent a hormonal trigger for the pyloric caeca, being the onset of vitellogenesis and gametogenesis (Voogt et al., 1985).

Johnson et al., (1988) described the inhibition of gonadal recrudescence and reduced levels of plasma oestradiol in female English sole, *Parophrys vetulus*, from a heavily contaminated area. Since both conditions were associated with elevated hepatic aryl hydrocarbon hydroxylase, it is tentatively concluded that the disposition of oestradiol and consequently the ovarian development is influenced via interference of xenobiotics with enzymes involved in steroid metabolism. Of the two classes of xenobiotics suspected, aromatic hydrocarbons (AHs) and PCBs, the AHs appeared to be most closely associated with the inhibited ovarian development and depressed plasma oestradiol. However, it is important to recognize that other contaminants could also be involved (Johnson et al., 1988).

This linkage between disrupted gonadal maturation and altered steroid level has been noted in other fish as well. In Atlantic cod, *Gadus morhua*, the hormone synthesizing ability of the testis was impaired by PCBs (Freeman et al., 1982). Truscott et al., (1983) observed decreases in blood testosterone in Winter flounder, *Pseudopleuronectus americanus*, exposed to crude oil. It was found that *in vivo* PCB exposed Atlantic cod caused an *in vitro* increase in metabolism of steroid hormones in kidney and liver. Furthermore it was found that the usual increase in plasma androgen levels correlated with the approach of functional sexual maturity, failed to occur. This indicates interference of PCBs with androgen production and/or utilization (Freeman et al., 1984).

The impairment of reproductive endocrine function by xenobiotics in female Atlantic croaker *Micropogonias undulatus*, was investigated by Thomas (1988). Significant decreases in plasma steroid levels, ovarian steroid secretion and ovarian growth occurred after exposure to lead, benzo[a]pyrene, and a PCB mixture, Aroclor 1254. All toxicants impaired ovarian growth but only upon exposure to benzo[a]pyrene and lead was there a significant decline in circulating oestradiol-17β levels. All three xenobiotics decreased plasma testosterone levels. It was concluded that the decreased ovarian growth may be a consequence of low plasma oestradiol levels. No evidence was obtained for a direct suppressive action of the chemicals on ovarian steroidogenesis.

In a later study the effects of cadmium and Aroclor 1254 were studied in greater detail (Thomas, 1990). In addition to reduced ovarian growth, decreased plasma oestradiol, lower vitellogenin levels and a lower hepatic oestrogen receptor concentration in Aroclor 1254 exposed fish, it was found that the total oestradiol production per ovary was decreased. These findings can be interpreted as lower plasma oestradiol levels being primarily due to smaller amounts of steroidogenic tissue present in PCB exposed animals. The decline in ovarian growth and steroidogenesis suggests an impairment of gonadotropin (GTH) secretion. This is supported by a significant decrease in spontaneous secretion of GTH from hemipituitaries incubated *in vitro* after *in vivo* PCB treatment.

Cadmium exerted opposite effects: increased ovarian growth, elevated plasma oestradiol concentrations and also marked increase in GTH from pituitaries of Cd-exposed fish *in vitro*. This study clearly demonstrates that pollutants can profoundly influence reproductive endocrine function of the hypothalamus-pituitary-gonadal-liver axis. The effects of both pollutants could result in the production of mature oocytes outside the hormonal spawning season when environmental and biotic conditions might not be optimal for larval survival.

Freeman and Sangalang (1977) studied the effects of methyl mercury (MeHg), cadmium, arsenic (As), selenium (Se) and a PCB mixture (Aroclor 1254) on adrenal and testicular steroidogenesis *in vitro* in the grey seal, *Halichoerus grypus*. Adrenal and testicular tissue from seals treated with each contaminant, was incubated with pregnenolone and progesterone. All contaminants except As and Se, stimulated the *in vitro* biosynthesis of testosterone in seal testicular incubates. However, in adrenal tissue, when treated with progesterone, less corticosterone and aldosterone, but more cortisol was produced, indicating interference at the progesterone-corticosterone level and not at the pregnenolone-progesterone level.

In a similar study with harp seals, *Phoca groenlandica*, the effects of *in vivo* methylmercury treatment on *in vitro* biosynthesis of steroid hormones were investigated (Freeman et al., 1984). Lowered biosynthesis of aldosterone and cortisol was found in the MeHg treated seal. There was stimulation of metabolites slightly more polar than 11-ketotestosterone and less polar than testosterone in the ovaries of the treated seal. It is tentatively concluded that this could indicate a stimulated oestrogen biosynthesis, since testosterone is an immediate precursor of oestrogens.

A decrease in testosterone levels in Dall's porpoises, *Phocoenoides dalli*, was associated with increased PCBs and DDE concentrations. The mechanism for this decrease could not be provided (Subramanian et al., 1987).

## BIOTRANSFORMATION

The central catalyst in the elimination of hydrophobic pollutants is the liver microsomal cytochrome P-450 system. The function of the more than 150 individual forms of P-450 is to catalyze biotransformation of organic xenobiotics into metabolites that are then more readily eliminated. Chemical processes involved are hydroxylation, epoxylation, and oxygenation. In addition to their roles in metabolization of xenobiotic compounds, they also function in synthesis and metabolism of endobiotics such as steroid hormones, fatty acids, prostaglandins and fat soluble vitamins (Parkinson and Safe, 1987). Some environmental pollutants, the chlorobiphenyls (CBs) such as PCBs and related compounds, interact with cytochrome P-450. They can act as inducers, substrate and inhibitors (Boon et al., 1992).

Each of the many isoenzymes in the cytochrome P-450 system exhibits substrate specificity for the metabolism of xenobiotic and endobiotic compounds. This implies that for different chemicals, different enzymes in the P-450 family are involved. In addition, organisms develop species specific profiles of cytochrome P-450 further complicating our understanding. An added factor is the developmentally related changes in P-450 content.

An alteration in the profile of cytochrome P-450 enzymes may be caused by induction of the drug-metabolizing enzyme systems by xenobiotics. This would lead to an imbalance of endobiotics since P-450 systems are involved in catalyzing biosynthesis of steroids. Furthermore xenobiotics could be in competition with steroids for cytochrome P-450. The latter may particularly be the case in lower organisms in which the number of isoenzymes is limited (Livingstone, 1990).

In order to understand the toxicity of xenobiotics it is essential to assess the composition and characteristics of the P-450 systems in target organisms and even in target organs (Safe, 1984; Goksøyr et al., 1988; Watanabe et al., 1989). CBs can also affect the toxicokinetics of other contaminants. It is via induction that reactive intermediates are formed which in turn can act in a synergistic or an antagonistic way (Conney, 1967; Baily et al., 1987).

As substrates, CBs themselves are biotransformed by hydroxylation and again the metabolites can be more toxic than the parent compound, leading to lower levels of thyroid hormones (Brouwer et al., 1989; Brouwer et al., 1990). The other possible mechanism for interference of xenobiotics with the P-450 systems is via their role as inhibitors of enzyme activity (O'Hara et al., 1985; Elskus et al., 1989; den Besten, 1991).

## DEVELOPMENTAL DISORDERS

Disturbances in the early phase of reproductive cycles in marine organisms, postulated to be linked to xenobiotics and hormonal imbalance, are amply documented. However, in many cases, no clear cut correlation between residue levels and the observed effect could be established and the mode of action is only partly explained. In this chapter classes of effects are grouped and described for several trophic levels and the mechanisms elucidated as far as available information allowed interpretation.

*Gametogenesis*
The synthesis of vitellogin, precursor protein of the yolk, is in all egg-laying vertebrates under the modulation of oestrogen. It is synthesized by the liver and deposited in oocytes. In sea stars (den Besten, 1991), cadmium and PCBs (Clophen A50) affected oogenesis at the start of vitellogenesis. The production of oocytes decreased in PCB-exposed females, presumably causing a reduction in ovary weight, whereas cadmium induced a delay in oocyte maturation. The effect on spermatogenesis appeared to be less compared to the effect on oogenesis. This difference was attributed to lower PCB and cadmium levels in the testes as a result of different lipid and protein metabolism. Significant reductions were observed in pyloric caeca of cadmium or PCB exposed female and male sea stars. In gonads no effect of cadmium on steroid level was observed. Since PCB exposure caused an increase in testicular and ovarian testosterone levels, it is possible that microsomal steroid conversion activities are reduced leading to reduced oestrogen levels. This hypothesis needs further testing.

In female Atlantic croaker, PCBs and cadmium caused changes in plasma oestradiol levels, which regulates vitellogenesis (Thomas, 1990) and in rainbow trout, PCBs and Mirex were found to cause reduction in serum vitellogin levels (Chen et al., 1986).

A field study showed that polychaetes, *Nereis virens*, failed to form gametes in the presence of high concentrations of polycyclic aromatic hydrocarbons. This was associated with increased mixed function oxygenase activity and cytochrome P-450 content (Fries and Lee, 1984).

In male follicles of the mussel *Mytilis edulis L.,* collected at a heavy metal and sulphuric acid polluted site in the Baltic, no spermatogenic elements existed and female gonads were filled with anomalous ova, granulocytes and cellular debris (Sunila, 1986).

*Gonadal and Embryonic Development*
Disrupted ovarian maturation cycles with follicles remaining in a regressed stage were found in female plaice, *Pleuronectes platessa*, from a site of the Amoco Cadiz oil spill (Stott et al., 1983).

Kluytmans et al., (1988) studied experimentally the effect of cadmium on the reproductive cycle in the mussel and showed that follicle development in both male and female gonads was significantly inhibited. Since spawning increased, but no data on fertilization success and viability of gametes and embryos were obtained, the ecological implications of the cadmium stress can not be assessed.

Sunila (1988) reported on the occurrence of phagocytosis of sperm in follicles and necrotic follicles in mussels, and suggested it to be pollution provoked. This was based on experimentally induced changes that also occurred at polluted sites. The experiment was carried out with both copper and cadmium and no specific data on pollutants in the field, other than heavy metal and sulphuric acid pollution, were provided. The observed effects can therefore not be solely attributed to the pollutants analyzed.

Aberrations in the early development of embryos in the sea star *Asterias rubens* were both cadmium and PCB related (den Besten, 1991). In the sea star *Patiria miniata* they were found to be related to crude oil water-soluble fractions (Davis et al., 1981), in the sea urchin *Strongylocentrotus intermedius* to be cadmium related (Khristoforova et al., 1984) and PCB related (Pagano et al., 1985).

*Zooplankton Egg Production*
In a model ecosystem experiment the effects of three xenobiotics on a zooplankton community were studied: tetrapropylene-benzenesulphonate and two PCB mixtures, Aroclor 1221 and Aroclor 1254. In all three cases, the copepod egg production was lower than in the controls (Kuiper, 1982). The underlying mechanisms remain unclear.

*Pseudohermaphroditism*
Pseudohermaphroditism or imposex—male genitalia imposed on females—in shoreline whelks, *Nucella* genus, is reported to occur globally (Ellis and Pattisina, 1990; Saavreda Alvarez and Ellis, 1990; Spence et al., 1990). The induction of male sex characters, including a penis and vas deferens on females, is principally caused by tributyltin (TBT) compounds leached from marine antifouling paints used on ships, boats and mariculture pen nets (Bryan et al., 1988). The syndrome causes females to become sterile when the superficial vas deferens overgrows the genital pore, thus preventing egg capsules from being liberated. It is considered to be a global environmental problem, since oysters and other bivalve mollusca are known to be affected by TBT (Stephenson et al., 1986).

Poor breeding success of Western gulls, *Larus occidentalis*, in southern California, was attributed to DDT induced feminization of gull embryos (Fry and Toone, 1981). Epidemiological findings, e.g., high concentrations of DDT in eggs, skewed sex ratio in favour of females and female-female pairing, were corroborated by experimental testing. Testicular changes accompanied by abnormal development of ovarian tissue and oviducts in male embryos was associated with the inability to breed as adults.

*Implantation Failure*
Reproductive failure in common seals, *Phoca vitulina*, from the Wadden Sea is attributed to PCBs and/or PCB-metabolites (Reijnders, 1986). Studies on hormonal profiles showed that the effect occurred at a stage of the reproductive process around implantation, since the follicular, luteal and post-implantation phase were not affected. Although the precise mechanism could not be tested with the information available, it was demonstrated that the impact was reversible (Reijnders, 1988b).

*Pathological Disorders*

Organochlorine pollution, in particular with PCBs and DDT, is prominently observed in pinnipeds. Bergman and Olsson (1985) concluded that PCBs and other organochlorines interfere with the endocrine system in female Baltic ringed seals, *Phoca hispida*, and grey seals, *Halichoerus grypus*. The observed symptoms, similar to those present in hyperadrenocorticism, are uterine stenoses and occlusions, bilateral adrenocortical hyperplasia and hormonal osteoporosis. It is suggested that these are part of a disease complex exerted particularly by PCBs on the brain-hypothalamic-hypophysis-adrenal and placental axis or directly on adrenals, and leading to disrupted reproductive performance.

Premature pupping in California sea lions (DeLong et al., 1973) and reproductive disorders in St. Lawrence beluga, *Delphinapterus leucas* (Martineau et al., 1985), are related to both PCBs and DDT. However, the possible xenobiotic effects could not be separated from the effects of some pathogens and other environmental stresses.

## EFFECTS ON HUMANS

Trace quantities of PCBs, PCDDs, PCDFs, DDT and other insecticides occur commonly in human populations. Even in areas where no industry or other sources of these agents are found they are present in human blood, adipose tissue or milk (Jensen and Sundström, 1974; Akiyama et al., 1975; van Hove Holdrinet et al., 1977; Slorach and Vaz 1985; Kannan et al., 1988; Jensen, 1989). The major pathway of general population exposure seems to be through the ingestion of foods (Safe, 1987; Kannan, 1988; Anderson, 1989), even though inhalation and skin exposure can play an important role as well (Anderson, 1989).

Aside from this "normal" intake some people have accidentally been exposed to higher concentrations of xenobiotics than the average. This can either have a chronic source caused by specific feeding habits or occupational exposure (manufacturing or processing) or an acute source as a result of catastrophes such as the Yusho and Yu-Cheng food oil poisoning in Japan and Taiwan (PCBs, PCDDs, PCDFs) or the Seveso accident in Italy (TCDD). These catastrophes make it possible to evaluate the effects of high dosages of contaminants on humans, as most of the research on toxicity of these contaminants was done on laboratory animals.

Symptoms found in patients that were contaminated either by chronic or acute exposure generally have not been directly related to hormonal disorders. However, effects on reproduction have been found. For example the offspring of women who regularly consumed fish from the contaminated waters of Lake Michigan were reported to have been adversely affected (Jacobson et al., 1990). Aside from shortened gestation, infants had reduced birth weight and smaller head circumference, but also showed compromised neuromuscular development. As they grew older the children were found to show retardation in several stages of development (Fein et al., 1984; Thomann et al., 1987; Jacobson et al., 1990).

The most extensive research on reproductive effects was done in Italy following the consequences of the release of TCDD caused by an explosion of a factory. In addition to a large scale medical monitoring programme that recorded the occurrence of chloracne, disrupted organ functions, cancer, and mortality, reproduction statistics and records of birth defects were collected from ± 90% (equals 50,300) of all exposed women in the area. No effects on reproduction could be related to the levels of contamination with 2,3,7,8-TCDD (Reggiani, 1989). However, no studies that monitor the sexual development as the children exposed *in utero* matured, have been done.

Unfortunately there has been no comprehensive study of fertility, fecundity or rates of spontaneous abortions in either Yusho nor Yu Cheng patients. As a result of these two accidents, during which people were exposed to high levels of PCBs, PCDFs and PCQs (polychlorinated quaterphenyls), only mild endocrine disorders were observed. Abnormal levels of steroids were found in the urine of Yusho patients (Kuratsune, 1989). In women, menstrual irregularities and abnormal patterns of basal body temperature were found. The latter could be indicative of insufficiency of corpus luteum and retarded follicular maturation. Children born to Yu Cheng women were shorter and lighter than normal and showed a number of abnormalities which were most consistent with a general disorder of ectodermal tissue, and developmental impairment (Rogan et al., 1988; Rogan, 1989).

The observed symptoms are similar to effects caused by high levels of PCBs. However, the levels in the formerly cited studies are relatively low. Furthermore, children of mothers who are occupationally exposed to PCBs but not to PCDFs show much lower toxicity, even though the levels of PCBs in the blood of the mothers are comparable to levels in Yusho and Yu Cheng patients. PCDFs are known to be toxic at much lower concentrations (Tanabe et al., 1989; Kannan et al., 1988). It is therefore assumed that at least part of the toxicity is due to the PCDFs detected in the contaminated cooking oil (Rogan et al., 1988). A comparative toxic evaluation of the contaminants, found in Yusho patient's adipose tissue based on "2,3,7,8-TCDD Toxic Equivalent Analysis" reveals that 2,3,4,7,8-PCDF was the principal causative agent in Yusho poisoning. It also reveals an accountable contribution from coplanar PCBs (Tanabe et al., 1989).

Effects on reproduction were also found in persons not exposed to high doses of xenobiotics. In the context of *in vitro* fertilization, pollutants were measured in human follicular fluid (Trapp et al., 1983; Baukloh et al., 1985). Direct effects of high concentrations of biocides on oocyte fertilization and embryonic development were not obvious, but there are indications that they could decrease the cleavage rate (Trapp et al., 1983). Other tests indicated that the development of the oocyte is not disturbed, but in an earlier stage the primordial oocyte could be disturbed (Baukloh et al., 1985). In men, an inverse correlation between PCB and p,p'-DDE concentrations, with sperm motility index in samples with a sperm count less than $20 \times 10^6$ cells/ml, was found (Bush et al., 1986). Further reproductive effects have recently been found: a possible correlation between miscarriges and levels of PCBs (Leoni et al., 1989) and a correlation seems to exist between late hemorrhagic diseases in newborn babies and organochlorines in mother's milk (Koppe et al., 1989).

It is very difficult to obtain causal relationships between exposure to xenobiotics and hormone related reproductive effects in humans. Clearly, a simple case of extrapolation of effects found in animals to humans, is not adequate. Specificity of certain enzymes and differences in composition of involved compounds, with different physicochemical properties in each organism, contribute to this lack of consistency.

## FUTURE GLOBAL OCEANIC PCB TRENDS

It can be deduced from the aforementioned sections that PCBs are among the most prominent pollutants to be concerned about. Therefore an estimate of future global oceanic levels is provided based on past and present levels.

It was estimated that 1.5 million tonnes of PCBs have been produced on a global basis since the 1930s (Marquenie and Reijnders, 1989). Calculations suggest that about 20%—30% of all produced PCBs in one way or the other have found their way into the environment, accumulated in dumpsites or in sediments of lakes and coastal zones (Tanabe, 1988). This portion of the PCBs is beyond control and a certain portion will gradually be found in organisms. Even though global production of PCBs has now stopped, more than 70% of the global production is still in use, or in stock, and could reach the environment in the future. If this very large pool of PCBs is not located and destroyed in a controlled way, the risk is substantial that serious ecotoxicological effects will happen in the marine environment. From the past we learned that adequate measures to reduce the production and use of PCBs could result in lower concentrations in biota. After measures by the Baltic countries, the concentrations of PCBs in both Baltic fish and fish predators are in some areas about 50% of the concentrations in the early 1970s. The decrease in concentrations started approximately seven years after the international bans on the production and use of PCBs (Olsson and Reutergårdh, 1986; Bignert et al., 1992). However, in the southern part of the Swedish Baltic no decrease was found, and today the further decrease in the other areas is slow, if present at all. There are reasons to assume a continuous output of PCBs at a lower level.

We have estimated to date that only $\pm 1\%$ of the total quantity of PCBs have reached the open ocean. If the observed rise in PCB concentrations in oceanic top predators continues at the same rate, it can be expected that, in marine mammals, the levels associated with insufficient recruitment may be exceeded within 200 years (Marquenie and Reijnders, 1989). Since zooplankton reproduction is also affected by PCBs, increasing PCB concentrations may generate large algal blooms. These blooms are caused by reduced zooplankton grazing and might explain the co-occurrence of increased PCB concentration in samples dominated by the microflagellate, *Phaeocystis globosa*, found during surveys in the North Sea (Knickmeyer and Steinhart, 1989).

## CONCLUDING REMARKS

Hormonal imbalance and associated developmental disorders induced by xenobiotics are observed throughout the entire marine ecosystem. In certain cases clear xenobiotic interference with the endocrine system, i.e., biosynthesis and biotransformation, can be demonstrated. However, it is proving difficult to link any observed effects with one given pollutant. In the suite of disturbances presented in this paper, hormonal changes could be associated with specific xenobiotics during the early phase of reproductive cycles, although the underlying mechanisms remain unclear.

A prominent role in controlling toxicity as well as hormone balance is carried out by the mixed function oxygenase system, including the hepatic microsomal cytochrome P-450 enzyme systems. Metabolization of xenobiotic and endobiotic compounds occurs via induction of the P-450 systems, with the many isoenzymes from that system exhibiting substrate specificity. This implies that for each compound, in each organism, and even in each organ, different isoenzymes are involved. Extreme caution is therefore needed to extrapolate results found for some compounds in some species to other compounds and/or other species. The major task of identifying those isoenzymes and corresponding enzyme profiles, might be facilitated by grouping compounds based on their structure-activity relationships (Goldstein and Safe, 1989).

As a consequence of the involvement of so many different isoenzymes, P-450 enzyme profiles are manifold as well. However, the existence of a specific enzyme profile for each compound in a given species/organ, could offer unique opportunities for environmental risk assessment, especially for the toxicity of organochlorine pollutants. In combination with continued search for target organisms, like whelks for effects of TBT, the essential elements to develop a more predictive concept to assess environmental impact of pollutants are provided as outlined for marine mammals in Reijnders (1988a).

Trace quantities of a large number of contaminants are found to occur commonly in humans. Compared to marine animals who carry much larger body burdens of the same contaminants, only moderate adverse effects of xenobiotics on endocrine functioning have been reported in humans. However, there are indications that reproductive disorders do occur.

Without ignoring the single and/or synergistic effects of other contaminants, organochlorines are—in the context of this chapter—considered to be the most immediate threat to marine organisms, as well as other wildlife, and humans. In particular PCBs concentrations, in different ecosystems will remain high, or continue to rise in the future. There is worldwide potential for PCBs to reach levels leading to seriously affected recruitment in fish-eating marine mammals and also to generate large algal blooms. Unless adequate retrieval and disposal of remaining PCBs in use is enforced, these noxious compounds will in the near future become an even larger global environmental problem than at present.

## REFERENCES

Akiyama, K., Ohi, G., Fujitani K., Yagyu H., Ogino M., and Kawana, T. (1975). Polychlorinated biphenyl residues in maternal and cord blood in Tokyo metropolitan area. *Bull. Environm. Contam. Toxicol.*, **14**, 588-592.

Anderson, H.A. (1989). General population exposure to environmental concentrations of halogenated biphenyls. In *Halogenated Biphenyls, Terphenyls, Naphthalenes, Dibenzodioxins and Related Products*, eds. R.D. Kimbrough and A.A. Jensen. Elsevier Amsterdam, New York, Oxford, pp. 345-380.

Bailey, G.S., Selivonchick, D., and Hendricks, J. (1987). Initiation, promotion, and inhibition of carcinogenesis in rainbow trout. *Environm. Health Persp.*, **71**, 147-153.

Baukloh, V., Bohnet, H.G., Trapp, M., Heeschen, W., Feichtinger, W., and Kemeter, P. (1985). Biocides in human follicular fluid. *In Vitro Fert. Embryo Trans.*, **442**, 240-250.

Bergman, A. and Olsson, M. (1985). Pathology of baltic grey seal and ringed seal females with special reference to adrenocortical hyperplasia: is environmental pollution the cause of widely distributed disease syndrome? *Finn. Game Res.*, **44**, 47-62.

Besten, den P.J. (1991). Effects of cadmium and PCBs on reproduction of the sea star *Asterias rubens*. Ph.D. Thesis, Univ. Utrecht, The Netherlands, pp. 148.

Bignert, A., Göthberg, A., Jensen, S., Litzén, K., Odsjö, T., Olsson, M., and Reutergårdh, L. (1992). The need for adequate biological sampling in ecotoxicological investigations. *Sci. Tot. Environm.*, (in press).

Boon, J.P., Arnhem, E., Jansen, S., Kannan, N., Petrick, G., Schulz, D., Duinker, J.C., Reijnders, P.J.H., and Goksøyr, A. (1992). The toxicokinetics of PCBs in marine mammals with special reference to possible interactions of individual congeners with the cytochrome P-450-dependent monooxygenase system--an overview. In *Persistent Pollutants In Marine Ecosystems*, eds. C.H. Walker and Livingstone. SETAC Spec. Publ. in press.

Brouwer, A., Reijnders, P.J.H., and Koeman, J.H. (1989). Polychlorinated biphenyl (PCB)-contaminated fish induces vitamin A and thyroid hormone deficiency in the common seal, *Phoca vitulina*. *Aq. Tox.*, **15**, 99-106.

Brouwer, A., Murk, A.J., and Koeman, J.H. (1990). Biochemical and physiological approaches in ecotoxicology. *Funct. Ecol.*, **4**, 275-281.

Bryan, G.W., Gibbs, P.E., and Burt, G.R. (1988). A comparison of the effectiveness of tri-N-butyltin chloride and five other organotin compounds in promoting the development of imposex in the dogwhelk, *Nucella lapillus*. *J. mar. biol. Ass. U.K.*, **68**, 733-744.

Bush, B., Bennet, A.H., and Snow, J.T. (1986). Polychlorobiphenyl congeners, p,p'-DDE and sperm function in humans. *Arch. Environm. Contam. and Toxicol.*, **15**, 333-341.

Chen, T.T., Reid, P.C., van Beneden, R., and Sonstegard, R.A. (1986). Effect of Aroclor 1254 and Mirex on estradiol-induced vitellogin production in juvenile Rainbow trout *Salmo gairdneri*. *Can J. Fish. Aq. Sci.*, **43**, 169-173.

Conney, A.H. (1967). Pharmacological implications of microsomal enzyme induction. *Pharmacol. Rev.*, **19**, 317-366.

Davis, P.H., Schultz, T.W., and Spies, R.W. (1981). Toxicity of Santa Barbara seep oil to starfish embryos: Part 2. The growth bioassay. *Mar. Environm. Res.*, **5**, 287-294.

DeLong, R.L., Gilmartin, W.G., and Simpson, J.G. (1973). Premature births in California sea lions: association with high organochlorine pollutant residue levels. *Science*, **181**, 1168-1170.

Ellis, D.V. and Pattisina, L.A. (1990). Widespread Neogastropod imposex: a biological indicator of global TBT contamination. *Mar. Poll. Bull.*, **21**, 248-253.

Elskus, A.A., Stegeman, J.J., Susani, L.C., Black, D., Pruell, R.J., and Fluck, S.J. (1989). Polychlorinated biphenyls concentration and cytochrome P-450E expression in winter flounder from contaminated environments. *Mar. Environm. Res.*, **28**, 25-30.

Fein, G.G, Jacobson, J.L., Jacobson, S.W., Schwartz, P.M., and Dowler, J.K. (1984). Prenatal exposure to polychlorinated biphenyls: Effects on birth size and gestational age. *J. Pediatr.*, **105**, 315 -320.

Freeman, H.C. and Sangalang, G.B. (1977). A study of the effects of methyl mercury, cadmium, arsenic, selenium, and a PCB (Aroclor 1254) on adrenal and testicular steroidogeneses *in vitro*, by the Grey seal *Halichoerus grypus. Arch. Environm. Contam. and Toxicol.*, **5**, 369-383.

Freeman, H.C., Sangalang, G.B., and Flemming, B. (1982). The sublethal effects of polychlorinated biphenyl (Aroclor 1254) diet on the Atlantic cod *Gadus morhua. Sci. Tot. Environm.*, **24**, 1-11.

Freeman, H.C., Sangalang, G.B., and Uthe, J.F. (1984). The effects of pollutants and contaminants on steroidogenesis in fish and marine mammals. *Adv. Environm. Sci. Technol.*, **16**, 197-211.

Fries, C.R. and Lee, R.F. (1984). Pollutant effects on the mixed function oxygenase (MFO) and reproductive systems of the marine polychaete *Nereis virens. Mar. Biol.*, **79**, 187-193.

Fry, D.M. and Toone, C.K. (1981). DDT-induced feminization of Gull embryos. *Science*, **213**, 922-924.

Goksøyr, A., Andersson, T., Förlin, L., Stenersen, J., Snowberger, E.A., Woodin, B.R., and Stegeman, J.J. (1988). Xenobiotic and steroid metabolism in adult and foetal Piked (Minke) whales *Balaenoptera acutorostrata. Mar. Environm. Res.*, **24**, 9-13.

Goldstein, J.A. and Safe, S. (1989). Mechanisms of action and structure-activity relationship for the chlorinated dibenzo-p-dioxins and related compounds. In *Halogenated Biphenyls, Terphenyls, Naphthalenes, Dibenzodioxins and Related Products*, eds. R.D. Kimbrough and A.A. Jensen. Elsevier Amsterdam, New York, Oxford, pp. 239-293.

Hove Holdrinet, van M., Braun, H.E., Frank, R., Stopps, G.J., Smout, M.S., and McWade, J.W. (1977). Organochlorine residues in human adipose tissue and milk from Ontario residents, 1969-1974. *Can. J. Publ. Health.*, **68**, 74-79.

Jacobson, J.L., Jacobson, S.W., and Humphrey, H.E.B. (1990). Effects of exposure to PCBs and related compounds on growth and activity in children. *Neurotox. Teratol.*, **12**, 319 -326.

Jensen, S. (1989). Background levels in humans. In *Halogenated Biphenyls, Terphenyls, Naphthalenes, Dibenzodioxins and Related Products*, eds. R.D. Kimbrough and A.A. Jensen. Elsevier Amsterdam, New York, Oxford, pp. 345-380.

Jensen, S. and Sundström, G. (1974). Structures and levels of most chlorobiphenyls in two technical PCB products and in human adipose tissue. *Ambio*, **3**, 70-76.

Johnson, L.L., Casillas, E., Collier, T.K., McCain B.B., and Varanasi, U. (1988). Contaminant effects on ovarian development in English sole *Parophrys vetulus*, from Pudget Sound, Washington. *Can. J. Fish. and Aq. Sci.*, **45**, 2133-2146.

Kannan, N., Tanabe, S., and Tatsukawa, R. (1988). Potentially hazardous residues of non-orthochlorine substituted coplanar PCBs in human adipose tissue. *Arch. Environm. Health.*, **43**, 11-14.

Khristoforova, N.K., Gnezdibova, S.M., and Vlasova, G.A. (1984). Effect of cadmium on gametogenesis and offspring of the sea urchin, *Strongylocentrotus intermedius*. *Mar. Ecol. Prog. Ser.*, **17**, 9-14.

Kluytmans, J.H., Brands, F., and Zandee, D.I. (1988). Interactions of cadmium with the reproductive cycle of *Mytilus edulis L. Mar. Environm. Res.*, **24**, 189-192.

Knickmeyer, R. and Steinhart, H. (1989). Cyclic organochlorines in plankton from the North Sea in spring. *Estuar. Coast. Shelf Sci.*, **28**, 117-127.

Koppe, J.G., Pluim, E., and Olie, K. (1989). Breastmilk, PCBs, dioxins and vitamin K deficiency: discussion paper. *J. Royal Soc. Med.*, **82**, 416-420.

Kuiper, J. (1982). The use of model ecosystems for the validation of screening tests for biodegradation and acute toxicity. TNO, The Hague, The Netherlands, Report Cl 82/01, pp. 101.

Kuratsune, M. (1989). Yusho, with reference to Yu-Cheng. In *Halogenated Biphenyls, Terphenyls, Naphthalenes, Dibenzodioxins and Related Products*, eds. R.D. Kimbrough and A.A. Jensen. Elsevier Amsterdam, New York, Oxford, pp. 401-416.

Leoni, V., Fabiani, L., Marinelli, G. Puccetti, G., Tarsitani, G.F., De Carolis, A., Vescia, N., Morini, A., Aleandri, V., Pozzi, V., Cappa, F., and Barbati, D. (1989). PCB and other organochlorine compounds in blubber of women with or without miscarriage: a hypothesis of correlation. *Ecotox. Environment. Safety*, **17**, 1-11.

Livingstone, D.R. (1990). Cytochrome P-450 and oxidative metabolism in invertebrates. *Biochem. Soc. Trans.*, **18**, 15-19.

Marquenie, J.M. and Reijnders, P.J.H. (1989). PCBs, an increasing concern for the marine environment. ICES: CM, 1989/N:12, pp 5.

Martineau, D., Béland, P., Desjardins C., and Vézina, A. (1985). Pathology, toxicology and effects of contaminants on the population of the St. Lawrence beluga *Delphinapterus leucas*, Quebec, Canada. ICES:CM, 1985/N:13.

O'Hara, S.C.M., Neal, A.C., Cornet, E.D.S., and Pulslord, A.L. (1985). Interrelationships of cholesterol and hydrocarbon metabolism in the shore crab *Carcinus maenas. J. mar. biol. Ass. U.K.*, **65**, 113-131.

Olsson, M. and Reutergardh, L. (1986). DDT and PCB pollution trends in the Swedish aquatic environment. *Ambio*, **15**, 103-109.

Pagano, M., Cipollaro, M., Corsale, G., Esposito, A., Ragucci, E., Giordano, G.G., and Trieff, N.M. (1985). Comparative toxicities of chlorinated biphenyls on sea urchin egg fertilization and embryogenesis. *Mar. Environm. Res.*, **17**, 240-244.

Parkinson, A. and Safe, S. (1987). Mammalian biologic and toxic effects of PCBs. In *Polychlorinated Biphenyls (PCBs): Mammalian and Environmental Toxicology*, ed. S. Safe. Springer, Berlin, pp. 49-75.

Reggiani, G.M. (1989). The Seveso accident: Medical survey of a TCDD exposure. In *Halogenated Biphenyls, Terphenyls, Naphthalenes, Dibenzodioxins and Related Products*, eds R.D. Kimbrough and A.A. Jensen. Elsevier Amsterdam, New York, Oxford, pp. 445-470.

Reijnders, P.J.H. (1986). Reproductive failure in common seals feeding on fish from polluted coastal waters. *Nature*, **324**, 456-457.

Reijnders, P.J.H. (1988a). Ecotoxicological perspectives in marine mammalogy: research principles and goals for a conservation policy. *Mar. Mamm. Sci.*, **4**, 91-102.

Reijnders, P.J.H. (1988b). Environmental impact of PCBs in the marine environment. In *Environmental Protection of the North Sea*. eds P.J. Newman and A.R. Agg. Heineman Professional Publ., Oxford, pp. 85-98.

Rogan, W.J. (1989). Yu-Cheng. In *Halogenated Biphenyls, Terphenyls, Naphthalenes, Dibenzodioxins and Related Products*, eds. R.D. Kimbrough and A.A. Jensen. Elsevier Amsterdam, New York, Oxford, pp. 401-416.

Rogan, W.J., Gladen, B.C., Hung, K.L., Koong, S.L., Shih, L.Y., Taylor, J.S., Wu, Y.C., Yang, D., Ragan, N.B., and Hsu, C.C. (1988). Congenital poisoning by polychlorinated biphenyls and their contaminants in Taiwan. *Science*, **241**, 334-336.

Safe, S. (1984). Polychlorinated biphenyls (PCBs) and polybrominated biphenyls (PBBs): Biochemistry, toxicology and mechanism of action. *CRC Crit. Rev. Toxicol.*, **13**, 319-393.

Safe, S. (1987). PCB and human health. In *Polychlorinated Biphenyls (PCBs): Mammalian and Environmental Toxicology*, ed. S. Safe. Springer. Berlin, pp. 133-145.

Saavreda Alvarez, M.M. and Ellis, D.V. (1990). Widespread *Neogastropod imposex* in the Northeast Pacific: implications for TBT contamination surveys. *Mar. Poll. Bull.*, **21**, 244-247.

Slorach, S.A. and Vaz, R. (1985). PCB levels in breast milk: data from the UNEP/WHO pilot project on biological monitoring and some other recent studies. *Environm. Health Perspect.*, **60**, 121-126

Spence, S.K., Bryan, G.W., Gibbs, P.E., Masters, D., Morris, L., and Hawkins, S.J. (1990). Effects of TBT contamination on *Nucella* populations. *Funct. Ecol.*, **4**, 425-432.

Stephenson, M.D., Smith, D.R., Goetzl, J., Ichikawa G., and Martin, M. (1986). Growth abnormalities in mussels and oysters from areas with high levels of Tributyltin in San Diego Bay. *Proc. Oceans*, **86**, 1246-1251.

Stott, G.G., Haensly, W., Neff, J., and Sharp, J. (1983). Histopathologic survey of ovaries of plaice *Pleuronectus platessa L.*, from AberWrac'h and Aber Benoit, Brittany, France, oil spills. *J. Fish Dis.*, **6**, 429-437.

Subramanian, A., Tanabe, S., Tatsukawa, R., Saito S., and Miyazaki, N. (1987). Reduction in the testosterone levels by PCBs and DDE in Dall's porpoises of northwestern North Pacific. *Mar. Poll. Bull.*, **18**, 643-646.

Sunila, I. (1986). Histopathological changes in the mussel *Mytilus edulis L.*, at the outlet from a titanium dioxide plant in Northern Baltic. *Ann. Zool. Fennici*, **23**, 61-70.

Sunila, I. (1988). Pollution-related histopathological changes in the mussel *Mytilus edulis L.* in the baltic Sea. *Mar. Environm. Res.*, **24**, 277-280.

Tanabe, S. (1988). PCB problems in the future: Foresight from current knowledge. *Environm. Poll.*, **50**, 5-28.

Tanabe, S., Kannan, N., Wakimoto, T., Tatsukawa, R., Okamoto, T., and Masuda, Y. (1989). Isomere specific determination and toxic evaluation of potentially hazardous coplanar PCBs, dibenzofurans and dioxins in the tissues of "Yusho" PCB poisoning victim and in the causal oil. *Toxicol. Environm. Chem.*, **24**, 215-231.

Thomann, R.V., Connolly, J.P., and Thomas, N.A. (1987). The Great Lakes ecosystem -Modeling the fate of PCBs. In *PCBs and the Environment. Vol. III*, ed. Waid J.S. CRC Press Inc., Boca Raton, Florida, pp. 153-180.

Thomas, P. (1988). Reproductive endocrine function in female Atlantic croaker exposed to pollutants. *Mar. Environm. Res.*, **24**, 179-183.

Thomas, P. (1990). Effects of Aroclor 1254 and cadmium on reproductive endocrine function and ovarian growth in Atlantic croaker. *Mar. Environm. Res.*, **28**, 499-503.

Trapp, M., Baukloh, V., Bohnet, H.G., and Heeschen, W. (1983). Pollutants in human follicular fluid. *Fertil. Steril.*, **42**, 146-148.

Truscott, B., Walsh, J., Burton, M., Payne, J., and Idler, D. (1983). Effect of acute exposure to crude oil petroleum on some reproductive hormones in salmon and flounder. *Comp. Biochem. Physiol.*, **75C**, 121-130.

Voogt, P.A., Broertjes, J.J.S., and Oudejans, R.C.H.M. (1985). Vitellogenesis in sea star: physiological and metabolic implications. *Comp. Biochem. Physiol.*, **80A**, 141-147.

Voogt, P.A., den Besten, P.J., Kusters, G.C.M., and Messing, M.W.J. (1987). Effects of cadmium and zinc on steroid metabolism and steroid level in the sea star *Asterias rubens L. Comp. Biochem. Physiol.*, **84B**, 83-89.

Watanabe, S., Shimada, T., Nakamura, S., Nishiyama, N., Yamashita, N., Tanabe S., and Tatsukawa, R. (1989). Specific profile of microsomal cytochrome P-450 in dolphin and whales. *Mar. Environm. Res.*, **27**, 51-65.

# MALE REPRODUCTIVE SYSTEM ONTOGENY: EFFECTS OF PERINATAL EXPOSURE TO 2,3,7,8-TETRACHLORODIBENZO-*p*-DIOXIN

### Richard E. Peterson[1]
School of Pharmacy and Environmental Toxicology Center,
University of Wisconsin, Madison, Wisconsin

### Robert W. Moore
School of Pharmacy and Environmental Toxicology Center,
University of Wisconsin, Madison, Wisconsin

### Thomas A. Mably[2]
School of Pharmacy, University of Wisconsin, Madison, Wisconsin

### Donald L. Bjerke
School of Pharmacy, University of Wisconsin, Madison, Wisconsin

### Robert W. Goy
Wisconsin Regional Primate Research Center,
University of Wisconsin, Madison, Wisconsin

In utero *and lactational exposure of male rats to 2,3,7,8-tetra-chlorodibenzo-*p*-dioxin (TCDD) profoundly affects ontogeny of the reproductive system. Anogenital distance is reduced, testis descent is delayed, and testis, epididymis, and accessory sex organ weights are reduced throughout sexual development. In addition, spermatogenesis is inhibited, sexual behavior is both demasculinized and feminized, and the regulation of luteinizing hormone (LH) secretion is feminized. The ED50 for these effects is approximately 0.16 µg/kg when TCDD is given as a single maternal dose on Day 15 of pregnancy. The effects of TCDD on the male reproductive system described above appear to be due, in part, to perinatal reductions in plasma testosterone concentrations. TCDD and structurally related compounds may similarly affect ontogeny of the male reproductive system in a variety of other species.*

## INTRODUCTION

2,3,7,8-TCDD is one of 75 possible chlorinated dibenzo-*p*-dioxin congeners. It is the most potent of the polychlorinated and polybrominated dibenzo-*p*-dioxins (PCDDs, PBDDs), dibenzofurans (PCDFs, PBDFs), and biphenyls (PCBs, PBBs) and as such serves as the prototype congener for toxicity elicited by these classes of chemicals. Reproductive and developmental toxicity is generally believed to be caused by the parent compound; there is no evidence that TCDD

1. Corresponding Author: Dr. Richard E. Peterson, School of Pharmacy, University of Wisconsin, 425 N. Charter Street, Madison, WI 53706.
2. Present address: Wyeth-Ayerst Research, Chazy, NY 12921.

metabolites are involved. The toxic potency of TCDD is due to the number and position of chlorine substitutions on the dibenzo-*p*-dioxin molecule. Dioxin and furan congeners not having chlorine or bromine substitutions at the lateral 2, 3, 7, and 8 positions, and congeners having chlorine and bromine substitutions at positions in addition to the 2, 3, 7, and 8 positions, are less potent than TCDD (Safe, 1990). Nevertheless, provided a high enough dose of a less potent congener is administered, all 2,3,7,8-substituted PCDD and PBDD congeners will produce toxicity. Further, the pattern of responses within animals of the same species, strain, sex and age will generally be similar to that of TCDD (McConnell and Moore, 1979; Poland and Knutson, 1982).

A mechanism of action which PCDD, PBDD, PCDF, and PBDF congeners substituted in the lateral positions have in common is that they bind to the Ah receptor (Poland et al., 1976; Poland and Knutson, 1982). PCB and PBB congeners substituted in the lateral positions but not in the *ortho* positions (coplanar PCBs and PBBs) also bind to this protein, as can some laterally substituted PCBs and PBBs with a single *ortho* halogen. The Ah receptor-ligand complex then binds to a translocating protein that carries it into the nucleus (Hoffman et al., 1991). These activated complexes bind to specific sequences of DNA referred to as dioxin-responsive elements, resulting in alterations in gene transcription (Whitlock, 1987). There is evidence that this Ah receptor mechanism is involved in the antiestrogenic action of TCDD (Safe et al., 1991) and in its ability to produce structural malformations in mice (Couture et al., 1990). However, the role of the Ah receptor in producing other signs of female reproductive toxicity (hormonal irregularities in the estrous cycle, reduced litter size, and reduced fertility), male reproductive toxicity (altered regulation of LH (defined in abstract) secretion, reduced testicular steroidogenesis, reduced plasma androgen concentrations, reduced testis and accessory sex organ weights, abnormal testis morphology, decreased spermatogenesis, and reduced fertility), and developmental toxicity (fetal/neonatal growth retardation and death) remains to be established.

Those PCDD and PCDF congeners that are generally believed to act through an Ah receptor mechanism are also the congeners that are preferentially bioaccumulated by fish, birds, and mammals (Stalling et al., 1983; Cook et al., 1991; U.S. EPA, 1991). Furthermore, coplanar PCBs and/or mono-*ortho* chlorine-substituted analogs of the coplanar PCBs which can also act through an Ah receptor mechanism bioaccumulate in fish, wildlife, and humans (Kannan et al., 1988; Mac et al., 1988; Tanabe, 1988; Kubiak et al., 1989; Smith et al., 1990). Sufficiently high cumulative body burdens of these halogenated aromatic hydrocarbons are of concern because a potential combined effect of the laterally substituted PCDD, PBDD, PCDF, PBDF, PCB, and PBB congeners which act through an Ah receptor mechanism is to decrease feral fish and wildlife populations secondary to developmental and/or reproductive toxicity (Gilbertson, 1989; Cook et al., 1991; Walker et al., 1991; Walker and Peterson, 1991). Humans are not exempt from the reproductive and developmental effects of complex halogenated aromatic hydrocarbon mixtures. Such mixtures which contain both TCDD-like congeners and non-TCDD-like congeners have been implicated in causing reproductive and developmental toxicity in the Yusho and Yu-Cheng poisoning incidents in Japan and Taiwan (Hsu et al., 1985; Kuratsune, 1989; Rogan, 1989). Thus, exposure to TCDD-like congeners during early development is of concern for humans as well as for domestic animals, fish and wildlife.

## RATIONALE FOR INVESTIGATING EFFECTS OF TRANSPLACENTAL AND LACTATIONAL TCDD EXPOSURE ON THE MALE REPRODUCTIVE SYSTEM

Since TCDD can decrease plasma androgen concentrations when given to adult rats (Moore et al., 1985, 1989), and since it can be transferred from mother to young *in utero* and during lactation (Moore et al., 1976; Van den Berg et al., 1987), TCDD is expected to have its greatest impact on the male reproductive system during early development (Mably et al., 1991). This is because testosterone and/or its metabolite 5α-dihydrotestosterone (DHT) are essential prenatally and/or early postnatally for imprinting and development of accessory sex organs (Chung and Raymond, 1976; Rajfer and Coffey, 1979; Coffey, 1988) and for initiation of spermatogenesis (Steinberger and Steinberger, 1989). In addition, aromatization of testosterone to 17β-estradiol within the central nervous system (CNS) is required perinatally for the imprinting of typical adult male patterns of reproductive behavior (Naftolin et al., 1975) and LH secretion (Barraclough, 1980). Thus, normal development of male reproductive organs and imprinting of typical adult sexual behavior patterns require sufficient testosterone be secreted by the testis at critical times in early development before and shortly after birth (MacLusky and Naftolin, 1981; Wilson et al., 1981) and requires that 17β-estradiol, derived from the aromatization of testosterone in the brain, be involved in mediating sexual differentiation of the CNS. TCDD may affect this CNS imprinting because it is known to decrease perinatal plasma testosterone concentrations (Mably et al., 1991; 1992a) and to exert an antiestrogenic effect in rats (Safe et al., 1991).

## DECREASES IN FETAL AND NEONATAL PLASMA TESTOSTERONE CONCENTRATIONS

To determine if perinatal exposure to TCDD produces an androgenic deficiency before and/or shortly after birth, Mably et al. (1991; 1992a) dosed pregnant rats with 1.0 μg TCDD/kg on Day 15 of gestation (Day 0 = sperm positive). Day 15 of gestation was chosen for TCDD treatment because most organogenesis in the fetus is complete by this time and because the hypothalamic/pituitary/testis axis is just beginning to function (Warren et al., 1975, 1984; Aubert et al., 1985). Plasma testosterone concentrations were greater in control male than in control female fetuses on Days 17-21 of gestation, particularly during the prenatal testosterone surge (Days 17-19). On Days 18-21 of gestation, TCDD exposure significantly reduced the magnitude of this sex-based difference. Postnatally, plasma testosterone concentrations peaked 2 hours after birth in control males, whereas in TCDD-exposed males the peak did not occur until 4 hours after birth and was only half as large. Thus, in male rats TCDD can produce both prenatal and early postnatal androgen deficiencies.

## OVERT FETAL AND MATERNAL TOXICITY

To determine how the ontogeny of the male reproductive system is affected by *in utero* and lactational TCDD exposure, Mably et al. (1991; 1992 a,b,c) treated pregnant rats with a single oral dose of TCDD (0.064, 0.16, 0.40, or 1.0 μg/kg) or vehicle on Day 15 of gestation. TCDD exposure of the pups, via the mother, ended at weaning (21 days after birth). The consequences of TCDD exposure for the male offspring were characterized at various stages of postnatal sexual development.

Mably and coworkers (1992a) found that TCDD treatment had no effect on maternal daily feed intake during pregnancy and the first 10 days after delivery. Nor did it have an effect on body weight of the dams on Day 20 of gestation or on Days 1, 7, 14 or 21 postpartum. Treating dams with graded doses of TCDD on Day 15 of gestation had no effect on the percentage of dams that delivered at least one live offspring, the length of gestation, or litter size. Except for an 8% decrease at the highest maternal dose, TCDD had no effect on live birth index (as determined by visual inspection of the litters). Neither the 4-day nor 21-day survival index was significantly affected by TCDD. In all dosage groups the number of dead offspring was evenly distributed between males and females. In TCDD-exposed offspring perinatal mortality was often associated with gastrointestinal hemorrhages; this sign of developmental toxicity was not observed in dead control fetuses and neonates. Of the females that failed to deliver litters, none were pregnant as evidenced by an absence of ammonium sulfide-stained implantation sites in the uteri. Signs of overt toxicity among the offspring were limited to the above mentioned 8% decrease in live birth index (highest dose only), initial 8-19% decreases in body weight (two highest doses), and initial 13-21% decreases in postweaning feed intake (measured for males only, two highest doses). The latter two effects disappeared by early adulthood. No male or female offspring with gross external malformations were found.

## DECREASES IN ANDROGENIC STATUS

Androgenic status of the male offspring includes such parameters as plasma androgen concentrations and androgen-dependent structures and functions. Anogenital distance, which is dependent on both circulating androgen concentrations and androgenic responsiveness (Neumann et al., 1970), was reduced in 1- and 4-day-old male pups, even when slight decreases in body length were considered. Testis descent, an androgen-mediated developmental event that normally occurs in rats between 20 and 25 days of age (Rajfer and Walsh, 1977), was delayed by up to 1.7 days. For the accessory sex organs to grow normally and respond fully to androgens in adulthood, there is a critical period which starts before birth and can last until puberty when adequate concentrations of androgens are necessary (Desjardins and Jones, 1970; Chung and Ferland-Raymond, 1975; Chung and Raymond, 1976; Rajfer and Coffey, 1979; Coffey, 1988). To determine if perinatal TCDD exposure affects postnatal growth of the accessory sex organs, one rat from each litter was sacrificed at 32, 49, 63, and 120 days of age (corresponding to juvenile, pubertal, postpubertal, and mature stages of sexual development, respectively). At each developmental stage dose-related decreases in seminal vesicle and ventral prostate weights were found that could not be explained by decreases in body weight. Trends for plasma testosterone and DHT concentrations to be decreased at these times, though not statistically significant, were also found, while plasma LH concentrations were generally unaffected. An exception was a 95% decrease in plasma LH concentration on Day 32 caused by a maternal TCDD dose of 1.0 µg/kg. The lowest maternal TCDD dose to affect androgenic status was 0.064 µg/kg (which significantly depressed ventral prostate weight at 32 days of age), while effects were commonly seen in response to 0.16 µg/kg. The reductions in seminal vesicle and ventral prostate weights may be due to modest concurrent reductions in plasma androgen concentrations and/or reductions in androgen responsiveness caused by incomplete perinatal imprinting of the accessory sex organs. These results, in combination with the finding that *in utero* TCDD exposure decreases plasma testosterone concentrations in males prior to birth, demonstrate that maternal TCDD treatment decreases the androgenic status of male rats from the fetal stage into adulthood. Table 1 summarizes the postnatal effects (Mably et al., 1991; 1992a).

## DECREASES IN SPERMATOGENESIS

Mably et al. (1991; 1992c) found that decreased spermatogenesis was among the most sensitive responses of the male rat reproductive system to perinatal TCDD exposure. Testis and epididymis weights and indices of spermatogenesis were determined on postnatal Days 32, 49, 63, and 120. Perinatal TCDD exposure caused dose-related decreases in testis and epididymis weights. Weights of the caudal portion of the epididymis, where mature sperm are stored prior to ejaculation, were decreased by as much as 53%. The number of sperm per cauda epididymis was decreased by 75% and 56% on Days 63 and 120, respectively; this decrease appeared to be the most sensitive effect of perinatal TCDD exposure on the male reproductive system. Daily sperm production was decreased by up to 43% at puberty (Day 49), but the decrease was less at sexual maturity (26% on Day 120). Seminiferous tubule diameter was decreased at all four developmental stages. Each effect of TCDD was dose-related and in all cases except testis weight a significant decrease was seen in response to the lowest maternal TCDD dose tested, 0.064 µg/kg, during at least one stage of sexual development. These results are summarized in Table 2 (Mably et al., 1991; 1992c).

In general, the magnitude of the decreases described above lessened with time, suggesting that perinatal TCDD exposure delays testicular development. Yet a

**TABLE 1.**   **Effects of *In Utero* and Lactational TCDD Exposure on Indices of Androgenic Status[a]**

| Index | Lowest effective maternal dose (µg TCDD/kg)[b] | Maximum effect[c] |
|---|---|---|
| Anogenital distance | 0.16 (Days 1 and 4) | 21% decrease (Day 1) |
| Time to testis descent | 0.16 | 1.7 day delay |
| Plasma testosterone concentration | n.s.[d] | 69% decrease (Day 32) |
| Plasma 5α-dihydrotestosterone concentration | n.s. | 59% decrease (Day 49) |
| Plasma luteinizing hormone concentration | 1.0 | 95% decrease (Day 32) |
| Seminal vesicle weight | 0.16 (Days 32 and 63) | 56% decrease (Day 49) |
| Ventral prostate weight | 0.064 (Day 32) | 60% decrease (Day 32) |

[a] Adapted, with permission, from Mably et al., (1991).
[b] The lowest dose of TCDD (given on Day 15 of gestation) that caused a significant ($p < 0.05$) effect in the male offspring and the day or days at which this dose caused such an effect are shown.
[c] The magnitude of the greatest change seen in response to maternal dosing with 1.0 µg TCDD/kg and the day at which this effect was seen are shown.
[d] n.s. indicates not statistically significant between 32 and 120 days after birth.

portion of the effect of TCDD on spermatogenesis also appears to be permanent. Daily sperm production in control rats reaches a maximum by 100-125 days of age (Robb et al., 1978), and spermatogenesis was still clearly affected by TCDD at 120 days of age, even in response to the lowest maternal dose tested (0.064 µg/kg). Furthermore, we recently found that a maternal TCDD dose of 1.0 µg/kg decreased daily sperm production in male rat offspring that were nearly 11 months old (Moore et al., 1992). It therefore appears that perinatal TCDD exposure both delays the development of spermatogenesis and permanently inhibits it.

## POTENTIAL MECHANISMS FOR DECREASED SPERMATOGENESIS

Severe preweaning and/or postweaning undernutrition can reduce sex organ weights and inhibit spermatogenesis in adult male rodents (Ghafoorunissa, 1980; Jean-Faucher et al., 1982a,b; Glass et al., 1986). However, reductions in sex organ weights, epididymal sperm reserves, and spermatogenesis occurred at the two lowest maternal TCDD doses, neither of which reduced feed intake, body weight, or crown-rump length of the male offspring. Only at the highest TCDD doses did decreases in feed consumption and body weight occur that could contribute to these reproductive system effects (Mably et al., 1992 a,c). Thus, undernutrition cannot account for the decreases in spermatogenesis observed at the lower maternal doses of TCDD, and it probably only accounts in part for the effects seen at higher doses.

---

**TABLE 2.**   **Effects of *In Utero* and Lactational TCDD Exposure on Indices of Spermatogenesis and Reproductive Capability[a]**

| Index | Lowest effective maternal dose ($\mu$g TCDD/kg)[b] | | Maximum effect[c] |
|---|---|---|---|
| Testis weight | 0.40 | (Day 32) | 17% decrease (Day 32) |
| Epididymis weight | 0.064 | (Days 49 and 120) | 35% decrease (Day 32) |
| Cauda epididymis weight | 0.064 | (Days 63 and 120) | 53% decrease (Day 63) |
| Sperm per cauda epididymis | 0.064 | (Days 63 and 120) | 75% decrease (Day 63) |
| Daily sperm production rate | 0.064 | (Days 63 and 120) | 43% decrease (Day 49) |
| Seminiferous tubule diameter | 0.064 | (Days 32, 49, 120) | 15% decrease (Day 32) |
| Leptotene spermatocyte: Sertoli cell ratio | n.s.[d] | | no dose-related effects |
| Sperm motility; percentage abnormal sperm | n.s. | | no dose-related effects |
| Fertility | n.s. | | 22% decrease (Day 70) |
| Gestation index; litter size; live birth index; pup survival | n.s. | | no dose-related effects |

[a] Adapted, with permission, from Mably et al., (1991).
[b] The lowest dose of TCDD (given on Day 15 of gestation) that caused a significant (p < 0.05) effect in the male offspring and the day or days at which this dose caused such an effect are shown.
[c] The magnitude of the greatest change seen in response to maternal dosing with 1.0 $\mu$g TCDD/kg and the day at which this effect was seen are shown.
[d] n.s. indicates not statistically significant.

---

Since follicle-stimulating hormone (FSH) and testosterone are essential for quantitatively normal spermatogenesis (Steinberger and Steinberger, 1989), an alternative explanation for the decreases in daily sperm production is a decrease in FSH and/or testosterone levels. In rats the duration of spermatogenesis is 52 days (Blazak et al., 1985; Amann, 1986; Working and Hurtt, 1987) so the slight decreases in plasma FSH concentrations observed in 32-day-old male offspring could contribute to the reductions of spermatogenesis when the rats were 49 and 63 days of age. However, this effect was transitory; no effect of perinatal TCDD exposure was found on plasma FSH levels when the offspring were 49, 63, and 120 days old. It was concluded that reduced spermatogenesis in 120-day-old male rats perinatally exposed to TCDD is not due to decreases in plasma FSH levels when the animals were 49-120 days of age (Mably et al., 1992c).

Mean plasma testosterone concentrations in the same rats were reduced up to 69% by perinatal TCDD exposure, yet intratesticular testosterone concentrations must be reduced by at least 80% in rats before spermatogenesis is impaired (Zirkin et al., 1989). Based on the magnitude of the reductions in plasma androgen concentrations, it was concluded that corresponding reductions in testicular testosterone concentrations in 32- to 120-day-old TCDD-exposed rats would probably not be severe enough to impair spermatogenesis (Mably et al., 1992a,c).

In explaining the decrease in spermatogenesis a key finding is that the ratio of leptotene spermatocytes to Sertoli cells in testes of 49-, 63-, or 120-day-old rats appeared to be unaffected by perinatal TCDD exposure (Mably et al., 1992c). This suggests two mechanisms for the decrease in daily sperm production: a decrease in spermatogenic efficiency and/or a decrease in Sertoli cell number. TCDD could decrease spermatogenic efficiency by increasing germ cell degeneration and/or by decreasing germ cell proliferation (meiosis). Furthermore, the lack of effect of TCDD on leptotene spermatocyte/Sertoli cell ratios indicates that decreased spermatogenic efficiency, if it occurs, must be subsequent to leptotene spermatocyte formation. Sertoli cells provide spermatogenic cells with functional and structural support and are essential for spermatogenesis (Bardin et al., 1988). Since each Sertoli cell supports a finite number of germ cells, the upper limit of daily sperm production depends on the number of Sertoli cells (Russell and Peterson, 1984). Thus, a TCDD-induced decrease in daily sperm production, without an effect on the leptotene spermatocyte/Sertoli cell ratio, is consistent with the possibility that the total number of Sertoli cells in the testes of rats exposed perinatally to TCDD might be decreased (Orth et al., 1988).

## LACK OF EFFECT ON SPERM MOTILITY AND MORPHOLOGY

The epididymis has two functions. In proximal regions spermatozoa mature, gaining the capacity for motility and fertility, whereas in distal regions mature sperm are stored before ejaculation (Robaire and Hermo, 1989). Mably et al. (1991; 1992c) found that motility and morphology of sperm taken from the cauda epididymis on postnatal Days 63 and 120 were unaffected by perinatal TCDD exposure. Thus, no effect of TCDD on epididymal function was detected. The dose-dependent reductions in epididymis and cauda epididymis weights in postpubertal rats (63 and 120 days old) can be accounted for, in part, by decreased sperm production. However, the decrease in weights of epididymal tissue in immature males (32 and 49 days of age) cannot be because sperm are not yet present in the epididymis. Since epididymal growth is androgen dependent (Setty and Jehan, 1977; Dhar and Setty, 1990), a TCDD-induced androgen deficiency and/or a decrease in androgen responsiveness of the epididymis could account for decreased size of the organ.

## LACK OF EFFECT ON REPRODUCTIVE CAPABILITY

To assess reproductive capability, male rats born to dams given TCDD (0.064, 0.16, 0.40, or 1.0 µg/kg) or vehicle on Day 15 of pregnancy were mated with control virgin females when the males were approximately 70 and 120 days of age (Mably et al., 1991; 1992c). The two highest maternal TCDD doses decreased the fertility index of male offspring by 11 and 22%, respectively (fertility index of the males is defined as the number of males impregnating females divided by the number of males that mated). However, these decreases were not statistically significant and at lower doses the fertility index was not affected. Gestation index, defined as the percentage of control females mated with TCDD-exposed males that delivered at least one live offspring, was also not affected by perinatal TCDD exposure. With respect to the progeny of these matings, there was no effect on litter size, live birth index, or 21-day survival index. When perinatal TCDD-exposed males were mated again at 120 days of age there was no effect on any of these same parameters. Thus, despite pronounced reductions in cauda epididymal sperm reserves at the times the TCDD-treated males were mated, perinatal TCDD exposure had little or no effect on fertility of male rats or on survival and growth of their offspring. These results (Mably et al., 1991; 1992c) are summarized in Table 2.

## POTENTIAL SIGNIFICANCE OF DECREASED SPERMATOGENESIS TO HUMANS

Since sexually mature rats produce and ejaculate ten times more sperm than are necessary for normal fertility and litter size (Aafjes et al., 1980; Amann, 1982), the absence of a reduction in fertility of male rats exposed perinatally to TCDD is not inconsistent with the substantial reductions in testicular spermatogenesis and epididymal sperm reserves. In contrast, reproductive efficiency in human males is very low, with the number of sperm per ejaculate being close to that required for fertility (Working, 1988). Thus, a percent reduction in daily sperm production in humans similar in magnitude to that observed in rats by Mably et al. (1991; 1992c) should reduce fertility in men. The finding that the developing reproductive system in male rats is exceptionally sensitive to TCDD suggests that reproductive function in human males might be more susceptible to TCDD than was previously believed.

## SEXUAL DIFFERENTIATION OF THE CENTRAL NERVOUS SYSTEM

Sexual differentiation of the CNS is dependent on the presence of androgens during early development. In rats the critical period for some aspects of CNS sexual differentiation, such as defeminization of the preovulatory LH surge system and masculinization of the morphology of the sexually dimorphic nucleus of the preoptic area in males, extends from late fetal life through the first week of postnatal life (MacLusky and Naftolin, 1981). In the absence of adequate circulating levels of testosterone during this time, adult rats display high levels of feminine sexual behavior (e.g., lordosis), low levels of masculine sexual behavior, and a cyclic (i.e., feminine) pattern of LH secretion (Gorski, 1974; Barraclough, 1980). In contrast, perinatal androgen exposure of rats will result in the masculinization of sexually dimorphic neural parameters including reproductive behaviors, regulation of LH secretion, and several morphological indices (Raisman and Field, 1973; Gorski et al., 1978). The mechanism by which androgens cause sexual differentiation of the CNS is not completely understood. In the rat it appears that 17β-estradiol, formed by the aromatization of testosterone within the CNS, is necessary for some aspects of CNS sexual differentiation, particularly defeminization (McEwen, 1978), however, androgens are also involved.

## DEMASCULINIZATION OF SEXUAL BEHAVIOR

Mably and coworkers (1991; 1992b) assessed sexually dimorphic functions in male rats born to dams given graded doses of TCDD or vehicle on Day 15 of pregnancy. Masculine sexual behavior was assessed at 60, 75 and 115 days of age by placing a male rat in a cage with a receptive control female and observing the first ejaculatory series and subsequent postejaculatory interval. The number of mounts and intromissions (mounts with vaginal penetration) before ejaculation were increased by a maternal TCDD dose as low as 0.064 and 1.0 μg/kg, respectively. The same males exhibited 12- and 11-fold increases in mount and intromission latencies, respectively, and a 2-fold increase in ejaculation latency. All latency effects were dose-related and were statistically significant at a maternal TCDD dose as low as 0.064 μg/kg (intromission latency) or 0.16 μg/kg (mount and ejaculation latencies). Copulatory rates (number of mounts + intromissions / time from first mount or intromission to ejaculation) were decreased up to 43%; this effect was dose-related and was statistically significant at maternal TCDD doses as low as 0.16 μg/kg. Postejaculatory intervals were increased up to 35%, an effect that was significant at maternal doses of TCDD as low as 0.40 μg/kg. Collectively, these results (Table 3) demonstrate that perinatal TCDD exposure demasculinizes sexual behavior.

Since perinatal exposure to a maternal dose of 1.0 μg TCDD/kg has no effect on the open field locomotor activity of adult male rats (Schantz et al., 1991), the increased mount, intromission, and ejaculation latencies appear to be specific for these masculine sexual behaviors, not secondary to a depressant effect of TCDD on motor activity. Mean postpubertal plasma testosterone and DHT concentrations in littermates of the rats evaluated for masculine sexual behavior were as low as 56 and 68% of control, respectively (Mably et al., 1991; 1992a). However, plasma testosterone concentrations only 33% of control are still sufficient to support masculine sexual behavior of adult male rats (Damassa et al., 1977). Therefore, the modest reductions in *adult* plasma androgen concentrations following perinatal TCDD exposure were not of sufficient magnitude, alone, to demasculinize sexual behavior.

Reductions in perinatal androgenic stimulation can inhibit penile development and subsequent sensitivity to sexual stimulation in adulthood (Nadler, 1969; Södersten and Hansen, 1978). Therefore, the demasculinization of sexual

**TABLE 3.** **Effects of *In Utero* and Lactational TCDD Exposure on Indices of Sexual Behavior and on the Regulation of LH Secretion in Adulthood[a]**

| Index | Lowest effective maternal dose (µg TCDD/kg)[b] | Maximum effect[c] |
|---|---|---|
| Masculine sexual behavior[d] | | |
| Mount latency | 0.16 | 1200% increase |
| Intromission latency | 0.064 | 1100% increase |
| Ejaculatory latency | 0.16 | 97% increase |
| Number of mounts | 0.064 | 130% increase |
| Number of intromissions | 1.0 | 38% increase |
| Copulatory rate (mounts + intromissions/min) | 0.16 | 43% decrease |
| Postejaculatory interval | 0.40 | 35% increase |
| | | |
| Feminine sexual behavior[e] | | |
| Lordosis quotient[f] | 0.16 | 200% increase |
| Lordosis intensity score | 0.40 | 50% increase |
| | | |
| Regulation of LH secretion | | |
| Progesterone-induced LH surge | 0.40 | 460% increase[g] |

[a] Adapted, with permission, from Mably et al., (1991).
[b] The lowest dose of TCDD (given on Day 15 of gestation) that caused a significant ($p < 0.05$) effect in the male offspring is shown.
[c] The magnitude of the change seen in response to maternal dosing with 1.0 µg TCDD/kg is shown (average of three trials for masculine behavior and two for feminine).
[d] Measured when the rats were approximately 60, 75, and 115 days of age.
[e] Feminine sexual behavior was measured following castration, estrogen priming, and progesterone administration. The rats were 170-185 days old.
[f] Number of times lordosis was displayed in response to a mount, divided by the number of times each rat was mounted, times 100.
[g] A percentage increase in this response cannot be calculated because control males do not respond to progesterone. This figure was calculated by comparing peak plasma LH concentrations in TCDD-exposed rats with plasma LH concentrations in control males at the same time.

behavior could, to some extent, be secondary to decreased androgen-dependent penile development. However, perinatal TCDD exposure had no effect on gross appearance of the rat penis. In addition, TCDD-exposed males exhibited deficits in such masculine sexual behaviors as mount latency and postejaculatory interval which do not depend on stimulation of the penis for expression (Sachs and Barfield, 1976). Thus, while some effects of TCDD, such as decreased copulatory rate and prolonged latency until ejaculation, could be due to reduced sensitivity of the penis to sexual stimulation, the 12-fold increase in mount latency and the increase in postejaculatory interval cannot be explained by this mechanism.

## FEMINIZATION OF SEXUAL BEHAVIOR

Mably et al. (1991; 1992b) determined whether the potential of adult male rats to display feminine sexual behavior was altered by perinatal TCDD exposure. Male offspring of dams treated on Day 15 of pregnancy with TCDD or vehicle were castrated at approximately 120 days of age and beginning at about 160 days of age were injected weekly for 3 weeks with 17β-estradiol benzoate, followed 42 hours later by progesterone. Four to six hours after the progesterone injection on weeks 2 and 3, each male was placed in a cage with a sexually excited control stud male. The frequency of lordosis in response to being mounted by the stud male was increased from 18% (control) to 54% by the highest maternal TCDD dose (1.0 μg/kg). Lordosis intensity in the males was also increased by perinatal TCDD exposure. Both effects were dose-related, and they were statistically significant at maternal TCDD doses as low as 0.16 μg/kg (increased lordotic frequency) and 0.40 μg/kg (increased lordotic intensity). Although severe undernutrition from 5 to 45 days after birth potentiates the display of lordosis behavior in adult male rats (Forsberg et al., 1985), the increased frequency of lordotic behavior was seen at a maternal TCDD dose (0.16 μg/kg) which had no effect on feed intake, body weight, or crown-rump length. It was concluded that perinatal TCDD exposure feminizes sexual behavior in adult male rats independent of undernutrition.

## FEMINIZATION OF THE REGULATION OF PITUITARY LH SECRETION

The effect of perinatal TCDD exposure on regulation of LH secretion by ovarian steroids was determined in male offspring at about 270 days of age. There is normally a distinct sexual dimorphism to this response. In rats castrated as adults, estrogen-primed females greatly increase their plasma LH concentrations when injected with progesterone, whereas similarly treated males fail to respond (Taleisnik et al., 1969). Progesterone had little if any effect on plasma LH concentrations in estrogen-primed control males, but significant increases were seen in males exposed to maternal TCDD doses of 0.40 and 1.0 μg/kg. Thus, perinatal TCDD exposure increases pituitary and/or hypothalamic responsiveness of male rats to ovarian steroids in adulthood, indicating that regulation of LH secretion is permanently feminized. Table 3 summarizes sexual behavior and LH secretion results (Mably et al., 1991; 1992b).

## TCDD APPEARS TO IMPAIR SEXUAL DIFFERENTIATION OF THE CENTRAL NERVOUS SYSTEM

The most plausible explanation for the demasculinization of sexual behavior and feminization of sexual behavior and LH secretion is that perinatal exposure to TCDD impairs sexual differentiation of the CNS. Neither undernutrition, altered locomotor activity, reduced sensitivity of the penis to sexual stimulation, nor modest reductions in *adult* plasma androgen concentrations of the male offspring can account for this effect (Mably et al., 1992b). On the other hand, exposure of the developing brain to testosterone, aromatization of testosterone to 17β-estradiol within the brain, and events initiated by the binding of 17β-estradiol to its receptor are all critical for sexual differentiation of the CNS. If TCDD interferes with any of these processes during late gestation and/or early neonatal life it could irreversibly demasculinize and feminize sexual behavior (Hart, 1972; McEwen et al., 1977; Whalen and Olsen, 1981) and feminize the regulation of LH secretion (Gogan et al., 1980, 1981) in adult male rats.

Treatment of dams on Day 15 of pregnancy with 1.0 μg TCDD/kg significantly decreases plasma testosterone concentrations in male rat fetuses on Days 18 through 21 of gestation and in male rat pups 2 hr postpartum (Mably et al., 1992a). Thus, the ability of maternal TCDD treatment to reduce prenatal and early postnatal plasma testosterone concentrations can account, in part, for the impaired sexual differentiation of male rats exposed perinatally to TCDD. Other mechanisms which may potentially contribute to the apparent TCDD-induced impairment in CNS sexual differentiation are (1) a decrease in the formation of 17β-estradiol from testosterone within the CNS that is independent of the decrease in plasma testosterone concentrations, (2) a reduction in responsiveness of the CNS to estrogen during the critical period of sexual differentiation, (3) and/or an increase in 17β-estradiol catabolism within the CNS. Each of these three mechanisms is consistent with the Ah receptor-mediated antiestrogen action of TCDD described for rat and mouse uterus, and for estrogen-responsive MCF-7 and Hepa 1c1c7 cells (Gierthy et al., 1987; Gierthy and Lincoln, 1988; Astroff and Safe, 1990; Harris et al., 1990; Spink et al., 1990; Zacharewski et al., 1991; Safe et al., 1991).

## POTENTIAL RELEVANCE OF IMPAIRED SEXUAL DIFFERENTIATION TO WILDLIFE AND HUMANS

The relevance of these findings to wildlife is that *in utero* and/or lactational exposure to TCDD and to structurally related chemicals may cause similar effects in wild mammalian species, such as nonhuman primates (Pomerantz et al., 1986; Thornton and Goy, 1986; Goy et al., 1988), in which reproductive system ontogeny is under androgenic control. With respect to humans, social factors account for much of the variation in sexually dimorphic behavior; however, there is evidence that prenatal androgenization influences the sexual differentiation of such behavior (Ehrhardt and Meyer-Bahlburg, 1981; Hines, 1982) and that human brain hypothalamic structure is sexually dimorphic, with homosexual men manifesting a feminine type of brain structure (LeVay, 1991). Thus, our findings in rats (Mably et al., 1991; 1992a,b,c) raise the possibility that TCDD and related Ah receptor agonists could potentially affect sexually dimorphic behavior and neural structure in wildlife and humans if TCDD exposure were to occur during perinatal development.

## ACKNOWLEDGEMENTS

We thank Dr. Frederick S. vom Saal, Dr. Stephen H. Safe and Dr. Stanley I. Dodson for peer reviewing this chapter prior to its acceptance for publication. This research was supported by NIH grant ES01332. This article is contribution 243, Environmental Toxicology Center, University of Wisconsin, Madison, WI 53706 and publication number 31-028 of the Wisconsin Regional Primate Research Center.

## REFERENCES

Aafjes, J.H., Vels, J.M., and Schenck, E. (1980). Fertility of rats with artificial oligozoospermia. *J. Reprod. Fertil.*, **58**, 345-351.

Amann, R.P. (1982). Use of animal models for detecting specific alterations in reproduction. *Fundam. Appl. Toxicol.*, **2**, 13-26.

Amann, R.P. (1986). Detection of alterations in testicular and epididymal function in laboratory animals. *Environ. Health Perspect.*, **70**, 149-158.

Astroff, B. and Safe, S. (1990). 2,3,7,8-Tetrachlorodibenzo-*p*-dioxin as an antiestrogen: Effect on rat uterine peroxidase activity. *Biochem. Pharmacol.*, **39**, 485-488.

Aubert, M.L., Begeot, M., Winiger, B.P., Morel, G., Sizonenko, P.C., and Dubois, P.M. (1985). Ontogeny of hypothalamic luteinizing hormone-releasing hormone (GnRH) and pituitary GnRH receptors in fetal and neonatal rats. *Endocrinology*, **116**, 1565-1576.

Bardin, C.W., Cheng, C.Y., Musto, N.A., and Gunsalus, G.L. (1988). The Sertoli cell. In *The Physiology of Reproduction*, ed. E. Knobil and J.D. Neill, Raven Press, New York, pp. 933-974.

Barraclough, C.A. (1980). Sex differentiation of cyclic gonadotropin secretion. In *Advances in the Biosciences*, Vol. 25, ed. A.M. Kaye and M. Kaye, Pergamon Press, New York, pp. 433-450.

Blazak, W.F., Ernst, T.L., and Stewart, B.E. (1985). Potential indicators of reproductive toxicity: Testicular sperm production and epididymal sperm number, transit time, and motility in Fischer 344 rats. *Fundam. Appl. Toxicol.*, **5**, 1097-1103.

Chung, L.W.K. and Ferland-Raymond, G. (1975). Differences among rat sex accessory glands in their neonatal androgen dependency. *Endocrinology*, **97**, 145-153.

Chung, L.W.K. and Raymond, G. (1976). Neonatal imprinting of the accessory sex glands and hepatic monooxygenases in adulthood. *Fed. Proc.*, **35**, 686.

Coffey, D.S. (1988). Androgen action and the sex accessory tissues. In *The Physiology of Reproduction*, ed. E. Knobil and J.D. Neill, Raven Press, New York, pp. 1081-1119.

Cook, P.M., Walker, M.K., Kuehl, D.W., and Peterson, R.E. (1991). Bioaccumulation and toxicity of TCDD and related compounds in aquatic ecosystems. In *Biological Basis for Risk Assessment of Dioxins and Related Compounds*, Banbury Report, Vol. 35, ed. M.A. Gallo, R.J. Scheuplein, and C.A. van der Heijden, Cold Spring Harbor Laboratory Press, Cold Spring Harbor, NY, pp. 143-167.

Couture, L.A., Abbott, B.D., and Birnbaum, L.S. (1990). A critical review of the developmental toxicity and teratogenicity of 2,3,7,8-tetrachlorodibenzo-*p*-dioxin: Recent advances toward understanding the mechanism. *Teratology*, **42**, 619-627.

Damassa, D.A., Smith, E.R., Tennent, B., and Davidson, J.M. (1977). The relationship between circulating testosterone levels and male sexual behavior in rats. *Horm. Behav.*, **8**, 275-286.

Desjardins, C. and Jones, R.A. (1970). Differential sensitivity of rat accessory-sex-tissues to androgen following neonatal castration or androgen treatment. *Anat. Rec.*, **166**, 299.

Dhar, J.D. and Setty, B.S. (1990). Changes in testis, epididymis and other accessory organs of male rats treated with Anandron during sexual maturation. *Endocr. Res.*, **16**, 231-239.

Ehrhardt, A.A. and Meyer-Bahlburg, H.F.L. (1981). Effects of prenatal sex hormones on gender-related behavior. *Science*, **211**, 1312-1318.

Forsberg, G., Abrahamsson, K., Södersten, P., and Eneroth, P. (1985). Effects of restricted maternal contact in neonatal rats on sexual behaviour in the adult. *J. Endocrinol.*, **104**, 427-431.

Ghafoorunissa. (1980). Undernutrition and fertility of male rats. *J. Reprod. Fertil.*, **59**, 317-320.

Gierthy, J.F. and Lincoln II, D.W. (1988). Inhibition of postconfluent focus production in cultures of MCF-7 human breast cancer cells by 2,3,7,8-tetrachlorodibenzo-*p*-dioxin. *Breast Cancer Res. Treat.*, **12**, 227-233.

Gierthy, J.F., Lincoln II, D.W., Gillespie, M.B., Seeger, J.I., Martinez, H.L., Dickerman, H.W., and Kumar, S.A. (1987). Suppression of estrogen-regulated extracellular tissue plasminogen activator activity of MCF-7 cells by 2,3,7,8-tetrachlorodibenzo-*p*-dioxin. *Cancer Res.*, **47**, 6198-6203.

Gilbertson, M. (1989). Effects on fish and wildlife populations. In *Halogenated Biphenyls, Terphenyls, Naphthalenes, Dibenzodioxins and Related Products*, 2nd edition, ed. R.D. Kimbrough and A.A. Jensen, Elsevier Science Publishers, Amsterdam, pp. 103-127.

Glass, A.R., Herbert, D.C., and Anderson, J. (1986). Fertility onset, spermatogenesis, and pubertal development in male rats: Effect of graded underfeeding. *Pediatr. Res.*, **20**, 1161-1167.

Gogan, F., Beattie, I.A., Hery, M., Laplante, E., and Kordon, C. (1980). Effect of neonatal administration of steroids or gonadectomy upon oestradiol-induced luteinizing hormone release in rats of both sexes. *J. Endocrinol.*, **85**, 69-74.

Gogan, F., Slama, A., Bizzini-Koutznetzova, B., Dray, F., and Kordon, C. (1981). Importance of perinatal testosterone in sexual differentiation in the male rat. *J. Endocrinol.*, **91**, 75-79.

Gorski, R.A. (1974). The neuroendocrine regulation of sexual behavior. In *Advances in Psychobiology*, Vol. 2, ed. G. Newton and A.H. Riesen, John Wiley and Sons, New York, pp. 1-58.

Gorski, R.A., Gordon, J.H., Shryne, J.E., and Southam, A.M. (1978). Evidence for a morphological sex difference within the medial preoptic area of the rat brain. *Brain Res.*, **148**, 333-346.

Goy, R.W., Bercovitch, F.B., and McBrair, M.C. (1988). Behavioral masculinization is independent of genital masculinization in prenatally androgenized female rhesus macaques. *Horm. Behav.*, **22**, 552-571.

Harris, M., Zacharewski, T., and Safe, S. (1990). Effects of 2,3,7,8-tetrachlorodibenzo-*p*-dioxin and related compounds on the occupied nuclear estrogen receptor in MCF-7 human breast cancer cells. *Cancer Res.*, **50**, 3579-3584.

Hart, B.L. (1972). Manipulation of neonatal androgen: Effects on sexual responses and penile development in male rats. *Physiol. Behav.*, **8**, 841-845.

Hines, M. (1982). Prenatal gonadal hormones and sex differences in human behavior. *Psychol. Bull.*, **92**, 56-80.

Hoffman, E.C., Reyes, H., Chu, F.F., Sander, F., Conley, L.H., Brooks, B.A., and Hankinson, B.A. (1991). Cloning of a factor required for activity of the Ah (dioxin) receptor. *Science*, **252**, 954-958.

Hsu, S.T., Ma, C.I., Hsu, S.K.H., Wu, S.S., Hsu, N.H.M., Yeh, C.C., and Wu, S.B. (1985). Discovery and epidemiology of PCB poisoning in Taiwan: A four-year followup. *Environ. Health Perspec.*, **59**, 5-10.

Jean-Faucher, C., Berger, M., de Turckheim, M., Veyssiere, G., and Jean, C. (1982a). The effect of preweaning undernutrition upon the sexual development of male mice. *Biol. Neonate,* **41**, 45-51.

Jean-Faucher, C., Berger, M., de Turckheim, M., Veyssiere, G., and Jean, C. (1982b). Effect of preweaning undernutrition on testicular development in male mice. *Int. J. Androl.*, **5**, 627-635.

Kannan, N., Tanabe, S., and Tatsukawa, R. (1988). Potentially hazardous residues of non-ortho chlorine substituted coplanar PCBs in human adipose tissue. *Arch. Environ. Health*, **43**, 11-14.

Kubiak, T.J., Harris, H.J., Smith, L.M., Schwartz, T., Stalling, D.L., Trick, J.A., Sileo, L., Docherty, D., and Erdman, T.C. (1989). Microcontaminants and reproductive impairment of the Forster's tern on Green Bay, Lake Michigan - 1983. *Arch. Environ. Contam. Toxicol.*, **18**, 706-727.

Kuratsune, M. (1989). Yusho, with reference to Yu-Cheng. In *Halogenated Biphenyls, Terphenyls, Naphthalenes, Dibenzodioxins and Related Products,* 2nd edition, ed. R.D. Kimbrough and A.A. Jensen, Elsevier Science Publishers, Amsterdam, pp. 381-400.

LeVay, S. (1991). A difference in hypothalamic structure between heterosexual and homosexual men. *Science*, **253**, 1034-1037.

Mably, T.A., Moore, R.W., Bjerke, D.L., and Peterson, R.E. (1991). The male reproductive system is highly sensitive to *in utero* and lactational TCDD exposure. In *Biological Basis for Risk Assessment of Dioxins and Related Compounds*, ed. M.A. Gallo, R.J. Scheuplein, and C.A. van der Heijden, Banbury Report Vol. 35, Cold Spring Harbor Laboratory Press, Cold Spring Harbor, New York, pp. 69-78.

Mably, T.A., Moore, R.W., and Peterson, R.E. (1992a). *In utero* and lactational exposure of male rats to 2,3,7,8-tetrachlorodibenzo-*p*-dioxin: 1. Effects on androgenic status. *Toxicol. Appl. Pharmacol.* **114**, 97-107.

Mably, T.A., Moore, R.W., Goy, R.W., and Peterson, R.E. (1992b). *In utero* and lactational exposure of male rats to 2,3,7,8-tetrachlorodibenzo-*p*-dioxin: 2. Effects on sexual behavior and the regulation of luteinizing hormone secretion in adulthood. *Toxicol. Appl. Pharmacol.*, **114**, 108-117.

Mably, T.A., Bjerke, D.L., Moore, R.W., Gendron-Fitzpatrick, A., and Peterson, R.E. (1992c). *In utero* and lactational exposure of male rats to 2,3,7,8-tetrachlorodibenzo-*p*-dioxin: 3. Effects on spermatogenesis and reproductive capability. *Toxicol. Appl. Pharmacol.*, **114**, 118-126.

Mac, M.J., Schwartz, T.R., and Edsall, C.C. (1988). Correlating PCB effects on fish reproduction using dioxin equivalents. *Soc. Environ. Toxicol. Chem.*, Ninth Annual Meeting Abstr., p. 116.

MacLusky, N.J. and Naftolin, F. (1981). Sexual differentiation of the central nervous system. *Science*, **211**, 1294-1303.

McConnell, E.E. and Moore, J.A. (1979). Toxicopathology characteristics of halogenated aromatics. *Ann. New York Acad. Sci.*, **320**, 138-150.

McEwen, B.S. (1978). Sexual maturation and differentiation: The role of the gonadal steroids. *Prog. Brain Res.*, **48**, 291-307.

McEwen, B.S., Lieburg, I., Chaptal, C., and Krey, L.C. (1977). Aromatization: Important for sexual differentiation of the neonatal rat brain. *Horm. Behav.*, **9**, 249-263.

Moore, J.A., Harris, M.W., and Albro, P.W. (1976). Tissue distribution of [$^{14}$C] tetrachlorodibenzo-*p*-dioxin in pregnant and neonatal rats. *Toxicol. Appl. Pharmacol.*, **37**, 146-147.

Moore, R.W., Potter, C.L., Theobald, H.M., Robinson, J.A., and Peterson, R.E. (1985). Androgenic deficiency in male rats treated with 2,3,7,8-tetrachlorodibenzo-*p*-dioxin. *Toxicol. Appl. Pharmacol.*, **79**, 99-111.

Moore, R.W., Parsons, J.A., Bookstaff, R.C., and Peterson, R.E. (1989). Plasma concentrations of pituitary hormones in 2,3,7,8-tetrachlorodibenzo-*p*-dioxin-treated male rats. *J. Biochem. Toxicol.*, **4**, 165-172.

Moore, R.W., Mably, T.A., Bjerke, D.L., and Peterson, R.E. (1992). *In utero* and lactational 2,3,7,8-tetrachlorodibenzo-*p*-dioxin (TCDD) exposure decreases androgenic responsiveness of male sex organs and permanently inhibits spermatogenesis and demasculinizes sexual behavior in rats. *The Toxicologist*, **12**, 81.

Nadler, R.D. (1969). Differentiation of the capacity for male sexual behavior in the rat. *Horm. Behav.*, **1**, 53-63.

Naftolin, F., Ryan, K.J., Davies, I.J., Reddy, V.V., Flores, F., Petro, Z., Kuhn, M., White, R.J., Takaoko, J., and Wolin, L. (1975). The formation of oestrogens by central neuroendocrine tissue. *Recent Prog. Horm. Res.*, **31**, 295-319.

Neumann, F., von Berswordt-Wallrabe, R., Elger, W., Steinbeck, H, Hahn, J.D., and Kramer, M. (1970). Aspects of androgen-dependent events as studied by antiandrogens. *Recent Prog. Horm. Res.*, **26**, 337-410.

Orth, J.M., Gunsalus, G.L., and Lamperti, A.A. (1988). Evidence from Sertoli cell-depleted rats indicates that spermatid number in adults depends on numbers of Sertoli cells produced during perinatal development. *Endocrinology*, **122**, 787-794.

Poland, A. and Knutson, J.C. (1982). 2,3,7,8-Tetrachlorodibenzo-*p*-dioxin and related halogenated aromatic hydrocarbons: Examination of the mechanism of toxicity. *Ann. Rev. Pharmacol. Toxicol.*, **22**, 517-554.

Poland, A., Glover, E., and Kende, A.S. (1976). Stereospecific, high affinity binding of 2,3,7,8-tetrachlorodibenzo-*p*-dioxin by hepatic cytosol. Evidence that the binding species is receptor for inducers of aryl hydrocarbon hydroxylase. *J. Biol. Chem.*, **251**, 4936-4946.

Pomerantz, S.M., Goy, R.W., and Roy, M.M. (1986). Expression of male-typical behavior in adult female pseudohermaphrodotic rhesus: Comparisons with normal males and neonatally gonadectomized males and females. *Horm. Behav.*, **20**, 483-500.

Raisman, G. and Field, P.M. (1973). Sexual dimorphism in the neurophil of the preoptic area of the rat and its dependence on neonatal androgen. *Brain Res.*, **54**, 1-29.

Rajfer, J. and Walsh, P.C. (1977). Hormonal regulation of testicular descent: Experimental and clinical observations. *J. Urol.*, **118**, 985-990.

Rajfer, J. and Coffey, D.S. (1979). Effects of neonatal steroids on male sex tissues. *Invest. Urol.*, **17**, 3-8.

Robaire, B. and Hermo, L. (1989). Efferent ducts, epididymis, and vas deferens: Structure, functions, and their regulation. In *The Physiology of Reproduction*, ed. E. Knobil and J.D. Neill, Raven Press, New York, pp. 999-1080.

Robb, G.W., Amann, R.P., and Killian, G.J. (1978). Daily sperm production and epididymal sperm reserves of pubertal and adult rats. *J. Reprod. Fertil.*, **54**, 103-107.

Rogan, W.J. (1989). Yu-Cheng. In *Halogenated Biphenyls, Terphenyls, Naphthalenes, Dibenzodioxins and Related Products*, 2nd edition, ed. R.D. Kimbrough and A.A. Jensen, Elsevier Science Publishers, Amsterdam, pp. 401-415.

Russell, L.D. and Peterson, R.N. (1984). Determination of the elongate spermatid-Sertoli cell ratio in various mammals. *J. Reprod. Fertil.*, **70**, 635-641.

Sachs, B.D. and Barfield, R.J. (1976). Functional analysis of masculine copulatory behavior in the rat. *Adv. Study Behav.*, **7**, 91-154.

Safe, S. (1990). Polychlorinated biphenyls (PCBs), dibenzo-*p*-dioxins (PCDDs), dibenzofurans (PCDFs), and related compounds: Environmental and mechanistic considerations which support the development of toxic equivalency factors (TEFs). *Crit. Rev. Toxicol.*, **21**, 51-88.

Safe, S., Astroff, B., Harris, M., Zacharewski, T., Dickerson, R., Romkes, M., and Biegel, L. (1991). 2,3,7,8-Tetrachlorodibenzo-*p*-dioxin (TCDD) and related compounds as antiestrogens: Characterization and mechanism of action. *Pharmacol. Toxicol.*, **69**, 400-409.

Schantz, S.L., Mably, T.A., and Peterson, R.E. (1991). Effects of perinatal exposure to 2,3,7,8-tetrachlorodibenzo-*p*-dioxin (TCDD) on spatial learning and memory and locomotor activity in rats. *Teratology*, **43**, 497.

Setty, B.S. and Jehan, Q. (1977). Functional maturation of the epididymis in the rat. *J. Reprod. Fertil.*, **49**, 317-322.

Smith, L.M., Schwartz, T.R., Feltz, K., and Kubiak, T.J. (1990). Determination and occurrence of AHH-active polychlorinated biphenyls, 2,3,7,8-tetra-chlorodibenzo-*p*-dioxin and 2,3,7,8-tetrachlorodibenzofuran in Lake Michigan sediment and biota. The question of their relative toxicological significance. *Chemosphere*, **21**, 1063-1085.

Södersten, P. and Hansen, S. (1978). Effects of castration and testosterone, dihydrotestosterone or oestradiol replacement treatment in neonatal rats on mounting behavior in the adult. *J. Endocrinol.*, **76**, 251-260.

Spink, D.C., Lincoln II, D.W, Dickerman, H.W., and Gierthy, J.F. (1990). 2,3,7,8-Tetrachlorodibenzo-*p*-dioxin causes an extensive alteration of 17β-estradiol metabolism in MCF-7 breast tumor cells. *Proc. Natl. Acad. Sci. (USA)*, **87**, 6917-6921.

Stalling, D.L., Smith, L.M., Petty, J.D., Hogan, J.W., Johnson, J.L., Rappe, C., and Buser, H.R. (1983). Residues of polychlorinated dibenzo-*p*-dioxins and dibenzofurans in Laurentian Great Lakes fish. In *Human and Environmental Risks of Chlorinated Dioxins and Related Compounds*, ed. R.E. Tucker, A.L. Young, and A.P. Gray, Plenum Press, New York, NY, pp. 221-240.

Steinberger, E. and Steinberger, A. (1989). Hormonal control of spermatogenesis. In *Endocrinology*, 2nd edition, ed. L.J. DeGroot, W.B. Saunders Co., Philadelphia, pp. 2132-2136.

Taleisnik, S., Caligaris, L., and Astrada, J.J. (1969). Sex difference in the release of luteinizing hormone evoked by progesterone. *J. Endocrinol.*, **44**, 313-321.

Tanabe, S. (1988). PCB problems in the future: Foresight from current knowledge. *Environ. Pollut.*, **50**, 5-28.

Thornton, J. and Goy, R.W. (1986). Female-typical sexual behavior of rhesus and defeminization by androgens given prenatally. *Horm. Behav.*, **20**, 129-147.

U.S. EPA (1991). Bioaccumulation of Selected Pollutants in Fish. A National Study, Vol.1. EPA 506/6-90/001a, Office of Water Regulations and Standards, Washington, DC, April, 1991.

Van den Berg, M., Heeremans, C., Veenhoven, E., and Olie, K. (1987). Transfer of polychlorinated dibenzo-*p*-dioxins and dibenzofurans to fetal and neonatal rats. *Fundam. Appl. Toxicol.*, **9**, 635-644.

Walker, M.K. and Peterson, R.E. (1991). Potencies of polychlorinated dibenzo-*p*-dioxins, dibenzofurans, and biphenyls, relative to 2,3,7,8-tetrachlorodibenzo-*p*-dioxin, for producing early life stage mortality in rainbow trout (*Oncorhynchus mykiss*). *Aquat. Toxicol.*, **21**, 219-238.

Walker, M.K., Spitsbergen, J.M., Olson, J.R., and Peterson, R.E. (1991). 2,3,7,8-Tetrachlorodibenzo-*p*-dioxin toxicity during early life stage development of lake trout (*Salvelinus namaycush*). *Can. J. Fish. Aquat. Sci.*, **48**, 875-883.

Warren, D.W., Huhtaniemi, I.T., Tapanainen, J., Dufau, M.L., and Catt, K.J. (1984). Ontogeny of gonadotropin receptors in the fetal and neonatal rat testis. *Endocrinology*, **114**, 470-476.

Warren, D.W., Haltmeyer, G.C., and Eik-Nes, K.B. (1975). The effect of gonadotrophins on the fetal and neonatal rat testis. *Endocrinology*, **96**, 1226-1229.

Whalen, R.E. and Olsen, K.L. (1981). Role of aromatization in sexual differentiation: Effects of prenatal ATD treatment and neonatal castration. *Horm. Behav.*, **15**, 107-122.

Whitlock, J.P. (1987). The regulation of gene expression by 2,3,7,8-tetrachlorodibenzo-*p*-dioxin. *Pharmacol. Rev.*, **39**, 147-161.

Wilson, J.D., George, F.W., and Griffin, J.F. (1981). The hormonal control of sexual development. *Science*, **211**, 1278.

Working, P.K. (1988). Male reproductive toxicology: Comparison of the human to animal models. *Environ. Health Perspect.*, **77**, 37-44.

Working, P.K. and Hurtt, M.E. (1987). Computerized videomicrographic analysis of rat sperm motility. *J. Androl.*, **8**, 330-337.

Zacharewski, T., Harris, M., and Safe, S. (1991). Evidence for the mechanism of action of the 2,3,7,8-tetrachlorodibenzo-*p*-dioxin-mediated decrease of nuclear estrogen receptor levels in wild-type and mutant Hepa 1c1c7 cells. *Biochem. Pharmacol.*, **41**, 1931-1939.

Zirkin, B.R., Santulli, R., Awoniyi, C.A., and Ewing, L.L. (1989). Maintenance of advanced spermatogenic cells in the adult rat testis: Quantitative relationship to testosterone concentration within the testis. *Endocrinology*, **124**, 3043-3049.

# TOXICITY OF POLYCHLORINATED DIBENZO-*p*-DIOXINS, DIBENZOFURANS, AND BIPHENYLS DURING EARLY DEVELOPMENT IN FISH

**Mary K. Walker**
Environmental Toxicology Center, University of Wisconsin, Madison, Wisconsin

**Richard E. Peterson**
School of Pharmacy, University of Wisconsin, Madison, Wisconsin

*Early life stages of fish are more sensitive than adults to the lethal effects of polychlorinated dibenzo-*p*-dioxins (PCDDs), dibenzofurans (PCDFs), and biphenyls (PCBs). Part per trillion concentrations of structurally related PCDD, PCDF, and PCB congeners in lake trout (Salvelinus namaycush) and rainbow trout (Oncorhynchus mykiss) eggs manifest toxicity by sac fry mortality associated with yolk sac edema and hemorrhages. In addition, selected PCDD and PCB congeners are more and less potent, respectively, in producing fish early life stage mortality than would be predicted based on their toxic potency in mammals, underscoring the need to determine fish-specific toxic potencies for individual PCDD, PCDF, and PCB congeners known to occur in fish in the environment. Although environmental levels of PCDDs, PCDFs, and PCBs do not produce overt lethality in adult fish, their combined presence in feral fish eggs may pose an increased risk to early life stage survival and, ultimately, to feral fish populations.*

## INTRODUCTION

Polychlorinated dibenzo-*p*-dioxins (PCDDs), dibenzofurans (PCDFs), biphenyls (PCBs), and related compounds belong to a family of lipophilic halogenated aromatic hydrocarbons that resist chemical and biological degradation, persist in the environment, and readily bioaccumulate in fish (Cook et al., 1991; U.S. EPA, 1991). During fish early development, the major route of exposure to halogenated aromatic hydrocarbons is not from contaminated food and water; rather, early life stages of fish are exposed to PCDDs, PCDFs, and PCBs by the deposition of these lipophilic chemicals from maternal tissues to the oocytes during vitellogenesis (Guiney et al., 1979; Niimi, 1983; Vodicnik and Peterson, 1985; Cook et al., 1991). This is of concern because early life stages of fish are more sensitive than adults to the lethal effects of halogenated aromatic hydrocarbons (Nebeker et al., 1974; McKim, 1977; DeFoe et al., 1978; Kleeman et al., 1988; Mehrle et al., 1988; Spitsbergen et al., 1991; Walker and Peterson, 1991; Walker et al., 1991, 1992).

1. Corresponding Author: Dr. Mary K. Walker, National Fisheries Research Center, P.O. Box 818, La Crosse, WI 54602-0818.

PCDDs, PCDFs, and PCBs have been detected in the eggs of fish species such as lake trout (*Salvelinus namaycush*), chinook salmon (*Oncorhynchus tshawytscha*), and coho salmon (*O. kisutch*) in the Great Lakes (Willford et al., 1969; Morrison et al., 1985; Giesy et al., 1986; Mac et al., 1988; DeVault et al., 1989; Smith et al., 1990; Mac and Edsall, 1991; Cook and Lodge, unpublished data); starry flounder (*Platichthys stellatus*) in San Francisco Bay (Spies and Rice, 1988); Atlantic salmon (*Salmo salar*), Baltic herring (*Clupea harengus*), and Baltic flounder (*Platichthys flesus*) in the Baltic Sea (Johansson, 1970; von Westernhagen et al., 1981; Hansen et al., 1985); whiting (*Merlangius merlangus*) in the North Sea (Cameron et al., 1986); and arctic char (*Salvelinus alpinus*) in Lake Geneva, Switzerland (Monod, 1985). In many of these same species, the concentrations of halogenated aromatic hydrocarbons in the eggs have been correlated with increases in early life stage mortality (Johansson, 1970; von Westernhagen et al., 1981; Hansen et al., 1985; Monod, 1985; Giesy et al., 1986; Mac et al., 1988; Spies and Rice, 1988; Mac and Edsall, 1991). Therefore, the combined presence of maternally-derived PCDDs, PCDFs, and PCBs in feral fish eggs may pose an increased risk to early life stage survival.

There are 75, 135, and 209 possible PCDD, PCDF, and PCB congeners, respectively; however, only 21 congeners are considered extremely toxic and these are structurally similar to the most potent congener, 2,3,7,8-tetrachlorodibenzo-*p*-dioxin (2,3,7,8-TCDD) (Poland and Knutson, 1982; Safe et al., 1985; Bellin and Barnes, 1989). These 2,3,7,8-TCDD-like congeners cause similar patterns of toxic responses, and are believed to share a common *Ah*-receptor mediated mechanism of action (Poland and Knutson, 1982). Thus, 2,3,7,8-TCDD serves as a prototype for other toxic PCDD, PCDF, and PCB congeners.

## 2,3,7,8-TCDD TOXICITY DURING FISH EARLY LIFE STAGE DEVELOPMENT

To determine the developmental toxicity of PCDDs, PCDFs, and PCBs in fish, newly fertilized lake trout eggs were exposed to vehicle or graded concentrations of waterborne 2,3,7,8-[$^3$H]TCDD for 48 hr and observed through the fry stage of development for 2,3,7,8-TCDD metabolism, elimination, and toxicity (Spitsbergen et al., 1991; Walker et al., 1991). 2,3,7,8-TCDD was not metabolized or eliminated by lake trout eggs or sac fry (post hatch), but was eliminated from fry ($t_{1/2}$ = 35-37 d) (Walker et al., 1991). 2,3,7,8-TCDD toxicity was manifested by some embryos dying half-hatched, but primarily by a dose-related increase in sac fry mortality preceded by fluid accumulation beneath the yolk sac epithelial membrane and subcutaneous hemorrhages (Figure 1), resembling blue-sac disease (Wolf, 1969; Spitsbergen et al., 1991; Walker et al., 1991). Egg 2,3,7,8-TCDD doses as low as 55 parts per trillion (pg 2,3,7,8-TCDD/g egg, ppt) significantly increased sac fry mortality, and 65 ppt produced 50% mortality above control ($LD_{50}$) (Walker et al., 1991).

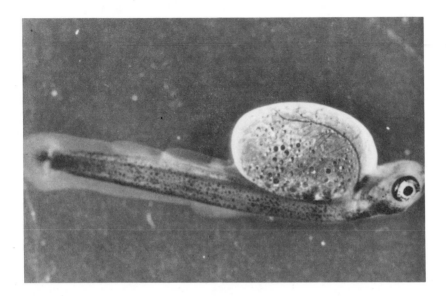

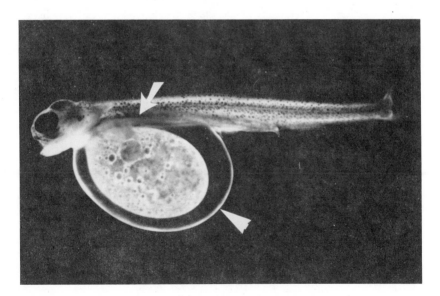

**FIGURE 1.** Representative lake trout sac fry approximately 3 wk post hatch exposed as a newly fertilized egg to either acetone in water (top panel) or to [$^3$H]TCDD dissolved in acetone in water (bottom panel, egg 2,3,7,8-TCDD dose of 200 ppt). 2,3,7,8-TCDD toxicity was manifested by fluid accumulation beneath the yolk sac epithelial membrane (arrow head) and subcutaneous hemorrhages (arrow).

## TOXICITY OF SELECTED PCDDS, PCDFS, AND PCBS DURING FISH EARLY DEVELOPMENT

To assess the toxicity of other PCDD, PCDF, and PCB congeners known to bioaccumulate in fish in the environment, newly fertilized rainbow trout eggs were injected with vehicle or graded doses of an individual PCDD, PCDF, or PCB congener (Walker and Peterson, 1991; Walker et al., 1992). Following injection, 2,3,7,8-TCDD; 1,2,3,7,8-PeCDD; 1,2,3,4,7,8-HxCDD; 2,3,7,8-TCDF, 1,2,3,7,8-PeCDF; 2,3,4,7,8-PeCDF; 1,2,3,4,7,8-HxCDF; 3,3',4,4'-TCB (IUPAC #77, Ballschmiter and Zell, 1980); or 3,3',4,4',5-PeCB (#126) manifested toxicity by some embryos dying half-hatched, but predominantly by a dose-related increase in sac fry mortality associated with blue-sac disease (Walker and Peterson, 1991; Walker et al., 1992).

## RATIONALE FOR DETERMINING TOXIC POTENCIES OF PCDDS, PCDFS, AND PCBS IN FISH

To assess the combined toxicity of a mixture of PCDDs, PCDFs, and PCBs in feral fish eggs, the toxic potency of individual congeners, relative to the most potent congener, 2,3,7,8-TCDD, must be known (Safe, 1990). The toxic equivalency factor (TEF), or relative toxic potency of an individual PCDD, PCDF, and PCB congener, is defined as the ratio 2,3,7,8-TCDD $ED_{50}$/congener $ED_{50}$. Multiplication of the concentration of a congener in a mixture by its respective TEF yields a 2,3,7,8-TCDD equivalent concentration (TEC) for that congener. The toxic potency of the entire mixture can then be expressed as an equivalent concentration of 2,3,7,8-TCDD by addition of the TECs for all the individual congeners in the mixture (Eadon et al., 1986; Bellin and Barnes, 1989). Congener-specific TEFs have been determined in mammals (Safe, 1990), and have been used to predict the combined toxicity of PCDDs, PCDFs, and PCBs to fish in the environment (Mac et al., 1988; Ankley et al., 1989; Smith et al., 1990). However, the toxic potencies of individual PCDD, PCDF, and PCB congeners, relative to 2,3,7,8-TCDD, may be quantitatively different between fish and mammals. Thus, fish-specific TEFs need to be determined for PCDD, PCDF, and PCB congeners known to occur in fish in the environment.

## "FISH-SPECIFIC" TOXIC EQUIVALENCY FACTORS (TEFS)

Following injection of rainbow trout eggs with vehicle or graded doses of 2,3,7,8-TCDD; 1,2,3,7,8-PeCDD; 1,2,3,4,7,8-HxCDD; 2,3,7,8-TCDF, 1,2,3,7,8-PeCDF; 2,3,4,7,8-PeCDF; 1,2,3,4,7,8-HxCDF; 3,3',4,4'-TCB (#77); or 3,3',4,4',5-PeCB (#126), $LD_{50}$s were determined based on percent mortality as a function of the egg congener dose (Walker and Peterson, 1991; Walker et al., 1992). TEFs were then calculated as 2,3,7,8-TCDD $LD_{50}$/congener $LD_{50}$ (Table 1) (Walker and Peterson, 1991). 2,3,7,8-TCDD was the most potent congener in producing rainbow trout early life stage mortality (TEF = 1.0). Other structurally related PCDD, PCDF, and PCB congeners were less potent in producing mortality (TEFs = 0.00016-0.730). Based on rainbow trout early life stage mortality, TEFs of PCDD congeners were 1.5-3 fold higher and PCB congeners were 1/20 - 1/62 lower than TEFs in mammals (Safe, 1990; Walker, and Peterson, 1991). In contrast, TEFs for PCDF congeners were similar in fish and mammals (Safe, 1990; Walker and Peterson, 1991). Therefore, the contribution of PCDDs to the combined toxicity of PCDDs, PCDFs, and PCBs in feral fish eggs may be greater than previously estimated using mammalian TEFs, while the contribution of PCBs may be significantly less.

**TABLE 1.**  **Toxic equivalency factors (TEFs) based on rainbow trout early life stage mortality and proposed for mammalian risk assessment[a].**

| Congener | Toxic Equivalency Factor | |
|---|---|---|
| | Rainbow Trout Early Life Stage Mortality | Mammalian Risk Assessment[b] |
| PCDDs | | |
| 2,3,7,8-TCDD | 1.0 | 1.0 |
| 1,2,3,7,8-PeCDD | 0.730 | 0.5 |
| 1,2,3,4,7,8-HxCDD | 0.319 | 0.1 |
| | | |
| PCDFs | | |
| 2,3,4,7,8-PeCDF | 0.359 | 0.5 |
| 1,2,3,4,7,8-HxCDF | 0.280 | 0.1 |
| 1,2,3,7,8-PeCDF | 0.034 | 0.05 |
| 2,3,7,8-TCDF | 0.028 | 0.1 |
| | | |
| PCBs | | |
| 3,3',4,4',5-PeCB (#126) | 0.005 | 0.1 |
| 3,3',4,4'-TCB (#77) | 0.00016 | 0.01 |

[a] Adapted, with permission, from Walker and Peterson, 1991.
[b] TEFs are values proposed for risk assessment based on a diverse spectrum of acute and subchronic toxicity tests in mammalian species (Safe, 1990).

## POTENTIAL RELEVANCE TO FERAL FISH POPULATIONS

Using fish-specific TEFs, and knowing the concentration of PCDD, PCDF, and PCB congeners in feral fish eggs, a 2,3,7,8-TCDD equivalent concentration (TEC) can be calculated. In order to assess the risk that PCDDs, PCDFs, and PCBs in feral fish eggs pose to fish early development, the calculated TEC must be compared to an acceptable level of risk, such as a lowest-observable-adverse-effect-level (LOAEL). In lake trout, for example, the LOAEL, based on the lowest egg 2,3,7,8-TCDD dose to significantly increase early life stage mortality ($p < 0.05$), was 40 ppt (Spitsbergen et al., 1991). If a calculated TEC in feral lake trout eggs equaled or exceeded 40 ppt, then the combined presence of PCDDs, PCDFs, and PCBs in feral lake trout eggs would increase the risk of early life stage mortality. Congener-specific concentrations of PCDDs, PCDFs, and PCBs in feral fish eggs, including lake trout, are relatively unknown, making it difficult to assess the risk that these contaminants pose to fish early development. However, given the fact that early life stages of fish are exposed to maternally-derived PCDDs, PCDFs, and PCBs in the environment, and that early life stages of fish are extremely sensitive to these contaminants, the combined presence of PCDDs, PCDFs, and PCBs in feral fish eggs likely increases the risk of early life stage mortality in many fish species, and may ultimately impact feral fish populations.

## ACKNOWLEDGEMENTS

We thank Dr. Mark E. Hahn and Dr. Glen Van Der Kraak for peer reviewing this chapter prior to its acceptance for publication. This research was funded in part by the University of Wisconsin Sea Grant Institute under a grant from the National Sea Grant College Program, National Oceanic and Atmospheric Administration, U.S. Department of Commerce and from the State of Wisconsin; Federal Grant NA90AA-D-SG469, University of Wisconsin Sea Grant Project R/MW-40; and in part by the Great Lakes Protection Fund FG6901038. M.K. Walker was supported in part by a Charles Stewart Mott Fellowship, awarded by the International Association for Great Lakes Research; and in part by the National Institute of Environmental Health Sciences training grant ES07015 awarded to the Environmental Toxicology Center, University of Wisconsin, Madison, Wisconsin; contribution 245.

## REFERENCES

Ankley, G.T., Tillitt, D.E., and Giesy, J.P. (1989). Maternal transfer of bioactive polychlorinated aromatic hydrocarbons in spawning chinook salmon (*Oncorhynchus tshawytscha*). *Mar. Environ. Res.*, **28**, 231-234.

Ballschmiter, K. and Zell, M. (1980). Analysis of polychlorinated biphenyls by capillary gas chromatography. *Fresenius J. Anal. Chem.*, **302**, 20-31.

Bellin, J.S. and Barnes, D.G. (1989). Interim procedures for estimating risks associated with exposure to mixtures of chlorinated dibenzo-*p*-dioxins and -dibenzofurans (CDDs and CDFs). EPA/625/3-89/016, Risk Assessment Forum, Washington, DC.

Cameron, P., von Westernhagen, H., Dethlefsen, V., and Janssen, D. (1986). Chlorinated hydrocarbons in North Sea whiting (*Merlangius merlangus*) and effects on reproduction. International Council for the Exploration of the Sea. Marine Environmental Quality Committee, **E:25**, 1-10.

Cook, P.M., Walker, M.K., Kuehl, D.W., and Peterson, R.E. (1991). Bioaccumulation and toxicity of TCDD and related compounds in aquatic ecosystems. In *Biological Basis for Risk Assessment of Dioxins and Related Compounds*, Banbury Report, Vol. 35., (M.A. Gallo, R.J. Scheuplein, C.A. van der Heijden, eds.) Cold Spring Harbor Laboratory Press, Cold Spring Harbor, NY, pp. 143-167.

DeFoe, D.L., Veith, G.D., and Carlson, R.W. (1978). Effects of Aroclor[R] 1248 and 1260 on the fathead minnow (*Pimephales promelas*). *J. Fish. Res. Board Can.*, **35**, 997-1002.

DeVault, D., Dunn, W., Bergqvist, P., Widberg, K., and Rappe, C. (1989). Polychlorinated dibenzofurans and polychlorinated dibenzo-*p*-dioxins in Great Lakes fish: A baseline and interlake comparison. *Environ. Toxicol. Chem.*, **8**, 1013-1022.

Eadon, G., Kaminsky, L., Silkworth, J., Aldous, K., Hilker, D., O'Keefe, P., Smith, R., Gierthy, J., Hawley, J., Kim, N., and DeCaprio, A. (1986). Calculation of 2,3,7,8-TCDD equivalent concentrations of complex environmental contaminant mixtures. *Environ. Health Perspec.*, **70**, 221-227.

Giesy, J.P., Newsted, J., and Garling, D.L. (1986). Relationships between chlorinated hydrocarbon concentrations and rearing mortality of chinook salmon (*Oncorhynchus tshawytscha*) eggs from Lake Michigan. *Internat. Assoc. Great Lakes Res.*, **12**, 82-98.

Guiney, P.D., Melancon, Jr., M.J., Lech, J.J., and Peterson, R.E. (1979). Effects of egg and sperm maturation and spawning on the distribution and elimination of a polychlorinated biphenyl in rainbow trout (*Salmo gairdneri*). *Toxicol. Appl. Pharmacol.*, **47**, 261-272.

Hansen, P.D., von Westernhagen, H., and Rosenthal, H. (1985). Chlorinated hydrocarbons and hatching success in Baltic herring spring spawners. *Mar. Environ. Res.*, **15**, 59-76.

Johansson, N. (1970). PCB-Indications of effects on fish. PCB Conference, Swedish Salmon Research Institute, Stockholm, Sweden, December 1970.

Kleeman, J.M., Olson, J.R., and Peterson, R.E. (1988). Species differences in 2,3,7,8-tetrachlorodibenzo-*p*-dioxin toxicity and biotransformation in fish. *Fundam. Appl. Toxicol.*, **10**, 206-213.

Mac, M.J. and Edsall, C.C. (1991). Environmental contaminants and the reproductive success of lake trout in the Great Lakes: An epidemiological approach. *J. Toxicol. Environ. Health*, **33**, 375-394.

Mac, M.J., Schwartz, T.R., and Edsall, C.C. (1988). Correlating PCB effects on fish reproduction using dioxin equivalents. *Soc. Environ. Toxicol. Chem.*, Ninth Annual Meeting Abstr. p. 116.

McKim, J.M. (1977). Evaluation of tests with early life stages of fish for predicting long-term toxicity. *J. Fish. Res. Board Can.*, **34**, 1148-1154.

Mehrle, P.M., Buckler, D.R., Little, E.E., Smith, L.M., Petty, J.D., Peterman, P.H., Stalling, D.L., DeGraeve, G.M., Coyle, J.J., and Adam, W.J. (1988). Toxicity and bioconcentration of 2,3,7,8-tetrachlorodibenzo-*p*-dioxin and 2,3,7,8-tetrachlorodibenzofuran in rainbow trout. *Environ. Toxicol. Chem.*, **7**, 47-62.

Monod, G. (1985). Egg mortality of Lake Geneva char (*Salvelinus alpinus* L.) contaminated by PCB and DDT derivatives. *Bull. Environ. Contam. Toxicol.*, **35**, 531-536.

Morrison, P.F., Leatherland, J.F., and Sonstegard, R.A. (1985). Proximate composition and organochlorine and heavy metal contamination of eggs from Lake Ontario, Lake Erie and Lake Michigan coho salmon (*Oncorhynchus kisutch* Walbaum) in relation to egg survival. *Aquat. Toxicol.*, **6**, 73-86.

Nebeker, A.V., Puglisi, F.A., and DeFoe, D.L. (1974). Effect of polychlorinated biphenyl compounds on survival and reproduction of the fathead minnow and flagfish. *Trans. Amer. Fish. Soc.*, **103**, 562-568.

Niimi, A.J. (1983). Biological and toxicological effects of environmental contaminants in fish and their eggs. *Can. J. Fish. Aquat. Sci.*, **40**, 306-312.

Poland, A. and Knutson, J.C. (1982). 2,3,7,8-Tetrachlorodibenzo-*p*-dioxin and related halogenated aromatic hydrocarbons: Examination of the mechanism of toxicity. *Ann. Rev. Pharmacol. Toxicol.*, **22**, 517-554.

Safe, S. (1990). Polychlorinated biphenyls (PCBs), dibenzo-*p*-dioxins (PCDDs), dibenzofurans (PCDFs), and related compounds: Environmental and mechanistic considerations which support the development of toxic equivalency factors (TEFs). *Crit. Rev. Toxicol.*, **21**, 51-88.

Safe, S., Bandiera, S., Sawyer, T., Robertson, L., Safe, L., Parkinson, A., Thomas, P.E., Ryan, D.E., Reik, L.M., Levin, W., Denomme, M.A., and Fujita, T. (1985). PCBs: Structure-function relationships and mechanism of action. *Environ. Health Perspec.*, **60**, 47-66.

Smith, L.M., Schwartz, T.R., Feltz, K., and Kubiak, T.J. (1990). Determination and occurrence of AHH-active polychlorinated biphenyls, 2,3,7,8-tetra-chlorodibenzo-*p*-dioxin and 2,3,7,8-tetrachlorodibenzofuran in Lake Michigan sediment and biota. The question of their relative toxicological significance. *Chemosphere*, **21**, 1063-1085.

Spies, R.B. and Rice, Jr., D.W. (1988). Effects of organic contaminants on reproduction of the starry flounder *Platichthys stellatus* in San Francisco Bay. *Mar. Biol.*, **98**, 191-200.

Spitsbergen, J.M., Walker, M.K., Olson, J.R., and Peterson, R.E. (1991). Pathologic alterations in early life stages of lake trout, *Salvelinus namaycush*, exposed to 2,3,7,8-tetrachlorodibenzo-*p*-dioxin as fertilized eggs. *Aquat. Toxicol.*, **19**, 41-72.

U.S. EPA (1991). Bioaccumulation of Selected Pollutants in Fish. A National Study, Vol.1. EPA 506/6-90/001a, Office of Water Regulations and Standards, Washington, DC, April, 1991.

Vodicnik, M.J. and Peterson, R.E. (1985). The enhancing effect of spawning on elimination of a persistent polychlorinated biphenyl from female yellow perch. *Fundam. Appl. Toxicol.*, **5**, 770-776.

von Westernhagen, H., Rosenthal, H., Dethlefsen, V., Ernst, W., Harms, U., and Hansen, P.D. (1981). Bioaccumulating substances and reproductive success in Baltic flounder *Platichthys flesus. Aquat. Toxicol.*, **1**, 85-99.

Walker, M.K. and Peterson, R.E. (1991). Potencies of polychlorinated dibenzo-*p*-dioxins, dibenzofurans, and biphenyls, relative to 2,3,7,8-tetrachlorodibenzo-*p*-dioxin, for producing early life stage mortality in rainbow trout (*Oncorhynchus mykiss*). *Aquat. Toxicol.*, **21**, 219-238.

Walker, M.K., Spitsbergen, J.M., Olson, J.R., and Peterson, R.E. (1991). 2,3,7,8-Tetrachlorodibenzo-*p*-dioxin (TCDD) toxicity during early life stage development of lake trout (*Salvelinus namaycush*). *Can. J. Fish. Aquat. Sci.*, **48**, 875-883.

Walker, M.K., Hufnagle, Jr., L.C., Clayton, M.K., and Peterson, R.E. (1992). An egg injection method for assessing early life stage mortality of polychlorinated dibenzo-*p*-dioxins, dibenzofurans, and biphenyls in rainbow trout (*Oncorhynchus mykiss*). *Aquat. Toxicol.*, **22**, 15-38.

Willford, W.A., Sills, J.B., and Whealdon, E.W. (1969). Chlorinated hydrocarbons in the young of Lake Michigan coho salmon. *Progr. Fish-Cult.*, **31**, 220.

Wolf, K. (1969). Blue-sac disease of fish. U.S. Fish and Wildlife Service, Fish Disease Leaflet #15. 4 p.

# CHEMICAL-INDUCED ALTERATIONS OF SEXUAL DIFFERENTIATION: A REVIEW OF EFFECTS IN HUMANS AND RODENTS

**Leon Earl Gray, Jr.**
Developmental Reproductive Biology Section, Reproductive Toxicology Branch,
DTD, HERL, US Environmental Protection Agency
Research Triangle Park, North Carolina

*During sexual differentiation there are a number of critical periods when the reproductive system is uniquely susceptible to chemically-induced perturbations. At these times an inappropriate chemical signal can result in irreversible lesions that often result in infertility, whereas similarly exposed young adults are only transiently affected. The serious reproductive abnormalities that resulted from human fetal exposure to DES, synthetic hormones and other drugs provide grim examples of the types of lesions that can be produced by interfering with this process. Furthermore, it is of concern that many of the abnormalities are not expressed during fetal and neonatal life and only become apparent after puberty. The present discussion will selectively review a wide range of chemically-induced abnormalities of sexual differentiation in mammals. The list of known developmental reproductive toxicants includes a broad spectrum of drugs, pesticides and toxic substances. Some of the xenobiotics, like the PCBs and dioxin, are of particular concern because they persist in the environment and bioaccumulate in the food chain. The fact that these toxicants alter sex differentiation through a wide variety of relatively well understood physiological mechanisms that are common to all mammals allows scientists to use rodent models to predict potential adverse outcomes in humans, domestic animals and wildlife.*

## INTRODUCTION

Twenty years ago, DES provided a grim example of how perinatal exposure to a chemical can seriously alter reproductive development in humans. Many of the effects of DES were not apparent until after puberty and the nature of the abnormalities could not be predicted from effects seen in DES or estrogen-exposed adults. Since then, scientific evidence has shown that a very wide range of drugs, toxic substances and pesticides can cause birth defects, infertility and

1. Corresponding Author: Leon Earl Gray, Jr., Developmental Reproductive Biology Section, Reproductive Toxicology Branch, DTD, HERL, US Environmental Protection Agency, MD - 72, Research Triangle Park, NC 27711.
2. Disclaimer: This paper has been reviewed by the Health Effects Research Laboratory, U.S. EPA, and approved for publication. Approval does not signify that the contents necessarily reflects the view and the policies of the U.S. EPA, nor does mention of trade names or commercial products constitute endorsement or recommendation for use.

abnormal reproductive development following exposure during critical developmental periods.

The fact that many of the basic mechanisms underlying this developmental process are homologous in all mammals, although the timing of certain events varies, indicates that chemicals that have adverse effects on reproductive development in rodents should be considered as potential human reproductive toxicants as well. Some of the developmental reproductive toxicants bind to and activate steroid hormone receptors and act as hormone agonists (DES, op DDT, a metabolite of methoxychlor, zearalenone), while others antagonize hormonal activity by competively binding to and inhibiting receptors (cyproterone acetate, tamoxifen). Still other chemicals act by altering hormone levels through inhibition of steroid hormone synthesis (finisteride, aminoglutethimide, alcohol) or stimulation of steroid hormone catabolism. Since hormonal activity is dependent upon mRNA and protein synthesis, acute exposure to chemicals that inhibit translational or transcriptional processes during critical stages of development can permanently alter sexual differentiation. In the CNS, sex differentiation also appears to be dependent upon hormonally induced changes in neurotransmitter activity because neurotransmitters act as morphogens in the fetal/neonatal CNS. Hence, drugs with adrenergic, serotonergic or opiate activity can alter sex differentiation. It appears, at least in mice, that prostaglandin synthesis may be required for masculinization of the external genitalia after endogenous or exogenous androgen exposure. For this reason, some inhibitors of prostaglandin synthesis inhibit differentiation of the male genitalia. Some other chemicals, like dioxin, may invoke multiple mechanisms, altering both hormone and hormone-receptor levels through interaction with the Ah-receptor, which leads to alterations in genetic expression, altered cell differentiation and reduced steroid hormone synthesis.

The first portion of this discussion will briefly review the process of normal mammalian sex differentiation, while the remainder will present selected examples of chemically induced alterations of sex differentiation. The intent is to represent the wide diversity of classes of chemicals that alter sex differentiation and the extensive variety of reasonably well understood physiological mechanisms that they alter. The author acknowledges that toxicants that permanently alter germ cell numbers during prenatal life, without altering phenotypic sex differentiation, are also important, because they too can produce infertility, but such effects were considered beyond the scope of this review. In addition, reproductive alterations induced during the infantile and pubertal stages of life were also not discussed because they result from exposures during different critical periods of life.

## SEX DETERMINATION AND DIFFERENTIATION

Aberrations of the chemical and genetic forces that regulate sex differentiation in mammals are relatively well understood since they generally are not lethal and are therefore amenable to study. Abnormal sexual development in man and rodents can be induced by drugs, chromosomal nondisjunction and single gene mutations. Sexual differentiation, the development of the male or female phenotype from an indifferent state, entails a complex series of events (Wilson, 1978). Genetic sex is determined at fertilization and this governs the expression of the "male factor" and the subsequent differentiation of gonadal sex. At this stage of embryonic development both sexes have bisexual potential with respect to the development of the duct system and external genitalia. Following gonadal sex differentiation, testicular secretions induce further differentiation of the male sexual phenotype and morphological and physiological development of males and females diverge, resulting in the formation of the male and female phenotypes. The development of phenotypic sex includes persistence of either the Wolffian (male) or Mullerian (female) duct system, and differentiation of the external genitalia and the central nervous system (CNS). Other organ systems, like the liver, are sexually "imprinted" as well. The male phenotype arises due to the action of testicular secretions, testosterone and Mullerian inhibiting substance. In the human embryo, the onset of testosterone synthesis by the testis occurs 65 days after fertilization. Testosterone induces the differentiation of the Wolffian duct system into the epididymis, vas deferens and seminal vesicles while its metabolite, 5-alpha-dihydrotestosterone (DHT), induces the development of the prostate and male external genitalia. It has generally been held that, in the absence of these secretions, the female phenotype is expressed (whether or not an ovary is present). However, the ovary secretes estrogens during development and recent studies have suggested that this hormone plays an important role in feminization of the female reproductive tract.

In the CNS, testosterone is aromatized (via the steroidogenic enzyme aromatase) to estradiol and reduced to DHT (via 5-alpha reductase), and it has been suggested for some species that all three hormones (T, DHT and $E_2$) play a role in the masculinization of the CNS. In the rat, mouse and hamster the aromatization of testosterone to estradiol is responsible, in part, for CNS sex differentiation. For example, in the hypothalamus the sexually dimorphic nucleus in the preoptic area (SDN-POA) of the rat is several-fold larger in male rats than in females due to the perinatal influence of estradiol. In other mammals, like the rhesus monkey, the role of estrogens in CNS sex differentiation process, if any, has yet to be defined and the androgenic (T and/or DHT) pathway is essential for CNS sex differentiation (McEwen, 1980).

In man, there are a number of genetic errors involving sex determining mechanisms including: complete and incomplete sex reversals (XX males and XY females) and sex chromosome anomalies (Polani, 1981); single gene defects resulting in a defect in a steroidogenic enzyme, which leads to reduced synthesis of sex steroids (20,22-desmolase; 17-ketosteroid reductase; and 5 alpha-reductase deficiency) or a defective steroid receptor, resulting in abnormal handling of androgens in the target tissues (complete testicular feminization; Reifensten syndrome) and various other genetic defects (LH deficiency and lack of responsiveness to human chorionic gonadotropin). In all, more than two dozen different genes regulate sexual development in man, and each mutation has a profound and, often unique, effect on the sexual phenotype (Polani, 1981). When similar congenital reproductive abnormalities have been detected in rodents they have dramatically facilitated our understanding of genetic errors of steroid metabolism and receptor function in man. For this reason, rodent models also have great utility for evaluating the potential of xenobiotics to alter human reproductive development.

## COMPOUND-INDUCED ALTERATIONS OF REPRODUCTIVE DEVELOPMENT: EFFECTS IN WOMEN

In humans, *in utero* exposure to a hormonally active chemical like DES, androgens or progestins results in morphological and pathological alterations of reproductive function. For example, DES causes cancer, infertility and serious morphological abnormalities, and alterations of reproductive and sex-linked nonreproductive behaviors have also been reported.

### DES
The pathological effects that develop in women as a consequence of *in utero* exposure to the potent estrogenic drug DES are well established. DES causes clear cell adenocarcinoma of the vagina, as well as gross structural abnormalities of the cervix, uterus and fallopian tube. These women are more likely to have an adverse pregnancy outcome, including spontaneous abortions, ectopic prenancies and premature delivery (Steinberger and Lloyd, 1985). It appears, however, that psychological and biological milestones of pubertal development in young women were not altered by prenatal DES exposure (Meyer-Bahlburg et al., 1984) and there have been no reports suggesting that DES accelerates reproductive senescence in women, as it does in rodents, although most affected women are still too young to assess this possibility.

In addition to DES, the use of other synthetic estrogens, like dienestrol and hexestrol, is contraindicated during pregnancy because they have the potential to induce delayed precancerous and cancerous changes in the reproductive tract.

### Androgens and Progestins
Women given androgens during pregnancy risk masculinization of the female offspring (Schardein, 1985). Masculinization has been associated with the androgens Danazol, methandriol, methyltestosterone, and normethandrone. The degree of masculinization appears related to the dosage of the drug administered, but, in general, the anomaly is less severe than that seen in pseudohermaphrodites with congenital virilizing adrenal hyperplasia. The type of anomaly is also correlated with the time of treatment during gestation. For example, treatment between the 8th and 13th week of gestation causes labioscrotal fusion, while phallic enlargement can result from exposure throughout mid-late pregnancy.

Virilization of the genital organs of infants whose mothers were treated with the formerly used anticonvulsant, aminoglutethimide, led to the withdrawal of this drug from the US market (Schardein, 1985). It is likely that this drug produces its androgenic effects in the fetal female by causing an accumulation of testosterone through inhibition of the aromatization of this steroid to estrogen by the cytochrome P-450 steroidogenic enzyme aromatase. Females are also masculinized by exposure to certain synthetic progestogens *in utero*, with ethisterone and norethindrone being the most active.

## CHEMICAL-INDUCED ALTERATIONS OF REPRODUCTIVE DEVELOPMENT: EFFECTS IN MEN

### *Effects of DES*
The potent estrogenic substance DES is a well known reproductive teratogen. Some of the pathological effects that develop in fetal males following DES exposure appear to result from an inhibition of androgens (hypospadias, underdevelopment or absence of the vas deferens, epididymis, and seminal vesicles) and antimullerian duct factor (persistence of the mullerian ducts) (Steinberger and Lloyd, 1985; Schardien, 1985; McLachlan, 1981). DES also causes epididymal cysts, hypotrophic testes and infertility in males. Some males have reduced ejaculate volume with reduced numbers of motile sperm, and may also experience difficulty in urination.

### *Effects of Progestins*
In addition to DES, progestins alter human male reproductive differentiation. These compounds include dimethisterone, hydroxyprogesterone, medroxyprogesterone, norethindrone, and progesterone. Effects reportedly include hypospadias, ambiguous genitalia and occasional testicular atrophy (Schardein, 1985). Similar effects have been obtained in male rodents and monkeys (Prahalada et al., 1985).

## POTENTIAL EFFECTS ON THE HUMAN CNS

The literature suggests that exposure to hormonally active chemicals during prenatal development can also induce changes in human behavior, as well as the reproductive tract (reviewed by Hines and Green, 1991). For example, sex-linked behavioral alterations are seen in women prenatally exposed to DES or androgens and in androgenized nonhuman primates. Meyer-Bahlburg et al., (1985) reported that women, exposed to DES *in utero*, were found to have less well established sex-partner relationships, and to be lower in sexual desire and enjoyment, sexual excitability, and coital functioning. In addition, Hines and Shipely (1984) found that DES-exposed women showed a more masculine pattern of cerebral lateralization on a verbal task than did their sisters. Such sex differences in specialization of the two hemispheres of the brain for different types of cognitive processing are well documented in humans, with men tending towards greater left-hemisphere specialization for verbal stimuli than women (McGlone, 1980). In addition, in the female rhesus monkey, prenatal testosterone or DHT administration defeminizes (Pomerantz et al., 1985) and masculinizes (Goy, 1978) some reproductive behaviors and rough-and-tumble play. The evidence suggests that physical energy expenditure by children during play is similarly influenced by prenatal androgens, albeit to a limited degree (Ehrhardt and Meyer-Bahlburg, 1981).

Along with these behavioral sex dimorphisms, structural differences in the CNS of normal men and women have been identified. Initially, sex differences in lateralization of the cortex and in the preoptic area of the hypothalamus were reported by Swaab and Fliers (1985). They found that the preoptic area of the human hypothalamus is 2.5 times larger in men than in women and contains 2.2 times as many cells; an effect that is reminiscent of the sex dimorphism present in the hypothalamus of the rat (Gorski et al., 1978). More recently, a quantitative analysis of the volume of 4 cell groups in the preoptic-anterior hypothalamic area (PO-AHA) and the supraoptic nucleus of 22 age matched men and women, found gender-related differences in two of four cell groups in the PO-AHA. The interstitial nuclei of the anterior hypothalamus (INAH), INAH-2 and INAH-3, were at least twice as large in the male brain as in the female brain (Allen et al., 1989). These authors suggest that functional sex differences in the CNS may be related to sex differences in neural structure like those seen in INAH-2 and 3. In the rat, this area of the hypothalamus contains a neuronal network that is essential for gonadotropin release and sexual behavior (Leranth et al., 1985). Interestingly, a recent report suggested that homosexual men have female-like INAH-3 structures, implying a biological basis may contribute to homosexuality (Le Vay, 1991).

The preceding discussion has presented scientific evidence demonstrating that prenatal exposure to hormonally active toxicants has resulted in dramatic abnormalities of human reproductive development. The alterations include morphological and pathological abnormalities of the reproductive system that were not apparent until well after childhood. One of these chemicals, DES, also appears to alter human CNS development as indicated by changes in sexually dimorphic behaviors. Many of the above abnormalities, seen in humans, are similar to experimentally induced alterations of sex differentiation in studies using rodents.

## EFFECTS IN RODENTS

In rodents, treatment with a hormonally active toxicants during perinatal life often induces multiple pathologies, some of which are similar to those seen in humans, while other effects are species specific. In female rats, mice and hamsters, perinatal treatment with steroidogenic chemicals can result in abnormal sex behavior, persistent vaginal cornification (PVC), and infertility via the Delayed Anovulatory Syndrome (DAS). Some of the classes of chemicals that have been shown to produce the aforementioned alterations include estrogens, anti-estrogens, DES, androgens, progestins, phytoestrogens and estrogenic pesticides.

When females develop PVC and the DAS they stop ovulating at a relatively young age, a condition that resembles neural and endocrine age-related changes in the hypothalamus. In male rodents, potent estrogens like estradiol and RU 2858, anti-estrogens, anti-androgens, and progestins alter morphological sex differentiation and cause infertility. Environmental compounds that are weakly estrogenic, like the estrogenic pesticides, appear to antagonize the action of testosterone on phenotypic sex differentiation. Sex differentiation in rodents is also altered by perinatal exposure to a wide range of toxicants devoid of hormonal activity. Such treatments include; polychlorinated biphenyls (PCBs), dioxin (TCDD), dibromochloropropane (DBCP), drugs that inhibit the 5-alpha reductase enzyme, the fungicide fenarimol, ethanol, phenobarbital, some neuroactive drugs, tetrahydrocannabinol (THC), monosodium glutamate (MSG), the herbicide nitrofen, and hexachlorophene, (Table 1).

---

**TABLE 1.**   Classes of chemicals that have been shown to alter sex differentiation in rodents.

---

Estrogens
    DES
    estradiol
    RU 2858
    chlordecone          Pesticide
    op DDT             Pesticide
    zearlenone         Fungal mycotoxin
    coumestrol         Plant estrogen
    methoxychlor      Pesticide
    some PCBs         Toxic substance

Androgens
    testosterone
    androstenedione
    DHT - (partial)

Progestins
    methyl acetoxyprogesterone
    medroxyprogesterone acetate
    progesterone

Anti-progestins
    mifepristone

Anti-estrogens (Receptor mediated mechanisms)
    tamoxifen
    clomiphene
    nafoxidine
    LY117018
    TCDD

---

**TABLE 1.**    (continued)

Anti-androgens (Receptor mediated mechanisms)
    testosterone
    cyproterone acetate
    flutamide
    spironolactone
    some fungicides

Steroid synthesis inhibitors (Enzyme mediated mechanisms)
| | |
|---|---|
| ethanol | inhibits T synthesis |
| some fungicides | inhibits T synthesis |
| aminoglutethimide | inhibits Estradiol synthesis (Human data) |
| fenarimol | inhibits Estradiol synthesis |
| finasteride | inhibits DHT synthesis |
| SK&F 105657 | inhibits DHT synthesis |
| TCDD | inhibits T synthesis |

Drugs with CNS activity/toxicity
| | |
|---|---|
| reserpine | block effects of sc T in female |
| chlorpromazine | block effects of sc T in female |
| pentobarbital | block effects of sc T in female |
| phenobarbital | block effects of sc T in female |
| pentylenetetrazol | blocked inhibitory action of pentobarbital |
| morphine | |
| lead | Toxic substance |
| THC | |
| monosodium glutamate | hypothalamic lesions |
| hexachlorophene | |

Other
| | | |
|---|---|---|
| stress | | |
| hydrocortisone | | |
| ACTH | | |
| aspirin | inhibitor of prostaglandin synthesis | |
| indomethacin | inhibitor of prostaglandin synthesis | |
| arachidonic acid | masculinized females | |
| PCBs | liver, some estrogenic | Toxic substance |
| PBBs | liver | Toxic substance |
| TCDD | Ah receptor-gene | Toxic substance |
| DBCP | | Pesticide |
| nitrofen | | Herbicide |

*Effects of DES/Estrogens on Female Rodents*
Transplacental exposure of the developing fetus to DES at critical periods leads to abnormalities of the urogenital tracts of both rodents and primates. Following DES exposure, the fetal anlagen of both sexes exhibit defective development such that both male and female rodents retain reproductive tract remnants of the opposite sex. The administration of DES to pregnant mice on days 9 to 16 of gestation reduces fertility and produces structural abnormalities of the oviduct, uterus, cervix and vagina (McLachlan et al., 1982; McLachlan, 1981; Newbold

et al., 1983). Ennis and Davies (1982) found two types of reproductive tract abnormalities in female rats treated neonatally with DES (3 μg, sc for 5 days). Squamous metaplasia is present in the uterus and part of the cervix was nonexistent in DES-treated female offspring. Huseby and Thurlow (1982) found that dietary administration of 0.2 μg of DES/gram diet during pregnancy reduced fertility and doubled the incidence of mammary carcinomas in the female offspring.

Some of the effects of DES administration can also be produced by exposure to other estrogenic substances. For example, neonatal injection of 20 μg of estradiol for 5 days also produces mammary gland abnormalities in female mice (Bern et al., 1983). In another study, prenatal exposure (administered on days 16-20 of gestation) to the synthetic estrogen, RU 2858 (moxestrol at 0.4, 2, 10, or 50 μg/rat) altered the genital tract of rat offspring more markedly than did estradiol itself (50, 250, or 1250 μg/rat) (Vannier and Raynaud, 1980). In this study, most treated females had a cleft clitorine urethra, while higher doses inhibited vaginal development, the ovaries were small and two females had persistent Wolffian ducts. Finally, both estrogens reduced fertility at lower dosage levels than those that caused morphological changes.

*Effects of Antiestrogens*
The administration of anti-estrogens is known to alter reproductive development in neonatal rodents. In the neonatal female rodent, a number of these "antiestrogens" actually act as estrogen receptor agonists, rather than antagonists, which confounds the interpretation of these data. For example, neonatal administration of the antiestrogens tamoxifen, clomiphene and nafoxidine to female mice results in estrogen-like growth of the columnar epithelium in cervicovaginal preparations, while MER-25, another anti-estrogen, was without affect (Forsberg, 1985). Although the mechanism of action of the anti-estrogens may be in question, due to their estrogenicity in neonates, it is clear that neonatal exposure to some of these chemicals, like tamoxifen, nafoxidine and clomiphene, causes gross abnormalities of reproductive development (Chamness et al., 1979; Clark and McCormack, 1977). Vaginal opening was accelerated, estrous cycles were absent at 4 months of age, the ovaries and uteri were atrophic and the oviducts showed squamous metaplasia. Similarly, female offspring, exposed *in utero* to the anti-estrogen LY117018, had cleft phallus and oviduct malformations as did DES and estradiol treated rats (Henry and Miller, 1986). Interestingly, perinatal treatment of female rats with the anti-estrogen tamoxifen resulted in permanent anovulatory sterility, however, it did not produce estrogen-like structural changes in the SDN-POA (Dohler et al., 1986).

*Effects of Environmental Estrogens*
*Estrogenic Pesticides.* Perinatal administration of a weakly estrogenic pesticide, like Kepone (chlordecone), DDT or methoxychlor, produces estrogen-like alterations of reproductive development. In general, weakly estrogenic chemicals accelerate vaginal opening, induce PVC and DAS in female rats, and they

masculinize sex-linked behaviors. For example, when op-DDT (1 mg) is administered sc on the second, third, and fourth days of life to female rat pups it advances vaginal opening by three days. op-DDT-treatment also induced PVC by 120 days of age. The ovaries of the treated females contained follicular cysts and lacked corpora lutea (Heinrichs et al., 1971).

Similar to the effects of op-DDT, Gellert (1978 a) found that sc administration of Kepone (0.2 or 1.0 mg/pup) advanced vaginal opening by more than ten days and accelerated the onset of PVC in a dose related manner. PVC was detected in some of the high-dose group rats as early as 4 months of age and in the low dosage group at 6 months. In this study, ovarian weight was reduced in the high dose group due to the lack of corpora lutea. When this pesticide was administered to the dam during gestation (days 14-20, 15 mg/kg/d) by gavage it induced PVC, anovulation, reduced ovarian weight and resulted in tonic serum levels of estradiol at 6 months of age in the female offspring (Gellert and Wilson, 1979).

The effects of neonatal exposure to Kepone have been studied in another rodent species, the hamster. When neonatal female hamsters are injected with Kepone or estradiol at 2 days of age, they displayed masculine sex behavior as adults, while the untreated females did not (Gray, 1982). These and other data indicate that, unlike the rat, female hamsters are not easily defeminized by neonatal estrogen administration. In this study, Kepone-treated female hamsters were not defeminized, they all displayed normal estrous cycles and feminine sex behavior even though they were masculinized by this chemical. Other studies using hamsters have shown that DAS, indicative of defeminization of the hypothalamus, is seen only at doses two orders of magnitude above those that masculinize females (Whitsett and Vandenbergh, 1975). It is interesting to note that the behavior and menstrual cyclicity of nonhuman primates, like hamsters, is not defeminized by treatments that do masculinize them.

Perinatal exposure to another weakly estrogenic pesticide produces a similar profile of reproductive alterations in the female rat offspring. Oral administration of methoxychlor *in utero* and during lactation to the dam at 50 mg/kg/d, accelerated vaginal opening by six days and induced PVC in female offspring (Gray et al., 1989). When the offspring were bred from weaning until 11 months of age, the treated pups all displayed PVC at ten months of age and they produced less than half as many pups as did control females.

*Estrogenic Toxic Substances.* A few PCBs have been shown *in vivo* to possess weak estrogenic activity. For example, the Aroclor mixtures 1221, produced a uterotropic response in female rats and permanently altered neuroendocrine reproductive function in treated females, while Aroclor 1224 did not (Gellert, 1978 b). Neonatal injection of 10 mg sc of Aroclor 1221 on the second and third days of life accelerated the age of vaginal opening, and increased the incidence of persistent vaginal estrus and anovulatory cycles. It has been proposed that some PCBs may be rendered estrogenic through metabolic hydoxylation, yielding polychlorinated hydroxybiphenyls (Korach et al., 1987). When a series of PCBs was compared for estrogenic activity, 4-hydroxy-2',4',6'-trichlorobiphenyl bound to the estrogen receptor with the greatest affinity *in vitro*, and stimulated uterine weight increase *in vivo*.

*Phytoestrogens and Fungal Mycotoxins.* In addition to pesticides and toxic substances, there are many other classes of "environmental estrogens" that have the potential to alter sex differentiation in an estrogen-like manner. This includes a number of plant estrogens and fungal toxins. For example, neonatal exposure to the fungal toxin, zearalenone, alters sex differentiation of the female rat and hamster reproductive system when administered as a single sc injection of 1.0 mg. Neonatal exposure to zearalenone at 3 or 5 d of age caused PVC in female rat later in life (Kumagai and Shimizu, 1982). Ovaries in these animals were smaller and contained many large follicles but not newly formed corpora lutea. PVC was observed in 6/9 rats injected at 5 days of age and in all rats dosed at 3 days of age. Irregular estrous cycles with prolonged estrus preceded the onset of PVC. In another study, neonatal female hamsters, injected at 2 days of age with 1 mg/pup of zearalenone, displayed accelerated vaginal opening as neonates and abnormal male-like sex behavior as adults. The treated females, however, were not defeminized and ovarian weights were normal (Gray et al., 1985 a). These data again indicate that hamsters differ from rats, in that the former are not easily defeminized.

In rats, neonatal exposure to the plant estrogen coumestrol (at 100 µg/d for the 5 d of life), or DES (0.08 µg) accelerated the age at vaginal opening, increased the incidence of PVC. Coumestrol-treated females also had hemorrhagic follicles (100 % at 40 days of age), an effect not seen in the DES group (Burroughs et al., 1985).

In summary, estrogenic substances produce a fairly uniform profile of abnormalities in female rodents after perinatal exposure, depending upon the species employed. Rats display accelerated vaginal opening, irregular estrous cycles and prolonged estrus, which may precede the onset of PVC and the DAS. In the female hamster, developmental exposure to estrogens will accelerate vaginal opening but they are not defeminized easily and are fertile and continue to cycle even though they have been behaviorally masculinized.

*Androgens*
Neonatal administration of testosterone to female rats produces effects on the CNS and behavior that resemble the effects of estrogen treatment while the morphological effects of androgens and estrogens on the reproductive tract differ greatly. For example, administration of testosterone to newborn pups, induces the development of PVC, polycystic ovaries, infertility, and, at low does, shortens the reproductive life span of the treated females (Gerall et al., 1980); all CNS-mediated alterations. These females develop PVC and stop ovulating at a relatively young age, a condition called the DAS, a condition that resembles neu-

ral and endocrine age-related changes in the hypothalamus (Swanson and van der Werff ten Bosch, 1964). Concurrent with the onset on DAS are changes in catecholaminergic system regulating GnRH secretion that occur in response to estradiol (Barraclough and Wise, 1982). DAS females do not show the dramatic changes in norepinephrine in the hypothalamus after ovariectomy and estrogen treatment that are seen in untreated females. The loss of cyclicity during normal aging has been related to changes in dopaminergic and noradrenergic systems. In addition, androgenized females have elevated serum levels of prolactin and estradiol and lower levels of progesterone than do untreated females (Mennin and Gorski, 1975).

Testosterone's effects on sexual differentiation of the CNS appear to resemble those of estradiol because, as indicated earlier, some of the effects of testosterone are dependent upon the aromatization of testosterone to estradiol. In the hypothalamus, the SDN-POA of the rat brain is several-fold larger in male rats than in females due to the perinatal influence of estradiol. While a single injection at 5 days of age of 5 μg of estradiol benzoate induces DAS in the rat (Gorski, 1963), and the aromatizable androgens testosterone and androstenedione induce PVC at doses of 200 μg and above (injected on days 2, 3, and 4), the nonaromatizable androgen DHT was ineffective (Luttge and Whalen, 1970). However, it appears that testosterone itself, or DHT, is responsible for the masculinization of the CNS for some other sexually dimorphic behaviors (Meany et al., 1983). For example, play behavior of female rats becomes more "male-like" after neonatal exposure to testosterone or DHT, but not estradiol (Meany and Stewart, 1981). In contrast to the effects on the CNS where DHT is only partially effective, T, DHT and androstenedione, all effectively masculinized the external genitalia of treated females (Luttge and Whalen, 1970).

Masculinization of the female rat appears to be incredibly sensitive to endogenous and exogenous hormones. In rats and mice, a naturally occurring phenomenon, termed the intrauterine-position phenomenon, results in the masculinization of females *in utero* (vom Saal and Finch, 1988). Female rodents that develop *in utero* between two male fetuses (2 M females) behave more like males, they are less fertile than 0 M females (a female located between two other females), and have longer estrous cycles. It appears that the 2 M females are masculinized and defeminized by the testicular secretions of the adjacent male siblings.

In conclusion, the administration of aromatizable androgens to neonatal female rats masculinizes and defeminizes the CNS in a manner that resembles the effects of administered estrogens. In contrast, the reproductive tract and external genitalia are masculinized by androgenic but not estrogenic treatments. Estrogenic compounds often produce unusual malformations of the female tract but these effects are not homologous to masculinization.

*Effects of Progestins*

It is known that exogenous progestins induce abnormal sexual differentiation. Fetal tissues contain progesterone receptors and exogenous administration of progestins during this period results in alterations of adult sex behavior, and genital morphology and estrous acyclicity (Hull, 1981). For example, when Kincl and Dorfman (1962) orally dosed pregnant rats with a synthetic progestin, methyl-acetoxyprogesterone, from d 15 to 20 of gestation, they found that the females were masculinized, displaying clitoral hypertrophy, increased anogenital distance, urethrovaginal fistulas and blind vaginas. Holzhausen et al. (1984) reported that medroxyprogesterone acetate (5 $\mu$g/g) given sc to lactating dams on postnatal day 1 defeminized the female offspring; they had altered proestrus LH surges after puberty.

*Effects of Neuroactive Drugs*

The sex steroids, discussed above, act on the developing CNS and promote growth and differentiation of responsive neurons, like the SDN-POA of the hypothalamus, through alterations of neurotransmitter and opiate systems in the sexually dimorphic areas. These changes lead to permanent alterations of neuronal patterning and activity (Mc Ewen, 1987) at this stage of development because the neurotransmitters can act as morphogens in the CNS during critical developmental periods. For example, neonatal alterations of monoaminergic activity modulate the organizing effect of testosterone, and chemicals that influence the activity of adrenergic receptors during this period of life also induce permanent changes in CNS sex differentiation (Jarzab, et al., 1987). Furthermore, Arai and Gorski (1968) found that neonatal treatment with the tranquilizing agents reserpine and chlorpromazine, partially blocked the sterilizing effect of testosterone on the female rat, while the barbiturates pentobarbital and phenobarbital provided marked protection against testosterone. They also found that coadministration of the antibarbiturate pentylenetetrazol blocked the protective action of pentobarbital. Similar to reserpine, chlorpromazine and the barbiturates, the alpha adenergic blocker phenoxy-benzamine blocks the effects of neonatal androgen administration, while the beta blocker propanolol cannot (Nishizuka, 1976).

In another study, prenatal morphine treatment disrupted reproductive function of the female rat, but had only minor effects on males (Vathy et al., 1985). When dams were exposed to morphine sulfate during gestational days 11-18 (5-10 mg/kg twice a day), their female offspring displayed precocious puberty and there was a substantial inhibition of feminine sexual behavior. This effect was linked to the emergence of opiate receptors in the fetal brain.

It is well established that steroid action requires binding of the steroid to a receptor, interaction of the steroid-receptor complex with DNA binding sites, increased translational and transcriptional processes, and subsequent increased protein synthesis. Hence, drugs that inhibit DNA, RNA or protein synthesis can antagonize the masculinizing action of exogenously administered androgens on

CNS sex differentiation. Inhibition of DNA synthesis for 24 h with 5-bromodeoxyuridine or hydroxyurea, or inhibition of protein synthesis with puromycin or cycloheximide for 6 h in the neonatal androgenized female rat prevents the formation of the DAS (Barnea and Linder, 1976; Gorski and Shryne, 1972). Furthermore, neonatal administration of inhibitors of RNA synthesis (amanitin and actinomycin D as well as puromycin) inhibit the effect of neonatal androgen treatment on the cyclic LH release in the female rat (Salaman and Birkett, 1974).

## CHEMICAL-INDUCED ALTERATIONS OF REPRODUCTIVE DEVELOPMENT: EFFECTS IN MALE RODENTS

*DES/Estrogens*
Effects seen in male animals, exposed *in utero* or neonatally to estrogens, resemble those seen in DES-exposed men. Male mice, given DES perinatally, develop epididymal cysts, hypospadias, phallic hypoplasia, inhibition of the growth and descent of the testes, and underdevelopment or absence of the vas deferens, epididymis and seminal vesicles (MacLachan, 1981). Similar effects are obtained using other potent estrogens like estradiol and RU 2858 (Vannier and Raynaud, 1980). In addition, in male mice, female structures derived from the Mullerian ducts persist after *in utero* administration of DES (Newbold and McLachlan, 1985; Newbold et al., 1987) and atypical gene expression is seen in seminal vesicles (Pentecost et al., 1988).

*Effects of Environmental Estrogens*
It is of concern that weakly estrogenic xenobiotics like o,p-DDT, chlordecone, zearalenone and methoxychlor could alter sex differentiation of the fetal male in an estrogen or DES-like manner. However, in general the effects that result from perinatal exposure to these substances are more variable and less severe in nature. For example, the effects of the pesticide methoxychlor appear to be dependent upon the route and timing of administration. Gellert et al., (1974) found that male rats, treated as neonates with methoxychlor or DDT, were unaffected, having normal reproductive organ weights as adults. In another study, fertility was unaffected in methoxychlor treated male offspring and epididymal cysts were not induced by this weak estrogen (Gellert and Wilson, 1979). However, when methoxychlor was administered to the dam throughout gestation and lactation, rather than injected directly into the pup, the males had slightly smaller testes, epididymides and lower sperm counts than did the controls (Gray et al., 1989; Gray, unpub.). The discrepancy between these studies may be due to the inability of the neonatal rodent, injected with methoxychlor, to metabolize it to its active estrogenic form.

Studies using hamsters, like those with rats, indicate that weakly estrogenic compounds may inhibit masculinization of the male reproductive tract in this species. As is the case in the rat, the effects, if detected, are subtle as compared to potent chemicals like DES. For example, a single injection of chlordecone

(Kepone) to neonatal hamsters reduced testicular and epididymal weights, without affecting male sexual behavior or inducing epididymal cysts (Gray, 1982), while the estrogenic mycotoxin zearalenone did not affect reproductive organ weights or male mating behavior in similarly treated males (Gray et al., 1985a).

It is noteworthy that adverse reproductive development has been reported in avian species that are not suceptible to eggshell thinning after *in ovo* exposure to environmental levels of estrogenic xenobiotics. For example, DDT and methoxychlor feminized the behavior, the gonads and reproductive tracts of the male California gull (Fry and Toone, 1981). The decline in the breeding success and local population levels of this species were attributed to the xenobiotic-induced reproductive alterations.

*Antiestrogens and Estrogen Synthesis Inhibitors*
Although the normal role of estrogens in the differentiation of the mammalian reproductive tract is only beginning to unfold, it is well established that estrogens are important in the development of sexual dimorphisms in the rodent CNS. Hence, numerous studies have shown that the administration of an anti-estrogen during the critical period of CNS sex differentiation profoundly affects differentiation of the brain of the male rodent. In one study, neonatal administration of the anti-estrogen tamoxifen demasculinized the sexually dimorphic nucleus of the preoptic area of the hypothalamus such that it was smaller in size, and hence, resembled that of the female rat (Dohler et al., 1984). Interestingly, perinatal treatment with this compound also drastically inhibited subsequent testicular development as the testes were aspermatozoic (Dohler et al., 1986).

Life-time dietary administration of the fungicide fenarimol, which inhibits ergosterol biosynthesis in fungi via effects on sterol demethylase (Hirsch et al., 1986), also causes a dose-related decrease in fertility and mating behavior in male rats. This chemical inhibits the activity of the steroidogenic enzyme aromatase, preventing the conversion of testosterone to estradiol. The authors proposed that the effect on fertility was most likely the result of inhibition of the synthesis of estradiol in the hypothalamus of the neonatal male rat, which would prevent masculinization of the CNS and result in a lack of mounting behavior and thus abnormal fertility. However, in contrast, we have found that the effects of fenarimol on male mating behavior and fertility are greater when administered to the males during adulthood rather than during the neonatal period of life (Gray et al., 1991). In addition, the role of testosterone in organizing mounting behavior in the male rat remains unclear, as some studies have found that adult females, exposed to testosterone as adults, can display normal male-like levels of this behavior although they rarely display the ejaculatory posture.

*Effects of Androgens*
As indicated earlier, testosterone is absolutely required for masculinization of the reproductive tract of the fetal male. With this in mind it is curious that

exogenously administered testosterone antagonizes the actions of endogenous androgens. Wilson and Wilson (1943) were the first to demonstrate that neonatal injections of testosterone adversely affect sexual differentiation in the male rodent. Male rats treated neonatally with high doses of testosterone had small testes with hypospermatogenesis and reduced accessory sex gland and epididymal weights. Such effects were subsequently attributed to a substantial decrease in the 5 alpha reductase activity in the prostate and epididymis of adult rats (Baranao et al., 1981). In addition, male rats exposed to another androgen, androstenedione, during pre- and/or neonatal development had reduced testes weights, while sexual behavior and accessory sex organ weights were not affected (Gilroy and Ward, 1978).

*Effects of Antiandrogens*
Exposure to antiandrogens during fetal development antagonizes the effects of endogenous testosterone and DHT in the male rat. For example, prenatal administration of the antiandrogen flutamide demasculinized sexual behavior and genitalia of the male rat (Clemens et al., 1978). Consequently, these rats were able to mount but had difficulty achieving intromission. Similar effects on the genitalia were obtained when male rats were treated prenatally with the antiandrogen cyproterone acetate. Treated males resembled females externally, lacking a penis or scrotum. The hypothalamus, in contrast, was not demasculinized by cyproterone acetate administration (Dohler et al., 1986). Interestingly, unlike the "textbook" examples the demasculinizing effects of these antiandrogens on the reproductive tract of rats and mice are not always complete. In these cases the Wolfian duct derivatives often persist after prenatal antiandrogen administration while the external genitalia are demasculinized to varing degrees (Fosberg, et al., 1968). Weakly antiandrogenic chemicals can also inhibit masculinization of the reproductive tract. Fetal exposure to spironolactone (40 mg/kg/d, d 13-21, orally), an aldosterone antagonist with antiandrogenic properties, also demasculinized male rats (Hecker et al., 1980). In another study, spironolactone treatment (10-20 mg/kg/d, d 14-20, sc) led to persistent endocrine dysfunctions (Jaussan et al., 1985). The treated males had decreased ventral prostate and seminal vesicles weights, and basal serum and pituitary prolactin levels were 50 % of control values. In contrast, LH, FSH, testosterone and DHT levels were normal in the treated males. The data on another weakly androgenic chemical are conflicting with respect to its ability to inhibit masculinization. Anand and Van Thiel (1982) claimed that exposing rats *in utero* and postnatally to a weak antiandrogen cimetidine, demasculinized the male pups and reduced their sexual performance as adults. However, Walker et al. (1987) were unable to replicate these effects.

*Effects of Steroidogenic Enzyme Inhibitors*
*5-Alpha Reductase Inhibitors.* While the chemicals discussed up to this point inhibit male sex differentiation via steroid hormone receptor-mediated mechanisms, the following are examples of chemicals that alter the hormonal milieu by inhibiting the activity of a steroidogenic enzyme. As indicated earlier, although

testosterone induces the differentiation of the Wolffian duct system into the epididymis, vas deferens and seminal vesicles, its metabolite, dihydrotestosterone (DHT), induces the development of the prostate and male external genitalia. For this reason, administration of 5-alpha reductase inhibitors, chemicals that prevent the conversion of testosterone to the more active androgen DHT, induce congenital abnormalities of the external genitalia of the male rodent. For example, administration of the 5 alpha reductase inhibitor finasteride to pregnant rats on gestational day 16 to 17 (at 3, 30, 100 or 300 µg/kg/d) caused hypospadias, decreased anogenital distance and weight of the sex accessory glands in the male offspring (Clark et al., 1990; Anderson and Clark, 1990). Similar effects were obtained by Weir et al., 1990, who administered another 5 alpha reductase inhibitor, SK&F 10567, to pregnant rats (0.01 to 100 mg/kg/d) on days 7-21 of gestation. In this study, anogenital distance was reduced at 1 mg/kg/d at birth, and hypospadias was seen at 10 mg/kg/d and above. Mating and fertility of male offspring without hypospadias was unaffected, but the sex accessory glands derived from the DHT-dependent urogenital sinus, the prostate and coagulating glands, were permanently reduced in size.

*Fetal Alcohol.* The fact that alcohol is a "functional" CNS teratogen in man and rodents is receiving considerable attention primarily due to the large human population at risk. Prenatal alcohol exposure leads to serious deficits in intellectual performance in exposed children and adolescents. In rodents, perinatal exposure to alcohol also alters neonatal testicular function and CNS sex differention. To date, however, similar alterations of human sex differentiation have not been considered. Male rats exposed to ethanol during the perinatal period display feminized play behavior as juveniles (Meyer and Riley, 1986) and demasculinized and feminized sexual behavior patterns as adults (Parker et al., 1984).

These behavioral alterations arise as a consequence of reduced androgen biosynthesis in the perinatal rat testis (Kelce et al., 1990a and b), which leads to permanent alterations in CNS sex differentiation. For example, *in utero* exposure to ethanol causes reductions in the volume of the sexually dimorphic nucleus of the preoptic area (Rudeen, 1986) and inhibits cerebral lateralization in male rats. Alcohol-exposed males showed a "feminized" asymmetry, as compared to six days old untreated male rats. In the normal male rat, the cerebral cortices in several regions are thicker on one side, usually the right, while females do not show asymmetry (Zimmerberg and Reuter, 1989). These results demonstrate that chemicals that inhibit steroidogenic enzymes, alter sexual differentiation of the reproductive system.

## Effects of Progestins
A number of studies have investigated the effects of progesterone on sex differentiation in the male rodent. Neonatal injections of progesterone induced slight changes in the development and function of the adrenal gland and the testis in the rat (Tapanainen et al., 1979) and interfered with behavioral

masculinization (Hull, 1981). Progestin-induced behavioral alterations appear to result from lowering fetal testicular testosterone synthesis (Pointis et al., 1984) and it binds to the androgen receptor, thus producing effects similar to the antiandrogens and inhibitors of androgen biosynthesis. While it has been proposed that the maternal progesterone treatment impairs fetal testosterone synthesis by inhibiting 3-beta-hydroxysteroid dehydrogenase, the precise mechanism of this effect has not been characterized. Similar effects of a progestin have been seen in nonhuman primates. Male cynomologus monkeys exposed in utero to medroxyprogesterone acetate had a short penis, hypospadias and small adrenals (Prahalada et al., 1985). These effects are quite similar to the effects of progestins on human sex differentiation.

Interestingly, neonatal administration of the anti-progestagenic drug mifepristone (1 mg sc every 2 days from day 1 to 15) permanently affected testicular develolment in the male, rat (van der Schoot and Baumgarten, 1990). Pubertal development in treated males was delayed and testis weight remained at 2/3 of control level. Sexual behavior was abnormal, treated males rarely ejaculated and, when they were injected with estradiol, they displayed abnormally high levels of female sexual behavior. While the mechanism of action for this effect was not defined in this study, this drug clearly inhibited masculinization of the CNS and reproductive tract.

*Effects of Prenatal Stress.* Stressing pregnant rats alters sexual differentiation of fetal males in a manner that also suggests inhibition of the masculinizing actions of androgens. The male offspring show aberrant sexual behavior in adulthood, shortened anogenital distance at birth and reduced testicular weight. These effects are presumably the consequence of the corticosteriods secreted by the stressed mother (Dahlof et al., 1977). Treatment of pregnant rats with hydrocortisone (1.5 or 3.0 mg/rat) from day 14 after conception until birth shortens anogenital distance and lowers testis weight in the offspring (Dahlof et al., 1978). Rhees and Flemming (1981) found that the copulatory behavior of male offspring from dams subjected to environmental stress (immobilization-illumination-heat), or injection of ACTH (20 IU/d im) was severly impaired. In a similar study, Stylianopoulou (1983) found that males born to dams treated with ACTH (8 IU/d sc) during the last third of gestation showed a decreased ability to perform sexually ( 42 % failed to mate as compared to 3 % of the control males).

## DRUGS

*Neuroactive Drugs*
Neuroactive and neurotoxic chemicals have been shown to alter sex differentiation in male rodents when administered during perinatal life. Reproductive dysfunction was noted in male rats following prenatal exposure to phenobarbital (Gupta et al., 1980). Anogenital distance was shorter, and fertility, seminal vesicle weights, serum testosterone and LH levels all were reduced. In addition, Clemens et al. (1979) reported that neonatal injections of pentobarbital

induced sexual behavior deficits in intact and castrated (testosterone suppl-mented) male rats.

Another drug, THC, the principal psychoactive component of marijuana, altered the hypothalamic-pituitary-gonadal axis and sexual behavior in male mice, exposed *in utero* (Dalterio and Bartke, 1979). Postnatal exposure to cannabinoids also decreased fertility in mice (Dalterio et al., 1982) and rats (Ahluwalia et al., 1985). Such alterations could result from disruption of the morphogenic activity of hypothalamic neurotransmitter systems during perinatal life.

In contrast to the above effects, MSG is cytotoxic and causes cell death when administered during neonatal and infantile stages of life. The injection of high doses of MSG induces numerous reproductive defects due to cell death in the arcuate nucleus of the hypothalamus. Male and female mice (Pizzi et al., 1977), rats (Bakke et al., 1978), and hamsters (Lamperti and Baldwin, 1982) exposed to MSG in this manner suffer endocrine dysfunction and are infertile. The hypothalamic regulation of the release of FSH and LH are altered, and thyroid function and growth hormone secretion are abnormal as well.

Hexachlorophene is another drug that causes CNS lesions during neonatal life. Infertility results from neonatal dermal application of this former topical antiseptic compound (Gellert et al., 1978). Eleven month old treated male rats were infertile even though testis weights, sperm motility and serum testosterone were normal. During an observation of their sexual behavior, it was apparent that the treated males mounted a receptive female but they could not ejaculate. In addition to these behavioral deficits, prostatic cysts were detected in treated males at necropsy.

*Other Drugs*
Recent evidence suggests that the stimulation of the arachidonic acid-prostaglandin pathway is involved in the action of testosterone on the external genitalia (Gupta and Goldman, 1986). Arachidonic acid administered during embryonic development masculinized the genitalia of female mice while the administration of aspirin, indomethacin and cortisone, agents which inhibit the arachidonic acid cascade, inhibited the masculine differentiation of the external genitalia in males. In support of the role of prostaglandins in sexual differentiation, Gupta (1989) found that prostaglandin (PG) levels were elevated two-fold in females exposed to testosterone, and treatment with an antiandrogen decreased PG levels in male fetuses. The author proposed that PGs may play a critical role in the masculinizing action of fetal testosterone. However, when three inhibitors (triamcinolone acetonide, aspirin and L-656,224) of the arachidonic acid cascade were given to pregnant rats during the critical period of morphogenesis of the external genitalia, they were largely ineffective (Wise et al., 1991). These authors concluded that prostaglandins were unlikely to be important mediators of androgen-induced masculinization in the Sprague-Dawley

rat, because the differentiation of the external genitalia was not seriously affected by administration of aspirin or glucocortocoids.

## NONESTROGENIC PESTICIDES AND TOXICANTS

In addition to the estrogenic pesticides, phytoestrogens and estrogenic PCBs, discussed previously, xenobiotics that are devoid of estrogenic activity also have been shown to alter sex differentiation, often dramatically. For example, the ubiquitous and persistent toxicant 2,3,7,8-tetrachlorodibenzo p-dioxin (TCDD) alters sexual behavior in male rats after perinatal administration at extremely low dosage levels (Mably et al., 1990). Male rats, born to females dosed with 0.0 to 1.0 μg of TCDD/kg on d 15 of pregnancy, display demasculinized and feminized sexual behaviors. There were dose-related increases in mount, intromission and ejaculation latencies and the number of mounts to ejaculation was increased. The TCDD-treated males also displayed dose related increases in the lordosis quotient and the quality of the lordotic response. Although there were no gross abnormalities of the external genitalia of TCDD-exposed pups, anogenital distance was reduced in male pups at birth. Furthermore, when these pups were examined at 32, 49, 63, and 120 days of age, testicular and accessory gland growth and sperm production were well below normal levels. In summary, TCDD-treatment creates a hypoandrogenic condition and may "down" regulate estrogen receptors in the CNS in fetal male rats, effects which interfer with sex differentiation of the reproductive tract and CNS. It is important to point out that the $ED_{50}$ for these effects in the developing male is about 0.16 μg/kg, a dose that is 100 fold lower than the $ED_{50}$ for reproductive effects in the adult.

It has been proposed that toxicant-induced changes in liver function during sex differentiation can indirectly inhibit sex differentiation by altering the internal hormonal/androgen milieu. For example, postnatal administration of a non-estrogenic PCB during the neonatal and juvenile periods, produces a hypo-androgenic condition by inducing the hepatic microsomal enzymes (Sager, 1983). As adults, these males had reduced reproductive capacity, and smaller sex accessory gland weights. Similarly, McCormack et al. (1979), reported that perinatal polybrominated biphenyls (PBBs) increased steroid catabolism in the male rat, reducing the effectiveness of exogenously administered steroid hormones.

The preceding environmental chemicals altered sex differentiation through effects on steroid hormone synthesis (TCDD), function or metabolism (PBB), and mimicked the action of steroid hormones (Kepone, op-DDT, a methoxychlor metabolite, plant and fungal estrogens). In contrast, toxicants that lack such biological activity can also produce surprising alterations of reproductive development through mechanisms that have yet to be defined. For example, prenatal administration of the nematocide DBCP profoundly effects both germ cell numbers and hormone dependent sex differentiation, resulting in some rather dramatic and novel alterations in rats. Males, whose dams were treated with

DBCP at 25 mg/kg on days 14 to 19 of gestation, had 90% reduced testis weight, androgen levels were decreased and the SDN-POA was reduced in size. In addition, none of the DBCP treated males displayed mounting behavior, and they all showed high levels of female sex behavior (lordosis). The most novel effect seen in this study, was the complete absence of seminiferous tubules in many of the males (Warren et al., 1988). In contrast to these developmental effects, this chemical does not produce direct reproductive endocrine alterations in adult male rats. The herbicide nitrofen is another example of a toxicant that produces unexpected alterations of sex differentiation. Prenatal exposure to nitrofen induces anomalous development of the para- and mesonephric duct derivatives in the hamster. Early gestational treatment causes uterus unicornis and occasional ipsilateral renal agenesis in the female, and unilateral agenesis of the vas and/or epididymis and seminal vesicular agenesis in the male. Male hamsters exposed to nitrofen later in gestation displayed lower levels of mounting behavior, reduced fertility and a high incidence of spermatic granulomas in the epididymis (Gray et al., 1985 b). These effects are of concern because they could not be predicted from the known biological activity of the chemicals. In spite of the fact that the mechanisms of mammalian sex differentiation are relatively well understood, serious reproductive abnormalities can result from exposure to chemicals like DBCP or nitrofen; effects that could not have been predicted from the effects of these chemicals in adult rodents or *in vitro*.

## CONCLUSIONS

The studies presented in this review indicate that perinatal exposure of the fetal human or neonatal rodent to a wide variety of chemicals can adversely affect reproductive development and fertility through a number of different mechanisms. In humans, exposure to DES, androgens and progestins during gestational development provides us with grim examples of the potential for environmental chemicals to induce morphological and pathological alterations of the reproductive tract of both men and women. It is quite clear that DES treatment causes cancer, infertility and serious morphological abnormalities in all species examined. Other studies have found that women exposed to DES *in utero* have altered sexual behaviors and show male-like cerebral lateralization of verbal cognitive function. In nonhuman primates, prenatal administration of androgens also masculinize females such that they show more male-like levels of some sex behaviors and aggressive play.

Studies using rats, mice and hamsters, have also found that perinatal treatment can alter neuroendocrine and hypothalamic sex differentiation as well as produce anatomical malformations. In the female rat, such alterations result in masculinization of the ducts and external genitalia, atypical sex and play behaviors, persistent vaginal cornification (PVC), and an acceleration of reproductive senescence (via the DAS) with, estrogens, antiestrogens, DES, androgens, and estrogenic pesticides.

In male rodents, potent estrogens, like estradiol and RU 2858, antiestrogens, anti-androgens, progestins, and anti-progestins alter morphological sex differentiation and cause infertility. Other compounds that are weak estrogens, or somehow antagonize the action of testosterone may not cause infertility, but they often reduce reproductive organ weights and sperm production.

A number of non-estrogenic drugs, pesticides and toxic substances have also been shown to adversely impact rodent sex differentiation. This list includes, PCBs, PBBs, TCDD, DBCP, inhibitors of arachadonic acid metabolism, MSG, lead, phenobarbital, morphine, THC, spironolactone, hydrocortisone, and ACTH.

In conclusion, the basic events of reproductive development are similar in all mammalian species, although, subtle but important differences exist. Perinatally induced alterations of this process, seen in studies using rodents, should be of concern because similar alterations may occur in man, domestic animals, and wildlife. Such developmental effects can only be detected in multigenerational studies that examine the reproductive function of offspring exposed during fetal and neonatal stages of life. For this reason, reproductive toxicity studies that include only an evaluation of the effects of a chemical on adult rodents may provide inadequate data for determination of a chemical's potential reproductive hazard to humans. In addition, it is clear that an evaluation of fertility alone is insufficient for hazard identification of developmental reproductive toxicants because serious effects can occur at doses below those that alter fertility.

## REFERENCES

Ahluwalia, B.S., Rajguru, S.U., and Nolan, G.H. (1985). The effect of Tetrahydrocannabinol *in utero* exposure on rat offspring fertility and ventral prostrate gland morphology. *J. Andrology,* **6**, 386-391.

Allen, L.S., Hines, M., Shryne, J.E., and Gorski R.A. (1989). Two sexually dimorphic cell groups in the human brain. *J. Neuroscience,* **9**(2), 497-506.

Anand, S. and Van Thiel, D.H. (1982). Prenatal and neonatal exposure to cimetidine results in gonadal and sexual dysfunction in adult males. *Science,* **218**, 493-494.

Anderson C.A. and Clark R.L. (1990). External genitalia of the rat: Normal development and the histogenesis of 5 alpha-reducatse inhibitor-induced abnormalities. *Teratology,* **42**, 483-496.

Arai, Y. and Gorski, R.A. (1968). Protection against neural organizing effect of exogenous androgen in the neonatal female rat. *Endocrinology,* **82**, 1005-1009.

Bakke, J.L., Lawrence, N., Bennet, J., Robinson, S., and Bowers, C.Y. (1978). Late endocrine effects of administering monosodium glutamate to neonatal rats. *Neuroendocrinology,* **26**, 220-228.

Baranao, J.L.S., Chemes, H.E., Tesone, M., Chiauzzi, V.A., Scacchi, P., Calvo, J.C., Faigon, M.R., Moguilevsky, J.A., Charreau, E.H., and Calandra, R.S. (1981). Effects of Androgen treatment of the neonate on rat testis and sex accessory organs. *Biology of Reproduction,* **25**, 851-858.

Barnea, A. and Linder. H. (1976). Short-term inhibition of macromolecular synthesis and androgen-induced sexual differentiation of the rat brain. *Brain Res,.* **45**, 479-487.

Barraclough, C.A. and Wise, P.M. (1982). The role of catecholamines in the regulation of pituitary luteinizing hormone and follicle stimulating hormone secretion. *Endocrine Reviews,* 3, 99-119.

Bern, H.A., Mills, K.T., and Jones, L.A. (1983). Critical period for neonatal estrogen exposure in occurrence of mammary gland abnormalities in adult mice. *Proceedings of the Society for Experimental Biology and Medicine,* 172, 239-242.

Burroughs, C.D., Bern, H.A., and Stokstad, E.L. (1985). Prolonged vaginal cornification and other changes in mice treated neonatally with coumestrol, a plant estrogen. *J.Toxicol.and Environ. Health,* 15, 51-61.

Chamness, G.C., Bannayan, G.A., Landry, L.A., Jr., Sheridan, and P.J., McGuire, W.L. (1979). Abnormal reproductive development in rats after neonatally administered antiestrogen (Tamoxifen). *Biology of Reproduction,* 21, 1087-1090.

Clark, J.H. and McCormack, S. (1977). Clomid or nafoxidine administered to neonatal rats causes reproductive tract abnormalities. *Science,* 197, 164-165.

Clark, R.L., C.A. Anderson, S. Prahalada, Y. M. Leonard, J. L. Stevens, and A.M. Hoberman. (1990). 5-alpha reductase inhibitor-induced congenital abnormalities in male rat external genitalia. *Teratology,* 41(5A), 544.

Clemens, L.G., Gladue, B.A., and Coniglio, L.P. (1978). Prenatal endogenous androgenic influences on masculine sexual behavior and genital morphology in male and female rats. *Hormones and Behavior,* 10, 40-53.

Clemens, L.G., Popham, T.V., and Ruppert, P.H. (1979). Neonatal treatment of hamsters with barbiturate alters adult sexual behavior. *Developmental Psychobiology,* 12, 49-59.

Dahlof, L.G., Hard, E., and Larsson, K. (1977). Influence of maternal stress on the development of the fetal genital system. *Physiology and Behavior,* 20, 192-195.

Dahlof, L.G., Hard. E., and Larsson, K. (1978). Sexual differentiation of offspring of mothers treated with cortisone during pregnancy. *Physiology and Behavior,* 21, 673-674.

Dalterio, S. and Bartke, A. (1979). Perinatal exposure to cannabinoids alters male reproductive functions in mice. *Science,* 205, 1420-1422.

Dalterio, S., Badr, F., Bartke, A., and Mayfield, D. (1982). Cannabinoids in male mice, Effects on fertility and spermatogenesis. *Science,* 216, 315-316.

Dohler, K.D., Srivastava, S.S., Shryne, J.E., Jarzab, B., Sipos, A., and Gorski, R.A. (1984). Differentiation of the sexually dimorphic nucleus in the preoptic area of the rat brain is inhibited by postnatal treatment with an estrogen antagonist. *Neuroendocrinology,* 38, 297-301.

Dohler, K.D., Coquelin, A., Davies, F., Hines, M., Shryne, J.E., Sickmoller, P.N., Jarzab, B., and Gorski, R.A. (1986). Pre-and postnatal influence of an estrogen antagonist on differentiation of the sexually dimorphic nucleus of the preoptic area of male and female rats. *Neuroendocrinology,* 42, 443-448.

Ehrhardt, A.A. and Meyer-Bahlburg, F.L. (1981). Effects of prenatal sex hormones on gender-related behavior. *Science,* 211, 1312-1318.

Ennis, B.W. and Davies, J. (1982). Reproductive tract abnormalities in rats treated neonatally with DES. *Am. J.Anatomy,* 164, 145-154.

Fosberg, J.G., Jacobsohn, D., and Norgren A. (1968). Modifications of reproductive organs in male rats influenced prenatally or pre- and post-natally by "antiandrogenic" steroid (cyproterone). *Z. Anat. Entwicklungsgesch,* 127, 175-186.

Forsberg, J.G. (1985). Treatment with different antiestrogens in the neonatal period and effects in the cervicovaginal epithelium and ovaries of adult mice: A comparison to estrogen-induced changes. *Bio. of Repro.,* 32, 427-441.

Fry, D.M. and Toone, T.K. (1981). DDT-Induced feminization of gull embryos. *Science*, **213**(21), 922-924.

Gellert, R. J., Heinrichs, W. L., and Swerdloff, R. (1974). Effects of neonatally-administered DDT homologs on reproductive function in male and female rats. *Neuroendocrinology*, **16**, 84-94.

Gellert, R.J. (1978a). Kepone, Mirex, Dieldrin and Aldrin: Estrogenic activity and the induction of persistent vaginal estrus and anovulation in rats following neonatal treatment. *Environmental Research*, **16**, 131-138.

Gellert, R.J. (1978b). Uterotrophic activity of polychlorinated biphenyls and induction of precocious reproductive aging in neonatally treated female rats. *Environ. Res,*. **16**, 123-130.

Gellert, R. J., Wallace, C.A., Wiesmeier, E.M., and Shuman, R.A. (1978). Topical exposure of neonates to hexachlorophene: Long-standing effects on mating behavior and prostatic development in rats. *Toxicol. and Appl. Pharmacol.*, **43**, 339-349.

Gellert, R.J. and Wilson, C. (1979). Reproductive function in rats exposed prenatally to pesticides and polychlorinated biphenyls (PCB). *Environ. Res.*, **18**, 437-443.

Gerall, A.A., Dunlap, J.L., and Sonntag, W.E. (1980). Reproduction in aging, normal and neonatally androgenized female rats. *J. Comp. and Physiol. Psych.*, **94**, 556-563.

Gilroy, A.F. and Ward, I.L. (1978). Effects of perinatal andostenedione on sexual behavior differentiation in male rats. *Behavioral Biology*, **23**, 243-248.

Gorski, R.A. (1963). Modification of ovulatory mechanisms by postnatal administration of estrogen to the rat. *Am. J. Physiol.*, **205**, 842-844.

Gorski, R.A. and J. Shryne. (1972). Intracerebral antibiotics and androgenization of the neonatal female rat. *Neuroendocrinology*, **10**, 109-120.

Gorski, R.A., Gordon, J.H. Shryne, J.E., and Southam, A.M. (1978). Evidence for a morphological sex difference within the medial preoptic area of the rat brain. *Brain Res.*, **148**, 333-346.

Goy, RW. (1978). Development of Play and Mounting Behavior in Female Rhesus Virilized Prenatally with Esters of Testosterone or Dihydrotestosterone. In: *Recent Advances in Primatology* (D.J. Chivers and J. Herbert, eds.) Academic Press, New York, pp. 449-462.

Gray, L.E., Jr. (1982). Neonatal chlordecone exposure alters behavioral sex differentiation in female hamsters. *Neurotoxicology*, **3**(2), 67-80.

Gray, L.E. Jr., Ferrell, J.M., and Ostby, J.S. (1985). Alteration of behavioral sex differentiation by exposure to estrogenic compounds during a critical neonatal period: Effects of Zearalenone, Methoxychlor, and Estradiol in hamsters. *Toxicol. and Appl. Pharmacol.*, **80**(1), 127-136.

Gray, L.E.Jr., Ferrell, J., and Ostby, J. (1985). Prenatal exposure to nitrofen causes anomalous development of para-and mesonephric duct derivatives in the hamster. *The Toxicologist*, **5**(1), 183.

Gray, L.E., Jr., Ostby, J., Ferrell, J., Rehnberg, G., Linder, R., Cooper, R., Goldman, J. Slott, V., and Laskey, J. (1989). A dose-response analysis of methoxychlor-induced alterations of reproductive development and function in the rat. *Fund. and Appl. Toxicol.*, **(12)** 92-108.

Gray, L.E., Jr.,Ostby , J.S., Sigmon, R., and Linder, R. (1991). A fungicide (Fenarimol) that inhibits fungal sterol synthesis also reduces mating behavior and fertility in male rats. *Bio. of Repro.*, **44** (suppl. 1), 132.

Gupta, C., Shapiro, B.H., and Sumner, J.Y. (1980). Reproductive dysfunction in male rats following prenatal exposure to phenobarbital. *Pediatric Pharmacology*, **1**, 55-62.

Gupta, C. and Goldman, A.S. (1986). The arachidonic acid cascade is involved in the masculinizing action of testosterone on embryonic external genitalia in mice. *Proc. Natl. Acad. Sci.,*. **83**, 4346.

Gupta C. (1989). The role of prostaglandins in masculine differentiation:' Modulation of prostaglandin levels in the diffentiating genital tract of the fetal mouse. *Endocrinology,* **124**(1), 129-133.

Hecker, A., Hasan, S.H., and Neumann, F. (1980). Disturbances of sexual differentiation of rat foetuses following spironolactone treatment. *Acta Endocrinologica,* **95**, 540-545.

Heinrichs, W.L., Gellert, R.J., Bakke, J.L., and Lawrence, N.L. (1971). DDT administered to neonatal rats induces persistent estrus syndrome. *Science,* **173**, 642-643.

Henry, E.C. and Miller, R.K. (1986). The antiestrogen LY117018 is estrogenic in the fetal rat. *Teratology* **34**, 59-63.

Hines, M. and Green, R. (1991). Human Hormonal and Neural correlates of sex-typed behaviors. *Rev. of Psych.,* **10**, 536-555.

Hines M. and Shipley, C. (1984). Prenatal exposure to diethylstilbestrol (DES) and the development of sexually dimorphic cognitive abilities and cerebral lateralization. *Develop. Psych.,* **20**(1), 81-94.

Hirsch, K.S., Adams, E.R., Hoffman, D.G., Markham, J.K., and Owen, N.V. (1986). Studies to elucidate the mechanism of fenarimol-infertility in the male rat. *Toxicol. and Appl. Pharmacol.,* **86**, 391-399.

Holzhausen C., Murphy S., and Birke L.I.A. (1984). Neonatal  exposure to a progestin via milk alters subsequent LH cyclicity in the female rat. *J. Endocr.* **100**, 149-154.

Hull, E.M. (1981). Effects of neonatal exposure to progesterone on sexual behavior of male and female rats. *Physiology and Behavior,* **26**, 401-405.

Huseby, R.A. and Thurlow, S. (1982). Effects of prenatal exposure of mice to "low-dose" diethylstilbestrol and the development of adenomyosis associated with the evidence of hyperprolactinemia. *Am. J. Obstet. and Gynecol.,* **144**(8), 939-949.

Jarzab, B., Sickmoller, P., Geerlings, H., and K. Dohler. (1987). Postnatal treatment of rats with adrenergic receptor antagonists influences differentiation of sexual behavior. *Hormones and Behavior,* **21**, 478-492.

Jaussan, V., Lemarchand-Beraud, T., and Gomez, F. (1985). Modifications of the gonadal function in the adult rat after fetal exposure to spironolactone. *Bio.of Repro.,* **32**(5), 1051-1061.

Kelce, W.R., Ganjam, V.K., and Rudeen, P.K. (1990a). Inhibition of testicular steroidogenesis in the neonatal rat following acute ethanol exposure. *Alcohol,* **7**, 75-80.

Kelce, W.R., Ganjam, V.K., and Rudeen, P.K. (1990b). Effects of fetal alcohol exposure on brain 5-alpha-reductase/aromatase activity. *J. Steroid Biochem.* **35**,103-106.

Kincl, F.A. and Dorfman, R.I. (1962). Influence of progestational agents on the genetic female foetus of orally treated pregnant rats. *Acta Endocrinologica* **41**, 274-279.

Korach, K.S., Sarver, P., Chae, K., McLachlan, J.A., and McKinney, J.D. (1988). Estrogen receptor-binding activity of polychlorinated hydroxybiphenyls: Conformationally restricted structural probes. *Molecular Pharmacology,* **33**, 120-126.

Kumagai, S. and Shimizu. (1982). Neonatal exposure to zearalenone causes persistent anovulatory estrus in the rat. *Arch. Toxicol.,* **50**, 270-286.

Lamperti, A.A., and Baldwin, D.M. (1982). Pituitary responsiveness to LHRH stimulation in hamsters treated neonatally with monosodium glutamate. *Neuroendocrinology,* **34**, 169-174.

Leranth, C.S., Sequra, L.M.G., Palkovits, M., MacLusky, N.J., Shanaburough, M., and Naftolin, F. (1985). The LH-RH containing neuronal network in the preoptic area of the rat: Demonstration of LH-RH containing nerve terminals in synaptic contact with LH- RH neurons. *Brain Res., 345*, 332-336.

Le Vay, S. (1991). A difference in hypothalamic structure between heterosexual and homosexual men. *Science, 253*, 1034-1037.

Luttge, W.G. and Whalen, R.E. (1970). Dihydrotestosterone, Androstenedione, Testosterone: Comparative effectiveness in masculenizing and defeminizing reproductive systems in male and female rats. *Hormones and Behavior, 1*, 265-281.

Mably, T.A. Moore, R.W., Bjerke, D.L., and Peterson, R.E. (1991). The male reproductive system is highly sensitive to *in utero* and lactational 2,3,7,8-tetrachlorodibenzo-*p*-dioxin exposure. In: *Biological Basis for Risk Assessment of Dioxins and Related Compounds*, (M.A. Gallo, R.J. Scheuplein, and C.A. van der Heijden, eds.) Banbury Report 35, Cold Spring Harbor Laboratory, Cold Spring Harbor, New York, pp. 143-167.

McCormack, K.M., Arneric, S.P., and Hook, J.B. (1979). Action of exogenously administered steroid hormones following perinatal exposure to polybrominated biphenyls. *J. Toxicol. and Environ. Health 5*, 1085-1094.

McEwen, B.S. (1980). Gonadal Steroid and Brain Development. *Bio. of Reprod., 22*, 43-48.

McEwen, B.S. (1987). External factors influencing brain development. In: NIDA Res. Monographs, Vol. 78. (D. Friedman and D. Clouet, eds.), pp. 1-14.

McGlone, J. (1980). Sex differences in human brain asymmetry: A critical survey. *Behavior and Brain Sciences, 3*, 215-263.

McLachlan, J.A. (1981). Rodent Models for Perinatal Exposure to Diethylstilbestrol and their Relation to Human Disease in the Male. In: "Developmental Effects of Diethylstilbestrol in Pregnancy" (A.L. Herbst and H.A. Bern, eds.) New York, Thieme-Stratton, Inc., pp. 48-157.

McLachlan, J.A., Newbold, R.R., Shah, H.C., Hogan, M.D., and Dixon, R.L. (1982). Reduced fertility in female mice exposed transplacentally to diethylstilbestrol (DES). *Fertility and Sterility, 38*(3), 364-371.

Meany, M.J. and Stewart, J. (1981). Neonatal androgens influence the social play of prepubescent rats. *Hormones and Behavior, 15*, 197-213.

Meany, M.J., Stewart, J., Poulin, P., and McEwen, B.S. (1983). Sexual differentiation of social play in rat pups is mediated by the neonatal androgen-receptor system. *Neuroendocrinology, 37*, 85-90.

Mennin, S.P. and Gorski, R.A. (1975). Effects of ovarian steroids on plasma LH in normal and persistant estrous adult female rats. *Endocrinology, 6*, 486-491.

Meyer, L.S. and Riley, E.P. (1986). Social play in juvenile rats prenatally exposed to alcohol. *Teratology, 34*, 1-7.

Meyer-Bahlburg H.F.L., Ehrhardt, A.A., Rosen, L.R., Feldman, J.F., Veridiano, N.P., Zimmerman, I., and McEwen, B.S. (1984). Psychosexual milestones in women prenatally exposed to diethylstilbestrol. *Hormones and Behavior, 18*, 359-366.

Meyer-Bahlburg, H.F.L., Ehrhardt, A.A., Feldman, J.F., Rosen, L.R., Veridiano, N.P., and Zimmerman, I. (1985). Sexual activity level and sexual functioning in women prenatally exposed to diethylstilbestrol. *Psychosomatic Medicine, 47*(6), 497-511.

Newbold, R.R., Tyrey, S., Haney, A.F., and McLachlan, J.A. (1983). Developmentally arrested oviduct: A structural and functional defect in mice following prenatal exposure to diethylstilbestrol. *Teratology, 27*, 417-426.

Newbold, R.R. and McLachlan, J.J. (1985). Diethystilbestrol-associated defects in murine genital tract development. In: *Estrogens in the Environment II: influences on development*, ed. J.J. McLachlan. Elsevier North-Holland, New York, pp. 288-318.

Newbold, R.R., Bullock, B.C, and McLachlan, J.A. (1987). Mullerian remnants of male mice exposed prenatally to diethystilbestrol. *Teratog. Carcinogen. Mutagen.,* **7**, 377-389.

Nishizuka, M. (1976). Neuropharmacological study on the induction of hypothalamic masculinization in female mice. *Neuroendocrinology,* **20**, 157-165.

Parker, S., Mahendra, U, Gavaler, J.S., and Van Thiel, D.H. (1984). Adverse effects of ethanol upon the adult sexual behavior of male rats exposed in utero. *Neurobehavioral Toxicol. and Teratol.,* **6**, 289-293.

Pentacost, B.T., Newbold, R.R., Teng, C.T., and McLachlan, J.A. (1988). Prenatal Exposure of male mice to diethylstilbestrol alters the expression of the lactotransferrin gene in seminal vesicles. *Molecular Endocrinology,* **2**, 1243-1248.

Pizzi W.J., Barnhart, J.E., and Fanslow, D.J. (1977). Monosodium Glutamate Administration to the Newborn Reduces Reproductive Ability in Female and Male mice. *Science,* **196**, 452-453.

Polani P.E. (1981). Abnormal Sex Development In: *Man. 1. Anomalies of Sex Determining Mechanisms. Mechanisms of Sex Differentiation in Animals and Man,* ed. R. Austin and R.G. Edwards. Academic Press, Inc, New York and London, pp. 465-547.

Pomerantz S.M., Roy, M.M., Thornton, J.E., and Goy, R.W. (1985). Expression of Adult Female Patterns of Sexual Behavior by Male, Female and Pseudohemorphroditic Female Rhesus Monkeys. *Bio. of Repro.,* **33**, 878-889.

Pointis, G., Latreille, M.T., Richard, M.O., Athis, P.D., and Cedard, P.D. (1984). Effect of maternal progesterone exposure on fetal testosterone in mice. *Biology of the Neonate,* **45**, 203-208.

Prahalada, S., Carroad, E., Cukierski. M., and Hendrick, A.G. (1985). Embryotoxicity of a single dose of medroxyprogesterone acetate (MPA) and maternal serum MPA concentrations in cynomolgus monkeys (Macaca fascicularis). *Teratology* **32**, 421-432.

Rhees, R.W. and Fleming, D.E. (1981). Effects of malnutrition, maternal stress or ACTH injections during pregnancy on sexual behavior of male offspring. *Physiology and Behavior,* **27**, 879-882.

Rudeen, P.K. (1986). Reduction of the volume of the sexually dimorphic nucleus of the preoptic area by *in utero* ethanol exposure. *Neuroscience Letters,* **72**, 363-368.

Sager, D.B. (1983). Effect of postnatal exposure to polychlorinated biphenyls on adult male reproductive function. *Environ. Res.,* **31**, 76-94.

Salaman, D.F. and Birkett, S. (1974). Androgen-induced sexual differentiation of the brain is blocked by inhibitors of DNA and RNA synthesis. *Nature,* **247**, 109-112.

Schardein J.L. (1985). Chemically Induced Birth Defects. Drug and Chemical Toxicology Series Vol. 2. Marcel Dekker, Inc., New York and Basel, p. 284.

Steinberger, E. and Lloyd, J.A. (1985). Chemicals affecting the development of reproductive capacity. In: *Reproductive Toxicology,* ed. R.L. Dixon. Raven Press, New York, pp. 1-20.

Stylianopoulou, F. (1983). Effect of maternal adrenocorticotropin injections on the differentiation of sexual behavior of the offspring. *Hormones and Behavior,* **17**, 324-331.

Swaab, D.F. and Fliers, E.A (1985). Sexually dimorphic nucleus in the human brain. *Science,* **228**, 1112-1114.

Swanson, H.H. and van der Werff ten Bosch, J.J. (1964). The early androgen syndrome: Differences in response to prenatal and postnatal administration of various doses of testosterone propinate in female and male rats. *Acta Endocrinologica,* **47**, 37-50.

Tapanainen, J., Penttinen, J., and Huhtaniemi, I. (1979). Effect of progesterone treatment on the development and function of neonatal rat adrenals and testes. *Biology of the Neonate,* **36,** 290-297.

van der Schoot P. and R. Baumgarten. (1990). Effects of treatment of male and female rats in infancy with mifepristone on reproductive function in adulthood. *J.Reprod. Fert.,* **90,** 255-266.

Vannier, B. and Raynaud, J.P. (1980). Long-term effects of prenatal oestrogen treatment on genital morphology and reproductive function in the rat. *J. Repro. and Fert.,* **59,** 43-49.

Vathy, I.U. Etgen, A.M., and Barfield, R.J. (1985). Effects of prenatal exposure to morphine on the development of sexual behavior in rats. *Pharmacol., Biochem. and Behav.,* **22,** 227-232.

vom Saal, F.S. and Finch, C.E. (1988). Reproductive senescence: Phenomena and mechanisms in mammals and selected vertebrates. In: *The Physiology of Reproduction,* ed. E. Knobil, J. Niell, et al., Chapter 60. New York, Raven Press.

Walker, T.F., Bott, J.H., and Bond, B.C. (1987). Cimetidine does not demasculinize male rat offspring exposed *in utero. Fund. and Appl. Toxicol.,* **8**(2), 118-197.

Warren, D.W., Ahmad, N., and Rudeen, P.K. (1988). The effects of fetal exposure to 1,2-Dibromo-3-Chloropropane on adult male reproductive function. *Bio. of Repro.* **39,** 707-716.

Weir, P.J., Conner, M., and Johnson, C.M. (1990). Abnormal development of male urogenital sinus derivatives produced by a 5alpha-reductase inhibitor. *Teratology,* **41**(5A), 599.

Wilson J.D. (1978). Sexual Differentiation. *Ann. Rev. Physiol.,* **40,** 279-306. **16,** 123-130.

Wilson, J.G. and Wilson, H.C. (1943). Reproductive capacity in adult rats treated prepubertally with androgenic hormone. *Endocrinology,* **33,** 353-350.

Wise, D.L, Vetter, C.M., Anderson, C.A., Antonello, J.M., and Clark, R.L. (1991). Reversible effects of triamcinolone and lack of effects with aspirin or L-656, 224 on external genitalia of male Sprague-Dawley rats exposed *in utero. Teratology,* **44,** 507-520.

Whitsett, J. M. and Vandenbergh, J.G. (1975). Influence of testosterone propionate administered neonatally on puberty and bisexual behavior in female hamsters. *J. Comp. and Physiol. Psych.,.* **88,** 248-255.

Zimmerberg, B. and Reuter, J.M. Sexually dimorphic behavioral and brain asymmetries in neonatal rats effects of prenatal alcohol exposure. *Develop. Brain Res.,* **46,** 281-290.

# THE INFLUENCE OF HORMONES AND HORMONE ANTAGONISTS ON SEXUAL DIFFERENTIATION OF THE BRAIN

**Klaus D. Döhler**
Pharma Bissendorf Peptide, Hannover, Germany

**Barbara Jarzab**
Clinic of General Surgery, Silesian Academy of Medicine, Bytom, Poland

## INTRODUCTION

The question about which factors may determine the fate of a developing fetus, causing it to become either male or female, has occupied many previous cultures and scientists. The "thermal hypothesis," put forth by the ancient Greek philosopher and scientist Empedokles of Akras (about 460 BC), claimed that temperature was an important factor in sex determination (Plato, translated by Jowett, 1953). Conception in a hot uterus would produce a male, in a cold uterus a female. Aristotle of Stagirus (384 to 322 BC) was convinced that sheep and goats would produce male offspring when warm winds were blowing from the south during copulation, but female offspring when cold winds were blowing from the north (Aristotle, translated by Cresswell, 1862).

The "thermal hypothesis" of Empedokles may actually not be that far off after all. It has been shown that frog larvae develop a male phenotype when raised at elevated water temperature, at low temperature they develop into females (Piquet, 1930). In some species of lizards, breeding of the eggs at temperatures below 26° C will prime the embryos for female development, whereas at temperatures above 26° C the embryos will develop into males (Short, 1982). In two species of turtles, *Emys orbicularis* and *Testudo graeca* the temperature effect on sexual differentiation is reversed. Male development is induced during breeding at temperatures below 28° C and female development is induced during breeding at above 32° C (Pieau, 1975).

Another environmental influence which may effect sexual differentiation is the concentration of potassium and calcium ions in the water. Three- to four-fold elevation of calcium ions in the water will stimulate the larvae of the toad *Discoglossus pictus* to develop into females. Five- to six-fold elevation of calcium ions will stimulate the same larvae to develop into males (Stolkovski and Bellec, 1960).

After the ancient times of the early Greek philosophers it took almost 2,500 years before the role of the Y-chromosome in masculinization of the gonads was discovered. Although differentiation of the mammalian gonads is under

1. Corresponding Author: Klaus D. Döhler, Pharma Bissendorf Peptide, Karl-Wiechert-Allee 3, D-3000 Hannover 61, Germany.

chromosomal control, differentiation of other sexual structures, like the reproductive tract, the external genitalia and the brain, is now known to be controlled by an imprinting action of hormones during fetal or neonatal life.

## SEXUALLY DIMORPHIC BRAIN STRUCTURES AND FUNCTIONS

A number of functions, which are controlled by the brain, are expressed differently in male and female organisms. These functions include the release of gonadotropic hormones from the pituitary gland, male and female sexual behavior, play and social behavior, agonistic behavior, learning behavior, gender role behavior, posture during urination, scent marking behavior, vocalization, regulation of food intake and body weight (Harlan et al., 1979; Goy and McEwen, 1980). The most obvious functional differences between male and female animals are those involved in reproductive physiology and reproductive behavior. The best-studied animal model in this respect is the rat. In the adult animal, the medial preoptic area of the brain has been implicated as a structure of central importance for the expression of reproductive functions. Studies using different experimental approaches such as lesions and electrical stimulation have implicated the medial preoptic area in the regulation of gonadotropic hormone release, and in masculine and feminine sexual behavior in several species (Van de Poll and van Dis, 1971; 1979; Hart, 1974; Kelley and Pfaff, 1978; Bermond, 1982).

Despite the well-known sex differences in brain functions, brain structure was for a long time believed to be essentially the same in males and females. The first anatomical sex differences, observed in the mammalian brain, were rather subtle. In rats Pfaff (1966) as well as Dörner and Staudt (1968) observed differences between the sexes in the size of nerve cell nuclei. Sex-linked differences in the pattern of neuronal connections were observed in rodents by Raisman and Field (1973), Dyer et al., (1976), Greenough et al., (1977), Matsumoto and Arai (1980), Nishizuka and Arai (1981), De Vries et al., (1981) and by Dyer (1984).

The first discovery of a gross sexual dimorphism of the brain was made by Nottebohm and Arnold (1976) on two species of song birds. During a reinvestigation of the male and female rat brain Gorski et al., (1978) observed a striking sexual dimorphism in gross morphology of the medial preoptic area (Fig. 1). The volume of an intensely staining area, now called the sexually dimorphic nucleus of the preoptic area (SDN-POA), is several times larger in adult male rats than in females (Gorski et al., 1978; 1980; Gorski, 1984a; Robinson et al., 1986). Analogous gross sexually dimorphic structures have subsequently been identified in a variety of other species such as the gerbil (Commins and Yahr, 1984a; 1984b; Yahr, 1988), guinea pig (Hines et al., 1985; Byne and Bleier 1987; Byne et al., 1987), ferret (Tobet et al., 1986), quail (Panzica et al., 1987), and also in the human (Swaab and Fliers, 1985; Swaab and Hofman, 1988; Hofman and Swaab, 1989; De Jonge et al., 1990). The development of this nucleus starts during late fetal life (Hsü et al., 1980;

Jacobson et al., 1980; 1981b) and depends on the hormonal environment during the critical period of sexual differentiation (Gorski et al., 1978; Jacobson et al., 1981a; Döhler et al., 1984a; 1984b; 1984c; 1986; Byne and Bleier 1987; Byne et al., 1987; Dodson et al., 1988).

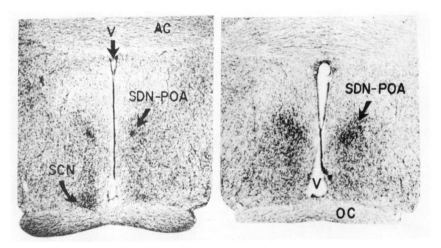

**FIGURE 1.** Representative coronal sections through the sexually dimorphic nucleus of the preoptic area (SDN-POA) in a normal adult female rat (left) and in a normal adult male rat (right). AC, anterior commissure; OC, optic chiasma; SCN, suprachiasmatic nucleus; V, third ventricle.

## SEXUAL DIFFERENTIATION OF BRAIN STRUCTURES AND FUNCTIONS

Sexual differentiation of the brain has most thoroughly been studied in the rat. In 1936 Pfeiffer presented evidence that there is a critical period during early postnatal development of the rat, during which differentiation of the pattern of anterior pituitary hormone secretion can be influenced permanently by testicular hormone action. He removed the testes of newborn male rats and replaced them with ovaries when the animals were adult. These male animals showed the female capacity to form corpora lutea in the grafted ovarian tissue. Newborn females, implanted with testes from littermate males, were unable to show estrous cycles or to form corpora lutea in their ovaries when adult.

Present knowledge of hormonal influences on the development of sexually dimorphic brain structures and functions is based on a great number of studies, most of which have been carried out in the last 30 years. The individual contributions to the field of sexual brain differentiation have been discussed in several excellent reviews (Booth, 1979; Goy and McEwen, 1980; Dörner, 1981; Gorski, 1987; Döhler, 1991). In summary, there is a sensitive developmental period during which sexual differentiation of neural substrates proceeds irreversibly under the influence of gonadal hormones. In the rat, this period starts a few days before birth and ends approximately 10 days after birth.

Female rats, treated during this sensitive period with androgens or estrogens, will permanently lose the capacity to release gonadotropin-releasing hormone (GnRH) in response to estrogenic stimulation, and will lose the capacity to show female lordosis behavior. The loss of female characteristics is termed "defeminization." Instead, female rats which are treated postnatally with androgens will develop the capacity to show the complete masculine sexual behavior pattern following administration of testosterone in adulthood. The acquisition of male characteristics is termed "masculinization."

If castrated perinatally, male rats become unable to display male sexual behavior patterns after treatment with testosterone in adulthood. The loss of male characteristics is termed "demasculinization." Instead, postnatally castrated male rats will develop the capacity to show lordosis behavior and to respond in adulthood with a positive GnRH feedback to estrogen treatment. The acquisition of female characteristics is termed "feminization."

These studies indicate that androgens and/or estrogens, whether released by the testis or applied exogenously during the perinatal period, will permanently defeminize and masculinize neural substrates controlling sexually dimorphic brain functions. The prevailing hypothesis indicates that androgens per se are not the primary stimulators of masculinization and defeminization of brain structure and functions. Instead, androgens seem to be a substrate, which has to be converted into estrogens before being able to influence sexual differentiation of the brain (for a more specialized review see Döhler, 1991).

*Differentiation of the Pattern of Gonadotropic Hormone Release*
Gonadotropic hormone (GTH) release from the pituitary gland is mainly controlled by the preoptic area and by the medial basal hypothalamus. The pattern of GTH release in adult females is cyclic, in adult males it is tonic. The decision for the differentiation of either the cyclic or the tonic pattern is made under the influence of gonadal hormones very early in life. Early postnatal gonadectomy of male or female rats will result in differentiation of the cyclic pattern of GTH release regardless of the genetic sex of the animals. Early postnatal implantation of testes into female rats or early postnatal treatment of female rats with aromatizable androgens or with high doses of estrogens has been shown to result in differentiation of the tonic pattern of GTH release (for review see Plapinger and McEwen, 1978; Booth, 1979; Goy and McEwen, 1980; Dörner, 1981; Döhler, 1991). Pre- and postnatal inhibition of androgenic activity by treatment of male rats with the androgen antagonist cyproterone acetate was shown to result in differentiation of the cyclic pattern of GTH release (Neumann and Elger, 1966; Neumann and Kramer, 1967).

The molecular mechanisms of steroid-induced structural and functional organization of the brain are still unknown. Evidence is accumulating that sex steroids act on the developing brain and promote growth of responsive neurons (Toran-Allerand, 1984). Steroids may also influence neurotransmitter metabolism, neuronal conductivity and synaptic connectivity of developing neurons, which may lead to permanent changes in synaptic transmission and overall neuronal activity (McEwen, 1987). It is well known that only neurons which form proper synaptic contacts are able to survive. Thus, growth promotion of neuronal processes may lead to completion of specific neural circuits and subsequent activation of neurotransmission may be essential for stabilization of these circuits (Wright and Smolen, 1985). As a consequence, permanent changes may be introduced by perinatal action of gonadal steroids which are responsible for the establishment of sexual differences in brain structure and function.

Interactions between steroids and neurotransmitters are widely investigated in adult animals (Nock and Feder, 1981) and have been described to operate also during the perinatal phase of sexual brain differentiation (Dörner, 1981; Jarzab and Döhler, 1984; Raum et al., 1984, Grossman et al., 1987; Jarzab et al., 1987). In early reports attention has been paid predominantly to the influence of the serotoninergic and adrenergic system in differentiation of neural centers. Perinatal treatment of rats with reserpine, which depletes the stores of catecholamines and serotonin in the brain, and postnatal treatment with monoamine oxidase (MAO) inhibitors revealed that alteration of monoaminergic activity modulates the organizing effect of testosterone and may even per se introduce changes in sexual differentiation of the brain (for review see Dörner, 1981). Alpha-adrenergic antagonists (see also Table 1) have been described to attenuate the testosterone-induced anovulatory syndrome (Nishizuka, 1976; Raum and Swerdloff, 1981) and it has been suggested, that this effect is mediated via increased stimulation of beta-adrenergic receptors (Raum et al., 1984). These studies awoke further interest in adrenergic participation of sexual differentiation of the brain since, in the adult animal, the adrenergic system is known to be essential for elicitation of sexual functions (Kalra and McCann, 1974; Dörner, 1981; Barraclough and Wise, 1982; Kalra and Kalra, 1983). Barraclough et al., (1984) concluded on the basis of extensive experiments (Rance et al., 1981; Wise et al., 1981; Lookingland and Barraclough, 1982; Lookingland et al., 1982) that the neural trigger for cyclic LH secretion, characteristic of female rats, resides within the catecholaminergic system and that defeminized animals lack the ability to generate this trigger. This conclusion was supported by Grossman et al., (1987) who proposed that during the postnatal period testosterone permanently alters adrenergic and opioid interactions, which control the cyclic pattern of LH release.

In a series of experiments we treated newborn rats for several days with compounds (Table 1) which stimulated or inhibited the alpha- and beta-adrenergic, the serotoninergic, or the cholinergic system (Jarzab and Döhler, 1984; Sickmöller, 1985; Sickmöller et al., 1985; Jarzab et al., 1986; 1987; 1989; 1990a; 1990b). All of these animals ovulated spontaneously at 3 months of age, but the ovaries of animals which had been treated with the beta-adrenergic agonists isoprenaline or salbutamol were significantly smaller than ovaries of control rats (Jarzab et al., 1989).

**TABLE 1.** Compounds used to influence neurotransmitter activity in neonatal rats

| Compound | Activity | Daily Dose (per animal) |
|---|---|---|
| saline | none (vehicle) | 50 µl |
| l-tryptophan | precursor for serotonin synthesis | 500 µg |
| para-chlorophenyl-alanine (p-CPA) | inhibitor of serotonin biosynthesis | 100 µg |
| clonidine | alpha$_2$-receptor agonist | 0.5 µg |
| prazosine | alpha$_1$-receptor antagonist | 25 µg |
| yohimbine | alpha$_2$-receptor antagonist | 6.25 µg |
| isoprenaline | general beta-receptor agonist | 50 µg |
| salbutamol | specific beta$_2$-receptor agonist | 25 µg |
| alprenolol | beta-receptor antagonist | 25 µg |
| physostigmine | acetylcholin-esterase inhibitor | 1 µg |
| atropine | muscarinic receptor antagonist | 250 µg |
| mecamylamine | nicotinic receptor antagonist | 25 µg |

Our results suggest that the adrenergic system is involved in differentiation of the gonadotropin release pattern, since the LH-release response to estradiol benzoate (EB) and progesterone in adult ovariectomized female rats, which resembles the preovulatory LH discharge, was intensified after postnatal blockade of alpha-adrenergic receptors and was reduced after postnatal blockade of beta-adrenergic receptors or after specific postnatal stimulation of beta$_2$-adrenergic receptors (Fig. 2). Also in normal adult animals the adrenergic system has been shown to have both stimulatory and inhibitory effects on gonadotropin secretion (Barraclough and Wise 1982). Whereas stimulation of muscarinic and

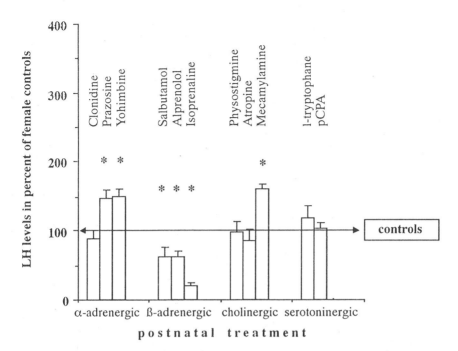

**FIGURE 2.** Influence of postnatal treatment of female rats with the alpha$_2$-receptor agonist clonidine, the alpha$_1$-receptor antagonist prazosine, the alpha$_2$-receptor antagonist yohimbine, the beta$_2$-receptor agonist salbutamol, the beta-receptor antagonist alprenolol, the beta-receptor agonist isoprenaline, the acetylcholinesterase inhibitor physostigmine, the muscarinic receptor antagonist atropine, the nicotinic receptor antagonist mecamylamine, the serotonin precursor l-tryptophan, or the inhibitor of serotonin biosynthesis para-chlorophenyl-alanine (pCPA) on LH release in response to treatment with estradiol benzoate (EB) and progesterone (P) in adulthood. Female rats, which had been treated with vehicle postnatally, served as controls. In order to make the results of different experiments comparable, LH levels of control rats in response to treatment with EB and P in adulthood were arbitrarily set as 100%. LH levels were always measured 5.5 to 6 hours after treatment with P. During this period LH-levels had been shown to be highest following treatment with EB + P. All results of experimental animals are presented in percent of the respective means of female control rats. Postnatal treatment is indicated by the name of the respective compound above each mean ± SEM result bar.
* $p < 0.05$. Data are redrawn from Jarzab et al. (1990b).

nicotinic receptors postnatally had no influence on the LH-release response in adulthood, inhibition of nicotinic receptors by mecamylamine (Fig. 2) resulted in permanent hypersensation of the positive feedback-mechanism (Sickmöller, 1985; Sickmöller et al., 1985; Jarzab et al., 1990b). Postnatal application of compounds which stimulate or inhibit the synthesis of serotonin (Fig. 2) had no influence on the LH-release response in adulthood (Jarzab and Döhler, 1984; Jarzab et al., 1990b).

### Differentiation of Sexual Behavior Patterns
Differentiation of male or female type of sexual behavior patterns is under

similar influence of gonadal hormones very early in life as is differentiation of the GTH release pattern. Early postnatal gonadectomy of male or female rats will result in differentiation of the capacity for female lordosis behavior regardless of the genetic sex of the animals. Early postnatal implantation of testes into female rats or early postnatal treatment of female rats with aromatizable androgens or estrogens has been shown to interfere with differentiation of lordosis behavior and to result in differentiation of the capacity for male mounting, intromission and ejaculatory behavior instead (for review see Plapinger and McEwen, 1978; Booth, 1979; Goy and McEwen, 1980; Dörner, 1981; Döhler, 1991). Pre- and postnatal inhibition of androgenic activity by treatment of male rats with the androgen antagonist cyproterone acetate was shown to result in differentiation of female behavior patterns (Neumann and Elger, 1966; Neumann and Kramer, 1967). Postnatal inhibition of estrogenic activity by treatment of male rats with the estrogen antagonists tamoxifen or LY 117018 was shown to interfere with differentiation of male sexual behavior patterns and to stimulate differentiation of female behavior patterns (Ganzemüller and Veit, 1988). It has previously been mentioned that androgens must be converted into estrogens before they can influence sexual differentiation of certain brain structures and functions.

Participation of adrenergic mechanisms in steroid-induced defeminization and masculinization of the brain was proposed in the early seventies (for reviews, see Booth, 1979 and Dörner, 1981). Most reports were focused on the differentiating mechanisms for sexually dimorphic secretion of gonadotropins. Treatment of newborn female rats with reserpine was reported to disturb the onset of puberty, ovarian cycles and female sexual behavior (Lehtinen et al., 1972, Dörner et al., 1977). Similar treatment of newborn male rats with reserpine was reported to augment (Lehtinen et al., 1972) or to inhibit (Dörner et al., 1976) the capacity for expression of male copulatory behavior in adulthood. The possible participation of the adrenergic system in sexual differentiation of the brain was also tested by postnatal treatment of male and female rats with the monoamine oxidase inhibitor pargyline. This treatment was shown to reduce the frequency of mounting behavior in adulthood in both sexes (Dörner et al., 1976; 1977). Reserpine and pargyline, however, are known to interact with several monoaminergic systems. Thus, it was not possible to draw final conclusions on the specific role of adrenergic neurotransmission during the organizing phase of neural structures controlling sexual functions.

In a series of experiments we used compounds with more specific stimulatory or inhibitory action (Table 1) on the alpha- and beta-adrenergic, the serotoninergic, or the cholinergic system (Jarzab and Döhler, 1984; Sickmöller, 1985; Sickmöller et al., 1985; Jarzab et al., 1986; 1987; 1989; 1990a; 1990b). Postnatal stimulation of serotonin synthesis by l-tryptophane inhibited the expression of lordosis behavior in female (Fig. 3) and in androgenized female rats (Fig. 4) in adulthood (Jarzab and Döhler, 1984; Jarzab et al., 1990b). Postnatal treatment with l-tryptophan also inhibited the expression of male mounting and intromission behavior in androgenized female rats after substitution with testosterone propionate in adulthood (Jarzab and Döhler, 1984). This organizational effect of serotonin resembles the inhibitory role of this neurotransmitter in activation of sexual behavior in adulthood (Meyerson, 1964; Malmnäs, 1973; Michanek and Meyerson, 1977).

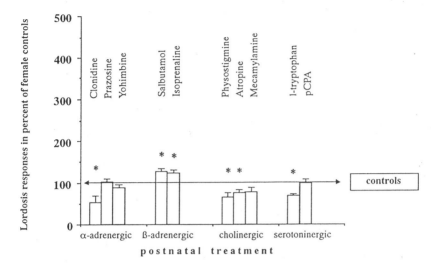

**FIGURE 3.** Influence of postnatal treatment of female rats with the alpha$_2$-receptor agonist clonidine, the alpha$_1$-receptor antagonist prazosine, the alpha$_2$-receptor antagonist yohimbine, the beta$_2$-receptor agonist salbutamol, the beta-receptor agonist isoprenaline, the acetylcholin-esterase inhibitor physostigmine, the muscarinic receptor antagonist atropine, the nicotinic receptor antagonist mecamylamine, the serotonin precursor l-tryptophan, or the inhibitor of serotonin biosynthesis para-chlorophenyl-alanine (p-CPA) on the capacity to perform female lordosis behavior in response to treatment with estradiol benzoate (EB) and progesterone (P) in adulthood. Female rats, which had been treated with vehicle postnatally, served as controls. In order,to make the results of different experiments comparable, lordosis frequency of control rats in response to treatment with EB and P in adulthood was arbitrarily set as 100%. Lordosis behavior was always observed 5 to 7 hours after treatment with P. All results of experimental animals are presented in percent of the respective means of female control rats. Postnatal treatment is indicated by the name of the respective compound above each mean ± SEM result bar. All results are presented as percentage increase or decrease of lordosis responses as compared to respective means ± SEM of female control rats.
* p<0.05. Data are redrawn from Jarzab et al. (1989; 1990b).

Subtle but statistically significant postnatal effects of adrenergic ligands were also observed on the expression of sexual behavior in adulthood. Administration of the alpha$_2$-adrenergic agonist clonidine postnatally resulted in reduced female sexual behavior of adult animals when compared with control rats (Fig. 3). Additional postnatal treatment with TP (Fig. 4) prevented the clonidine-induced reduction of lordosis behavior (Jarzab et al., 1986; 1987; 1990b). The results suggest that postnatal stimulation of alpha$_2$-adrenergic binding sites inhibits differentiation of female sexual behavior and that testosterone postnatally

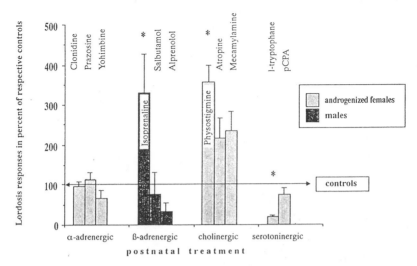

**FIGURE 4.** Influence of postnatal treatment of androgenized female rats with the alpha$_2$-receptor agonist clonidine, the alpha$_1$-receptor antagonist prazosine, the alpha$_2$-receptor antagonist yohimbine, the acetylcholin-esterase inhibitor physostigmine, the muscarinic receptor antagonist atropine, the nicotinic receptor antagonist mecamylamine, the serotonin precursor l-tryptophan, or the inhibitor of serotonin biosynthesis para-chlorophenyl-alanine (p-CPA), and postnatal treatment of male rats with the beta-receptor agonist isoprenaline, the beta$_2$-receptor agonist salbutamol, or the beta-receptor antagonist alprenolol, on the capacity to perform female lordosis behavior in response to treatment with estradiol benzoate (EB) and progesterone (P) in adulthood. Androgenized female rats, which had been treated with testosterone propionate postnatally, and male rats, which had been treated with vehicle postnatally, served as respective controls. In order to make the results of different experiments comparable, lordosis frequencies of male and androgenized female control rats in response to treatment with EB and P in adulthood were arbitrarily set as 100%. Lordosis behavior was always observed 5 to 7 hours after treatment with P. All results of experimental animals are presented in percent of the respective means of androgenized female or male control rats. Postnatal treatment is indicated by the name of the respective compound above each mean ± SEM result bar. All results are presented as percentage increase or decrease of lordosis responses as compared to respective means ± SEM of androgenized female or male control rats. * p<0.05. Data are redrawn from Jarzab et al. (1990b).

prevents this alpha$_2$-mediated inhibition. Postnatal treatment with prazosine or yohimbine (Fig. 3 and 4) had no significant effects on the lordotic response in adulthood (Jarzab et al., 1986; 1987; 1990b). Postnatal stimulation or inhibition of the alpha-adrenergic system had no significant influence on differentiation of male sexual behavior patterns (Jarzab et al., 1987).

The beta-adrenergic system seems to protect differentiation of female lordosis behavior in female rats from subtle defeminizing influences because postnatal treatment of female rats with the beta-receptor agonists salbutamol or isoprenaline increased the capacity for lordosis behavior in adulthood (Fig. 3).

Even in male rats postnatal stimulation of beta-adrenergic receptors augmented lordosis behavior (Fig. 4) after priming in adulthood with EB and progesterone (Jarzab et al., 1989; 1990b). Postnatal inhibition of beta-adrenergic receptors inhibited differentiation of ejaculatory behavior in male rats (Jarzab et al., 1989).

The cholinergic system also seems to be involved in differentiation of lordosis behavior. Postnatal inhibition of muscarinic receptors by atropine or postnatal stimulation of both muscarinic and nicotonic receptors by physostigmine resulted in decreased capacity for lordosis behavior in adulthood (Fig. 3). Simultaneous postnatal treatment with TP (Fig. 4) prevented the physostigmine-induced reduction of lordosis behavior (Sickmöller, 1985; Sickmöller et al., 1985; Jarzab et al., 1990b).

*Development and Differentiation of the Sexually Dimorphic Nucleus of the Preoptic Area (SDN-POA)*
*The influence of gonadal steroids on development and differentiation of the SDN-POA.* Development of the SDN-POA was shown to start during late fetal life and to extend throughout the first ten days of postnatal life (Hsü et al., 1980; Jacobson et al., 1980; 1981b). This developmental period is identical with the period when sexual differentiation of brain function proceeds under the influence of gonadal hormones.

A series of studies was performed during recent years in order to test the influence of hormones perinatally on development and differentiation of the SDN-POA. Neonatal castration of male rats (Fig. 5) reduced the volume of the SDN-POA permanently (Gorski et al., 1978; Jacobson et al., 1981a). Reimplantation of a testis or treatment with a single injection of testosterone propionate (TP) (Fig. 5) one day (Jacobson et al., 1981a), or up to four days after neonatal castration restored SDN-POA volume in male rats to normal (Rhees et al., 1990). Treatment of female rats with a single injection of TP postnatally (Gorski et al., 1978; Jacobson et al., 1981a) increased SDN-POA volume significantly, however, the volume of the SDN-POA in these animals was still significantly smaller than that of normal male rats. Only the extended pre- and postnatal treatment of female rats with TP (Fig. 5) resulted in SDN-POA differentiation equivalent to that of normal males (Döhler et al., 1984a). The treatment of male rats pre- and postnatally with TP (Fig. 5) did not increase the size of their SDN-POA above normal (Döhler et al., 1984a). Rhees et al., (1990) observed that the SDN-POA of female or postnatally gonadectomized male rats was susceptible to TP-treatment for up to day 5 after birth, but it became insensitive to TP-treatment after day 5.

Although pre- and postnatal treatment of rats with TP was shown to substitute fully for testicular activities in stimulating SDN-POA development, the prime candidates for the control of SDN-POA differentiation do not seem to be androgens as such, but rather estrogens. This conclusion is supported by several observations:

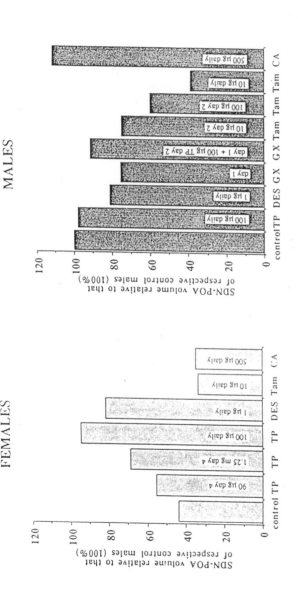

**FIGURE 5.** Schematic representation of the hormonal environment perinatally on development and differentiation of the sexually dimorphic nucleus of the preoptic area (SDN-POA) in female (left) and male (right) rats. Female rats received treatment with either a single injection of 90 μg or 1.25 mg testosterone propionate (TP) on day 4 after birth, or daily treatment with TP, diethylstilbestrol (DES), the estrogen antagonist tamoxifen (Tam), or the androgen antagonist cyproterone acetate (CA) from day 16 of fetal life until day 10 after birth. Two groups of male rats were gonadectomized (GX) on the day of birth, one group received a single injection of 100 μg TP one day after GX. Two groups of male rats received a single injection of either 10 μg or 100 μg TP on day 2 after birth. Four groups of male rats received daily treatment with TP, DES, Tam, or CA respectively from day 16 of fetal life until day 10 after birth. SDN-POA volume is indicated in percent as compared to SDN-POA volume of normal adult male rats (100 percent) from several different experiments (Döhler et al., 1984a; 1986; Gorski et al., 1978; Jacobson et al., 1982).

a.  Female rats, which had been treated pre- and postnatally with the synthetic estrogen, diethylstilbestrol (Fig. 5), developed a significantly enlarged SDN-POA which was similar in volume to that of control males (Döhler et al., 1984a). This observation indicates that estrogens can stimulate SDN-POA development directly. The treatment of male rats pre- and postnatally with diethylstilbestrol did not increase the size of their SDN-POA above normal (Döhler et al., 1984a).

b.  Male rats, treated pre- and postnatally with the androgen antagonist cyproterone acetate (Fig. 5), developed female genitalia, but the volume of their SDN-POA was not reduced (Döhler et al., 1986).

c.  Male rats, treated pre- and postnatally with the estrogen antagonist tamoxifen, developed male genitalia, but the volume of their SDN-POA was significantly reduced (Fig. 5) and was similar to that of control female rats (Döhler et al., 1986). The normal development of male genitalia in these animals and the observation that pre- and postnatal treatment of male rats with tamoxifen did not influence serum levels of testosterone (Döhler et al., 1986), indicate that tamoxifen did not act via inhibition of testosterone release from the testes. Instead, the growth inhibiting influence of the estrogen antagonist on the SDN-POA, a brain area with known sensitivity to estrogens (Stumpf et al., 1975; Gorski et al., 1980; Döhler et al., 1984a), seems most likely to be due to local interference with the activity of estrogens, which may have derived via enzymatic conversion from circulating androgens.

In the adult organism tamoxifen is known to bind to intracellular estrogen receptors and to prevent estrogen uptake as it inhibits cytosol receptor replenishment (Nicholson et al., 1976; Jordan et al., 1977; 1980). Tamoxifen may act similarly in the developing organism. After aromatization of testicular androgens into estrogens tamoxifen may have interfered with estrogen uptake into cell nuclei of the SDN-POA by occupying intracellular estrogen receptors. The inhibitory effect of pre- and postnatal tamoxifen on growth and differentiation of the SDN-POA in male rats indicates that structural differentiation of the male rat brain may be dependent on aromatization of testicular androgens into estrogens and the subsequent interaction of these estrogens with the cell nuclear material. The observation that the androgen antagonist, cyproterone acetate, did not interfere with growth and differentiation of the SDN-POA indicates, that androgens are not the primary stimulators of SDN-POA differentiation. Androgens seem to be the substrate, which has to be converted into estrogens before being able to activate SDN-POA differentiation.

*The influence of neurotransmitters on development and differentiation of the SDN-POA.* The SDN-POA is sexually dimorphic not only in terms of its volume but also in terms of neurochemicals present in the cell-bodies of neurons comprising this nucleus and in the fibers innervating the nucleus and its vicinity

(Commins and Yahr, 1984a; Simerly et al., 1986). These differences are established during the critical pre- and postnatal period (Simerly et al., 1985) when sexual differentiation of the SDN-POA takes place. Thus, it seems that during the perinatal period gonadal steroids act not only as differentiation signals for morphological and functional parameters of the brain, but also influence neurotransmitter activity in the developing brain.

The mechanisms of steroid-neurotransmitter interaction in the developing brain are not well investigated. Testosterone has been described to influence neurotransmitter and neuropeptide content in the brain (Giulian et al., 1973; Hardin, 1973; Reznikov and Nosenko, 1983; Diez-Guerra et al., 1987; Grossman et al., 1987). Compounds which change neurotransmitter activity have been reported to influence postnatal sexual differentiation of the brain and to interfere with the effects of steroids during this process (Reznikov et al., 1979; Raum and Swerdloff, 1981; Hull et al., 1984; Jarzab and Döhler, 1984; Raum et al. 1984; Sickmöller, 1985; Sickmöller et al., 1985; Jarzab et al., 1986; 1987; 1989; 1990a; 1990b).

Concerning the SDN-POA, it was shown by Simerly et al., (1986) that in adult rats this nucleus is innervated by adrenergic fibers. In a series of studies we demonstrated that alteration of serotoninergic or adrenergic neurotransmission postnatally has profound effects on development and differentiation of the SDN-POA (Jarzab et al., 1990a; 1990b). Both, stimulation and inhibition of serotonin synthesis postnatally, provided a stimulus for SDN-POA morphogenesis in female rats (Fig. 6). Postnatal treatment with TP (Fig. 6) potentiated the stimulatory effect of the serotonin precursor l-tryptophan (Jarzab et al., 1990b). The fact that stimulation, as well as inhibition, of serotonin synthesis postnatally exerts similar morphogenetic influences on SDN-POA development remains unexplained, in particular since the SDN-POA in adult animals of both sexes is practically devoid of serotoninergic innervation (Simerly et al., 1983; 1986). Trophic effects of serotonin on developing neurons have been documented by Lauder (1983) in the rat foetus. Handa et al. (1986) described an increase in SDN-POA volume of one-day old female rats after prenatal administration of pCPA. The results of Jarzab et al. (1990b) indicate that the same stimulatory effect on SDN-POA development can be induced postnatally and remains permanent into adulthood.

Adrenergic effects on differentiation of the SDN-POA are mediated mainly by alpha$_2$- and beta$_2$-adrenergic receptors (Jarzab et al., 1990a; 1990b). The alpha$_2$-receptor agonist clonidine was shown to augment the stimulatory effect of TP on SDN-POA differentiation in female rats (Fig. 6) and the beta$_2$-receptor agonist salbutamol causes the volume of the SDN-POA to increase in both female and male rats (Fig. 6). The observed effects are independent from postnatal levels of circulating testosterone, as judged in male rats on day 3 of life (Jarzab et al., 1990a).

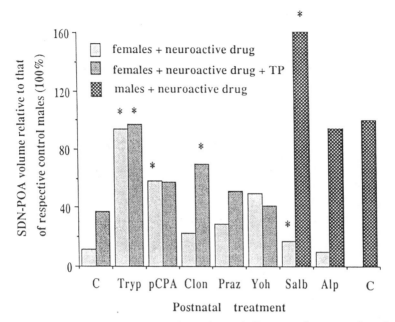

**FIGURE 6.** Schematic representation of the influence of neuroactive drugs postnatally on development and differentiation of the sexually dimorphic nucleus of the preoptic area (SDN-POA) in male, female, and postnatally with testosterone propionate (TP) androgenized female rats. Postnatal treatment with the serotonin precursor l-tryptophan (Tryp) or with the inhibitor of serotonin biosynthesis para-chlorophenyl-alanine (p-CPA) stimulated SDN-POA volume in female rats. Postnatal treatment with the alpha$_2$-receptor agonist clonidine (Clon) stimulated SDN-POA volume in androgenized female rats, treatment with the beta$_2$-receptor agonist salbutamol (Salb) stimulated SDN-POA volume in female and in male rats. Postnatal treatment of female rats with the alpha$_1$-receptor antagonist prazosine (Praz), the alpha$_2$-receptor antagonist yohimbine (Yoh), and postnatal treatment of male or female rats with the beta-receptor antagonist alprenolol (Alp) had no influence on SDN-POA differentiation. SDN-POA volume is indicated in percent as compared to SDN-POA volume of normal adult male rats (100 percent) from several different experiments (Jarzab et al., 1989; 1990a; 1990b).
* $P < 0.05$ as compared to the respective male, female, or androgenized female control group (C).

Hammer (1988) reported higher levels of opiate binding in the area of the SDN-POA of five-day-old female rats than in males of same age. Postnatal treatment of female rats with the non-aromatizable androgen DHT inhibited opiate binding in the SDN-POA, postnatal treatment of male rats with the androgen antagonist flutamide stimulated opiate binding in the SDN-POA. No changes were observed in opiate binding when females or males were treated postnatally with the estrogen antagonist tamoxifen (Hammer, 1988).

Possible mechanisms of steroid-induced SDN-POA formation, as discussed by Gorski (1984b; 1987), are the stimulation or prolongation of neurogenesis, protection from neuronal cell death, stimulation of migration of neurons from their origin in the ependymal lining of the third ventricle to the region of the

SDN-POA (Jacobson et al., 1981b), aggregation of these neurons into the distinct nucleus, perhaps through alteration of the cell-surface recognition process, or by influencing the specification of neurons destined to form the SDN-POA by activating or suppressing certain genes. The proposed mechanisms may also be applicable to the observed effects of adrenergic and serotoninergic compounds.

Beta-adrenergic binding sites were shown to be present in the rat brain during the period of SDN-POA development and differentiation (Bruinink and Lichtensteiger, 1984; Bruinink et al., 1983; Ribary et al., 1986). Ascending catechlamine fibers were shown to reach the anterior diencephalon by day 15 of fetal development and they reach the preoptic area by day 16 (Lichtensteiger and Schlumpf, 1981). An influence of salbutamol on neurogenesis seems unlikely since the number of dividing neurons in the SDN-POA diminishes rapidly during the last days of fetal development (Jacobson et al., 1981a). However, it is worth mentioning that psychotropic drugs, which alter noradrenaline metabolism, may influence replication of neurons even after birth (Patel et al., 1981). Stimulation of adrenergic receptors, located on neurons which form or are able to form the SDN-POA, may promote migration of the neurons to the center of the medial preoptic area. The stimulated neurons may be prevented from cell death during migration or after reaching the center of the preoptic area.

The influence of salbutamol on differentiation of the SDN-POA may also be conveyed indirectly via stimulation of neurons which innervate the SDN-POA. This indirect stimulation may increase the number of synaptic contacts within the SDN-POA. Since only neurons which form and receive proper synaptic contacts are able to survive, this mechanism would lead to an increase in neuronal survival rate and, thus, to an increase in SDN-POA volume. Transsynaptic influences are thought to play a critical role in regulation of the expression of neurotransmitter-related characteristics and may be responsible for the development of sexually dimorphic structure and function of the preoptic area (Changeux and Danchin, 1976; Smolen et al., 1985). Influences on neurotransmission may be some of the organizational mechanisms by which steroids induce sexual differentiation of the brain.

The effects of salbutamol treatment on SDN-POA differentiation are more distinct in male rats than in females (Jarzab et al., 1990a). It seems, therefore, that SDN-POA differentiation depends on adrenergic-steroid interaction. In adult rats many adrenergic effects have been described which modulate the action of steroids (Nock and Feder, 1981), but few investigations have been done on neonatal animals. Stimulation of beta-adrenergic receptors was shown to decrease the amount of testosterone-derived estradiol accumulation in the nuclei of developing hypothalamic neurons (Raum et al., 1984). This mechanism, however, does not explain the salbutamol-induced increase of SDN-POA volume.

Beta$_1$- and beta$_2$-receptors, although structurally closely related, differ in their affinity to various adrenergic agonists (Stiles et al., 1984). Norepinephrine is believed to stimulate mainly beta$_1$-adrenergic receptors, while epinephrine is potent at both beta$_1$- and beta$_2$-binding sites. Beta$_1$-adrenergic receptors are thought to be more closely related to neuronal functions than beta$_2$-receptors and their postsynaptic location has been confirmed. Exact cellular localisation of beta$_2$-receptors is still controversial. Some of them may be localized presynaptically where they stimulate noradrenaline release into the synaptic cleft. Some may also be localized outside the synapse and may respond to endocrine or paracrine signals. It should be mentioned that neurotransmitters with affinity exlusively to beta$_2$-adrenoreceptors do not seem to exist endogenously. Thus, the influence of salbutamol on differentiation of SDN-POA volume may be pharmacological and may not represent any physiological mechanism.

Based on their studies that perinatal administration of *para*-chlorophenylalanine, a serotonin synthesis inhibitor, increased the volume of the SDN-POA in one-day old female rats, without changing neonatal levels of testosterone or estradiol Handa et al., (1986) proposed that changes in postnatal neurotransmitter activity may directly influence the development of sexually dimorphic structures in the rodent brain. This proposition is supported by the results of our own studies (Jarzab et al., 1990a; 1990b) and it is conceivable that both adrenergic and serotoninergic inputs influence differentiation of the SDN-POA.

## WHICH FUNCTIONS ARE CONTROLLED BY THE SDN-POA?

Because of the sex difference in volume, its afferent and efferent connections (Simerly and Swanson, 1986; 1987), and its presence within the medial preoptic area, the SDN-POA has been hypothesized to be particularly involved in the regulation of reproductive functions. Conclusive data on functional aspects of the SDN-POA are rather scarce, however. Arendash and Gorski (1983) reported that small discrete lesions of the SDN-POA were unsuccessful in disrupting copulatory behavior in sexually experienced male rats. Lesions of the lateral sexually dimorphic area of adult male gerbils interfered with open field scent marking and decreased mating behavior (Commins and Yahr, 1984c). Preslock and McCann (1987) made discrete lesions in the area of the SDN-POA of male rats and observed attenuation of the post-castration rise in LH and FSH levels and a significant decrease in the serum levels of prolactin. Hennessey et al., (1986) observed an increase in the capacity to show lordosis behavior after adult male rats had received lesions of the SDN-POA. The ventromedial hypothalamus and the midbrain central gray are suggested to stimulate lordosis behavior (Barfield and Chen, 1977; Pfaff and Sakuma, 1979a; 1979b; Hennessey et al., 1986). Hennessey et al., (1986) concluded that cells of the preoptic area, which project to the ventromedial hypothalamus and from there to the midbrain central gray (Morrell and Pfaff, 1982), exert a tonic inhibition over the display of lordosis which is terminated after destruction of the medial preoptic area.

Our own studies with the androgen antagonist cyproterone acetate (Döhler et al., 1986) indicate that the SDN-POA may not be involved in the control of female lordosis behavior or the cyclic mechanism of gonadotropin release. Pre- and postnatal treatment of male rats with cyproterone acetate had previously been shown to stimulate differentiation of lordosis behavior and cyclic release of gonadotropins (Neumann and Elger, 1966; Neumann and Kramer, 1967). Our results demonstrate, however, that this same pre- and postnatal treatment did not "feminize" the SDN-POA (Döhler et al., 1986). Another finding which would speak against the SDN-POA being possibly involved in the control of lordosis behavior is the observation that beta-adrenergic stimulation postnatally increases both the volume of the SDN-POA and the capacity for lordosis behavior (Jarzab et al., 1989; 1990a; 1990b). Although our data suggest that the neurons of the SDN-POA are not involved in the control of lordosis behavior, they do not exclude the possibility that fibers, originating in other brain areas and passing through the preoptic area may be part of a lordosis inhibiting neural circuit. The interruption of such fibers, due to lesions in the preoptic area, may then result in increased capacity of lordosis behavior.

In conclusion, although many data concerning the perinatal influence of hormones and neurotransmitters on development and differentiation of the SDN-POA have been generated, very little is still known about the function of this nucleus and about its connection with other brain areas.

## SEXUAL DIFFERENTIATION OF THE BRAIN IS INFLUENCED BY STEROID-NEUROTRANSMITTER INTERACTIONS

The results of the studies presented and discussed in this review demonstrate that gonadal steroids and neurotransmitters are both involved in structural and functional differentiation of the brain. Molecular mechanisms of sexual differentiation of the brain are still not fully understood, which leaves plenty of room for speculation. There are various possibilities of interaction between neurotransmitters and gonadal steroids during development, which might influence sexual brain differentiation. Steroids are known to mediate neurotransmitter activities and neurotransmitters are known to modulate actions of steroids. Neurotransmitters have been shown to influence the number of steroid receptors (Carrillo and Sheridan, 1980; Cardinali et al., 1983) and to influence practically every biochemical step of steroid action, such as uptake of the steroid into the cell body (Nagle et al., 1973), concentration of cytoplasmic (Nock and Feder, 1981) and nuclear steroid receptors (Cardinali, 1977), and steroid-induced protein synthesis (Nagle et al., 1973; Cardinali et al., 1976).

Estradiol and diethylstilbestrol (DES) were observed to elevate cyclic AMP levels in rat hypothalamus, an effect which is prevented by both alpha- and beta-adrenoreceptor blocking drugs (Gunaga and Menon, 1973; Gunaga et al., 1974; Weissman and Skolnick, 1975; Weissman et al., 1975). Steroids have been shown to influence number and sensitivity of neurotransmitter-receptors, such as adrenergic (Wilkinson, 1978; Wagner et al., 1979; Wilkinson et al., 1979; Vacas and Cardinali, 1980; Wilkinson and Herdon, 1982), serotoninergic (Biegon et al., 1980; Kendall et al., 1981; Goetz et al., 1983), cholinergic (Rainbow et al., 1980; Dohanich et al., 1982), dopaminergic (Nausieda et al., 1979; Hruska et al., 1980; Goetz et al., 1983), GABAergic (Goetz et al., 1983) and opiate receptors (Hahn and Fishman, 1979). Steroids have also been shown to influence neurotransmitter synthesis, metabolism, and breakdown (Beattie and Soyka, 1973; Luine et al., 1975; 1980), as well as release and reuptake of neurotransmitters in synaptosomes (Janowsky and Davis, 1970; Wirz-Justice et al., 1974).

There is a great redundancy in the developing nervous system regarding the possibility of neuronal connections. Only those synapses will be stabilized which are being activated during the phase of central nervous differentiation, resulting in selective stabilization of neuronal circuits (Changeux and Danchin, 1976). Steroid-specific activation of neurons, which compete with other neurons for synaptic contacts during development, may stimulate differentiation of sexually dimorphic patterns of synaptic connections (Keyser, 1983). Neurons which are not activated during development will degenerate.

In summary, a number of studies have shown that not only estrogenic and androgenic steroids and their antagonists influence sexual differentiation of the brain but also drugs which stimulate or inhibit the adrenergic (Nishizuka, 1976; Reznikov et al., 1979; Dörner, 1981; Raum and Swerdloff, 1981; Reznikov and Nosenko, 1983; Jarzab et al., 1986; 1987; 1989; 1990a; 1990b), the serotoninergic (Jarzab and Döhler, 1984; Wilson et al., 1986; Jarzab et al., 1990b), the cholinergic (Sickmöller, 1985; Sickmöller et al., 1985; Jarzab et al., 1990b), or the dopaminergic system (Hull et al., 1984) in the developing brain.

## SUMMARY AND CONCLUSION

A number of brain structures and a great number of brain functions have been shown to be sexually dimorphic. It has also been shown that development and differentiation of these structures and functions proceed during a critical pre- and postnatal period of increased susceptibility and are controlled by gonadal steroids and neurotransmitter substances. Defeminization and masculinization of brain functions seem to be established during interaction of the developing nervous system with androgens, which have to be converted, at least in part, into estrogens. Structural differentiation of the male brain, e.g., the sexually dimorphic nucleus of the preoptic area (SDN-POA), seems to be exclusively estrogen dependent during differentiation of male brain functions, however, estrogens may be supportive, rather than directive, to the primary action of androgens (Döhler, 1991).

The molecular mechanisms of sexual differentiation of the brain are not yet fully understood. It seems, however, that the priming action of gonadal steroids during the period of increased susceptability is either mediated by neurotransmitters, or neurotransmitters modulate the priming action of gonadal steroids. In particular the adrenergic, the serotoninergic, the cholinergic, and possibly the dopaminergic system were shown to have strong influences on sexual differentiation of brain structure and functions. In contrast to the great number of available studies on the influence of gonadal steroids on sexual differentiation of the brain, there are rather few studies available concerning the influence of neurotransmitter systems. The available results are partly contradictory, so that an interpretation must be done with caution and will leave plenty of room for speculation.

Postnatal application of compounds which stimulate or inhibit adrenergic activity mainly affected the neural control of gonadotropin secretion, and had only minor influences on differentiation of behavior patterns. It seems, however, that adrenergic participation in the differentiation of the center for cyclic gonadotropin release is very complex and stimulatory and inhibitory components may operate simultaneously. Activation or inhibition of beta-adrenergic receptors during postnatal development was shown to impair the responsiveness of the center for cyclic gonadotropin release to gonadal steroids and impairs the expression of ejaculatory behavior in male rats. Activation of beta-adrenergic receptors postnatally has a stimulatory effect on the expression of female lordosis behavior in male and female rats, and stimulates development and differentiation of the SDN-POA in both sexes.

Hypothalamic concentrations of serotonin during postnatal development were shown by different groups of researchers to be higher in female rats, than in males or in androgenized females. Postnatal treatment with drugs which stimulate or inhibit serotoninergic activity gave, however, contradictory results. Some of the available data suggest that serotonin may prevent the defeminizing action of postnatal androgens on differentiation of the ovulation-inducing mechanism and on female sexual behavior, other data suggest that serotonin may inhibit differentiation of the cyclic LH-surge mechanism and of female lordosis behavior. Differentiation of the SDN-POA was shown to be enhanced postnatally by serotoninergic stimulation and by serotoninergic inhibition.

Very few data exist on the influence of the cholinergic and the dopaminergic systems on sexual differentiation of the brain. Both, stimulation and inhibition of dopaminergic activity pre- and postnatally, reduced the capacity for masculine sexual behavior in male rats, but had no influence on female rats. Cholinergic stimulation postnatally increased the capacity for male sexual behavior in male rats, inhibited differentiation of lordosis behavior in female rats, but attenuated the defeminizing activity of postnatal treatment with testosterone on differentiation of lordosis behavior. Inhibition of nicotinic receptors postnatally increased the sensitivity of the LH-surge mechanism in adulthood, which may be an indication for a longer than normal reproductive period of cyclicity.

The present knowledge on the possible participation of neurotransmitter systems in sexual differentiation of the brain and their mode of interaction in this process postnatally with gonadal steroids is still rather limited. Sexual differentiation of the central nervous system is a complex integrated process, which relies on proper chronological and quantitative interaction of various endocrine and neuroendocrine mediators. Any disturbance of this delicate endogenous hormonal balance during ontogenetic development, by means of environmental influences, can result in permanent manifestation of anatomic and functional sexual deviations.

## REFERENCES

Arendash, G.S. and Gorski, R.A. (1983). Effects of discrete lesions of the sexually dimorphic nucleus of the preoptic area or other medial preoptic regions on the sexual behavior of male rats. *Brain Research Bull.*, **10**, 147-154.

Aristotle (1862). In *History of Animals*, Book VI, Chapter XIX/2, (translated by R. Cresswell), H.G. Bohn, London, pp. 165.

Barfield, R.J. and Chen, J.J. (1977). Activation of estrous behavior in ovariectomized rats by intracerebral implants of estradiol benzoate. *Endocrinology*, **101**, 1716-1725.

Barraclough, C.A. and Wise, P.M. (1982). The role of catecholamines in the regulation of pituitary luteinizing hormone and follicle-stimulating hormone secretion. *Endocrine Rev.*, **3**, 91-119.

Barraclough, C.A., Lookingland, K.J., and Wise, P.M. (1984). Role of hypothalamic noradrenergic system in sexual differentiation of the brain. In *Sexual Differentiation: Basic and Clinical Aspects*, eds. M. Serio, M. Motta, M. Zanisi, and L. Martini. Raven Press, New York, pp. 99-106.

Beattie, C.W. and Soyka, L.F. (1973). Influence of progestational steroids on hypothalamic tyrosine hydroxylase activity *in vitro*. *Endocrinology*, **93**, 1453-1455.

Bermond, B. (1982). Effects of medial preoptic hypothalamus anterior lesions on three kinds of behavior in the rat: Intermale aggressive, male-sexual, and mouse-killing behavior. *Aggress. Behav.*, **8**, 335-354.

Biegon, A., Bercovitz, H. and Samuel, D. (1980). Serotonin receptor concentration during the estrous cycle of the rat. *Brain Research*, **187**, 221-225.

Booth, J.E. (1979). Sexual differentiation of the brain. In *Oxford Reviews of Reproductive Biology*, ed. C.A. Finn. Clarendon Press, Oxford, Vol. 1, pp. 58-158.

Bruinink, A. and Lichtensteiger, W. (1984). Beta-adrenergic binding sites in fetal rat brain. *J. Neurochem.*, **43**, 578-581.

Bruinink, A., Lichtensteiger, W., and Schlumpf, M. (1983). Ontogeny of diurnal rhythms of central dopamine, serotonin and spirodecanone binding sites and of motor activity in the rat. *Life Science*, **33**, 31-38.

Byne, W. and Bleier, R. (1987). Medial preoptic sexual dimorphisms in the guinea pig. I. An investigation of their hormonal dependence. *J. Neurosci.*, **7**, 2688-2696.

Byne, W., Warren, J.T., and Siggelkow, I. (1987). Medial preoptic sexual dimorphisms in the guinea pig. II. An investigation of medial preoptic neurogenesis. *J. Neurosci.*, **7**, 2697-2702.

Cardinali, D.P. (1977). Nuclear receptor estrogen complex in the pineal gland. Modulation by sympathetic nerves. *Neuroendocrinology*, **24**, 333-346.

Cardinali, D.P., Gómez, E., and Rosner, J.M. (1976). Changes in ($^3$H) leucine incorporation into pineal proteins following estradiol or testosterone administration: involvement of the sympathetic superior cervical ganglion. *Endocrinology* , **94**, 849-858.

Cardinali, D.P., Vacas, M.I., Ritta, M.N., and Gejman, P.V. (1983). Neurotransmitter-controlled steroid hormone receptors in the central nervous system. *Neurochem. Internat.*, **5**, 185-192.

Carrillo, A.J. and Sheridan, P.J. (1980). Estrogen receptors in the medial basal hypothalamus of the rat following complete deafferentiation. *Brain Research*, **186**, 157-164.

Changeux, J.P. and Danchin, A. (1976). Selective stabilization of developing synapses as a mechanism for the specification of neuronal networks. *Nature*, **264**, 705-712.

Commins, D. and Yahr, P. (1984a). Acetylcholinesterase activity in the sexually dimorphic area of the gerbil brain: sex differences and influences of adult gonadal steroids. *J. Comp. Neurol.*, **224**, 123-131.

Commins, D. and Yahr, P. (1984b). Adult testosterone levels influence the morphology of a sexually dimorphic area in the mongolian gerbil brain. *J. Comp. Neurol.*, **224**, 132-140.

Commins, D. and Yahr, P. (1984c). Lesions of the sexually dimorphic area disrupt mating and marking in male gerbils. *Brain Research Bull.*, **13**, 185-193.

De Jonge, F.H., Swaab, D.F., Ooms, M.P., Endert, E., and Van de Poll, N.E. (1990). Developmental and functional aspects of the human and rat sexually dimorphic nucleus of the preoptic area. In *Hormones, Brain and Behaviour in Vertebrates*. I. Sexual Differentiation, Neuroanatomical Aspects, Neurotransmitters and Neuropeptides. Comp. Physiol., ed. J. Balthazart. Karger, Basel, Vol. 8, pp. 121-136.

De Vries, G.J., Buijs, R.M., and Swaab, D.F. (1981). Ontogeny of the vasopressinergic neurons of the suprachiasmatic nucleus and their extrahypothalamic projection in the rat brain—presence of a sex difference in the lateral septum. *Brain Research*, **218**, 67-78.

Diez-Guerra, F.J., Bicknell, R.J., Mansfield, S., Emson, P.C., and Dyer, R.G. (1987). Effect of neonatal testosterone upon opioid receptors and the content of $\beta$-endorphin, neuropeptide Y and neurotensin in the medial preoptic and the mediobasal hypothalamic areas of the rat brain. *Brain Research*, **424**, 225-230.

Dodson, R.E., Shryne, J.E., and Gorski, R.A. (1988). Hormonal modification of the number of total and late-arising neurons in the central part of the medial preoptic nucleus of the rat. *J. Comp. Neurol.*, **275**, 623-629.

Dohanich, G.P., Witcher, J.A., Weaver, D.R., and Clemens, L.G. (1982). Alteration of muscarinic binding in specific brain areas following estrogen treatment. *Brain Research*, **241**, 347-350.

Döhler, K.D. (1991). The pre-and postnatal influence of hormones and neurotransmitters on sexual differentiation of the mammalian hypothalamus. *Int. Rev. Cytology*, **131**, 1-57.

Döhler, K.D., Coquelin, A., Davis, F., Hines, M., Shryne, J.E., and Gorski, R.A. (1984a). Pre- and postnatal influence of testosterone propionate and diethylstilbestrol on differentiation of the sexually dimorphic nucleus of the preoptic area in male and female rats. *Brain Research*, **302**, 291-295.

Döhler, K.D., Hancke, J.-L., Srivastava, S.S., Hofmann, C., Shryne, J.E., and Gorski, R.A. (1984b). Participation of estrogens in female sexual differentiation of the brain; neuroanatomical, neuroendocrine and behavioral evidence. In *Progress in Brain Research*, eds. G.J. De Vries, J.P.C. de Bruin, H.B.M. Uylings, and M.A. Corner. Elsevier Science Publ., Amsterdam, **Vol. 61**, pp. 99-117.

Döhler, K.D., Srivastava, S.S., Shryne, J.E., Jarzab, B., Sipos, A., and Gorski, R.A. (1984c). Differentiation of the sexually dimorphic nucleus in the preoptic area of the rat brain is inhibited by postnatal treatment with an estrogen antagonist. *Neuroendocrinology*, **38**, 297-301.

Döhler, K.D., Coquelin, A., Davis, F., Hines, M., Shryne, J.E., Sickmöller, P.M., Jarzab, B., and Gorski, R.A. (1986). Pre- and postnatal influence of an estrogen antagonist and an androgen antagonist on differentiation of the sexually dimorphic nucleus of the preoptic area in male and female rats. *Neuroendocrinology*, 42, 443-448.

Dörner, G. (1981). Sexual differentiation of the brain. *Vitam. Horm.*, 38, 325-381.

Dörner, G. and Staudt, J. (1968). Structural changes in the preoptic anterior hypothalamic area of the male rat, following neonatal castration and androgen substitution. *Neuroendocrinology*, 3, 136-140.

Dörner, G., Hecht, K., and Hinz, G. (1976). Teratopsychogenetic effects apparently produced by nonphysiological neurotransmitter concentrations during brain differentiation. *Endokrinologie*, 68, 1-5.

Dörner, G., Staudt, J., Wenzel, J., Kventnansky, R., and Murgas, K. (1977). Further evidence of teratogenic effects apparently produced by neurotransmitters during brain differentiation. *Endokrinologie*, 70, 326-330.

Dyer, R.G. (1984). Sexual differentiation of the forebrain-relationship to gonadotrophin secretion. In *Progress in Brain Research*, eds. G.J. De Vries, J.P.C. de Bruin, H.B.M. Uylings, and M.A. Corner. Elsevier Science Publ., Amsterdam, Vol. 61, pp. 223-236.

Dyer, R.G., MacLeod, N.K., and Ellendorf, F. (1976). Electrophysiological evidence for sexual dimorphism and synaptic convergence in the preoptic and anterior hypothalamic areas of the rat. *Proc. R. Soc. London (Biol.)*, 193, 421-440.

Ganzemüller, C. and Veit, C. (1988). Die Bedeutung der Östrogene in der perinatalen Periode für die Differenzierung sexualdimorpher Gehirnfunktionen bei der Ratte-die Effekte von Antiöstrogenen. *Dissertation*, University of Hannover, School of Medicine, Hannover, Germany.

Giulian, D., Pohorecky, L.A., and McEwen, B.S. (1973). Effects of gonadal steroids upon brain 5-hydroxytryptamine levels in neonatal rat. *Endocrinology*, 93, 1329-1335.

Goetz, C., Bourgoin, S., Cesselin, F., Brandt, A., Bression, D., Martinet, M., Peillon, F., and Hamon, M. (1983). Alterations in central neurotransmitter receptor binding sites following estradiol implantation in female rats. *Neurochem. Int.*, 5, 375-383.

Gorski, R.A. (1984a). Critical role of the medial preoptic area in the sexual differentiation of the brain. In *Progress in Brain Research*, eds. G.J. De Vries, J.P.C. de Bruin, H.B.M. Uylings, and M.A. Corner. Elsevier Science Publ., Amsterdam, Vol. 61, pp. 129-146.

Gorski, R.A. (1984b). Sexual differentiation of brain structure in rodents. In *Sexual Differentiation: Basic and Clinical Aspects*, eds. M. Serio, M. Motta, M. Zanisi, and L. Martini. Raven Press, New York, pp. 65-77.

Gorski, R.A. (1987). Sex differences in the rodent brain: their nature and origin. In *Masculinity/Feminity, Basic Perspectives*, eds. J.M. Reinisch, L.A. Rosenblum, and S.A Sanders. Oxford University Press, New York, pp. 37-67.

Gorski, R.A., Gordon, J.H., Shryne, J.E., and Southam, A.M. (1978). Evidence for a morphological sex difference within the medial preoptic area of the rat brain. *Brain Research*, 148, 333-346.

Gorski, R.A., Csernus, V.J., and Jacobson, C.D. (1980). Sexual dimorphism in the preoptic area, In *Advances in Physiological Sciences; Reproduction and Development*, eds. B. Flerkó, G. Sétáló, and L. Tima. Pergamon Press and Akadémia Kiadó Press, Budapest, Vol. 15, pp. 121-130.

Goy, R.W. and McEwen, B.S. (1980). *Sexual Differentiation of the Brain*. The MIT Press, Cambridge, Massachusetts.

Greenough, W.T., Carter, C.S., Steerman, C., and De Voogt, T.J. (1977). Sex differences in dendritic patterns in hamster preoptic area. *Brain Research*, 126, 63-72.

Grossman, R., Diez-Guerra, F.J., Mansfield, S., and Dyer, R.G. (1987). Neonatal testosterone modifies LH secretion in the adult female rat by altering the opioid-noradrenergic interaction in the medial preoptic area. *Brain Research*, **415**, 205-210.

Gunaga, K.P. and Menon, K.M.J. (1973). Effect of catecholamines and ovarian hormones on cyclic AMP accumulation in rat hypothalamus. *Biochem. biophys. Res. Commun.*, **54**, 440-448.

Gunaga, K.P., Kawano, A., and Menon, K.M.J. (1974). *In vivo* effect of estradiol benzoate on the accumulation of cyclic AMP in rat hypothalamus. *Neuroendocrinology*, **16**, 273-281.

Hahn, E.F. and Fishman, J. (1979). Changes in rat brain opiate receptor content upon castration and testosterone replacement. *Biochem. biophys. Res. Commun.*, **90**, 819-823.

Hammer, R.P. (1988). Opiate receptor ontogeny in the rat medial preoptic area is androgen-dependent. *Neuroendocrinology*, **48**, 336-341.

Handa, R.J., Hines, M., Schoonmaker, J.N., Shryne, J.E., and Gorski, R.A. (1986). Evidence that serotonin is involved in the sexually dimorphic development of the preoptic area in the rat brain. *Dev. Brain Research*, **30**, 278-282.

Hardin, C.M. (1973). Sex differences and the effect of testosterone injections on biogenic amine levels of neonatal rat brain. *Brain Research*, **59**, 437-439.

Harlan, R.E., Gordon, J.H., and Gorski, R.A. (1979). Sexual differentiation of the brain: implications for neuroscience. In *Reviews of Neuroscience*, ed. D.M. Schneider. Raven Press, New York, **Vol. 4**, pp. 31-71.

Hart, B.L. (1974). Medial preoptic-anterior hypothalamic area and the socio-sexual behavior of male dogs: A comparative neuropsychological analysis. *J. Comp. Physiol. Psychol.*, **86**, 328-349.

Hennessey, A.C., Wallen, K., and Edwards, D.A. (1986). Preoptic lesions increase the display of lordosis by male rats. *Brain Research*, **370**, 21-28.

Hines, M., Davis, F.C., Coquelin, A., Goy, R.W., and Gorski, R.A. (1985). Sexually dimorphic regions in the medial preoptic area and the bed nucleus of the stria terminalis of the guinea pig brain: a description and an investigation of their relationship to gonadal steroids in adulthood. *J. Neurosci.*, **5**, 40-47.

Hofman, M.A. and Swaab, D.F. (1989). The sexually dimorphic nucleus of the preoptic area in the human brain: a comparative morphometric study. *J. Anat.*, **164**, 55-72.

Hruska, R.E., Ludmer, L.Y., and Silbergeld, E.K. (1980). Characterization of the striatal dopamine receptor supersensitivity produced by estrogen treatment of male rats. *Neuropharmacology*, **19**, 923-926.

Hsü, H.K., Chen, F.N., and Peng, M.T. (1980). Some characteristics of the darkly stained area of the medial preoptic area of rats. *Neuroendocrinology*, **31**, 327-330.

Hull, E.M., Nishita, J.K., Bitran, D., and Dalterio, S. (1984). Perinatal dopamine-related drugs demasculinize rats. *Science*, **224**, 1011-1013.

Jacobson, C.D., Shryne, J.E., Shapiro, F., and Gorski, R.A. (1980). Ontogeny of the sexually dimorphic nucleus of the preoptic area. *J. Comp. Neurol.*, **193**, 541-548.

Jacobson, C.D., Csernus, V.J., Shryne, J.E., and Gorski, R.A. (1981a). The influence of gonadectomy, androgen exposure or a gonadal graft in the neonatal rat on the volume of the sexually dimorphic nucleus of the preoptic area. *J. Neurosci.*, **1**, 1142-1147.

Jacobson, C.D., Davis, F.C., Freiberg, E., and Gorski, R.A. (1981b). Formation of the sexually dimorphic nucleus of the preoptic area of the female rat brain. *Soc. Neurosci. Abstr.*, **7**, 286.

Janowsky, D.S. and Davis, J.N. (1970). Progesterone-estrogen effects on uptake and release of norepinephrine by synaptosomes. *Life Sci.*, **9**, 525-531.

Jarzab, B. and Döhler, K.D. (1984). Serotoninergic influences on sexual differentiation of the rat brain. In *Progress in Brain Research*, eds. G.J. De Vries, J.P.C. De Bruin, H.B.M Uylings, and M.A. Corner. Elsevier Science Publ., Amsterdam, **Vol. 61**, pp. 119-126.

Jarzab, B., Lindner, G., Lindner, T., Sickmöller, P.M., Geerlings, H., and Döhler, K.D. (1986). Adrenergic influences on sexual differentiation of the rat brain. In *Systemic Hormones, Neurotransmitters and Brain Development*, eds. G. Dörner, S.M. McCann and L. Martini. Karger, Basel, pp. 191-196.

Jarzab, B., Sickmöller, P.M., Geerlings, H., and Döhler, K.D. (1987). Postnatal treatment of rats with adrenergic receptor agonists or antagonists influences differentiation of sexual behavior. *Horm. Behav.*, **21**, 478-492.

Jarzab, B., Gubala, E., Achtelik, W., Lindner, G., Pogorzelska, E., and Döhler, K.D. (1989). Postnatal treatment of rats with beta-adrenergic agonists or antagonists influences differentiation of sexual brain functions. *Exp. Clin. Endocrinol.*, **94**, 61-72.

Jarzab, B., Kaminski, M., Gubala, E., Achtelik, W., Wagiel, J., and Döhler, K.D. (1990a). Postnatal treatment of rats with the $beta_2$-adrenergic agonist salbutamol influences the volume of the sexually dimorphic nucleus in the preoptic area. *Brain Research*, **516**, 257-262.

Jarzab, B., Kokocińska, D., Kaminski, M., Gubala, E., Achtelik, W., Wagiel, J., and Döhler, K.D. (1990b). Influence of neurotransmitters on sexual differentiation of the brain: relationship between the volume of the SDN-POA and functional characteristics. In *Hormones, Brain and Behaviour in Vertebrates*. I. Sexual Differentiation, Neuroanatomical Aspects, Neurotransmitters and Neuropeptides. Comp. Physiol., ed. J. Balthazart. Karger, Basel, pp. 41-50.

Jordan, V.C., Dix, C.J., Rowsby, L., and Prestwich, G. (1977). Studies on the mechanism of action of the nonsteroidal antiestrogen tamoxifen in the rat. *Mol. cell. Endocrinol.*, **7**, 177-192.

Jordan, V.C., Prestwich, G., Dix, C.J., and Clark, E.R. (1980). Binding of anti-estrogens to the estrogen receptor, the first step in anti-estrogen action. In *Pharmacological Modulation of Steroid Action*, eds. E. Genazzani, F. DiCarlo, and W.I.P. Mainwaring. Raven Press, New York, pp. 81-98.

Kalra, P.S. and Kalra, S.P. (1983). Neural regulation of luteinizing hormone secretion in the rat. *Endocrine Rev.*, **4**, 311-351

Kalra, S.P. and McCann, S.M. (1974). Effects of drugs modifying catecholamine synthesis on plasma LH and ovulation in the rat. *Neuroendocrinology*, **15**, 79-91.

Kelley, D.B. and Pfaff, D.W. (1978). Generalizations from comparative studies on neuroanatomical and endocrine mechanisms of sexual behaviour. In *Biological Determinants of Sexual Behavior*, ed. J.B. Hutchison. Wiley, New York, pp. 225-254.

Kendall, D.A., Stancel, G.M., and Enna, S.J. (1981). Imipramine: effect of ovarian steroids on modifications in serotonin receptor binding. *Science*, **211**, 1183-1185.

Keyser, A. (1983). Basic aspects of development and maturation of the brain: embryological contributions to neuroendocrinology. *Psychoneuroendocrinology*, **8**, 157-181.

Lauder, J.M. (1983). Hormonal and humoral influences on brain development. *Psychoneuroendocrinology*, **8**, 121-155.

Lehtinen, P., Hyyppä, M., and Lampinen, P. (1972). Sexual behavior of adult rats after a single neonatal injection of reserpine. *Psychopharmacology*, **23**, 171-179.

Lichtensteiger, W. and Schlumpf M. (1981). Steroids and neurotransmitter mechanisms in the prenatal period. In Steroid Hormone Regulation of the Brain, eds. K. Fuxe, J.A. Gustafsson and L. Wetterberg. Pergamon, Oxford, pp. 161-172.

Lookingland, K.J. and Barraclough, C.A. (1982). Changes in plasma hormone profiles and in hypothalamic catecholamine turnover rates in neonatally androgenized rats during the transition phase from cyclicity to persistent estrus (delayed anovulatory syndrome). Biol. Reprod., 27, 282-299.

Lookingland, K.J., Wise, P.M., and Barraclough, C.A. (1982). Failure of the hypothalamic noradrenergic system to function in adult androgenized rats. Biol. Reprod., 27, 268-281.

Luine, V.N., Khylchevskaya, R.I., and McEwen, B.S. (1975). Effect of gonadal steroids on activity of monoamine oxidase and cholin acetylase in rat brain. Brain Research, 86, 293-306.

Luine, V.N., Oark, D., Joh, T., Reis, D., and McEwen, B.S. (1980). Immunochemical demonstration of increased choline acetyltransferase concentration in rat preoptic area after estradiol administration. Brain Research, 191, 273-277.

Malmnäs, C.O. (1973). Monoaminergic influence on testosterone activated copulatory behavior in the castrated male rat. Acta Physiol. Scand. Suppl., 395, 1-128.

Matsumoto, A. and Arai, Y. (1980). Sexual dimorphism in "wiring pattern" in the hypothalamic arcuate nucleus and its modification by neonatal hormone environment. Brain Research, 190, 238-242.

McEwen, B.S. (1987). External factors influencing brain development. In NIDA Res. Monographs, eds. D. Friedman and D. Clouet. Vol. 78, pp.1-14.

Meyerson, B.J. (1964). Central nervous monoamines and hormone induced estrus behavior in the spayed rat. Acta Physiol. Scand. Suppl., 241, 1-32.

Michanek, A. and Meyerson, B.J. (1977). A comparative study of different amphetamines on copulatory behavior and stereotype activity in the female rat. Psychopharmacologia, 53, 175-183.

Morrell, J.I. and Pfaff, D.W. (1982). Characterization of estrogen concentrating hypothalamic neurons by their axonal projections. Science, 217, 1273-1276.

Nagle, C.A., Cardinali, D.P., and Rosner, J.M. (1973). Uptake of estradiol by the rat pineal organ. Effects of cervical sympathectomy, stage of the estrous cycle and estradiol treatment. Life Sci., 13, 1089-1103.

Nausieda, P.A., Koller, W.C., Weiner, W.J., and Klawans, H.L. (1979). Modification of postsynaptic dopaminergic sensitivity by female sex hormones. Life Sci., 25, 521-526.

Neumann, F. and Elger, W. (1966). Permanent changes in gonadal function and sexual behavior as a result of early feminization of male rats by treatment with an antiandrogenic steroid. Endokrinologie, 50, 209-224.

Neumann, F. and Kramer, M. (1967). Female brain differentiation of male rats as a result of early treatment with an androgen antagonist. In Hormonal Steroids, eds. L. Martini, F. Fraschini and M. Motta. Excerpta Medica, Amsterdam, pp. 932-941.

Nicholson, R.I., Golder, M.P., Davies, P., and Griffiths, K. (1976). Effects of oestradiol-17β and tamoxifen on total and accessible cytoplasmic oestradiol-17β receptors in DMBA-induced rat mammary tumours. Eur. J. Cancer, 12, 711-717.

Nishizuka, M. (1976). Neuropharmacological study on the induction of hypothalamic masculinization in female mice. Neuroendocrinology, 20, 157-165.

Nishizuka, M. and Arai, Y. (1981). Sexual dimorphism in synaptic organization in the amygdala and its dependence on neonatal hormone environment. Brain Research, 212, 31-38.

Nock, B. and Feder, H.H. (1981). Neurotransmitter modulation of steroid action in target cells that mediate reproduction and reproductive behavior. *Neurosci. Biobehav. Res.*, **5**, 437-447.

Nottebohm, F. and Arnold, A.P. (1976). Sexual dimorphism in vocal control areas of the songbird brain. *Science*, **194**, 211-213.

Panzica, G.C., Viglietti-Panzica, C., Calacagni, M., Anselmetti, G.C., Schumacher, M., and Balthazart. J. (1987). Sexual differentiation and hormonal control of the sexually dimorphic medial preoptic nucleus in the quail. *Brain Research*, **416**, 59-68.

Patel, A.J., Barochovsky, O., and Lewis, P.D. (1981). Psychotropic drugs and brain development: effects on cell replication *in vivo* and *in vitro*. *Neuropharmacology*, **20**, 1243-1249.

Pfaff, D.W. (1966). Morphological changes in the brains of adult male rats after neonatal castration. *J. Endocrinol.*, **36**, 415-416.

Pfaff, D.W. and Sakuma, Y. (1979a). Facilitation of the lordosis reflex of female rats from the ventromedial nucleus of the hypothalamus. *J. Physiol. (London)*, **288**, 189-202.

Pfaff, D.W. and Sakuma, Y. (1979b). Deficit in the lordosis reflex of female rats caused by lesions in the ventromedial nucleus of the hypothalamus. *J. Physiol. (London)*, **288**, 203-210.

Pfeiffer, C.A. (1936). Sexual differences of the hypophysis and their determination by the gonads. *Am. J. Anat.*, **58**, 195-226.

Pieau, C. (1975). Temperature and sex differentiation in embryos of two chalonians, Emys orbicularis L. and Testudo graeca L. In *Intersexuality in the Animal Kingdom*, ed. R. Reinboth. Springer, New York, pp. 332-339.

Piquet, J. (1930). Détermination de sexe chez les batraciens en fonction de la température. *Rev. Suisse Zool.*, **37**, 173-281.

Plapinger, L. and McEwen, B.S. (1978). Gonadal steroid-brain interactions in sexual differentiation. In *Biological Determinants of Sexual Behaviour*, ed. J.B. Hutchison. John Wiley and Sons, New York, pp. 153-218.

Plato (1953). Symposium. In *The Dialogues of Plato*, Vol. I, 4th ed., 189d-190a, translated by B. Jowett. Clarendon Press, Oxford, pp. 521.

Preslock, J.P. and McCann, S.M. (1987). Lesions of the sexually dimorphic nucleus of the preoptic area: effects upon LH, FSH and prolactin in rats. *Brain Research Bull.*, **18**, 127-134.

Rainbow, T.C., DeGroff, V., Luine, V.N., and McEwen, B.S. (1980). Estradiol-17β increases number of muscarinic receptors in hypothalamic nuclei. *Brain Research*, **198**, 239-243.

Raisman, G. and Field, P.M. (1973). Sexual dimorphism in the neuropil of the preoptic area of the rat and its development on neonatal androgen. *Brain Research*, **54**, 1-29.

Rance, N., Wise, P.M., Selmanoff, M.K., and Barraclough, C. (1981). Catecholamine turnover rates in discrete hypothalamic areas and associated changes in median eminence luteinizing hormone-releasing hormone and serum gonadotropins on proestrous and diestrous day 1. *Endocrinology*, **108**, 1795-1801.

Raum, W.J. and Swerdloff, R.S. (1981). The role of hypothalamic adrenergic receptors in preventing testosterone-induced androgenization in the female rat brain. *Endocrinology* , **109**, 273-278.

Raum, W.J., Marcano, M., and Swerdloff, R.S. (1984). Nuclear accumulation of estradiol derived from the aromatization of testosterone is inhibited by hypothalamic beta-receptor stimulation in the neonatal female rat. *Biol. Reprod.*, **30**, 388-396.

Reznikov, A.G. and Nosenko, N.D. (1983). It is possible that noradrenaline is the biogenic monoamine responsible for androgen-dependent sexual brain differentiation. *Exp. Clin. Endocrinol.*, **81**, 91-93.

Reznikov, A.G., Nosenko, N.D., and Demkiv, L.P. (1979). New evidences for participation of monoamines in androgen-dependent sexual differentiation of hypothalamic control of gonadotropin secretion in rats. *Endokrinologie*, **73**, 11-19.

Rhees, R.W., Shryne, J.E., and Gorski, R.A. (1990). Termination of the hormone-sensitive period for differentiation of the sexually dimorphic nucleus of the preoptic area in male and female rats. *Dev. Brain Research*, **52**, 17-23.

Ribary, U., Schlumpf, M., and Lichtensteiger, W. (1986). Analysis of HPLC-EC metabolites of monoamines in fetal and postnatal rat brain. *Neuropharmacology*, **25**, 981-986.

Robinson, S.M., Fox, T.O., Dikkes, P., and Pearlstein, R.A. (1986). Sex differences in the shape of the sexually dimorphic nucleus of the preoptic area and suprachiasmatic nucleus of the rat: 3-D computer reconstructions and morphometrics. *Brain Research*, **371**, 380-384.

Short, R.V. (1982). Sex determination and differentiation. In *Reproduction in Animals*, **Vol. 2**, eds. C.R. Austin and R.V. Short. Cambridge University Press, Cambridge, pp. 70-113.

Sickmöller, P.M. (1985). Cholinerge Einflüsse auf die sexuelle Differenzierung des Gehirns. *Dissertation*, University School of Medicine, Hannover, Germany.

Sickmöller, P.M., Jarzab, B., and Döhler, K.D. (1985). Cholinergic influence on sexual differentiation of the LH release mechanism in rats. *Acta Endocrinol.*, **108**, Suppl. 267, 110-111.

Simerly, R.B. and Swanson, L.W. (1986). The organization of neural inputs to the medial preoptic nucleus of the rat. *J. Comp. Neurol.*, **246**, 312-342.

Simerly, R.B. and Swanson, L.W. (1987). The distribution of neurotransmitter-specific cells and fibers in the anteroventral periventricular nucleus: implications for the control of gonadotropin secretion. *Brain Research*, **400**, 11-34.

Simerly, R.B., Swanson, L.W., and Gorski, R.A. (1983). Demonstration of a sexual dimorphism in the distribution of serotonin immunoreactive fibers in the medial preoptic nucleus of the rat. *Anat. Rec.*, **205**, 185A-186A.

Simerly, R.B., Swanson, L.W., and Gorski, R.A. (1985). Reversal of the sexually dimorphic distribution of serotonin immunoreactive fibers in the medial preoptic nucleus by treatment with perinatal androgen. *Brain Research*, **340**, 91-98.

Simerly, R.B., Gorski, R.A., and Swanson, L.W. (1986). Neurotransmitter specificity of cells and fibers in the medial preoptic nucleus: an immunohistochemical study in the rat. *J. comp. Neurol.*, **246**, 343-363.

Smolen, A.J., Beaston-Wimmer, P., Wright, L.L., Lindley, T., and Cader, C. (1985). Neurotransmitter synthesis, storage and turnover in neonatally deafferented sympathetic neurons. *Dev. Brain Research*, **23**, 211-218.

Stiles, G.L., Caron, M.G., and Lefkowitz, R.J. (1984). Beta-adrenergic receptors: Biochemical mechanisms of physiological regulation. *Physiol. Rev.*, **64**, 661-743.

Stolkovski, J. and Bellec, A. (1960). Influence du rapport potassium/calcium du milieu d'élevage sur la distribution des sexes chez Discoglosus pictur (Otth). *C.R. Acad. Sci. Paris*, **251**, 1669-1671.

Stumpf, W.E., Sar, M., and Keefer, D.A. (1975). Atlas of estrogen target cells - rat brain. In *Anatomical Neuroendocrinology*, eds. W.E. Stumpf and L.D. Grant. Karger, Basel, pp. 104-119.

Swaab, D.F. and Fliers, E. (1985). A sexually dimorphic nucleus in the human brain. *Science*, **228**, 1112-1115.

Swaab, D.F. and Hofman, M.A. (1988). Sexual differentiation of the human hypothalamus: ontogeny of the sexually dimorphic nucleus of the preoptic area. *Dev. Brain Research*, **44**, 314-318.

Tobet, S.A., Zahniser, D.J., and Baum, M.J. (1986). Sexual dimorphism in the preoptic/anterior hypothalamic area of ferrets: effects of adult exposure to sex steroids. *Brain Research*, **364**, 249-257.

Toran-Allerand, C.D. (1984). On the genesis of sexual differentiation of the central nervous system: Morphogenetic consequences of steroidal exposure and possible role of alpha-fetoprotein. In *Progress in Brain Research*, **Vol. 61**, eds. G.J. De Vries, J.P.C. de Bruin, H.B.M. Uylings and M.A. Corner. Elsevier Science Publ., Amsterdam, pp. 63-98.

Vacas, M.I. and Cardinali, D.P. (1980). Effect of estradiol on $\alpha$- and $\beta$-adrenoreceptor density in medial basal hypothalamus and pineal gland of ovariectomized rats. *Neurosci. Lett.*, **17**, 73-77.

van de Poll, N.E. and van Dis, H. (1971). Sexual motivation and medial preoptic selfstimulation in male rats. *Psychon. Sci.*, **25**, 137-138.

van de Poll, N.E. and van Dis, H. (1979). The effect of medial preoptic-anterior hypothalamic lesions on bisexual behavior of the male rat. *Brain Research Bull.*, **4**, 505-511.

Wagner, H.R., Crutcher, K.A., and Davis, J.N. (1979). Chronic estrogen treatment decreases $\beta$-adrenergic responses in rat cerebral cortex. *Brain Research*, **171**, 147-151.

Weissman, B.A. and Skolnick, P. (1975). Stimulation of cAMP in rat hypothalamus by estrogenic compounds: relationship to biologic potency and blockade by antiestrogens. *Neuroendocrinology*, **18**, 27-34.

Weissman, B.A., Daly, J.W., and Skolnick, P. (1975). Diethylstilbestrol-elicited accumulation of cyclic AMP in incubated rat hypothalamus. *Endocrinology*, **97**, 1559-1566.

Wilkinson, M. (1978). Pharmacological and physiological correlates of variable receptor sensitivity. *Biochem. Soc. Trans.*, **6**, 853-858.

Wilkinson, M. and Herdon, H.J. (1982). Diethylstilbestrol regulates the number of alpha- and beta-adrenergic binding sites in incubated hypothalamus and amygdala. *Brain Research*, **248**, 79-85.

Wilkinson, M., Herdon, H.J., Pearce, M., and Wilson, C.A. (1979). Radioligand binding studies on hypothalamic noradrenergic receptors during the estrous cycle or after steroid injection in ovariectomized rats. *Brain Research*, **168**, 652-655.

Wilson, C.A., Pearson, J.R., Hunter, A.J., Tuchy, P.A., and Payne, A.P. (1986). The effect of neonatal manipulation of hypothalamic serotonin levels on sexual activity in the adult rat. *Pharmac. Biochem. Behav.*, **24**, 1175-1183.

Wirz-Justice, A., Hackman, E., and Lichtensteiger, M. (1974). The effect of estradiol dipropionate and progesterone on monoamine uptake in rat brain. *J. Neurochem.*, **22**, 187-189.

Wise, P.M., Rance, N., and Barraclough, C.A. (1981). Effects of estradiol and progesterone on catecholamine turnover rates in discrete hypothalamic regions in ovariectomized rats. *Endocrinology*, **108**, 2186-2191.

Wright, L.L. and Smolen, A.J. (1985). Synaptogenic effects of neonatal estradiol treatment in rat superior cervical ganglia. *Dev. Brain Research*, **21**, 161-165.

Yahr, P. (1988). Pars compacta of the sexually dimorphic area of the gerbil hypothalamus: Postnatal ages at which development responds to testosterone. *Behav. Neural. Biol.*, **49**, 118-124.

# SURROUNDED BY ESTROGENS? CONSIDERATIONS FOR NEUROBEHAVIORAL DEVELOPMENT IN HUMAN BEINGS

Melissa Hines

Department of Psychiatry and Biobehavioral Sciences, School of Medicine, University of California, Los Angeles, California

## INTRODUCTION

From the viewpoint of a neuroendocrinologist, the presence of estrogens in the environment at higher than normal levels is cause for concern. In experimental animals, prenatal or neonatal exposure to higher than normal levels of estrogenic hormones has dramatic and permanent influences on brain structure and behavior. Although similar pervasive influences of estrogens on human development have not been demonstrated, at least to date, some behavioral alterations have been reported in the offspring of women treated with estrogens during pregnancy. In addition, many important behaviors that might be hypothesized to be influenced by estrogen have not been studied carefully in estrogen-exposed human offspring. Also, there is no information on the behavioral consequences of neonatal (as opposed to prenatal) estrogen exposure in human beings or on possible changes in human brain structure following either prenatal or neonatal estrogen exposure. This chapter will describe the consequences of estrogen treatment for neurobehavioral development in experimental animals, will review the available evidence regarding the possibility of similar effects in human beings and will suggest directions for future research.

## ESTROGEN AND NEUROBEHAVIORAL DEVELOPMENT IN EXPERIMENTAL ANIMALS

Genetic female rats, mice, hamsters and guinea pigs exposed to the synthetic estrogen, diethylstilbestrol (DES), or to other estrogens during late prenatal or early postnatal development experience lifelong alterations in behaviors related to reproduction. For instance, the male reproductive behavior, mounting, is increased in estrogen-treated females and the female reproductive behavior, lordosis, is decreased (see Hines et al., 1987; Hines and Goy, 1985; Paup et al., 1974; Whalen and Nadler, 1963). Non-reproductive behaviors that show sex differences, such as juvenile "rough and tumble" play, aggression and maze learning, have also been reported to be altered by early estrogen exposure. In all cases, the behavioral pattern is more masculine in the estrogen-exposed females (Edwards and Herndon, 1970; Hines et al., 1982; Williams et al., 1990).

It is thought that the permanent behavioral changes induced by hormonal manipulations during development are caused by hormone-induced changes in

---

1. Corresponding Author: Melissa Hines, Department of Psychiatry and Biobehavioral Sciences, School of Medicine, 760 Westwood Plaza, University of California, Los Angeles, Los Angeles, CA. USA 90024-1759.

brain structure, and, in keeping with this hypothesis, the early hormone treatments that influence behavioral differentiation also influence neural differentiation. For example, treatment of genetic female rodents with estrogen during prenatal or neonatal development permanently masculinizes a subregion of the preoptic/anterior hypothalamic area of the rodent brain, called the sexually dimorphic nucleus of the preoptic area (SDN-POA; Döhler et al., 1984; Hines et al., 1987). This nucleus is several times larger in normal male rats than in normal females, and prolonged treatment with DES during development increases the volume of the SDN-POA in genetic females to the size typical of genetic males (Döhler et al., 1984). Of particular relevance to this review, the environmental estrogens, genistein and zearalenone, when injected in high doses during neonatal development, have been found to have the same influence on the SDN-POA as does DES (Faber and Hughes, 1991).

Estrogenic influences on neural and behavioral development in male rodents appear to be more variable than in females. My colleagues and I have seen no influences of DES on brain or behavior in males given prolonged prenatal and/or neonatal hormone treatment (Döhler et al., 1984; Hines et al., unpublished data; Hines and Goy, unpublished data). In addition, the same prolonged neonatal treatments with environmental estrogens or DES that influence SDN-POA volume in genetic females, do not influence the SDN-POA in genetic males (Faber and Hughes, 1991). However, shorter durations of estrogen exposure have been reported to impair masculine-typical behavior and promote feminine-typical behavior in rats (Diamond et al., 1973; Tilson and Lamartiniere, 1979). One possible explanation of the apparent differences in the consequences of short versus long duration treatment is that, following estrogen treatment, feedback mechanisms produce a reduction in testicular androgen production (see Brown-Grant et al., 1975). This reduction may be offset by long-term, but not short-term, treatment.

It may seem surprising that estrogen, a hormone produced abundantly by the adult female ovary, promotes masculine-typical development in genetic female animals. However, although there is some evidence that small amounts of estrogen may be needed for normal female development in rodents (see Gerall et al., 1972; Hines et al., 1985), it is well-documented that prenatal or neonatal administration of higher doses of estrogen produces neural and behavioral masculinization (increases in male characteristics) and defeminization (decreases in female characteristics). It appears that during normal male development testosterone from the male testes is converted within certain regions of the brain to estrogen, and estrogen then interacts with neural receptors to produce the cellular events that lead to masculine development (see Goy and McEwen, 1980). Thus, administering estrogen to genetic females mimics processes that occur during normal male development.

Several details about estrogenic influences on brain development and behavior in experimental animals are relevant to understanding possible influences of estrogens on human development.

First, gonadal hormone influences on the developing brain appear to contribute not only to sex differences in behavior, but also to individual differences in behavior within each sex. For instance, the male sex behavior, mounting, is seen far more frequently, on the average, in male rodents than in females. However, some females show more male-typical mounting than others and these females appear to be those exposed to relatively high levels of androgens prenatally from nearby male littermates (Clemens et al., 1978; Meisel and Ward, 1981; vom Saal and Bronson, 1980).

Second, hormones do not necessarily have a consistent influence on the full range of sex-typed characteristics, but can influence some characteristics without influencing others. Because of this capacity for selective influences, there are circumstances that produce "sexual mosaics," or animals in which some characteristics are masculine and some are feminine. One such circumstance involves the timing of hormone exposure. Organizational influences of gonadal steroids are exerted during critical periods of development, corresponding to times when peripheral blood levels of androgens are normally elevated in developing males. However, the timing of hormone exposure within the overall critical period is important for the expression of specific sex-linked characteristics. For example, in the rat, the critical period for development of the female sexual behavior, lordosis, is slightly earlier than the critical period for the male sex behavior, mounting (Christensen and Gorski, 1978). Similarly, in the rhesus monkey, separate critical periods have been documented for hormonal influences on different individual behavioral traits associated with males, including mounting of peers versus "rough and tumble" play behavior (Goy et al., 1988). Thus, unless hormone exposure extends throughout the critical period, a "sexual mosaic" may be formed. Another mechanism for producing mixed masculine and feminine outcomes relates to the dosage of hormone. For example, in studies that Robert Goy and I conducted with guinea pigs, we found that high doses of DES during prenatal development both increased male-typical mounting and decreased female-typical lordosis behavior in genetic females. However, exposure to a low dose of DES increased mounting without reducing lordosis, thus creating animals that exhibited both male and female sexual behavior (Hines et al., 1987; Hines and Goy, 1985). A third way to create a "sexual mosaic" is by manipulating the two major, active metabolites of testosterone (estradiol, or other estrogens, and dihydrotestosterone (DHT)) independently. As mentioned above, in rodents, treatment with estrogen can mimic the consequences of testosterone exposure, because testosterone is normally converted to estradiol in some neural regions before acting to masculinize or defeminize these regions and the behaviors they regulate. However, this is not true for all neural regions and all behaviors, nor is it true for the external genital structures, which depend on DHT for masculine development. Similarly, in the rat, the SDN-POA depends on estrogen for masculine development, whereas a sexually dimorphic portion of the rat spinal cord, the spinal nucleus of the bulbocavernosus, depends on DHT (Arnold and Gorski, 1984). Thus, administering either estrogen alone or DHT alone can create an animal characterized by a mixture of masculine and feminine characteristics.

Third, although androgens or estrogens have been found to masculinize and defeminize developing females in all species studied to date, including song birds, amphibians, rodents, dogs, sheep, cattle and rhesus monkeys (Goy and McEwen, 1980), there are some species differences in hormonal effects. For instance, the role of DHT in neurobehavioral development in rats is small in comparison to that of estrogen. In contrast, in rhesus monkeys, DHT has dramatic influences on the development of sexual behavior. Although there are data suggesting that developmental exposure to DES can have long-term effects on neuroendocrine regulation in rhesus monkeys (Fuller et al., 1981), estrogenic influences on neurobehavioral sexual differentiation are largely unexplored in primates. However, the difference in the role of DHT in the rhesus versus the rat suggests that data from studies of estrogenic influences on sexual differentiation in rodents can not be extrapolated directly to human development. Rather, results from animal studies provide hypotheses that can be supported or not supported by data from studies of hormone-exposed people.

Finally, the behaviors influenced by gonadal steroids include sexual behaviors themselves, as well as behaviors that bear no obvious relation to reproduction, but which show sex differences, or differ for males and females of the species. In fact, the neural characteristics and behaviors influenced by gonadal steroids are limited to those showing sex differences. In practical terms this suggests that estrogenic influences on human development would be hypothesized to be specific to sex-linked characteristics. Thus, for example, estrogen exposure would not be expected to influence general intelligence, which is comparable for males and females, but might be predicted to influence specific cognitive abilities that show sex differences, such as certain types of visuospatial ability and verbal fluency (for information on cognitive sex differences, see Halpern, 1987; Hines, 1990; Maccoby and Jacklin, 1974). Similarly, estrogen would not be expected to have a generally positive or negative influence on emotional development, but might be hypothesized to influence certain personality traits or interests that have been linked to gender.

## STUDIES OF BEHAVIOR IN HUMAN BEINGS EXPOSED PRENATALLY TO DES OR OTHER ESTROGENS

One problem in determining whether DES, or any hormone, influences human neurobehavioral development is that ethical considerations generally prohibit conducting experiments. DES was widely prescribed to pregnant women in the 1950s and 1960s for pregnancy maintenance, and it is estimated that between 1 and 5 million pregnant women in the United States were treated with DES during this period (Heinonen, 1973; Herbst and Bern, 1981; Noller and Fish, 1974). Data indicating that DES increased the risk of vaginal and cervical adenocarcinoma in female offspring, and that it was not effective for pregnancy maintenance, caused most medical uses of DES during pregnancy in the United States to cease in 1972. Thus, information on possible behavioral effects of prenatal DES exposure has been obtained largely from studies of the offspring of women who had medical conditions (e.g., diabetes or threatened miscarriage) for which DES was prescribed prior to 1972. In addition to these studies derived from clinical populations, there are two behavioral studies of the offspring of women randomly assigned to be treated with DES or placebo as part of studies examining its efficacy for pregnancy maintenance.

Most studies of the consequences of prenatal estrogen exposure have not been experimental and have not involved random assignment or placebo-treated controls. Therefore, their results must be interpreted cautiously. For instance, the possibility that differences between DES-exposed offspring and controls are caused by factors associated with DES treatment (e.g., membership in a particular socioeconomic group, obtaining the services of a certain type of obstetrician, concern about the success of the pregnancy), rather than by DES itself, must be considered. Also, in clinical follow-up studies, DES treatment is not controlled by the researcher, and can vary widely in dosage and duration from subject to subject. In addition, the precise dosage and duration of treatment may not be known, because of the difficulty of obtaining complete medical records. Thus, DES-treated offspring may not represent a homogeneous treatment group, even within a given study. In addition, it may not be possible to determine the degree of variability within the DES-exposed group. Finally, in interpreting both experimental and clinical studies, it is important to consider the medical consequences of DES exposure. For instance, DES is associated with an increased risk of vaginal and cervical adenocarcinoma and with increased fertility problems. These medical consequences may have psychological sequelae independent of direct effects of DES on the developing brain, and results of behavioral studies need be interpreted in this context.

Some of the methodological problems associated with studies of DES-exposed offspring are common to clinical studies, and particularly to studies of other groups exposed to unusual hormone environments prenatally, and several strategies have been developed to ameliorate the problems (see, e.g., Hines, 1982; Reinisch and Gandelman, 1978). One is the use of same-sexed siblings as controls, in order to minimize differences in factors such as genetic and socioeconomic background between hormone-exposed and unexposed individuals. A second strategy is the use of animal models to predict specific behavioral effects. Using this approach, differences between DES and control groups that would not be predicted from animal studies are viewed as less likely to result directly from the hormone exposure. Because animal studies indicate that estrogens selectively influence neural and behavioral characteristics that show sex differences, this strategy suggests that DES-associated changes in behaviors that do not show sex differences are unlikely to result directly from the hormone.

With these considerations in mind, what are the data regarding behavior in DES-exposed offspring? Research to be reviewed can be divided into categories of: 1. sexual orientation; 2. "gender-role" behaviors, including parenting interest and sex-typed play activity; 3. cognitive abilities and hemispheric lateralization; and 4. personality and psychopathology. Research in each of these areas will be discussed separately. In addition, research in each category will be discussed from the perspective of predictions based on animal models. Thus, in girls or women, the predicted direction of DES-related behavioral influences is toward increased masculine behavior and decreased feminine behavior. For boys and men predictions are less clear, given that prenatal estrogen treatment in animals sometimes feminizes or demasculinizes, but sometimes is without effect.

*DES and Sexual Orientation*
Sexual orientation shows a sex difference in that men are more likely to be sexually attracted to women, whereas women are more likely to be attracted to men. Like all sex differences in human behavior, this difference is not absolute. According to Kinsey, approximately 10% of men resemble women in that they are attracted sexually to men, and 3 to 5% of women resemble men in that they are attracted sexually to women (Kinsey et al., 1948; Kinsey et al., 1953). Nevertheless, even with this overlap between the sexes, sexual orientation shows the most dramatic sex difference of any behavior that has been studied relative to prenatal estrogen exposure.

Because of the large sex difference, and because sexual orientation relates directly to reproduction, it might be considered the most likely behavior to show a relationship to prenatal hormone levels. Consistent with this expectation, the best evidence supporting a relationship between prenatal estrogen exposure and human behavior comes from studies of sexual orientation in DES-exposed women. In one study, sexual orientation was assessed in 30 DES-exposed women between the ages of 17 and 30, in 30 female controls with abnormal PAP smear findings (a condition associated with prenatal DES-exposure) recruited from the same medical clinic as the DES-exposed women, and in 12 unexposed sisters of the DES-exposed women. All women were Caucasian and middle to upper class. Semi-structured interviews were used to assess sexual orientation on a 7 point heterosexual to homosexual continuum (Kinsey scales; Kinsey et al., 1948; Kinsey et al., 1953). Results suggested that prenatal DES exposure was associated with an increase in bisexuality and homosexuality (Ehrhardt et al., 1985). Approximately 24% of the DES group indicated a lifelong sexual orientation that was bisexual or homosexual, compared to none of the women in the PAP control group. Looking only at the 12 pairs of sisters, 42% of the DES-exposed group, versus 8% of the unexposed sisters indicated a life-long bisexual orientation. In a second study, 30 additional DES-exposed women were compared to 30 demographically-matched controls, without a history of DES exposure or abnormal PAP smears. Although a full report of the results of this second study has not yet been published, they are summarized in a review article (Ehrhardt et al., 1987). The results appear to be similar to those of the first study, about a third of the DES-exposed women, versus about 10% of the matched controls, reporting bisexual or homosexual responsiveness since puberty.

Although these data suggest increased bisexual or homosexual orientation in DES-exposed women, most DES-exposed women in the studies were primarily heterosexual. One might speculate that dose or duration of DES exposure relates to the likelihood of a behavioral influence, but information on dose and duration of exposure is not provided, and may not have been available. Alternatively, the relationship between DES exposure and sexual orientation may not be deterministic. Prenatal exposure to DES may alter brain development in a manner that predisposes, but does not always result in, a bisexual or homosexual orientation. It is also possible that the relationship between prenatal DES exposure and sexual orientation does not reflect a direct effect of DES on brain development. As noted in other chapters, DES exposure has consequences for physical health and fertility. In addition, it may alter the social or psychological milieu in as yet unspecified ways that could influence sexual orientation. Regardless of mechanism, however, the available data suggest that prenatal exposure to higher than normal levels of estrogen in the form of DES increases the likelihood of bisexual activity and interest in adulthood.

Studies to date suggest that prenatal exposure to DES does not influence sexual orientation in males. In one study, 17 men exposed prenatally to DES alone (age range 18 to 30) and 22 men exposed to DES plus natural progesterone (age range 24 to 29) were compared to controls matched for sex, age and maternal age. Interviews were used to assess heterosexual and homosexual dating and sexual experiences. In addition, sexual fantasies were rated on a 7 point, heterosexual to homosexual continuum. No differences were seen between either group of hormone-exposed subjects versus controls (Kester et al., 1980). In a second set of studies, two groups of DES-exposed men were compared with matched controls. The first group included 31 DES-exposed men matched to 29 unexposed controls recruited from an obstetrical practice that had prescribed DES to the mothers of the exposed men. The second group was 34 DES-exposed men (15 with documented prenatal DES exposure and 19 without documentation, but claiming DES exposure) and 15 controls recruited from one urology practice. Although a full report on these samples has not been published, results have been summarized in a review article (Meyer-Bahlburg et al., 1987). Data on sexual orientation were obtained via interviews, as described above for studies of DES-exposed women. No consistent differences were seen in sexual orientation for either group of DES-exposed men versus controls.

*"Gender-role" Behaviors*
The same groups of DES-exposed women and matched controls for whom data on sexual orientation were reviewed above, were also interviewed to assess

"gender-role" behavior. The interview schedule included questions on: 1. parenting interests; 2. physical energy expenditure; 3. gender-role enactment; and 4. aggression and delinquency. An interview schedule similar to that administered to daughters was given to mothers of the DES-exposed and unexposed women. In addition, daughters completed the Bem Sex Role Inventory (BSRI). In an initial study, the authors reported an apparent DES-associated difference in parenting interests, 30 DES-exposed women showing less interest than 30 PAP controls. However, no differences were seen in the other 3 categories of "gender role" behavior, and no significant differences were seen on the BSRI (Ehrhardt et al., 1989). In addition, a second study, comparing 30 DES-exposed women to 30 matched controls, did not replicate the difference in parenting interest and again found no systematic differences in the other "gender-role" behaviors, or on the BSRI (Lish et al., 1991).

The authors suggest that the failure to observe relationships between DES and "gender-role" behaviors is not caused by a lack of experimental power, since they have used the same measures in studies of girls exposed to androgens prenatally, and have found hormone-behavior relationships (Lish et al., 1991). However, the dose and duration of estrogen exposure and androgen exposure in the two types of studies can not be assumed comparable. In addition, power analysis (Cohen, 1988) suggests that sample sizes of 30 provide only a 47% probability of detecting effects of moderate size, even assuming that all 30 women were exposed to sufficient amounts of DES during the appropriate critical period. The sensitivity of the measures used may also have constrained the ability to detect effects. Each behavioral category was targeted by only a few interview questions and responses were limited to a 3 or 5 point scale. Finally, many questions referred to behaviors that occurred 15 to 20 years earlier, adding error to the responses. Hence, it is premature to rule out the possibility that prenatal exposure to estrogen could influence the behaviors in question, although research to date does not support such influences.

Another study assessed "gender role" behaviors in DES-exposed men. The same men studied by Kester et al. (1980) for sexual orientation were interviewed to assess child, adolescent and adult activities related to sex role. These included, among others, favorite games and toys, peer group composition, "rough-and-tumble" play, aggression, sports, reading, television viewing, experience being called a sissy, popularity among girls and boys, current activities and leisure time expenditures. Subjects also completed the BSRI, the Guilford Zimmerman Temperament Survey (GZTS: a personality scale which includes a masculine-feminine rating scale), and the Strong Vocational Interest Blank (SVIB: a measure of vocational interests). Although there were some significant differences between exposed and unexposed men on individual questionnaire items, no clear pattern of differences was evident (e.g., DES-exposed men reported less fighting as boys, but more interest in aggressive television shows as adults). Similarly, DES-exposed men showed elevated scores on some subscales of the SVIB, but these did not correspond to a pattern of masculinity or femininity (e.g., they showed elevated scores on technical supervisor and on social service). The only consistent difference was a reduced score on the masculine subscale of the GZTS in both men exposed to DES and those exposed to DES plus progesterone. However, even this result is difficult to interpret in light of the large number of variables analyzed and the consequent potential increase in chance results. In addition, data were analyzed for effects of trimester of exposure as well as presence vs. absence of exposure, further increasing the possibility of chance results. On the other hand, real differences between DES-exposed men and controls may have been undetected in this study for reasons similar to those described above for the studies of "gender role" behaviors in DES-exposed women (e.g., relatively insensitive measures and the need to rely on retrospective reports).

*Cognitive Abilities and Hemispheric Lateralization*
Although there are no differences between men and women in general intelligence, there are sex differences in certain specific cognitive abilities. Notably, men excel compared to women on tests of visuospatial abilities, whereas women excel on measures of verbal fluency (Halpern, 1987; Hines, 1990; Maccoby and Jacklin, 1974). In addition, men and women differ in language lateralization, men showing a greater reliance on their dominant hemisphere than do women (see, e.g., McGlone, 1980). None of these sex differences is absolute. Distributions of scores for men and women overlap. To put the differences in perspective, all are smaller than the sex difference in height. Nevertheless, the sex differences have been documented repeatedly and can be measured reliably and objectively using well-validated, standardized tests. For this reason, they are good measures for assessing possible hormonal influences on human neurobehavioral development (see, e.g., Hines, 1990; Hines and Shipley, 1984).

*Cognitive Abilities*
A study of 71 children (age range 5 to 17 years) exposed to estrogen plus progesterone prenatally found no differences from sibling controls in overall performance on the Wechsler Intelligence Scales or in performance on subscales of the Wechsler tests (Reinisch and Karow, 1977). Even after *post hoc* division of the hormone-exposed children into those exposed to 1. predominantly estrogen; 2. predominantly progestin; and 3. mixed estrogen and progestin regimens; no differences were seen. However, several factors reduced the likelihood of observing differences between hormone-exposed and unexposed children in this study: 1. hormone-exposed children were not matched to *same-sexed* siblings; 2. data were not examined separately for males and females (remember, evidence from experimental animal models suggests that effects of estrogen on the two sexes would be expected to differ); and 3. most of the children were not old enough to show sex differences on Wechsler subscales.

A study investigating possible influences of DES on sex-linked cognitive abilities in females compared 25 women who had been exposed prenatally to

DES to 25 of their sisters who had not been exposed (Hines and Shipley, 1984). Only women past the age of puberty (mean age = 24 years) were studied, because sex differences in cognitive abilities are seen most reliably after puberty (Maccoby and Jacklin, 1974). In addition, because the prenatal critical period for hormonal influences on human sexual differentiation is not known with certainty, only women with a long duration of exposure (at least 20 weeks of gestation) and including the entire second trimester, were studied. The 25 sister pairs completed a measure of visuospatial ability (requiring mental rotation of 2-dimensional shapes) and a measure of verbal fluency (requiring generation of words beginning with specified letters). Based on patterns of sex differences observed in prior research, it was predicted that DES-exposed women would show a more masculine cognitive pattern than their unexposed sisters, that is increased visuospatial ability and reduced verbal fluency. However, no such differences were observed. The scores of the DES-exposed women and their sisters were comparable on both tests.

A more recent and more powerful study investigated a different type of sex-linked cognitive performance in DES-exposed offspring (Wilcox et al., in press). This study involved offspring of 1646 pregnant women from a randomized, double-blind, placebo-controlled clinical trial of DES, conducted between 1950 and 1952. Approximately half of the pregnant women (840) received DES, beginning at their first prenatal visit (the 12th week of gestation on average and always by the 20th week) and approximately half (806) received placebos. Treatment continued through the 35th week of gestation. Offspring available for study included 820 males (405 DES-exposed and 415 unexposed) and 783 females (402 exposed and 381 unexposed). American College Testing (ACT) Scores were available for 42% of these offspring (175 DES-exposed women, 172 DES-exposed men, 150 unexposed women and 175 unexposed men). The ACT measures performance in four academic areas: English, mathematics, social sciences and natural sciences. Females scored significantly higher than males on the English subtest, and significantly lower on the other three subtests. The most obvious prediction from studies of the effects of DES exposure in experimental animals, would be more masculine-typical performance in DES-exposed women (that is, reduced scores on the English test and increased scores on the mathematics and science tests). However, no significant differences were seen on any of the subtests between DES-exposed women and unexposed female controls. An unexpected difference was seen between DES-exposed and unexposed men on the social science subtest, DES-exposed men attaining slightly higher scores. However, this difference was small, would not be predicted from animal research and was considered a type 1 error (a chance result, rather than a consequence of DES exposure).

Results of this large scale, placebo-controlled, experimental study reinforce the conclusion that long-term prenatal DES exposure does not influence cognitive function in women. However, the results for men contrast with results from two of three smaller, clinical studies in which estrogen exposure was not experimental and in which no placebo-exposed controls were available. Two such studies suggest demasculinization of cognitive function in estrogen-exposed males, whereas one does not. In the first study, 19 boys (age range 16 to 17), exposed prenatally to estrogen and progesterone as part of treatment for maternal diabetes, performed less well on a disembedding task (the embedded figures test, a timed test which requires the subject to identify simple figures embedded in more complex designs) than 8, 16 year old, sons of diabetic women not treated with hormones, and 14 normal controls of similar age and socioeconomic class (Yalom et al., 1973). In the second study, 10 boys and young men (age range 8 to 20) exposed prenatally to DES, were compared to 10 unexposed brothers. The DES-exposed group showed reduced scores on a composite spatial ability scale derived from the Picture Completion, Block Design and Object Assembly subtests of the Wechsler Intelligence Scales (Wechsler Intelligence Scale for Children (WISC) and the Wechsler Adult Intelligence Scale (WAIS)) (Reinisch and Sanders, 1992). In a third study, 17 young men exposed to DES prenatally and 22 exposed to DES plus natural progesterone were compared to equivalent numbers of matched controls, and no differences were seen on the embedded figures test (Kester et al., 1980).

What might explain these inconsistent results? One possibility is that some parents treat boys born of estrogen-treated pregnancies in ways that could affect their cognitive function. For instance, diabetic mothers who used estrogen during pregnancy may be more protective of their sons and discourage them from playing in rough, active ways typical of other boys. Since male styles of play have been associated with disembedding ability (Sprafkin et al., 1983), this could hypothetically lead to less masculine performance on measures of this specific ability. The ACT subtests do not provide measures of disembedding ability or other abilities that show the largest sex differences. In addition, the disembedding test used in the Yalom et al. study, unlike the ACT, has been found to be sensitive to early hormone influences in other studies (Hier and Crowley, 1982). Thus, differences between the kinds of cognitive abilities measured in the studies may explain the differences in results. Finally, as outlined above, animal studies in which estrogens are administered to developing males have also produced inconsistent results, and suggest that short-term and long-term treatment may have different consequences. Subjects in the placebo-controlled study were enrolled early and treated through week 35 of gestation. Such long-term treatment is generally without effect in studies of male animals. In contrast, 9 of the 10 DES-exposed subjects in the Reinisch and Sanders study were exposed for 10 weeks or less, early in gestation. Although the duration of DES treatment in the Yalom et al. study showing reduced disembedding ability is not specified, it is also likely to have been of shorter duration than that used in the placebo-controlled study. Thus, in human males, it is possible that estrogen exposure at certain times produces defeminization of specific cognitive functions, as has been demonstrated for other behavioral characteristics in experimental animals.

*Hemispheric Lateralization*

In addition to differing on average in verbal fluency and visuospatial abilities, men and women differ on average in language lateralization, or degree of left hemisphere dominance for processing or producing verbal material. Men show greater reliance on the left hemisphere for verbal tasks than do women. This sex difference in lateralization has been demonstrated by examining the consequences of neurological insult to the left hemisphere, as well as by presenting lateralized input to the two hemispheres in normal individuals (see, e.g., McGlone, 1980). The tests that show the most reliable sex differences in normals are verbal dichotic listening tasks composed of consonant-vowel nonsense syllables (Bryden, 1982). In these tasks, subjects are presented with two syllables (e.g., ba and da) simultaneously, one in each ear, and asked to report what they have heard. Most people correctly report more of the syllables presented to the right than the left ear, reflecting left hemisphere dominance for language, and, on the average, men show a larger discrepancy between the two ears than do women (Bryden, 1982; Hines and Shipley, 1984).

One study has investigated whether this sex difference relates to the early hormone environment. In the study, DES-exposed women and their unexposed sisters completed a verbal dichotic listening test, composed of consonant-vowel nonsense syllables. Data from 13 sister pairs (a subgroup of the 25 pairs in whom cognitive ability was assessed) indicated a more masculine pattern of language lateralization in the DES-exposed group (Hines and Shipley, 1984), a result that was predicted based on studies of DES exposure in experimental animals. There are no other published studies examining language lateralization in DES-exposed women. However, the same study described above as reporting DES-related changes in spatial ability in 10 DES-exposed boys and young men compared to 10 unexposed brothers also reported reduced lateralization in the DES-exposed group, as reflected in performance on a dichaptic shapes task (Reinisch and Sanders, 1992). In contrast to dichotic listening measures of language lateralization, patterns of sex differences on the dichaptic shapes task have not been clearly defined. Thus, the results are difficult to interpret in the context of models of sexual differentiation. Finally, a third reflection of neural lateralization, hand preferences for writing, was examined in 25 DES-exposed women and their 25 unexposed sisters by Hines and Shipley in their study of cognitive abilities. Because more men than women are left-handed, and because women are more likely than men to be strongly right-handed (e.g., to use their right hand consistently across a variety of tasks (see, e.g., Annett, 1970), it was predicted that more DES-exposed than unexposed women would be left-handed. However, no significant difference was observed between the two groups (Hines, 1981), a result that may not be surprising, given the relatively small sample and relatively insensitive measure of hand preference (simply the hand used for writing) used.

*Personality and Psychopathology*

Three studies examined general personality traits in estrogen-exposed offspring. Two used the Cattell Personality Questionnaires and the third used the GZTS. The first study was described above as showing estrogen-related differences in performance on an embedded figures task in 16 year old boys. In the same study, 20 estrogen-exposed boys and 22 controls completed the Cattell 16 Personality Factors Questionnaire. No differences were seen between the groups in any of the 16 personality dimensions measured (Yalom et al., 1973). However, a variety of other measures (e.g., questionnaires and self-ratings) suggested that the estrogen-exposed boys might be less aggressive and less assertive than controls. Similarly, in the same study, 20 6-year-old estrogen-exposed boys, were found to be less assertive, as judged by teacher ratings of behavior, than 17 unexposed boys of similar age (Yalom et al., 1973). A second study (Reinisch and Karow, 1977), also described above in the section on cognitive abilities, examined personality in 69 hormone-exposed children and 70 sibling controls using the Cattell Personality Questionnaires (The Early School Personality Questionnaire for subjects 5 to 7 years of age (n = 22), the Children's Personality Questionnaire for subjects 8 to 11 years of age (n = 50), The High School Personality Questionnaire for subjects 12 to 17 years of age (n = 61) and the 16 Personality Factors for subjects 18 or older (n = 6)). Data were reported for 12 of the 16 primary factors and for 4 second order factors derived from the Cattell questionnaires. Planned comparisons of all hormone-exposed children to all controls revealed no significant differences. However, there were some differences between *post hoc* subgroups of estrogen-exposed children and controls. A group exposed primarily to estrogen was less individualistic and less self-sufficient, and a group exposed to approximately equal amounts of estrogen and progestins was less sensitive than controls. No data were presented suggesting that control boys and girls in the study differed on these specific personality dimensions, nor is such data available elsewhere in the literature. In addition, the same problems that hampered interpretation of data on cognition in this study (e.g., lack of sex-matching of hormone-exposed and unexposed children and lack of separate data analyses for male and female groups) make these results difficult to interpret in the context of sexual differentiation. The third study, described above in the sections on "gender role" behaviors and in the section on cognitive abilities, included 17 men exposed to DES, 22 men exposed to DES plus natural progesterone and 39 matched controls. No differences were observed between either group of hormone-exposed men versus unexposed men on most of the general subscales of the GZTS, although the DES plus progesterone group scored higher on the reflective scale, and, as noted above, were more feminine on the masculinity-femininity scale (Kester et al., 1980). Also, in contrast to the results of the Yalom et al. study, suggesting reduced aggression in DES-exposed boys, DES exposure in this study did not show a consistent relationship to aggression, some variables being increased (e.g., aggressive television), some being decreased (e.g., fighting in childhood) and some unchanged (e.g., aggressive themes and stories) in DES-exposed males.

A subsequent study investigated possible influences of estrogens specifically on sex-linked aspects of personality, comparing 25 women who had been exposed prenatally to DES to 25 of their sisters who had not been exposed (Hines, 1981). (The same 25 pairs of sisters described above in the section on cognitive abilities). The women completed paper-and-pencil measures of the personality characteristics of dominance, arousability and pleasure. These characteristics were selected for study based on evidence of sex differences, men typically showing higher levels of dominance and lower levels of arousability and pleasure than women (Mehrabian, 1977; Mehrabian, 1978; Mehrabian and Hines, 1978). Like sex differences in other behavioral characteristics, these sex differences are not absolute. Distributions of scores for men and women overlap. Nevertheless, when groups of men and women are tested, sex differences in mean scores are seen. Despite the sex differences documented in prior studies, no significant differences in any of the three personality dimensions were seen between the 25 DES-exposed women and their 25 unexposed sisters.

*Psychopathology*
A follow up of a randomized, double-blind, placebo-controlled study of the efficacy of prenatal treatment with DES for pregnancy maintenance, suggests an association with psychiatric disease, particularly depression and anxiety (Vessey et al., 1983). The study of DES efficacy was conducted in London, England in the early 1950s. Participants were assigned to receive either DES or placebo beginning as near as possible to week 6 of pregnancy and no later than week 16 (average = week 12) and continuing until week 35. The dose began at 5 mg/day and increased gradually to 125 mg/day by week 35. The follow up study, conducted in the late 1970s and early 1980s, involved the offspring of 650 women. Records indicating assignment to either treatment group A or group B were available for each of the 650 women, but records indicating which treatment group was DES and which was placebo were not. However, based on a higher incidence of spontaneous abortion in group B, a higher incidence of vaginal and cervical abnormalities in group B and the memory of one of the investigators involved in the original study, it was surmised that group B was treated with DES. For fear of arousing anxiety, DES-exposed individuals were not contacted directly. Rather, data were derived from medical records of general practitioners who had treated the offspring. Records were obtained for 530 individuals (151 sons and 130 daughters treated with DES and 135 sons and 152 daughters treated with placebo). Results indicated an unanticipated rise in psychiatric disorders in DES-exposed offspring compared to controls, particularly in depression, anxiety, anorexia nervosa and phobic neurosis. Numbers for DES-exposed women for these four disorders were 8, 4, 3, and 0 individuals (of 130), respectively, compared to 4, 1, 0 and 1 individuals (of 152) placebo-treated women. Thus, for women, depression, anxiety and anorexia nervosa appeared to be associated with DES. For men, numbers suffering the same disorders were 3, 4, 0 and 2 (of 151) for the DES-exposed group, respectively, compared to 2, 2, 1 and 0 (of 135) for the control group. Thus, for men, anxiety and phobic neurosis may be associated with DES.

A second series of studies also suggests an association between prenatal DES exposure and psychiatric disorders, particularly depression (Ehrhardt et al., 1987; Meyer-Bahlburg and Ehrhardt, 1987; Meyer-Bahlburg et al., 1985). These studies involved three samples of DES-exposed men and women and controls, similar to those described above for studies of sexual orientation. Sample 1 included 30 DES-exposed women and 30 controls with abnormal PAP smears. Sample 2 included 15 DES-exposed men, 19 men who thought they were DES-exposed, but for whom documentation was unavailable, and 15 unexposed men, all recruited from the same urological practice. Sample 3 included 17 DES-exposed men and 17 unexposed men selected from maternal records of one obstetrics practice. Control groups in samples 1 and 2 were selected to match for clinic referral and thus for possible concern over medical conditions. Current depression and history of major depression were assessed using the Schedule for Affective Disorders and Schizophrenia, Life-time Version (SADS-L; Endicott and Spitzer, 1978). In regard to current depression, there were no differences between any of the DES-exposed groups and unexposed controls. However, differences were seen in lifetime history of major depression. Fifty percent of the DES-exposed women (Sample 1), 40% of the verified and 39% of the unverified DES-exposed men from the urological practice (Sample 2), and 71% of the DES-exposed men from the obstetrical practice (Sample 3) had experienced major depression. Major depression was defined as a period of life dominated by a dysphoric mood and at least three associated symptoms lasting 1 week or more, and including either seeking or being referred for help, taking medication for the depression, or having notably impaired social functioning at home, work or school. The rates of major depression in the DES-exposed offspring are surprisingly high. In addition, two of the three control groups also showed surprisingly high rates of major depression. Both the female PAP controls (Sample 1) and the male urological controls (Sample 2) showed a 67% rate of lifetime depression. In contrast, only 12% of the controls identified from obstetrical records (Sample 3) had experienced major depression in their lifetimes, and this group was the only one that differed significantly from the DES-exposed group to which they were matched. The authors point out that although the elevated depression rates for DES-exposed individuals are not higher than those for control groups with medical problems similar to those associated with DES, they are higher than community norms which suggest that approximately 25% of women and 10% of men in the age range studied would be expected to have a history of major depression (Vernon and Roberts, 1982; Weissman and Myers, 1978).

As illustrated by the data on community norms, major depressive disorder shows a sex difference, women being more likely sufferers than men. Although there is a debate as to whether higher rates of depression in women reflect social or biological factors, the sex difference suggests that possible associations between depression and hormonal factors, such as prenatal exposure to DES, merit investigation. However, as pointed out by the authors of the second series of studies on DES and depression, the direction of results observed (increased depression in both men and women exposed to DES) is not consistent with animal models. Therefore, those authors posit a teratological origin, involving estrogen-induced neural damage, rather than an origin related to processes of sexual differentiation (Meyer-Bahlburg and Ehrhardt, 1987). An alternative possibility is that high rates of depression reflect psychological responses to medical or other consequences of DES exposure. The DES-exposed offspring in the Vessey et al. study were unaware of the exposure. However, the increase in depression in that study was clear only for women, and the DES-exposed women in the study showed increases in cervical lesions, and in infertility and unfavorable pregnancy outcomes (Vessey et al., 1983). Thus, medical problems associated with DES exposure could have contributed to depression without the women being aware of their exposure. This explanation would also be consistent with the high rates of depression in the second series of studies in controls who were not exposed to DES, but who were selected because they had medical problems usually associated with DES exposure (Ehrhardt et al., 1987; Meyer-Bahlburg and Ehrhardt, 1987; Meyer-Bahlburg et al., 1985).

## CONCLUSIONS AND DIRECTIONS FOR FUTURE RESEARCH

Research on women exposed to DES prenatally, because their mothers were prescribed this hormone during pregnancy, suggests estrogen-associated increases in bisexuality and in major depressive disorder. Alterations in each of these two categories of behavior have been observed in at least two studies of individuals exposed prenatally to DES. In the case of depression, one of the studies was experimental, involving random assignment, a double-blind procedure and placebo-treated controls. In the case of sexual orientation, data have been derived only from clinical studies, but the increase in bisexuality has been seen in comparing DES-exposed women to their unexposed sisters, as well as to matched controls, thus reducing the possibility that differences in background factors between the two groups account for the behavioral difference. In both cases, it is not yet known whether DES-associated behavioral changes reflect direct influences of estrogen on the developing brain, or result from other DES-associated sequelae (e.g., medical problems). Nevertheless, they suggest caution in assuming that increasing levels of estrogen in our environment would be without consequences for human well-being.

In addition to these consistent relationships between prenatal estrogen and behavior, there is also some evidence that estrogen exposure may influence several other categories of behavior, including aggression, visuospatial ability, language lateralization and the psychiatric disorders of anxiety, anorexia nervosa and phobic neurosis, although evidence in these areas is far from conclusive. Additional behaviors, such as parenting and others described under the rubric of "gender role" behaviors, have not been investigated sufficiently to rule out estrogenic influences.

Thus, there is surprisingly little information on the behavioral consequences of prenatal exposure to estrogens in human beings, given the dramatic consequences of estrogen exposure in other species. Recent suggestions of high levels of estrogenic substances in the environment underline the importance of obtaining such information. Individuals exposed to DES or other estrogens, because their mothers were prescribed these hormones during pregnancy, provide a valuable resource for estimating the potential human toll of adding estrogens to the environment. There are clear hypotheses based on animal models and a potentially large estrogen-exposed human population in which to test them. Increased attention to the neural and behavioral development of individuals who were exposed to DES prenatally is needed.

Studies of possible estrogenic influences on brain development would also be of interest. There are several reports of sex differences in human brain structure. Notably, a potential human analogue of the SDN-POA has been described in the human brain (Allen et al., 1989) and has recently been reported to relate to sexual orientation (LeVay, 1991). Similarly, the splenium, a portion of the corpus callosum (the main fiber tract connecting the two cerebral hemispheres) has been reported to differ on average in women versus men (de Lacoste-Utamsing and Holloway, 1982), and has been found to relate to sexually dimorphic cognitive traits (Hines et al., 1992). This last study was conducted using magnetic resonance imaging, a technology that allows visualization of brain structure in healthy individuals. Thus, it may be possible to investigate not only how estrogen exposure relates to behavior, but also how estrogen exposure relates to aspects of brain structure that could underlie estrogen-induced behavioral changes.

Finally, studies examining the effects of estrogen exposure during the early postnatal period are needed. Studies of prenatal exposure to DES and other estrogens used for pregnancy maintenance will not fully determine the potential consequences of creating an environment in which we are "surrounded by estrogens". Testosterone is elevated in developing human males both prenatally, from approximately week 8 to week 24 of gestation, and postnatally, from approximately the second to the sixth month of life (Smail et al., 1981). Thus, there appear to be critical periods for human sexual differentiation during the early postnatal period, as well as prenatally. Because the cerebral cortex develops late relative to other neural regions, these postnatal critical periods may be of particular importance for cognitive development, and other aspects of behavior that are mediated cortically. Thus, consequences of estrogen exposure during infancy, such as might result from increases in environmental estrogens, might differ from those seen following prenatal exposure. In addition, these postnatal influences might be particularly important, since they would be more likely to involve the cerebral cortex, the organ that most distinguishes our human nature.

## ACKNOWLEDGEMENTS

This work was supported in part by United States Public Health Service Grant HD 24542. I thank Gerianne Alexander, Marcia Collaer, Theo Colborn and Kim Wallen for comments on the manuscript of this article.

## REFERENCES

Allen, L. S., Hines, M., Shryne, J. E., and Gorski, R. A. (1989). Two sexually dimorphic cell groups in the human brain. *The Journal of Neuroscience*, **9**, 497-506.

Annett, M. (1970). A classification of hand preference by association analysis. *British Journal of Psychology*, **61**, 303-321.

Arnold, A. P. and Gorski, R. A. (1984). Gonadal steroid induction of structural sex differences in the central nervous system. *Annual Review of Neuroscience*, **7**, 413-442.

Brown-Grant, K., Fink, G., Greig, F., and Murray, M. A. F. (1975). Altered Sexual development in male rats after oestrogen administration during the neonatal period. *Journal of Reproduction and Fertility*, **44**, 25-42.

Bryden, M. P. (1982). *Laterality: Functional asymmetry in the intact brain*. Academic Press, San Diego.

Christensen, L. W. and Gorski, R. A. (1978). Independent masculinization of neuroendocrine systems by intracerebral implants of testosterone or estradiol in the neonatal female rat. *Brain Research*, **146**, 325-340.

Clemens, L. G., Gladue, B. A., and Coniglio, L. P. (1978). Prenatal endogenous androgenic influences on masculine sexual behavior and genital morphology in male and female rats. *Hormones and Behavior*, **10**, 40-53.

Cohen, J. (1988). *Statistical power analysis for the behavioral sciences* (2 ed.). Lawrence Erlbaum Associates, Hillsdale, N.J.

de Lacoste-Utamsing, C. and Holloway, R. L. (1982). Sexual dimorphism in the human corpus callosum. *Science*, **216**, 1431-1432.

Diamond, M., Llacuna, A., and Wong, C. L. (1973). Sex behavior after neonatal progesterone, testosterone, estrogen, or antiandrogens. *Hormones and Behavior*, **4**, 73-88.

Döhler, K.D., Coquelin, A., Davis, F., Hines, M., Shryne, J. E., and Gorski, R. A. (1984). Pre- and postnatal influence of testosterone propionate and diethylstilbestrol on differentiation of the sexually dimorphic nucleus of the preoptic area in male and female rats. *Brain Research*, **302**, 291-295.

Edwards, D. A. and Herndon, J. (1970). Neonatal estrogen stimulation and aggressive behavior in female mice. *Physiology and Behavior*, **5**, 993-995.

Ehrhardt, A. A., Feldman, J. F., Rosen, L. R., Meyer-Bahlburg, H. F. L., Gruen, R., Veridiano, N. P., Endicott, J., and Cohen, P. (1987). Psychopathology in prenatally DES-exposed females: Current and lifetime adjustment. *Psychosomatic Medicine*, **49**, 183-196.

Ehrhardt, A. A., Meyer-Bahlburg, H. F. L., Rosen, L. R., Feldman, J. F., Veridiano, N. P., Elkin, E. J., and McEwen, B. S. (1989). The development of gender-related behavior in females following prenatal exposure to diethylstilbestrol (DES). *Hormones and Behavior*, **23**, 526-541.

Ehrhardt, A. A., Meyer-Bahlburg, H. F. L., Rosen, L. R., Feldman, J. F., Veridiano, N. P., Zimmerman, I., and McEwen, B. S. (1985). Sexual orientation after prenatal exposure to exogenous estrogen. *Archives of Sexual Behavior*, **14**, 57-77.

Ehrhardt, A. A., Meyer-Bahlburg, H. F. L., and Veridiano, N. P. (1987). Women with a history of prenatal exposure to diethylstilbestrol (DES): Sexual functioning and reproductive concerns. In *Proceedings of the Workshop on Psychosexual and Reproductive Issues Affecting Patients with Cancer*, ed. American Cancer Society, New York, pp. 54-57.

Endicott, J. and Spitzer, R. L. (1978). A diagnostic interview. The schedule for affective disorders and schizophrenia. *Archives of General Psychiatry*, **35**, 837-844.

Faber, K. A. and Hughes, C. L. J. (1991). The effect of neonatal exposure to diethylstilbestrol, genistein, and zearalenone on pituitary responsiveness and sexually dimorphic nucleus volume in the castrated adult rat. *Biology of Reproduction*, **45**, 649-653.

Fuller, G. B., Yates, D. E., Helton, E. D., and Hobson, W. C. (1981). Diethylstilbestrol reversal of gonadotropin patterns in infant rhesus monkeys. *Journal of Steroid Biochemistry*, **15**, 497-500.

Gerall, A. A., Dunlap, J. L., and Hendricks, S. E. (1972). Effect of ovarian secretions on female behavior potentiality in the rat. *Journal of Comparative and Physiological Psychology*, **82**, 449-465.

Goy, R. W., Bercovitch, F. B., and McBrair, M. C. (1988). Behavioral masculinization is independent of genital masculinization in prenatally androgenized female rhesus macagues. *Hormones and Behavior*, **22**, 552-571.

Goy, R. W. and McEwen, B. S. (1980). *Sexual Differentiation of the Brain*. MIT Press, Cambridge, Massachusetts.

Halpern, D. F. (1987). *Sex differences in cognitive abilities*. Erlbaum, Hillsdale, N.J.

Heinonen, O. P. (1973). Diethylstilbestrol in pregnancy: Frequency of exposure and usage patterns. *Cancer*, **31**, 573-577.

Herbst, A. L. and Bern, H. A. (Ed.). (1981). *Developmental effects of diethylstilbestrol (DES) in pregnancy*. New York: Thieme-Stratton.

Hier, D. B. and Crowley, W. F. (1982). Spatial ability in androgen-deficient men. *The New England Journal of Medicine*, **306**, 1202-1205.

Hines, M. (1981). *Prenatal diethylstilbestrol (DES) exposure, human sexually dimorphic behavior and cerebral lateralization.* doctoral dissertation, University of California, Los Angeles.

Hines, M. (1982). Prenatal gonadal hormones and sex differences in human behavior. *Psychological Bulletin*, **92**, 56-80.

Hines, M. (1990). Gonadal hormones and human cognitive development. *Comparative Physiology*, **8**, 51-63.

Hines, M., Alsum, P., Roy, M., Gorski, R. A., and Goy, R. W. (1987). Estrogenic contributions to sexual differentiation in the female guinea pig: Influences of diethylstilbestrol and tamoxifen on neural, behavioral and ovarian development. *Hormones and Behavior*, **21**, 402-417.

Hines, M., Chiu, L., McAdams, L. A., Bentler, P. M., and Lipcamon, J. (1992). Cognition and the corpus callosum: Verbal fluency, visuospatial ability, and language lateralization related to midsagittal surface areas of callosal subregions. *Behavioral Neuroscience*, **106**, 3-14.

Hines, M., Davis, F. C., Coquelin, A., Goy, R. W., and Gorski, R. A. (1985). Sexually dimorphic regions in the medial preoptic area and the bed nucleus of the stria terminalis of the guinea pig brain: A description and an investigation of their relationship to gonadal steroids in adulthood. *The Journal of Neuroscience*, **5**, 40-47.

Hines, M., Dohler, K. D., and Gorski, R. A. (1982). Rough play in female rats following pre- and postnatal treatment with diethylstilbestrol or testosterone. *Abstracts: Conference on Reproductive Behavior*, **14**, 66.

Hines, M., Döhler, K. D., and Gorski, R. A. (unpublished data). Rough and tumble play behavior in male rats exposed to diethylstilbestrol during prenatal and neonatal critical periods for sexual differentiation. .

Hines, M. and Goy, R. W. (1985). Estrogens before birth and development of sex-related reproductive traits in the female guinea pig. *Hormones and Behavior*, **19**, 331-347.

Hines, M. and Goy, R. W. (unpublished data). Sexual behavior in male guinea pigs exposed to estradiol or diethylstilbestrol during prenatal critical periods for sexual differentiation.

Hines, M. and Shipley, C. (1984). Prenatal exposure to diethylsttilbestrol (DES) and the development of sexually dimorphic cognitive abilities and cerebral lateralization. *Developmental Psychology*, **20**, 81-94.

Kester, P., Green, R., Finch, S. J., and Williams, K. (1980). Prenatal 'female hormone' administration and psychosexual development in human males. *Psychoneuroendocrinology*, **5**, 269-285.

Kinsey, A., Pomeroy, W., and Martin, C. (1948). *Sexual Behavior in the Human Male*. Saunders, Philadelphia.

Kinsey, A., Pomeroy, W., and Martin, C. (1953). *Sexual Behavior in the Human Female*. Saunders, Philadelphia.

LeVay, S. (1991). A difference in hypothalamic structure between heterosexual and homosexual men. *Science*, **253**, 1034-1037.

Lish, J. D., Ehrhardt, A. A., Meyer-Bahlburg, H. F. L., Rosen, L. R., Gruen, R. S., and Veridiano, N. P. (1991). Gender-related behavior development in females exposed to diethylstilbestrol (DES) *in utero*: An attempted replication. *Journal of the American Academy of Child and Adolescent Psychiatry*, **30**, 29-37.

Maccoby, E. E. and Jacklin, C. N. (1974). *The psychology of sex differences*. Stanford University Press, Stanford, CA.

McGlone, J. (1980). Sex differences in human brain asymmetry: A critical survey. *Behavior and Brain Sciences*, **3**, 215-263.

Mehrabian, A. (1977). A questionnaire measure of individual differences in stimulus screening and associated differences in arousability. *Environmental Psychology and Nonverbal Behavior*, **1**, 89-103.

Mehrabian, A. (1978). Measures of individual differences in temperament. *Educational and Psychological Measurement*, **38**, 1105-1117.

Mehrabian, A. and Hines, M. (1978). A questionnaire measure of individual differences in dominance submissiveness. *Educational and Psychological Measurement*, **38**, 479-484.

Meisel, R. L. and Ward, I. L. (1981). Fetal female rats are masculinized by male littermates located caudally in the uterus. *Science*, **213**, 239-242.

Meyer-Bahlburg, H. F. L. and Ehrhardt, A. A. (1987). A prenatal-hormone hypothesis for depression in adults with a history of fetal DES exposure. In Hormones and Depression, ed. U. Halbreich. Raven Press, New York, pp. 325-338.

Meyer-Bahlburg, H. F. L., Ehrhardt, A. A., Endicott, J., Veridiano, N. P., Whitehead, E. D., and Vann, F. H. (1985). Depression in adults with a history of prenatal DES exposure. *Psychopharmacology Bulletin*, **21**, 686-689.

Meyer-Bahlburg, H. F. L., Ehrhardt, A. A., Whitehead, E. D., and Vann, F. H. (1987). Sexuality in males with a history of prenatal exposure to diethylstilbestrol (DES). In *Psychosexual and Reproductive Issues Affecting Patients with Cancer*, ed. American Cancer Society, New York.

Noller, K. L. and Fish, C. R. (1974). Diethylstilbestrol usage: Its interesting past, important present and questionable future. *Medical Clinics of America*, **58**, 793-810.

Paup, D. C., Coniglio, L. P., and Clemens, L. G. (1974). Hormonal determinants in the development of masculine and feminine behavior in the female hamster. *Behavioral Biology*, **10**, 353-363.

Reinisch, J. M. and Gandelman, R. (1978). Human research in behavioral endocrinology: Methodological and theoretical considerations. In *Hormones and brain development,* ed. G. Dörner and M. Kawakami. Elsevier/North Holland Biomedical Press, Amsterdam,

Reinisch, J. M. and Karow, W. G. (1977). Prenatal exposure to synthetic progestins and estrogens: Effects on human development. *Archives of Sexual Behavior,* 6, 257-288.

Reinisch, J. M. and Sanders, S. A. (1992). Effects of prenatal exposure to diethylstilbestrol (DES) on hemispheric laterality and spatial ability in human males. *Hormones and Behavior,* 26, 62-75.

Smail, P. J., Reyes, F. I., Winter, J. S. D., and Faiman, C. (1981). The fetal hormone environment and its effect on the morphogenesis of the genital system. In *Pediatric Andrology,* ed. S. J. Kogan and E. S. E. Hafez. Martinus Nijhoff, The Hague, pp. 9-20.

Sprafkin, C., Serbin, L. A., Denier, C., and Connor, J. M. (1983). Sex-differentiated play: Cognitive consequences and early interventions. In *Social and Cognitive Skills,* ed. M. B. Liss. Academic Press, New York, pp. 167-192.

Tilson, H. A. and Lamartiniere, C. A. (1979). Neonatal exposure to diethylstilbestrol affects the sexual differentiation of male rats. *Neurobehavioral Toxicology,* 1, 123-128.

Vernon, S. W. and Roberts, R. E. (1982). Use of the SADS-RDC in a tri-ethnic community survey. *Archives of General Psychiatry,* 39, 47-52.

Vessey, M. P., Fairweather, D. V. I., Norman-Smith, B., and Buckley, J. (1983). A randomized double-blind controlled trial of the value of stilboestrol therapy in pregnancy: long-term follow-up of mothers and their offspring. *British Journal of Obstetrics and Gynaecology,* 90, 1007-1017.

vom Saal, F. S. and Bronson, F. H. (1980). Sexual characteristics of adult female mice are correlated with their blood testosterone levels during prenatal development. *Science,* 208, 597-599.

Weissman, M. M. and Myers, J. K. (1978). Affective disorders in a US urban community. *Archives of General Psychiatry,* 35, 1304-1311.

Whalen, R. E. and Nadler, R. D. (1963). Suppression of the development of female mating behavior by estrogen administered in infancy. *Science,* 14, 273-274.

Wilcox, A. J., Maxey, J., and Herbst, A. L. Prenatal hormone exposure and performance on college entrance examinations. *Hormones and Behavior,* (in press).

Williams, C. L., Barnett, A. M., and Meck, W. A. (1990). Organizational effects of early gonadal secretions on sexual differentiation in spatial memory. *Behavioral Neuroscience,* 104, 84-97.

Yalom, I. D., Green, R., and Fisk, N. (1973). Prenatal exposure to female hormones: Effect on psychosexual development in boys. *Archives of General Psychiatry,* 28, 554-561.

# DISEASE PATTERNS AND ANTIBODY RESPONSES TO VIRAL ANTIGENS IN WOMEN EXPOSED *IN UTERO* TO DIETHYLSTILBESTROL

**Phyllis B. Blair**
Department of Molecular and Cell Biology,
University of California, Berkeley, California

**Kenneth L. Noller**
Department of Obstetrics and Gynecology,
University of Massachusetts, Worchester, Massachusetts

**Judith Turiel**
DES Action, San Francisco, California

**Bagher Forghani**
Viral and Rickettsial Disease Laboratory, Division of Laboratories,
California State Department of Health Services, Berkeley, California

**Shirley Hagens**
Viral and Rickettsial Disease Laboratory, Division of Laboratories,
California State Department of Health Services, Berkeley, California

## INTRODUCTION

As documented in this volume and elsewhere, there is increasing evidence that prenatal exposure to a variety of agents may have long-term consequences, both morphologic and functional, which may not be evident at birth. The effect of diethylstilbestrol (DES) on the developing human fetus is one example of this.

Studies in experimental animals have provided convincing evidence that perinatal exposure to diethylstilbestrol (DES) can significantly and permanently affect the immune system; as adults, perinatally exposed mice exhibit altered immune responses to viral infections and to experimental inoculations of antigens which can be detected throughout the life of the animals. Some changes may even become more severe as the animals age (Blair, 1981). Observations on immune reactivity in humans after prenatal exposure to DES are limited but suggest that changes occur in this species also. In two experimental studies involving a limited number of subjects, altered function of T cells and of natural killer cells in DES-exposed women has been reported (Ford et al., 1983; Ways et al., 1987). In addition, two analyses of questionnaire responses have demonstrated an increase in the lifetime prevalence of autoimmune diseases in DES-exposed individuals compared with that observed in the general population (Turiel and

1. Corresponding Author: Phyllis B. Blair, 461 LSA, University of California, Berkeley, CA 94720.
2. This research was supported by funds from the University of California and by grant CA 36873 from the National Cancer Institute, National Institutes of Health, Public Health Service.

Wingard, 1988) or in a control group of non-exposed women participating in the National Cooperative Diethylstilbestrol Adenosis (DESAD) Project (Noller et al., 1988).

Using two different groups of DES-exposed women, with an appropriate control group for each, we have examined disease and infection patterns (by analysis of questionnaire responses and by determination of serum antibody titers to viral pathogens) to determine if immune alterations in humans prenatally exposed to DES might be expressed by changes in responses to microbial pathogens. No differences were observed in the prevalence or titer of antibodies to any of six common viruses, or in the prevalence of five common infectious diseases and six less common ones. However, one disease, rheumatic fever, which is a later occurring immunologic aberration of a previous infection with streptococcus, occurred significantly more frequently in DES-exposed individuals than in controls.

## RESPONSES TO DESAD QUESTIONNAIRES

In 1974 women exposed before birth to DES and unexposed controls were recruited for participation in the DESAD Project, a large prospective multicenter epidemiologic project designed in a manner which minimized self-selection and other common biases. The details of participant recruitment have been described previously (Labarthe et al., 1978). Since the termination of the examination phase of the DESAD Project in 1983, the participants have been contacted yearly by questionnaire. The 1986 questionnaire included inquiries regarding general immune status, occurrence of common diseases, and occurrence of specific autoimmune diseases. Responses from two of the study groups, a group of 1711 DES-exposed individuals identified by review of obstetric records and a group of 922 unexposed individuals identified at the same time from the same record sources, have been analyzed. Over 97% of the women originally enrolled in these two groups have continued to participate by completion of the questionnaires, despite the long-term nature of the study. The increased occurrence of autoimmune disease in the DES-exposed cohort, compared with the control group, has already been reported (Noller et al., 1988).

Responses to questionnaires returned by individuals in the record review groups (control and DES-exposed) of the DESAD Project have now been analyzed for information on the occurrence of various infectious diseases. Some questions were not answered by all study participants returning the questionnaires, but no significant differences were observed between the control and DES-exposed groups in the response rate for each question. Response rates were highest for the more common diseases (measles, mumps, rubella, chickenpox, and strep throat), ranging from 75% to 94%. Somewhat lower response rates were observed for the less common diseases, ranging from 65% to 76%. Comparisons of reported diseases between the control and the DES-exposed groups are presented here in two ways, (a) as percent reporting the disease of those who responded to the question, and (b) as percent reporting the disease of those who returned the questionnaire (Table 1). No differences were observed between the DES-exposed and the control groups in the lifetime history of common childhood diseases (measles, mumps, rubella, chickenpox, and strep throat). Similarly, reports of the less common diseases (mononucleosis, oral herpes, pneumonia, appendicitis, and hepatitis) were essentially the same in the two groups. In some infections, multiple episodes of the disease are possible, and questionnaire responses were analyzed to determine if differences existed in such disease patterns. No differences were observed.

**TABLE 1.**   **Percent reporting specific disease occurrence on the DESAD Project questionnaire.**

| Disease history | All returned questionnaires | | All responses | |
|---|---|---|---|---|
| | Controls | Exposed | Controls | Exposed |
| Measles | 62 | 59 | 81 | 75 |
| Mumps | 61 | 60 | 74 | 72 |
| Rubella | 54 | 50 | 72 | 67 |
| Mononucleosis | 21 | 22 | 29 | 29 |
| Oral herpes | 21 | 20 | 28 | 27 |
| Pneumonia | 20 | 22 | 27 | 29 |
| Appendicitis | 7 | 7 | 10 | 10 |
| Hepatitis | 3 | 3 | 5 | 4 |
| Chickenpox | 88 | 87 | 94 | 93 |
| Shingles | 4 | 3 | 6 | 5 |
| Strep throat | 62 | 60 | 78 | 75 |
| Rheumatic Fever | 0.4 | 1.4* | 0.6 | 2* |

*Difference is statistically significant by Chi square, p=<0.05.

Two of the diseases, shingles and rheumatic fever, represent sequelae afflicting a limited number of individuals who have previously developed common infections. Shingles results from the reemergence of the varicella-zoster virus after a period of latency. A few of the individuals in each of the two groups reported this disease, but there was no difference between the two groups. Rheumatic fever occurs after infection with streptococcus A (strep throat), and bacteria may not be detectable at the time the disease symptoms occur (Wannamaker, 1981). The disease represents an immunologic complication of the response to the bacterial infection which manifests itself as a response against tissue antigens. The reported occurrence of strep throat in the controls and in the DES-exposed groups was similar, but a significant difference in the frequency of the later immunologic complication, rheumatic fever, was seen. The disease was rare in both groups, but more than three times as many DES-exposed individuals as controls reported it. This difference is statistically significant not only in calculations involving only those responding to the question but also in calculations involving all those returning the questionnaire (Table 1).

## PREVALENCE AND TITER OF ANTIBODIES
## TO SIX VIRUSES

A second, smaller study involved women recruited more recently in the San Francisco Bay Area, with the cooperation of DES Action, an organized consumer action group. Participants in this group responded to a letter sent to the DES Action mailing list, to posters, or to presentations in classes on the Berkeley campus. Each participant completed a questionnaire and donated a sample of blood. Based on responses to questions regarding the use of medications such as DES by their mothers during their pregnancies, the participants were grouped into those exposed to DES *in utero*, those not exposed, and those unsure of their status with regard to DES exposure. Data from individuals in the first two groups only were used in these analyses, with recognition that there might be some errors in classification because of the absence in most cases of pertinent medical records, and also with recognition that the DES-exposed group was self-selected and might not be representative of the DES-exposed population as a whole. The two groups were further limited to include only white females aged 25-35 years, which yielded a group of 33 DES-exposed individuals and a group of 21 unexposed controls.

Serum samples obtained from individuals in the Bay Area study were analyzed for the prevalence and titer of antibodies to six human viruses: measles, varicella-zoster, rubella, cytomegalovirus, influenza A, and herpes simplex (Table 2). These six were chosen to provide information on antibody titers to common pathogens (measles, rubella, varicella-zoster, influenza A) to which most of the individuals should have been exposed naturally or by immunization, and to pathogens (cytomegalovirus and herpes simplex) for which exposure is less common but for which the frequency of infection typically increases with age (Dworsky et al., 1983). Antibodies to cytomegalovirus, herpes simplex virus, varicella-zoster virus, and measles virus were determined by enzyme immunoassay (Cremer et al., 1985); viral antigens were prepared from virus-infected cell lysates and control antigens from uninfected cell lysates. Antibodies to influenza A virus were determined by microtiter complement fixation test (Hawkes, 1979); viral antigen was prepared from virus-infected egg allantoic fluid, and control antigen from uninfected egg allantoic fluid. Antibodies to rubella virus were determined using the commercial "Rubazyme" kit (Abbott Laboratories, Illinois) following the recommended procedures of the manufacturer. Antibodies to viruses causing the three typical childhood diseases (measles, rubella, and chickenpox) were common and no significant differences in either prevalence or titer between the control and the DES-exposed groups were observed. Similarly, antibodies to influenza virus were common and significant differences were not detected. For all four viruses, antibody titers were slightly but not significantly higher in the DES-exposed group. The sera were also analyzed for the prevalence and titer of antibodies to two additional viruses, herpes simplex and cytomegalovirus, for which the occurrence of infection is less common. No differences in either prevalence or titer were observed between the control and the DES-exposed groups. The frequencies were slightly higher, and the titers slightly lower, for both viruses in the DES-exposed group, but these differences were not statistically significant.

**TABLE 2.** **Percent and average titer of antibodies to six viruses in the Bay Area study group.\***

| Virus | Controls | | DES-exposed | |
|---|---|---|---|---|
| | Percent Positive | Average Titer # | Percent Positive | Average Titer |
| Measles | 100 | 9.77 | 100 | 10.66 |
| Rubella | 95 | 2.33 | 91 | 2.39 |
| Varicella | 95 | 8.44 | 94 | 9.09 |
| Influenza | 94 | 10.82 | 88 | 13.45 |
| Herpes simplex | 52 | 8.94 | 67 | 8.70 |
| Cytomegalovirus | 38 | 8.88 | 48 | 8.37 |

\* Test results are reported for 21 controls and 33 DES-exposed individuals for analyses of antibodies to measles, rubella, varicella, herpes simplex and cytomegalovirus, and for 18 controls and 25 DES-exposed for influenza virus.
# Reciprocal of endpoint dilution of serum showing significant reaction with antigen.

## DISCUSSION

We infer from these data that, in general, individuals exposed to DES prenatally do not exhibit severe defects in immune function, and that their responses to microbial pathogens are probably within normal limits. Nevertheless, we did find an increased prevalence in DES-exposed women of a relatively rare immunologic hyperreactivity, rheumatic fever, subsequent to microbial infection (strep throat). Thus, both our previous report on the increased prevalence of autoimmune disease (Noller et al., 1988) and this report concern defects at the level of immune regulation. We recognize that in a survey of a large number of diseases a statistically significant difference in one might occur by chance, but the fact that both of the differences detected involve problems in the regulation of immune self reactivity suggests that the observations may be biologically relevant. A study of the specific characteristics of the immune response to streptococcus A in DES-exposed individuals may provide confirmation of the observation.

## REFERENCES

Blair, P.B. (1981). Immunologic consequences of early exposure of experimental rodents to diethylstilbestrol and steroid hormones. In *Developmental Effects of Diethylstilbestrol (DES) in Pregnancy*, (A. Herbst and H.A. Bern, eds.) Thieme-Stratton, New York, pp. 167-178.

Cremer, N.E., Cossen, C.K., Sell, G., Diggs, J., Gallo, D., and Schmidt, N. (1985). Enzyme immunoassay versus plaque neutralization and other methods for determination of immune status to measles and varicella-zoster virus and versus complement fixation for serodiagnosis. *J. Clin. Microbiol.*, **21**, 869-874.

Dworsky, R., Paganini-Hill, A., Arthur, M., and Parker, J. (1983). Immune responses of healthy humans 83-104 years of age. *J. Natl. Cancer Inst.*, **71**, 265-268.

Ford, C.D., Johnson, G.H., and Smith, W.G. (1983). Natural killer cells in *in utero* diethylstilbestrol-exposed patients. *Gynecol. Oncol.*, **16**, 400-404.

Hawkes, R.A. (1979). General principles underlying laboratory diagnosis of viral infections. In *Diagnostic Procedures for Viral, Rickettsial and Chlamydial Infections*, (5th ed.) (E.H. Lennette and N.J. Schmidt, eds.) American Public Health Association, Washington, DC, pp. 35.

Labarthe, D., Adam, E., Noller, K.L., O'Brien, P.C., Robboy, S.J., Tilley, B.C., Townsend, D., Barnes, A.B., Kaufman, R.H., Decker, D.G., Fish C.R., Herbst, A.L., Gundersen, J., and Kurland, L.T. (1978). Design and preliminary observations of National Cooperative Diethylstilbestrol Adenosis (DESAD) Project. *Obstet. Gynecol.*, **51**, 453-458.

Noller, K.L., Blair, P.B., O'Brien, P.C., and Mellon, L.J. (1988). Increased occurrence of autoimmune disease among women exposed *in utero* to diethylstilbestrol. *Fertil. Steril.*, **49**, 1080-1082.

Turiel, J. and Wingard, D.L. (1988). Immune response in DES-exposed women. *Fertil. Steril.*, **49**, 928.

Wannamaker, L.W. (1981). Immunology of streptococci. In *Immunology of Human Infection, part I: Bacteria, Mycoplasmae, Chlamydiae, and Fungi*, (A.J. Nahmias and R.J. O'Reilly, eds.) Plenum Medical Book Company, New York, pp.47-92.

Ways, S.C., Mortola, J.F., Zvaifler, N.J., Weiss, R.J., and Yen, S.S.C. (1987). Alterations in immune responsiveness in women exposed to diethylstilbestrol *in utero*. *Fertil. Steril.*, **48**, 193-197.

# IMMUNOLOGIC STUDIES OF WOMEN EXPOSED *IN UTERO* TO DIETHYLSTILBESTROL

**Phyllis B. Blair**
The Department of Molecular and Cell Biology,
University of California, Berkeley California

## INTRODUCTION

Data available from studies of women prenatally exposed to diethylstilbestrol (DES) provide a clear example of the types of long-term morphologic and functional changes which prenatal exposure to an agent may induce and which may not be evident at birth. First recognized was the long-term effect on the reproductive system, documented both in the human and also in the mouse model system (reviewed in Herbst and Bern, 1981). Other studies demonstrated that long-term alterations in immune function are a consequence of prenatal exposure to DES in experimental animals (reviewed in Blair, 1981) and in human females (Ford et al., 1983; Ways et al., 1987). Although infection patterns and antibody responses to common pathogens appear to be normal in DES-exposed women (Adler-Storthz et al., 1985; Blair et al., 1991), evidence is accumulating which indicates that there is an increase in diseases which are a consequence of problems in immune regulation. Prenatal exposure to DES can lead to small but significant increases in the prevalence of autoimmune diseases (Turiel and Wingard, 1988; Noller et al., 1988) and of rheumatic fever, a relatively rare immunological aberration occurring subsequent to infection with streptococcus (Blair et al., 1991). It is thus pertinent to examine DES-exposed and control women for immunologic changes which might be indicative of potential problems in immune regulation, or which might precede clinical detection of an autoimmune or other regulatory disease.

## EXPERIMENTAL OBSERVATIONS

The analysis reported here was undertaken because autoimmune diseases are often accompanied by serologic changes such as the development of heterophile antibodies and rheumatoid factors, or changes in titer of immunoglobulin classes such as IgA. A set of serum samples which had been collected for a collaborative study in which the sera were examined for the incidence and titer of antibodies to six common viral pathogens (Blair et al., 1991) was available for this pilot study.

The groups of DES-exposed and non-exposed women were selected from those who had participated in a research study in the San Francisco Bay Area by

1. Corresponding Author: Phyllis B. Blair, 461 LSA, University of California, Berkeley CA, 94720.
2. These studies were supported by funds from the University of California, Berkeley CA.

completing a questionnaire and donating a sample of blood (Blair et al., 1991). Based on responses to questions regarding the use of medications such as DES by their mothers during their pregnancies, the participants were grouped into those exposed to DES *in utero*, those not exposed, and those unsure of their status. Data for individuals in the first two groups only were used in the serum analyses, with recognition that there might be some errors in classification because of the absence in most cases of pertinent medical records, and also with recognition that the DES-exposed group because of the element of self-selection might not be representative of the DES-exposed population as a whole. White females 25 to 35 years of age were studied, 33 exposed to DES, and 21 unexposed controls.

Aliquots of the sera were examined for the presence of factors often associated with autoimmune diseases, using commercially available kits and the procedures recommended by the manufacturers; SLE Rythrotex (ICL Scientific, Fountain Valley, CA) for antinucleoprotein factors, Mono-diff (Wampole Laboratories, Cranbury, NJ) for heterophile antibodies, and Rheumanosticon Dri-Dot (Organon Teknika Corp., Morris Plains, NJ) for rheumatoid factors. In the latter two tests, the sera were also used undiluted, to determine if lower concentrations of the pertinent factors or antibodies might be detectable. Antibody titers to human red blood cell (RBC) A and B antigens were determined by microtiter hemagglutination (Ways et al., 1980). Levels of immunoglobulin were determined using the commercial Accuplate Radial Immunodiffusion System (ICL Scientific, Fountain Valley, CA) following the recommended procedures of the manufacturer.

All sera were negative in the tests to antinucleoprotein factors associated with SLE, for heterophile antibodies, and for rheumatoid factors, although sera from two of the DES-exposed females did react in the rheumatoid factor assay when tested undiluted. Using the serum samples as a source of antibodies to the human RBC antigens A and B, individuals were typed as A, B, AB, or O, and the sera then appropriately tested for titer of antibodies to the A or to the B antigen (Table 1). In each of the two tests, the incidence of high titers of antibody was greater in the DES-exposed females than in the controls. Further, when the data were combined and the incidence of individuals demonstrating a high titer of antibodies against at least one of the two antigens (A and/or B) was determined, the difference was statistically significant (38% of the DES-exposed females compared to 11% of the controls).

The serum samples were also examined for relative levels of the immunoglobulin classes IgM, IgG, and IgA. No significant differences between the DES-exposed and control groups in titers of IgM or IgG were detected. In this assay normal values of IgM are 82-246 international units (I.U.); titers ranged from 174 to 404 I.U. in the DES-exposed women and from 122 to 404 I.U. in the controls. Some women in each of the groups had titers higher than expected normal values, but the difference between the two groups was not significant. Normal values of IgG in this assay are 80-195 I.U.; titers ranged from 99 to 273 I.U. in the DES-exposed women and from 115 to 202 in the controls. Again, some women in each of the groups had titers higher than expected normal values, but the difference between the two groups was not significant. Normal values of IgA in this assay are 40-200 I.U. IgA titers ranged from 66 to 222 in the DES-exposed and from 58 to 142 I.U. in the controls. A statistically significant number of DES-exposed women (8 of 25, 32%) had titers greater than the upper end of the normal range (142 I.U.) whereas none of the controls had such high titers (Table 1).

**TABLE 1.**  **Antibody responses to human red blood cell antigens A and B and titers of IgA.**

| Antigen or Ig | Response | DES-exposed Number | Percent | Controls Number | Percent | Signif ^ |
|---|---|---|---|---|---|---|
| A | High titer* | 6 | 30% | 1 | 14% | n s |
|  | Total tested | 20 |  | 7 |  |  |
| B | High titer* | 8 | 30% | 2 | 12% | n s |
|  | Total tested | 27 |  | 17 |  |  |
| A or B | High titer* | 12 | 38% | 2 | 11% | 0.05 |
|  | Total tested | 32 |  | 19 |  |  |
| IgA | High titer # | 8 | 32% | 0 | 0% | 0.01 |
|  | Total tested | 32 |  | 20 |  |  |

^ significance determined by Chi square: ns = not significant
* greater than 1:8
# greater than 142 I.U.

## DISCUSSION

Thus, reports to date indicate that, in general, humans exposed prenatally to DES do not exhibit severe defects in basic immune function, but their propensity to develop autoimmune and other diseases associated with defects in immune regulation is increased. The data reported here strengthen these conclusions by demonstrating higher titers of antibodies to human RBC antigens and higher levels of the immunoglobulin class IgA, which can be indicative of immunoregulatory problems, in DES-exposed women.

Problems in the regulation of immune self reactivity typically increase with age (Kay, 1980), and in this regard it is pertinent to briefly comment on the results of studies in the mouse regarding the effect on the immune system of perinatal exposure to DES (reviewed in Blair, 1981; Blair 1991). In the mouse the reproductive tract and the immune system are still developing late in gestation and also in the neonate, and mice treated with DES during this time have been used in a number of immunologic studies as an experimental model of the human exposed prenatally to DES. These studies have demonstrated that immune capabilities can be permanently altered after perinatal DES exposure. Major changes have been found in the functioning of T cells and B cells, both in specific immune responses and in responses to mitogens, and also in the functioning of natural killer (NK) cells, which are part of the non-specific immune defense system. Although the majority of the reports, from a number of different laboratories, document decreases in immune function as a consequence of DES exposure, there are also reports of no changes, or of increased reactivity, depending on the strain used. Thus, genetic factors may play a significant role in the expression of the immunologic changes.

From these experimental studies, two observations with potential significance for the human population of DES-exposed individuals emerge. First, although no major impact on general health and survival has been observed, it has been reported in several studies, some of which were designed for other purposes, that DES-exposed mice may be less able to withstand the stress of experimental manipulations, such as surgery (Ways et al., 1984), the inoculation of carcinogens (Kalland and Forsberg, 1981) or heterologous proteins (Ways et al., 1984), or the transplantation of tumors (Blair, 1987), and may be more susceptible to the development of tumors (Kalland and Forsberg, 1981; Ways, 1982). Second, the severity of the immune defects detected often increases with age, and, in fact, changes in immune capability may not be detectable in young adult mice but only later in life (Ways et al., 1980; Blair, 1991).

Individuals (men and women) exposed prenatally to DES are now in their 30s, 40s, and 50s, and may be increasingly subject to a variety of problems, including those involving immune regulation, as they continue to age.

## REFERENCES

Adler-Storthz, K., Dreesman, G.R., Kaufman, R.H., Melnick, J.L., and Adam, E. (1985). A prospective study of herpes simplex virus infection in a defined population in Houston, Texas. *Am. J. Obstet. Gynecol.*, **151**, 582-586.

Blair, P.B. (1981). Immunologic consequences of early exposure of experimental rodents to diethylstilbestrol and steroid hormones. In *Developmental Effects of Diethylstilbestrol (DES) in Pregnancy*, ed. A Herbst and H.A. Bern. Thieme-Stratton, New York, pp. 167-178.

Blair, P.B. (1987). Abnormalities in immunologic development induced by perinatal exposure to hormones. *Fed. Proc.*, **46**, 1517.

Blair, P.B. (1991). Immunologic consequences of early exposure of mice to diethylstilbestrol (DES). *Clin. Pract. Gynecol.*, **2**, 91-108.

Blair, P.B., Noller, K.L., Turiel, J., Forghani, B., and Hagens, S. (1992). Disease patterns and antibody responses to viral antigens in women exposed *in utero* to diethylstilbestrol. In *Chemically-Induced Alterations in Sexual and Functional Development: The Wildlife/Human Connection*, eds. T. Colborn and C. Clement, Princeton Scientific Publishing Co., pp. 283-288.

Ford, C.D., Johnson, G.H., and Smith, W.G. (1983). Natural killer cells in *in utero* diethylstilbestrol-exposed patients. *Gynecol. Oncol.*, **16**, 400-404.

Herbst, A. and Bern, H.A. (eds) (1981). *Developmental Effects of Diethylstilbestrol (DES) in Pregnancy.* Thieme-Stratton, New York.

Kalland, T. and Forsberg, J.G. (1981). Natural killer cell activity and tumor susceptibility in female mice treated neonatally with diethylstilbestrol. *Cancer Res.*, **41**, 5134-5140.

Kay, M.M.B. (1980). Aging and the decline of immune responsiveness. In *Basic and Clinical Immunology*, ed. H.H. Fudenberg, D.P. Stites, J.L. Caldwell and J.V. Wells. Lange Medical Publications, Los Altos, CA, pp. 327-342.

Noller, K.L., Blair, P.B., O'Brien, P.C., and Mellon, L.J. (1988). Increased occurrence of autoimmune disease among women exposed *in utero* to diethylstilbestrol. *Fertil. Steril.*, **49**, 1080-1082.

Turiel, J. and Wingard, D.L. (1988). Immune response in DES-exposed women. *Fertil. Steril.*, **49**, 928.

Ways, S.C. (1982). Local induction of fibrosarcomas by diethylstilbestrol. *Internat. Res. Comm. Sys.*, **10**, 796-797.

Ways, S.C., Bern, H.A., and Blair, P.B. (1984). Effect of immunosuppression on neonatally diethylstilbestrol-induced genital tract lesion and tumor development in female mice. *J. Natl. Cancer Inst.*, **73**, 863-870.

Ways, S.C., Blair, P.B., Bern, H.A., and Staskawicz, M.O. (1980). Immune responsiveness of adult mice exposed neonatally to diethylstilbestrol, steroid hormones, or vitamin A. *J. Environ. Path. and Toxicol.*, **3**, 207-220.

Ways, S.C., Mortola, J.F., Zvaifler, N.J., Weiss, R.J., and Yen, S.S.C. (1987). Alterations in immune responsiveness in women exposed to diethylstilbestrol *in utero.* *Fertil. Steril.*, **48**, 193-197.

# AN "IN CULTURE" BIOASSAY TO ASSESS THE ESTROGENICITY OF XENOBIOTICS (E-SCREEN)

**Ana M. Soto**
Tufts University, School of Medicine,
Department of Anatomy and Cellular Biology, Boston, Massachusetts

**Tien-Min Lin**
Tufts University School of Medicine, Boston, Massachusetts

**Honorato Justicia**
Tufts University School of Medicine, Boston, Massachusetts

**Renée M. Silvia**
Tufts University School of Medicine, Boston, Massachusetts

**Carlos Sonnenschein**
Tufts University School of Medicine, Boston, Massachusetts

*An "in culture" bioassay was developed to assess the estrogenicity of xenobiotics using human breast estrogen-sensitive MCF7 cells. The assay compares the cell yield achieved after 6 days of culture in medium supplemented with 10% charcoal-dextran stripped human serum in the presence or absence of estradiol ($10^{-13}$ to $10^{-9}M$), and with diverse concentrations of xenobiotics suspected of being estrogenic. Among the chemicals tested (pesticides, phytoestrogens, polychlorobiphenyls, alkylphenols and phytohormones), the bioassay confirmed the estrogenicity of compounds previously shown to be estrogenic in rodent models; no false positives were found. In addition, a case of estrogen contamination due to the shedding of estrogenic xenobiotics by polystyrene labware was solved using this assay. This bioassay has the following advantages over those currently used: a) it is easy to perform; it requires a standard cell culture facility and a human estrogen-sensitive cell line; b) it is relevant to humans, since it relies on the responses of a human cell line growing in human serum-supplemented media, and c) it is sensitive since it detects 10 pg/ml estradiol-17β. This assay may also be used to determine the presence of estrogenic xenobiotics in soil, water, human foods and animal feeds. Among the foods and feeds tested, a soy bean drink and a laboratory rat chow were shown to be estrogenic. We believe that the adoption of this bioassay by industry and regulatory agencies may provide a rigorous tool to identify estrogenic xenobiotics.*

1. Corresponding Author: Ana M. Soto, Department of Anatomy and Cellular Biology, Tufts University School of Medicine, 136 Harrison Ave., Boston, MA, 02111.
2. Key words: xenobiotic, *in vitro*, cell proliferation, estrogens, bioassay.

## INTRODUCTION

Environmental xenobiotics are suspected to play a causative role in human infertility and cancer. Similar concerns have been raised over their effect on wildlife reproduction. However, an objective causal relationship between these detrimental effects and their presumed etiology is tempered by: a) the lack of appropriate technology to explore this subject, and b) the uncertainty of predicting reproductive toxicity by glancing at the chemical structure of xenobiotics.

Estrogens promote cell proliferation and hypertrophy of female secondary sex organs and induce the synthesis of cell type-specific proteins (Hertz, 1985). Xenobiotics of widely diverse chemical structure have estrogenic properties. This diversity makes it difficult to predict the estrogenicity of xenobiotics solely on structural bases. To overcome this shortcoming, their identification as estrogens relies on rodent bioassays. However, these assays measure either vaginal cornification or the increase of uterine weight; the latter is not a specific estrogen response (Clark et al., 1980). In addition, these assays are costly and time-consuming. The lack of accurate, sensitive, discriminatory, and easy to perform bioassays to identify estrogens hinders efforts to prevent the release of estrogenic xenobiotics into the environment; for example, estrogenic effects of DDT and chlordecone (kepone) were reported long after these compounds were released for use as pesticides (Kupfer, 1975; Bulger et al., 1978; Palmiter and Mulvihill, 1978; Hammond et al., 1979; Guzelian, 1982). In addition to these synthetic compounds, natural substances produced by fungi and plants have also been reported to cause reproductive impairment in farm animals (Shutt, 1976; Stangroom and Smith, 1984); the suspected estrogenicity of these compounds has not yet been documented in humans. Moreover, with the exception of DDT, the impact of these or other estrogenic xenobiotics in the food chain has not received adequate attention. The evidence of reproductive impairment and altered sexual development gathered from wildlife monitoring programs presented at this meeting indicates the need for further study of these issues, and probably a change in public policy restricting the use of chemicals strongly suspected to cause these detrimental health effects.

The proliferative effect of natural estrogens on the female genital tract is considered the hallmark of estrogen action; Hertz (1985) proposed that this property should be adopted to determine whether or not a substance is an estrogen. This requires measuring the increase of mitotic activity in tissues of the rodent female genital tract after estrogen administration. Although reliable, this method is not suitable for large scale screening of suspected chemicals. Here, we propose instead the use of an easily performed, biologically equivalent assay, based on the estrogen-induced proliferation of human breast MCF7 cells. The estrogen sensitivity of this MCF7 cell line is demonstrated by its estrogen dependency to grow as a palpable tumor in athymic mice (Soule and McGrath, 1980; Soto and Sonnenschein, 1985).

Extensive studies done on estrogen control of cell proliferation served as background to develop the bioassay described herein. Human estrogen-sensitive cell lines are inhibited from proliferating when exposed to medium supplemented with charcoal-dextran stripped human serum (CDHuS) (Soto and Sonnenschein, 1984; Soto and Sonnenschein, 1985; Sonnenschein et al., 1985) or bovine serum (Darbre et al., 1983; Berthois et al., 1986). While the effect of bovine serum may vary from batch to batch (Darbre et al., 1983), CDHuS supplemented medium consistently inhibited the proliferation of these cells. Only natural and synthetic estrogens release this inhibition and induce maximal cell proliferation. In this report, we describe this reliable bioassay and propose its use for the detection of estrogenic xenobiotics prior to their release into the environment, as well as for their detection in feeds, foods and plastics.

## MATERIAL AND METHODS

*Cell Line and Cell Culture Conditions*
Human breast cancer estrogen-sensitive MCF7 cells were obtained from the Michigan Cancer Foundation, Detroit, MI (Soule et al., 1973). For routine maintenance, cells were grown in Dulbecco's modification of Eagle's Medium (DME) (GIBCo, Grand Island, NY) supplemented with 5% fetal bovine serum (FBS) (Hyclone, Logan, Utah) in an atmosphere of 5% $CO_2$/95% air under saturating humidity at 37°C. Other bona-fide estrogen-sensitive cell lines may be used (i.e., human breast cancer cells T47D and ZR75; rat pituitary cell lines $GH_3$ and 9RAP); however, MCF7 cells are recommended for their reproducible and stable estrogen-sensitivity.

*Serum Collection*
Venous blood was obtained from healthy adult volunteers. Blood was drawn by venipuncture, and allowed to clot in glass centrifuge tubes for 2-4 hours to obtain serum. Serum was clarified by centrifugation (3000 rpm x 10 min), aliquoted and stored in glass tubes at -20 °C. Serum was then heat-inactivated (56 °C for 30 minutes), centrifuged and stored at -20 °C until use. In addition, charcoal-dextran stripped mammalian (horse, fetal bovine, etc.) sera (Soto and Sonnenschein, 1984) may be used as well; it should be noted, however, that the inhibitory effect of these sera may vary from batch to batch (Darbre et al., 1983).

*Removal of Sex Steroids by Charcoal-Dextran Treatment of Serum*
Charcoal (Norit A, acid washed, Sigma Chemical Co, St. Louis, MO) was washed twice with cold sterile water immediately before using. A 0.5% charcoal -0.05% dextran T70 (Pharmacia-LKB, Upsala, Sweden) suspension was prepared. Charcoal-dextran suspension aliquots of a volume similar to the serum aliquots to be processed were centrifuged at 2,500 rpm for 10 min. Supernatants were aspirated and serum aliquots were mixed with the charcoal pellets. This charcoal-serum mixture was maintained in suspension by rolling at 4 cycles/min at 37°C for 1 hour. This suspension was centrifuged at 2,500 rpm for 20 min. The supernatant was then filtered through a 0.45 µm Nalgene filter. Over 99% of

serum sex steroids were removed by this treatment (Soto and Sonnenschein, 1985). CD sera were stored at -20 °C until needed; samples kept for one year in the freezer maintained their inhibitory properties on the proliferation of human estrogen-sensitive breast tumor MCF7 cells. Ten percent CDHuS was used to supplement the culture media for these assays.

### Cell Proliferation Experiments in Culture

Cloned MCF7 cells were trypsinized and plated into 12-well plates (Costar, Cambridge, MA) at initial concentrations of approximately $10^4$ cells per well (Soto and Sonnenschein, 1985). Cells were allowed to attach for 24 hours; then, the seeding medium (5% FBS in DME) was removed and replaced by the experimental medium (10% heat-inactivated human serum rendered estrogenless by charcoal dextran treatment supplemented to phenol red-free DME). To this medium, a range of concentrations of the test compound was added. The bioassay was terminated on the 6th day (late exponential phase) by removing the media from the wells, adding a cell lysing solution [10% ethylhexadecyl-dimethylammonium bromide (Eastman Kodak Co., Rochester, NY) in 0.5% Triton X100, 2 mM $MgCl_2$, 15 mM NaCl, 5 mM phosphate buffer pH 7.4] and counting the nuclei in a Coulter Counter Apparatus, Model $Zf_i$ (Coulter Electronics, Hialeah, FL).

### Steroids and Xenobiotics Tested

Estradiol-17β ($E_2$) was obtained from Calbiochem, Richmond, CA. Zearalenol, zearalenone, coumestrol and p,p'-DDT were obtained from Sigma Chemical Co., St. Louis, MO. Arochlor 1221, chlordane, α-chlordane, 1-hydroxy-chlordene, chlordecone (kepone), heptachlor, mirex, and o,p'-DDD were obtained from the United States Environmental Protection Agency Pesticides and Industrial Chemicals Repository Program. Alkylphenols were obtained from Aldrich Chemical Co, Milwaukee, WI, and technical grade nonylphenol was obtained from Fluka Chemical Co, Ronkonkoma, NY. All steroids and xenobiotics were stored as a $3 \times 10^{-3}$ M and $3 \times 10^{-2}$ M respectively in ethanol stock solutions at -20 °C, except for chlordane and its α isomer that were kept in dimethylsulfoxide (DMSO); they were all diluted to desired concentrations with DME immediately before using. The final solvent concentration in culture media did not exceed 0.1%.

### Crude Substances Tested

Rat chow was from Agway Prolab (formula R-M-H 3200 meal). Soybean drink premixture (China National Cereals, Oils and Foodstuffs I/E Corp., Wuzhou, Guangxi, China) and sweet rice (Koda Farms, Inc., So. Dos Palos, CA) were purchased from a local grocery store. Sewage pellets were obtained at a Massachusetts Horticulture Society show. These substances were homogenized and extracted with 10 mM sodium acetate (pH 5.2, 4 ml/3 g); these extracts were then treated with 4,000 units β-glucuronidase per ml (EC 3.2.1.31) (Sigma Chemical Co., St. Louis, MO) for 16 hours at 37°C to cleave conjugates. The extracts were centrifuged for 15 minutes at 3,000 rpm. Next, the supernatant was

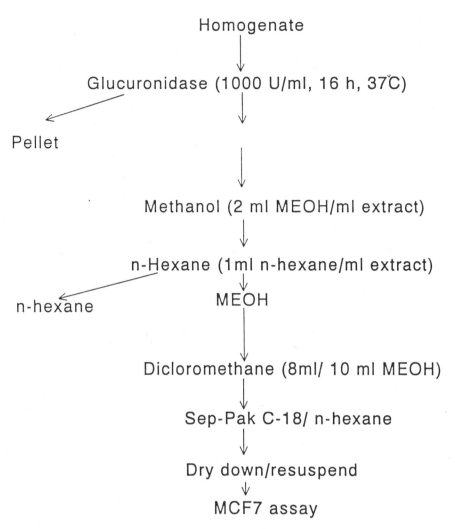

**FIGURE 1.** Xenobiotic Extraction

extracted with methanol (2 ml methanol/ml of extract); these methanolic extracts were toxic for MCF7 cells. The following clean-up procedure significantly decreased the toxicity of the extracted material while removing lipids. Each methanol extract was mixed with equal volume of n-hexane; the n-hexane phase was discarded. Next, xenobiotics in 10 ml of the methanol phase were extracted with 8 ml dichloromethane; the dichloromethane phase was passed through Sep-Pak C-18 cartridges (Waters Assoc., Milford, MA) to clean up the sample. Xenobiotics were eluted through these cartridges with 2 ml of n-hexane; eluates were dried down and resuspended in 10% CDHuS (Figure 1). They were sterilized by filtering through 0.45 μm Millex filters (Millipore Co., Bedford, MA). A 1 ml stock solution was prepared from each gram of crude substance. The recovery yield of added $^3$H-E$_2$ was $53.38 \pm 4.23\%$.

*Isolation of Estrogenic Contaminants from Polystyrene*
"Modified" (Corning glass Co., catalogue number 25310-15) and "unmodified" (Falcon Plastics, catalogue number 2095) polystyrene tubes were filled with 5 ml methanol and extracted at 37°C for 2 h in a roller apparatus (6 cycles/min). The extract was dried under a nitrogen stream, and the residue was resuspended in 10% CDHuS, made sterile by filtration and added to MCF7 cells as described above. Polystyrene pellets were weighed, transferred to glass tubes, and extracted as described above with 5 ml methanol/g of polystyrene.

## RESULTS

*Experimental Design*
The E-SCREEN assay is based on the following premises: a) a human serum-borne molecule specifically inhibits the proliferation of human estrogen-sensitive cells; and b) estrogens induce cell proliferation by cancelling this inhibitory effect (Soto and Sonnenschein, 1987). Non-estrogenic steroids and growth factors do not abolish the proliferative inhibition by human serum (Soto and Sonnenschein, 1984; 1985; Sonnenschein et al., 1985). In contrast, contradictory reports have been published regarding the effect of growth factors in charcoal-dextran stripped fetal bovine serum supplemented medium (van der Burg et al., 1988; Daly et al., 1990).

The best estimate of the proliferative behavior of a cell population is $t_D$ or doubling time. "$t_D$" is the time interval in which an exponentially growing culture doubles its cell number. Determining $t_D$ requires measuring the cell number at several time intervals during the exponential phase. A less cumbersome alternative to measuring proliferation rates is comparing the cell yield achieved by similar cell inocula harvested simultaneously during the exponential phase of proliferation. The proliferative effect (PE) is measured as the ratio between the highest cell yield obtained with the test chemical and the hormone-free control. Under these experimental conditions, cell yield represents a reliable estimate of the relative proliferation rate achieved by similar inocula exposed to different proliferation regulators; in our experimental design MCF7 cell yields were measured 6 days after $t_0$. However, significant differences between control and estrogen-treated cultures are apparent after 4 days.

The estrogenic activity of xenobiotics was assessed by: a) determining their relative proliferative potency (RPP); this is the ratio between the minimal concentration of $E_2$ needed for maximal cell yield at 6 days and the minimal dose of the test compound to achieve similar effect, and b) measuring their relative proliferative effect (RPE); this is 100 x the ratio between the highest cell yield obtained with the chemical and with $E_2$. The RPE indicates whether or not the compound being tested induces 1) a proliferative response quantitatively similar to the one obtained with $E_2$, that is, a full agonist (RPE=100), or 2) a proliferative yield significantly lower than the one obtained with $E_2$, that is, a partial agonist (Figure 2).

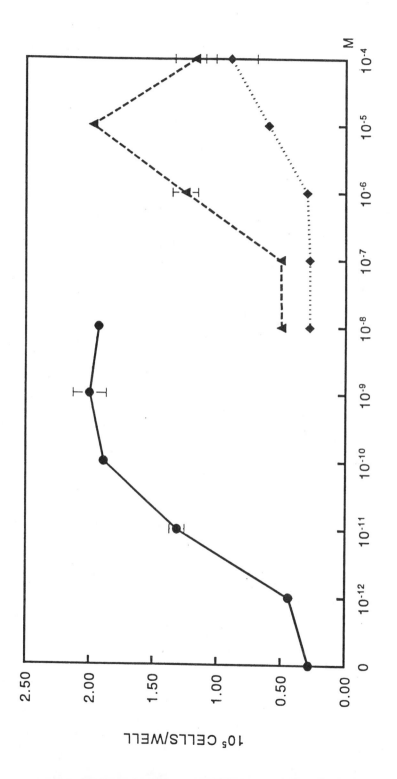

**FIGURE 2.** Effect of estradiol (●——●), 6-Bromonaphthol (◆-----◆) and 4-pentylphenol (▲------▲) on the proliferation of MCF7 cells grown in 10% CDHuS for 6 days. Values are mean ±SD.

**TABLE 1.**   Estrogenic   response   of   MCF7   cells   to insecticides, phytoestrogens   and   phytohormones

| Compound | Concentration* | PE*** | RPE (%) # | RPP (%) ## |
|---|---|---|---|---|
| Estradiol | 30 pM | 6.7 | 100 | 100 |
| Kepone | 30 μM | 5.6 | 81 | 0.0001 |
| Mirex | 30 μM | 0.6 | — | — |
| DDT,p,p' | 30 μM | 5.0 | 70 | 0.0001 |
| DDD,o,p' | 30 μM | 5.8 | 84 | 0.0001 |
| 1-hydroxychlordene | 30 μM** | 3.1 | 37 | 0.0001 |
| Chlordene | 30 μM** | 1.2 | 4 | — |
| Heptachlor | 30 μM** | 1.5 | 8 | — |
| Arochlor 1221 | 30 μM** | 1.4 | 7 | — |
| Giberellic acid | 30 μM** | 1.2 | 4 | — |
| Chlordane | 30 μM** | 1.3 | 5 | — |
| Zearalenone | 3nM | 6.0 | 88 | 1 |
| Zearalenol | 3nM | 6.3 | 93 | 1 |
| Coumestrol | 3 μM | 6.3 | 93 | 0.001 |

*       indicates the lowest concentration needed for maximal cell yield.
**     indicates the highest concentration tested in culture.
***   proliferative effect is expressed as the ratio between the highest cell yield obtained with the test chemical and the hormone-free control.
#       Relative proliferative effect, is calculated as $100 \times (PE-1)$ of the test compound/(PE-1) of $E_2$. A value of 100 indicates that the compound tested is a full agonist; a value of 0 indicates that the compound lacks estrogenicity at the doses tested, and intermediate values suggest that the xenobiotic is a partial agonist.
##    Relative proliferative potency is the ratio between the dose of $E_2$ and that of the xenobiotic needed to produce maximal cell yields x 100.

*Proliferative Effect of Xenobiotics Known to be Estrogenic in Animal Models*
$E_2$ induced maximal cell yields at $3 \times 10^{-11}$M. Compounds reported to have estrogenic activity (Meyers et al., 1977; Palmiter and Mulvihill, 1978; Hammond et al., 1979) or suspected to be estrogens because of their molecular structure were tested by the above described assay (Table 1). Among them, the mycotoxins zearalenol and zearalenone have been used as anabolic feed additives for cattle and sheep; they are potent stimulators of MCF7 cell proliferation (RPP=1% of $E_2$)(Table 1). The phytoestrogen coumestrol was effective with an RPP=0.001% of $E_2$, as were the pesticides p,p'-DDT and o,p'-DDD, a main metabolite of DDT (RPP=0.0001%) (Table 1). The pesticide chlordecone (kepone) was as estrogenic as DDT (Table 1). Doisynolic, allenolic and 4-(p-hydroxyphenyl)-2,2,6,6 tetramethyl cyclohexanecarboxylic acids, which are estro-

genic in rodents (Meyers et al., 1977), were also estrogenic in the MCF7 assay (Table 2). In sum, the results in Table 1 strongly indicate the reliability of this in culture assay.

**TABLE 2.** **Response of MCF7 cells to natural and synthetic estrogens**

| Compound | Concentration* | PE*** | RPE (%) # | RPP (%) ## |
|---|---|---|---|---|
| Estradiol | 100 pM | 4.7 | 100 | 100 |
| Diethylstilbestrol | 10pM | 5.1 | 112 | 1,000 |
| 11β-Chloromethyl-estradiol | 10pM | 5.1 | 110 | 1,000 |
| Dehydrodoisynolic acid | 10nM | 4.8 | 103 | 1 |
| Dichloro-doisynolic acid | 100nM | 4.6 | 97 | 0.1 |
| Allenolic acid | 10nM | 4.9 | 105 | 1 |
| Hydroxyphenyl-cyclohexanoic acid | 10nM | 4.9 | 105 | 1 |

*     indicates the lowest concentration needed for maximal cell yield.
**    indicates the highest concentration tested in culture.
***   proliferative effect is expressed as the ratio between the highest cell yield obtained with the test chemical and the hormone-free control.
#      Relative proliferative effect, is calculated as 100 x (PE-1) of the test compound/(PE-1) of $E_2$. A value of 100 indicates that the compound tested is a full agonist; a value of 0 indicates that the compound lacks estrogenicity at the doses tested, and intermediate values suggest that the xenobiotic is a partial agonist.
##    Relative proliferative potency is the ratio between the dose of $E_2$ and that of the xenobiotic needed to produce maximal cell yields x 100.

*Estrogenic Effect of Xenobiotics not Previously Known to be Estrogenic*
Submaximal estrogenic activity by 1-hydroxychlordene (RPE=37) was obtained at $3 \times 10^{-5}$ M (Table 1); higher concentrations were cytotoxic as defined by the presence of vacuoli, shrivelling and floating cells. This pesticide was previously unknown to be estrogenic. Other pesticide derivatives (such as chlordane α isomer, chlordane, heptachlor and mirex), a phytohormone (gibberellic acid) and polychlorobiphenyls (arochlor 1221 and 4,4'-dichlorobenzaphenone) had no estrogenic activity (Table 1).

*Proliferative Effect of Xenobiotics Shed from Polystyrene Tubes*
Charcoal-dextran stripped human serum stored in "modified" polystyrene tubes (Corning Glass Co., Cat.No. 25310-15) failed to inhibit the proliferation of MCF7 cells, while storage in glass or polystyrene tubes (Falcon Plastics, Cat. No. 2095) preserved the inhibitory activity. Methanol extracts obtained from "modified" polystyrene tubes induced the proliferation of MCF7 cells. After pu-

rification by flash chromatography and reverse phase HPLC, the estrogenic compound was identified by gas chromatography-mass spectrometry as a p-nonylphenol isomer. This nonylphenol was a full estrogen for MCF7 cells (RPE=100; RPP=0.0003 %, Table 3). Nonylphenol also increased the mitotic index of the endometrial epithelium in adult ovariectomized rats. As expected from a genuine estrogen, it also induced progesterone receptor in MCF7 cells (Soto et al., 1991).

**TABLE 3.   Estrogenic effect of alkylphenols in the MCF7 cell model**

| Compound | Concentration* | PE*** | RPE(%) # | RPP (%) ## | $^3$H-E$_2$ displacement + |
|---|---|---|---|---|---|
| Estradiol | 30pM | 6.8 | 100 | 100 | 100 |
| Phenol | 10 µM** | 1.0 | 0 | — | 0 |
| 4-ethylphenol | 10 µM** | 1.3 | 5 | — | — |
| 4-propylphenol | 10 µM | 2.0 | 17 | — | — |
| 4-sec-Butylphenol | 10 µM | 5.4 | 76 | 0.0003 | 50 |
| 4-tert-Butylphenol | 10 µM | 5.1 | 71 | 0.0003 | — |
| 4-tert-pentylphenol | 10 µM | 7.1 | 105 | 0.0003 | 65 |
| 4-isopentylphenol | 10 µM | 6.4 | 93 | 0.0003 | 100 |
| 4-butoxyphenol | 10 µM** | 0.7 | 0 | — | — |
| 4-hexyloxyphenol | 10 µM** | 1.0 | 0 | — | — |
| 4-hydroxybyphenyl | 10 µM | 6.0 | 87 | — | — |
| 4,4'dihydroxy-biphenyl | 10 µM | 5.9 | 84 | 0.0003 | 100 |
| 1-naphthol | 10 µM** | 1.0 | 0 | — | 90 |
| 2-naphthol | 10 µM** | 1.0 | 0 | — | 105 |
| 5,6,7,8,tetrahydro-naphthol-2 | 10 µM** | 1.0 | 0 | — | 100 |
| 6-bromo-naphthol-2 | 10 µM | 3.2 | 38 | — | 90 |
| 4-nonylphenol | 10 µM | 6.8 | 100 | 0.001 | — |

| * | indicates the lowest concentration needed for maximal cell yield. |
|---|---|
| ** | indicates the highest concentration tested in culture. |
| *** | proliferative effect is expressed as the ratio between the highest cell yield obtained with the test chemical and the hormone-free control. |
| # | Relative proliferative effect, is calculated as 100 x (PE-1) of the test compound/(PE-1) of E$_2$. A value of 100 indicates that the compound tested is a full agonist; a value of 0 indicates that the compound lacks estrogenicity at the doses tested, and intermediate values suggest that the xenobiotic is a partial agonist. |
| ## | Relative proliferative potency is the ratio between the dose of E$_2$ and that of the xenobiotic needed to produce maximal cell yields x 100. |
| + | indicates % activity; 100% is the activity observed with 50 µg/ml of tetrahydronaphthol. These data were taken from Mueller and Kim (1978). |

*Proliferative Effect of Other Alkylphenols*

The estrogenicity of alkylphenols was unexpected. p-nonylphenol is as potent an estrogen as kepone and DDD, and it mimics both the proliferative and inductive properties of natural estrogens. Some of these compounds had been shown to displace $^3$H-E$_2$ bound to the estrogen receptor (Mueller and Kim, 1978); however, their interaction with estrogen receptors was interpreted to be at sites different from that of the estrogen-binding. Pentylphenols were reported to induce estrogenic response in rats (Dodds and Lawson, 1938). Table 3 compares the proliferative potency of these compounds with their ability to displace $^3$H-E$_2$ from the receptor; receptor data are taken from Mueller and Kim. These data suggest that the ability to displace $^3$H-E$_2$ from the estrogen receptor is not a reliable indicator of estrogenicity. In addition, these data revealed that to evoke an estrogenic response from an alkylphenol the following conditions need to be fulfilled: a) the alkyl chain must have at least 3 carbons, b) the backbone of the alkylchain must be formed by C-C bonds; C-O bonds destroy the estrogenic activity, c) fused rings containing a phenol are inactive in spite of their ability to displace $^3$H-E$_2$ from the estrophilin binding site and their being an integral part of the A and B rings of natural estrogens. In contrast to the lack of activity of naphthols, certain fused ring derivatives such as 6-bromo 2-naphthol and allenolic acid are active. It is not clear whether these substitutions render fused rings estrogenic due to a "bulk" effect or because of their electronegativity. In addition, polyalkylated phenols like Irganox 1640 (Ciba-Geigy) and butylated hydroxytoluene are not estrogenic, although they are powerful antioxidants (not shown).

*Proliferative Effect of Crude Food/Feed Extracts*

Once this assay was proven to detect estrogenic xenobiotics reliably, an extraction method was devised to test for the presence of estrogenic activity in feeds and foods. Of the items tested so far only a rat chow and a soybean drink were estrogenic in this bioassay. Estrogenic activity in these extracts was detected at concentrations corresponding to 31 mg of starting material/ml of culture medium. Estrogens were also present in sewage pellets used as fertilizers (Table 4).

## DISCUSSION

Assays currently used to detect estrogenic compounds rely either on the molecular identification of the compound or on the detection of estrogenic activity by means of a bioassay. On the one hand, gas chromatography-mass spectrometry (GC-MS) methods are useful to assess the presence and concentration of specific xenobiotics previously known to be estrogenic. GC-MS is indeed the choice method when screening for banned chemicals, like DES, DDT and kepone (Covey et al., 1988). On the other hand, bioassays are choice methods when 1) assessing whether or not a purified chemical is estrogenic, and 2) when trying to identify the cause of a suspected estrogen contamination. Animal bioassays using chicken, rat or mouse are costly and

**TABLE 4.**  **Estrogenic effect of extracts obtained from sewage pellets, foods and feeds**

| Extract dilutions* | Cell number x $10^3$ | | | | 10% CDHuS | |
|---|---|---|---|---|---|---|
| | 1:8 | 1:16 | 1:32 | 1:64 | $-E_2$ | $+E_2$ |
| Sewage pellets | 271±8 | 505±7 | 620±12 | 707±6 | 170±2 | 726±8 |
| Soybean drink | 385±4 | 729±2 | 865±13 | ND | 110±2 | 946±36 |
| Rat chow | 900±5 | 898±5 | 922±2 | ND | 110±2 | 946±36 |

* Serial dilutions were made from a stock solution prepared from 1g of starting material/ml of 10% CDHuS. ND: not determined.

laborious techniques which may not predict human toxicity reliably. It has been documented that estrogen-like molecules may behave differently in different species (Martin, 1980). The most widely used rodent bioassay measures the increase of uterine wet weight; this is only a crude estimate of estrogen action because it represents the combination of three separate effects, namely, water imbibition, hypertrophy, which is also produced by estrogen antagonists, and hyperplasia (Clark et al., 1980).

To obviate problems inherent to animal testing, bioassays using cells in culture are being developed. For example, the induction of prolactin in primary sheep pituitary cell culture has been proposed as a measure of estrogen action (Lieberman et al., 1978). In this model, estrogens induce protein synthesis but are ineffective at inducing cell proliferation. The limitations of this assay are that results obtained may not be applicable to human toxicology, and that most of the estrogen-inducible proteins could also be induced by non-estrogenic substances. For example, prolactin synthesis could also be induced by epidermal growth factor, thyrotropin releasing factor, and phorbol esters (Ramsdell and Tashjian, 1985). Another estrogen inducible marker, ovalbumin synthesis, is also stimulated by other steroids such as progesterone and glucocorticoids (Palmiter, 1975).

The human bioassay described in this paper has several advantages over those currently used. They are: 1) Results obtained with this method may be applied reliably to predict estrogenic effects on human health because target cells and serum are of human origin. 2) This assay is highly sensitive to detect $3 \times 10^{-11}$M $E_2$ or comparable estrogen activity. And 3) this assay is easy to perform and it allows the screening of multiple compounds in a wide range of doses. The E-SCREEN assay is specific; all of the tested compounds which are known to elicit estrogenic effects in the live animal were estrogenic in our "in culture" bioassay. PCBs were not active in this bioassay; it has been claimed that these compounds become estrogenic upon metabolic activation in liver (Metzler, 1985; Blaich et al., 1987). It follows that incubation of PCBs with liver microsomes will generate estrogenic compounds that can then be detected by the E-SCREEN assay.

Thus far, we have not obtained false positive results. In addition, this assay was instrumental in identifying an estrogenic xenobiotic, p-nonylphenol, present in modified polystyrene; its estrogenicity was confirmed in the rat uterus (Soto et al., 1991). This finding led us to explore the structure-activity relationship of a series of alkylphenols and naphthols. The following pattern emerged from these studies: a) the alkyl chain must at least have three carbons, b) only the p-isomers of alkylphenols are estrogenic (Soto et al., 1991), c) fused rings such as 2-naphthol and 2-tetrahydronaphthol are inactive, d) fused ring derivatives such as 6-Br-2 naphthol and allenolic acid are active; it is uncertain whether activity is due to a "bulk" effect or to electronegativity, and e) polyalkylated phenols are inactive.

In summary, the E-SCREEN assay is suited for the screening of xenobiotics before they are released into the environment. Also, it detects estrogenic activity in animal feeds, human foods, water and soil. It is anticipated that upon development of a method to selectively extract steroidal estrogens, the E-SCREEN assay may also be used to detect the presence of estrogenic xenobiotics in biological fluids and tissues.

## ACKNOWLEDGEMENTS

We wish to thank Drs. M.F. Olea-Serrano and N. Olea for their helpful advice. This work was supported by grants E.P.A. CR813481, NIH-CA13410, NSF-DCB 8711746 and NSF-DCB 9105594.

## REFERENCES

Berthois, Y., Katzenellenbogen, J.A., and Katzenellenbogen, B.S. (1986). Phenol red in tissue culture media is a weak estrogen: implications concerning the study of estrogen-responsive cells in culture. *Proc. Natl. Acad. Sci. USA*, **83**, 2496-2500.

Blaich, G., Pfaff, E., and Metzler, M. (1987). Metabolism of diethystilbestrol in hamster hepatocytes. *Biochem. Pharmacol.*, **36**, 3135-3140.

Bulger, W.H., Mucitelli, R.M., and Kupfer, D. (1978). Studies on the *in vivo* and *in vitro* estrogenic activities of methoxychlor and its metabolites. Role of hepatic mono-oxygenase in methoxychlor activation. *Biochem. Pharmacol.*, **27**, 2417-2423.

Clark, J.H., Watson, C., Upchurch, S., McCormack, S., Padykula, H., Markaverich, B., and Hardin, J.W. (1980). Estrogen action in normal and abnormal cell growth. In *Estrogens in the Environment*, ed. J.A. McLachlan. Elsevier/North-Holland, New York/Amsterdam/Oxford, pp. 53-67.

Covey, T.R., Silvestre, D., Hoffman, M.K., and Henion, J.D. (1988). A gas chromatographic/mass spectrometric screening, confirmation, and quantification method for estrogenic compounds. *Biomed. Environ. Mass. Spectrom.*, **12**, 274-287.

Daly, R.J., King, R.J.B., and Darbre, P.A. (1990). Interaction of growth factors during progression towards steroid independence in T47D human breast cancer cells. *J. Cell Biochem.*, **43**, 199-211.

Darbre, P.A., Yates, J., Curtis, S., and King, R.J.B. (1983). Effect of estradiol on human breast cancer cells in culture. *Cancer Research* , **43**, 349-354.

Dodds, E.C. and Lawson, W. (1938). Molecular structure in relation to oestrogenic activity. Compounds without a phenanthrene nucleus. *Proc. Roy. Soc. B*, **125**, 222-232.

Guzelian, P.S. (1982). Comparative toxicology of chlordecone (kepone) in humans and experimental animals. *Annu. Rev. Pharmacol. Toxicol.*, **22**, 89-113.

Hammond, B., Katzenellenbogen, B.S., Kranthammer, N., and McConnell, J. (1979). Estrogenic activity of the insecticide chlordecone (kepone) and interaction with uterine estrogen receptors. *Proc. Natl. Acad. Sci., USA*, **76**, 6641-6645.

Hertz, R. (1985). The estrogen problem--retrospect and prospect. In *Estrogens in the Environment II- Influences on Development*, ed. J.A. McLachlan. Elsevier, New York/Amsterdam/Oxford, pp. 1-11.

Kupfer, D. (1975). Effects of pesticides and related compounds on steroid metabolism and function. *CRC Crit. Rev. Toxicol.*, **4**, 83-124.

Lieberman, M.E., Maurer, R.A., and Gorski, J. (1978). Estrogen control of prolactin synthesis *in vitro*. *Proc. Natl. Acad. Sci. USA*, **75**, 5946-5949.

Martin, L. (1980). Estrogens, anti-estrogens and the regulation of cell proliferation in the female reproductive track *in vivo*. In *Estrogens in the Environment*, ed. J.A. McLachlan. Elsevier/North-Holland, New York/Amsterdam/Oxford, pp. 103-130.

Metzler, M. (1985). Role of metabolism in determination of hormonal activity of estrogens: introductory remarks. In *Estrogens in the Environment II- Influences on Development* ed. J.A. McLachlan. Elsevier, New York/Amsterdam/Oxford, pp. 187-189.

Meyers, C.Y., Matthews, W.S., Ho, L.L., Kolb, V.M., and Parady, T.E. (1977). Carboxylic acid formation from kepone. In *Catalysis in Organic Synthesis*, ed. G.W. Smith. Academic Press, New York, pp. 213-215, 253-255.

Mueller, G. and Kim, U.H. (1978). Displacement of estradiol from estrogen receptors by simple alkylphenols. *Endocrinology*, **102**:1429-1435.

Palmiter, R.D. (1975). Quantitation of parameters that determine the rate of ovalbumin synthesis. *Cell*, **4**, 189-197.

Palmiter, R.D. and Mulvihill, E.R. (1978). Estrogenic activity of the insecticide kepone on the chicken oviduct. *Science*, **201**, 356-358.

Ramsdell, J.S. and Tashjian, A.H. (1985). Thyrotropin-releasing hormone and epidermal growth factor stimulate prolactin synthesis by a pathway(s) that differs from that used by phorbol esters: dissociation of actions by calcium dependency and additivity. *Endocrinology*, **117**, 2050-2060.

Shutt, D.A. (1976). The effects of plant estrogens on animal reproduction. *Endeavour*, **35**, 110-113.

Soto, A.M. and Sonnenschein, C. (1984). Mechanism of estrogen action on cellular proliferation: evidence for indirect and negative control on cloned breast tumor cells. *Biochem. Biophys. Res. Commun.*, **122**, 1097-1103.

Sonnenschein, C., Papendorp, J.T. and Soto, A.M. (1985). Estrogenic effect of tamoxifen and its derivatives on the proliferation of MCF7 human breast tumor cells. *Life Sciences*, **37**, 387-394.

Soto, A.M. and Sonnenschein, C. (1985). The role of estrogens on the proliferation of human breast tumor cells (MCF-7). *J. Steroid Biochem.*, **23**, 87-94.

Soto, A.M. and Sonnenschein, C. (1987). Cell proliferation of estrogen-sensitive cells: the case for negative control. *Endocrine Reviews*, **8**, 44-52.

Soto, A.M., Justicia, H., Wray, J.W., and Sonnenschein, C. (1991). p-nonylphenol: An estrogenic xenobiotic released from "modified" polystyrene. *Environm. Health Perspectives*, **92**, 167-173.

Soule, H.D., Vazquez, J., Long, A., Albert, S., and Brennan, M.J. (1973). A human cell line from a pleural effusion derived from a breast carcinoma. *J. Natl. Cancer Inst.*, **51**, 1409-1413.

Soule, H.D. and McGrath, C.M. (1980). Estrogen responsive proliferation of clonal human breast carcinoma cells in athymic mice. *Cancer Lett.*, **10**,177-189.

Stangroom, K.E. and Smith, T.K. (1984). Effect of whole and fractionated alfalfa meal on zearalenone toxicosis and metabolism in rat and swine. *Can. J. Physiol. Pharmacol.*, **62**, 1219-1224.

van der Burg, B., Rutteman, G.R., Bloukenstein, M.A., de Laat, S.W., and van Zoelen, E.J.J. (1988). Mitogenic stimulation of human breast cancer cells in a growth factor-defined medium: synergestic action of insulin and estrogen. *J. Cell Physiol.*, **134**, 101-108.

# CHEMICAL REVOLUTION TO SEXUAL REVOLUTION: HISTORICAL CHANGES IN HUMAN REPRODUCTIVE DEVELOPMENT

### Patricia L. Whitten
Laboratory of Reproductive Ecology and Environmental Toxicology,
Department of Anthropology, Emory University, Atlanta, Georgia

*The chemical revolution has left a legacy of environmental pollutants with steroidal activity. The well-documented role of steroids in the sexual differentiation of the reproductive tract and central nervous system raises the possibility that these chemicals might be influencing human sexual development. This paper tests this possibility by examining the history of some developmental parameters in the aftermath of the chemical and dietary revolutions that have occurred over the past century. Demographic data and historical trends in sexual behavior are examined in light of data on sexual differentiation in rodents and primates. This comparison demonstrates that DZ twinning rates and age of menarche change in a coordinated fashion over the last century with a periodicity of 25-50 years. These trends coincide with changes in diet and chemical production, and suggest that some fundamental shifts in human reproductive development have occurred.*

## INTRODUCTION

Periodically, our gonads secrete a tiny pulse of steroids into the bloodstream. Within minutes, these small, cholesterol-derived hormones have entered target tissues and initiated the enzymatic events that govern our reproductive function, physical appearance, and even our behavior. Sex steroids produce these effects, in large part, by binding to regulatory proteins, called receptors, within the nuclei of steroid-responsive cells. Once bound by steroid, the receptor undergoes a change in physical structure that allows it, in turn, to bind to regulatory sequences on the chromosomes, initiating gene transcription and translation. This function endows sex steroids with the ability not only to activate a wide range of physiological events in adult life, but also to irreversibly organize tissue-specific functions in development.

Sexual differentiation in mammals appears to be controlled by a fairly simple genetic switch. A single gene, now thought to be SRY (McLaren, 1990), on the Y chromosome induces the differentiation of the gonads and secretion of the testicular hormones, Mullerian inhibiting substance and testosterone (Wilson et al., 1981). These hormones induce a cascade of developmental events in the reproductive tract and central nervous system that culminates in the male

1. Corresponding Author: Patricia L. Whitten, Laboratory of Reproductive Ecology and Environmental Toxicology, Department of Anthropology, Emory University, Atlanta, GA 30322.

phenotype (Jost and Magre, 1984). In the absence of a testes, the female phenotype develops. Thus the basic mammalian developmental program appears to be female. Although this view of development has been challenged in the brain, where steroids may also play a role in inducing the female phenotype (Dohler et al., 1984), there is no doubt that testicular secretions are potent masculinizing factors. Consequently, exogenous substances that resemble androgens or their estrogen metabolites can themselves alter sexual development.

The wide-ranging effects of sex steroids make reproductive function particularly vulnerable to disruption by environmental substances (McLachlan and Newbold, 1987). Many organic chemicals, both natural and synthetic, resemble steroids in structure, enabling them to bind to steroid receptors or steroid metabolizing enzymes, thereby altering steroid action (McLachlan, 1985). The deleterious effects of these chemicals on wildlife became widely known with the publication of Rachel Carson's *Silent Spring* in 1962, but their implications for human health did not come to public attention until the late 1970s when the Love Canal scandal made cleanup of toxic dump sites a national priority (Brown, 1981). The carcinogenic and neurological effects of environmental toxins were the most immediately obvious consequences of human exposure, but there are more subtle and potentially far more devastating consequences of exposure. Because of the important developmental roles of steroids, xenobiotics with steroidal action can disrupt a variety of developmental processes, particularly those related to the sexual differentiation of the reproductive tract and central nervous system (McLachlan, 1985; Whitten and Naftolin, in press).

These developmental effects have raised concern about the steadily increasing concentration of organic chemicals in our environment. If many of these chemicals can drastically alter sexual differentiation, what are the likely consequences of exposure for human development? We can attempt to generate some predictions based on experimental studies of development in animal models, on the responses of wildlife to environmental pollutants, and on clinical studies of humans exposed inadvertently to these chemicals. These investigations are described in the rest of this volume. Here I describe an additional source of information, one gained by examining historical patterns of human sexual development to determine if any relationships can be discerned to historical changes in exposure to organic chemicals.

## DEVELOPMENTAL TOXICANTS

*The Chemical Revolution And Environmental Pollutants*
Over the last century, human populations have been increasingly exposed to organic chemicals. In the latter part of the eighteenth century, the Industrial Revolution created a demand for chemical products and the means to produce them in mass quantities (Taylor and Sudnick, 1984). Beginning in the nineteenth century with the production of aromatic chemicals tied to the textile industry (Aftalion, 1991), the chemical industry grew into a multi-billion dollar enterprise produc-

ing hundreds of millions of tons of organic chemicals per year (Caplan, 1990). One of the earliest technological developments that may have produced organic pollutants on a large scale was the introduction of gas lamps at the turn of the nineteenth century. From 1800-1880, coal distillation was used to generate gas for street lamps, leaving a tarry residue of aromatic chemicals (Aftalion, 1991). Because estrogen also has an aromatic ring, many aromatic substances exhibit estrogenic properties. The production of these chemicals was reduced after 1880 when the use of higher gasification reduced coal tar production. Another potential source of pollutants was the synthesis of phenolic chemicals as dyes and their use in the textile industry beginning in the 1850s (Taylor and Sudnik, 1984). Coal tar residues fostered the development of dye production initially, and dye manufacturers later turned to steelworks for sources of aromatics (Aftalion, 1991). Although France and Britain were early leaders in this area, Germany accomplished a rapid growth in dye production after 1885 and had captured most of the world market by the turn of the century (Taylor and Sudnik, 1984). Meanwhile, chemical production in the US centered on the development of fertilizers and nitrate explosives, and the explosive industry received a major impetus from the First World War (Taylor and Sudnik, 1984). These developments stimulated marked increases in the production of phenolic chemicals that may have produced new sources of developmental toxicants.

The burgeoning chemical industry fostered a "chemical revolution" characterized by increasing industrial dependence on chemicals and a steady rise in the production of organic chemicals (Brown, 1981; Worldwatch Institute, 1988). Over the past four decades, the production and use of organic chemicals has risen more than ten-fold (Worldwatch Institute,1988). The environmental burdens of this century include industrial by-products such as the PCBs and dioxin (Smith et al., 1990) and, beginning in World War II, potent chemical insecticides such as DDT (Dunlap, 1981). While this chemical revolution has transformed our daily lives, it has left a legacy of environmental pollutants that endanger animal and human development.

*Natural Sources Of Developmental Toxicants*
There also are a number of natural products with steroid-like action. Some phenolic plant products exhibit estrogenic action (Whitten and Naftolin, 1991). The resorcylic acid lactones are reproductive hormones produced by fungi of the genus *Fusarium* and are common contaminants of improperly stored grain known to produce some reproductive disturbances in humans. The isoflavonoids are defensive chemicals produced by legumes that are common in many human food staples. My own research has shown that these chemicals can alter the sexual differentiation of gonadotropin secretion (Whitten and Naftolin, 1991) and sexual behavior (Whitten, 1992) in rodents. In addition, a number of structurally related chemicals, the flavonoids, are inhibitors of steroid biosynthesis (Kellis and Vickery, 1984) and ligands for progestin and glucocorticoid receptors (Whitten and Naftolin, 1991). These latter chemicals are widely distributed in vegetable products and exhibit many enzymatic activities characteristic of

steroids, but their *in vivo* actions are as yet unknown (Whitten and Naftolin, 1991). All of these substances provide a dietary source of hormonally active chemicals with the potential to alter human sexual development (Whitten and Naftolin, in press).

The Industrial Revolution brought with it not only new sources of synthetic chemicals but also major changes in the distribution and lifestyle of human populations. Rapid urbanization was accompanied by increasing inequities in wealth and shifts in food consumption (Fogel, 1986). Adoption of a "Westernized diet," characterized by increased meat consumption and reduced dependence on vegetable protein, has been a major feature of industrial development. (Trowell and Burkitt, 1983). These dietary changes have several known consequences. First, fat and fiber alter the intestinal resorption of estrogen, resulting in higher circulating estrogen levels on a high-fat diet and lower estrogen levels on a high fiber diet (Adlercreutz, 1990). Secondly, reductions in vegetable consumption reduce exposure to isoflavonoids and diminish concentrations of the sex-hormone binding globulin that sequesters endogenous sex steroids (Adlercreutz, 1990). Thus increasing meat, and reducing vegetable consumption would result in higher endogenous estrogen levels that are more available to steroid-responsive tissues while concentrations of less potent, and perhaps estrogen-inhibitory, isoflavonids would decline. Historically, these dietary shifts are associated with increases in the incidence of estrogen-dependent "Western diseases," suggestive of increasing exposure to sex steroids (Trowell and Burkitt, 1983). Although explanations for these trends have focused on the activational effects of estrogens (Adlercreutz, 1990), developmental consequences must also be considered.

*Symptoms Of Exposure To Developmental Toxicants*
Experimental studies of sexual differentiation in rodents and primates and clinical studies of humans suggest some potential consequences of intrauterine exposure to steroid-like substances. Although there are a number of problems in extrapolating the available experimental models to human sexual function, they can be used to make some general predictions about changes in human reproductive development that might ensue from organic chemical exposure. These predictions are compared to available data on historical trends in some aspects of human reproductive function in the United States and other industrialized countries over the last century.

Experimental, field, and clinical investigations, reviewed extensively in other chapters in this volume, indicate that developmental exposure to androgenic or estrogenic substances produces a syndrome of reproductive traits reflecting the disruption of ontogenetic events. In the reproductive tract, this ontogenetic disruption syndrome is characterized by cervico-vaginal cancer, undescended testes, and gonadal lesions and cysts, a consequence of altered differentiation of the Mullerian and Wolffian ducts (Newbold and McLachlan,1985). In the immune system, symptoms include changes in lymphocyte responses and autoimmune disease, a consequence of altered development of the thymus and lymphoidal organs (Blair, 1981; Noller et al., 1988). In the central nervous system, symptoms include changes in the normal sex-linked pattern of cyclic vs. acyclic gonadotropin release and in altered thresholds of responsiveness to gonadal steroid elicitation of sex-typical behaviors, a consequence of changes in neuronal number, synaptic connections, and cell responsiveness (Whitten and Naftolin, in press).

These symptoms provide a set of physiologic and behavioral endpoints that might be useful for assessing exposure of human populations to developmental toxicants. To evaluate the utility of these endpoints for assessing human exposure, we can compare endpoints observed in rodents and wildlife to the available data on the steroidal regulation of reproductive development in humans and nonhuman primates. Consistent endpoints can then be evaluated for their ability to be adapted to population level monitoring systems. For example, cervicovaginal cancer appears to be a predictable endpoint in both rodents and humans of developmental exposure to the synthetic estrogen diethylstilbestrol (DES) (Bern, 1991). The natural plant estrogens, coumestrol and zearalenone, produce similar alterations in reproductive tract morphology (Williams et al., 1989; Burroughs et al., 1990, suggesting that rates of cervicovaginal cancer could provide a useful index of population-wide exposure to environmental estrogens. This endpoint would be of limited utility, however, in non-Westernized populations where medical care and medical records are not widely available. We face a similar problem of reportage in attempting to take an historical view. Data on many of the endpoints that would be useful in clinical settings are simply not available in historical records. In fact, records that might be useful for assessing secular trends, that is, historical changes over a century, are available only for demography and sexual behavior. In the sections that follow I will evaluate the utility of these data for assessing human sexual development and attempt to derive some general conclusions about secular changes in human reproductive function.

## USING DEMOGRAPHIC DATA TO ASSESS THE HYPOTHALAMIC-PITUITARY-GONADAL AXIS

One of the better understood aspects of sexual differentiation in the central nervous system is the development of the secretion of gonadotropins, the pituitary hormones governing gonadal function. Mammalian females are distinguished from males by the ability to periodically exhibit positive feedback regulation of gonadotropin secretion, in which rising estrogen levels stimulate a preovulatory surge of luteinizing hormone (LH). The locus of estrogen action appears to be the arcuate nucleus of the hypothalamus, which generates a periodic signal stimulating the pulsatile secretion of LH-releasing hormone (LHRH) by LHRH neurons into the pituitary portal vessels.

During certain "critical periods" in development, and perhaps throughout life, sex steroids can alter the neuroarchitecture of the hypothalamus to abolish the cyclic reproductive pattern of females and enable the tonic reproductive pattern of males (McLachlan and Newbold, 1987; Naftolin et al., 1990; Whitten and Naftolin, in press). In rodents, estrogens or androgens abolish or reduce female ability to respond to estradiol stimulation with an LH surge; antiestrogens or aromatase inhibitors result in male retention of surge ability (MacLusky and Naftolin, 1981). Unless the doses are high, changes in LH secretion are evident only following a period of exposure to ovarian hormones. Disruption of function is therefore not abrupt but occurs incrementally as basal LH levels rise, and periovulatory LH levels fall, over a prolonged period of time (Gorski, 1968; Lu et al., 1979; Naftolin et al., 1990).

In primates, males appear to retain the ability to respond to estrogen treatment with an LH surge (Karsch et al., 1973; Barbarino et al., 1979). However, gonadotropin secretion in primates does not appear to be entirely immune to the organizational effects of estrogen. Morphologic studies indicate that similar sex differences in neuronal ultrastructure can be seen in rats and primates and that these differences can be induced by estradiol (Naftolin et al., 1990). Moreover, prenatal treatment with the synthetic estrogen diethylstilbestrol (DES) changes gonadotropin responses in immature rhesus monkeys (Fuller et al., 1981), and chronic elevations of serum estradiol abolish positive feedback responses in adult rhesus monkeys (Billiar et al., 1985).

Clinical use of DES to sustain pregnancy between 1945-1971 provides a population of human women exposed to DES *in utero*. The variable doses and times of exposure, combined with the young ages of these women, complicate the interpretation of these data; however, they do indicate a higher rate of menstrual irregularities (Wu et al., 1980), and anovulation (Williamson and Satterfield, 1976) among these women. Testosterone levels are significantly higher in DES-exposed women, and basal LH levels are higher in a subpopulation who exhibit hirsutism and irregular cycles (Peress et al., 1982). All of these changes are indicative of changes in the hypothalamic-pituitary-gonadal axis, suggesting that estrogens may also participate in the organization of human gonadotropin function.

Demographic data provide two types of information potentially useful for evaluating gonadotropin function: 1) birth rates according to zygosity and 2) menarcheal age.

### Dizygotic Twinning

Dizygous, or fraternal twins, result from a double ovulation, an event associated with elevated gonadotropin secretion (Milham, 1964). Stimulation of ovulation with high dose LH or LHRH analogues frequently results in multiple ovulation (Wyshak and White, 1965). Moreover, elevated gonadotropin levels are associated with dizygotic (DZ) twinning in individual women, and populations with very high rates of twinning, such as the Nigerian Ibo, have higher gonadotropin levels than populations with low rates of twinning, such as the Japanese, while both twinning rates and gonadotropin levels are intermediate in European women (Nylander, 1973). These differences among human populations are interesting in light of the data indicating that Japanese women are exposed to much higher dietary levels of isoflavonoids than are European women (Adlercreutz, 1990) and suggest a possible link between developmental exposure to estrogens and reductions in DZ twinning. Further evidence of differences in hormone function is provided by the lower rates of menstrual disorders (Bonnelykke, 1989) among mothers of DZ twins (Wyshak, 1981; Bonnelykke, 1989).

*Menarcheal Age*
Menarche is a human reproductive milestone that, like vaginal opening in the rat, marks the entryway to fertile adult reproductive function. Moreover, we know that the onset of puberty in humans and other mammals is accompanied by a fundamental shift in neuroendocrine function: basal levels of LH begin to rise and secretion becomes more pulsatile, apparently due to maturation of the hypothalamic LHRH releasing system (Boyar et al., 1972; Terasama et al., 1984; Urbanski and Ojeda, 1985). This change may reflect the completion of synaptic connections (Matsumoto and Arai, 1977) of the hypothalamic neurons impinging upon LHRH-secreting neurons, since pulsatile administration of either LH-releasing hormone (LHRH) or an LHRH releaser stimulates precocious puberty in both rodents (Urbanski and Ojeda, 1987) and primates (Wildt et al., 1980; Plant et al., 1987).

Estrogen alters or accelerates these processes in rodents. Perinatal (Gorski, 1968; Hines et al., 1987) or peripubertal (Ramirez and Sawyer, 1965) estrogen hastens vaginal opening and first estrous and accelerates hypothalamic synaptogenesis (Matsumoto and Arai, 1977; 1980). Although androgens also stimulate vaginal opening, they do not alter the time of first ovulation and apparently act through local stimulation of estrogen biosynthesis in the vaginal epithelium (Lephart et al., 1989).

In primates, the picture is less clear. Prenatal androgen treatment delays the onset of menarche if the treatment occurs early enough in development (Goy and Resko, 1972; Goy et al., 1988). A significantly alerted age of menarche has not been reported among DES-exposed women (Wu et al., 1980), but again the lack of effect may be a function of the variable timing and dosage of treatment.

*General Conclusions*
In sum, the rodent models provide some good reasons for interest in gonadotropin function in human populations. The paucity of data on the responses of non-human primates and humans to perinatal exposure to steroid-like compounds make it difficult to generate exact predictions, other than to suggest that some changes in the regulation of gonadotropin secretion may occur. What we know of the physiological basis of DZ twinning and menarcheal age suggest that these data might provide a measure of such changes, if they in fact occur. In the next sections, I demonstrate that there are some clear secular trends in both end-

points and that these trends occur synchronously in a number of populations, suggesting some change in the organization of gonadotropin secretion.

## HISTORICAL TRENDS

### Historical Changes in DZ Twinning

Over the past three decades, DZ twinning rates have declined throughout the world (James, 1972; 1982; see Fig. 1). These changes are confined to DZ twinning (James, 1972; 1982) and cannot be explained by changes in maternal age or parity (James,1975). These trends first became apparent in the late 1950s and, in most countries, continued over the next two decades with an annual decline of 1-2% in age-specific rates, stabilizing by the late 1970s (James, 1986). In the United States, reductions in DZ twinning were first observed earlier, around 1933, and continued to 1959 (Jeanneret and MacMahon, 1962). This decline appears to have ceased in the 1960s, and reverted to an increase in the 1970s (James, 1982).

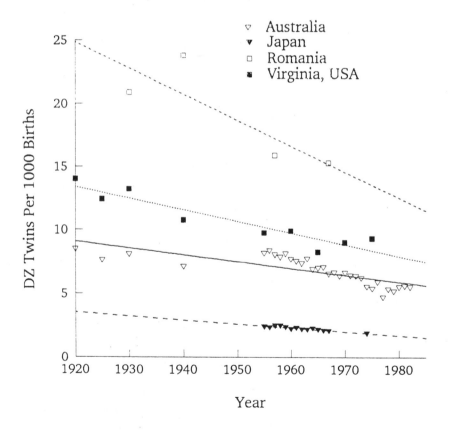

**FIGURE 1.** Historical decline in rates of dizygous twinning. Data from Doherty and Lancaster, 1986; Inouye and Imaizumi, 1981; Mosteller *et al.*, 1981.

In Scandinavia, Italy, and Australia, where longer term data are available, it appears that the decline in DZ twinning was preceded by a gradual elevation between 1910-1953 (Doherty and Lancaster, 1986). In Utah, Morman birth records available from 1815 also indicate two periods of decline: the first from 1860-1880, and the second from 1920-1950, with an elevation in twinning rates between 1880 and 1910 (Carmelli et al., 1980).

Age-specific rates indicate that changes in twinning occurred among women born roughly between 1915-1940 in Western Europe and Australia and 1925-1950 in Eastern Europe. Earlier elevations occur in women born between 1880-1915. In the US, the declines occurred in women born 1805-1830 and 1880-1915 while elevations occurred in women born between 1830-1880. Thus the secular changes in the US parallel the changes observed in Europe but are initiated approximately 25 years earlier.

There is no evidence that these changes are due to increases in spontaneous abortion rates or reductions in coital rate (James, 1982). Although contraceptive use has been proposed as a possible factor in changing ovulation rates (McGillivray, 1979), the onset of the DZ twinning decline (late 1950s) predates the commercial introduction of the birth control pill in the early 1960s, and declines have been substantial in countries where the pill has not been commonly used (James, 1982). The synchrony and ubiquity of these changes suggest that some environmental agent, such as pesticides or stilboestrol, may be responsible (James, 1972; 1982) and provide some support for historical changes in the development of gonadotropin secretion.

*Historical Trends in Menarcheal Age*
Records of menarcheal age have been kept for more than two centuries in many Western countries and indicate that menarcheal age has declined over the past century. (Marshall and Tanner, 1986). Beginning around 1880, menarcheal age declined about 0.3 years per decade in most modern, industrialized countries until the 1960-70s (Tanner, 1973; Marshall and Tanner, 1986). In Oslo, Norway menarcheal age fell from 1860-1880, leveled off until 1920, and thereafter declined steeply until 1960, when it leveled off again (Brudevall et al., 1979). The year of birth is a better predictor of these trends than occupation, marital status, or geographic origin (Rosenberg, 1991). Reductions in menarcheal age were observed among cohorts born 1830-1885 and 1905-1940 (Rosenberg, 1991). A similar but steeper decline occurred over the same period in the Norwegian city of Bergen while in the city of Trondheim, the second period of decline was delayed and occurred in cohorts born between 1925-1940 (Rosenberg, 1991). In Poland, the Netherlands, and Japan, the major secular decline was observed in cohorts born after the Second World War, between 1940-1965 (van Wieringen, 1986). In the United States, menarcheal age declined at a rate of 3.2 months per decade in cohorts born 1910-1940 (Wyshak, 1983; Goodman, 1983).

**TABLE 1.**    **Historical trends in reproductive parameters**

| | USA | | Scandinavia | |
|---|---|---|---|---|
| Age of Birth | DZ Twinning | Menarcheal Age | DZ Twinning | Menarcheal Age |
| 1800-1830 | Declines | Height increases | | |
| 1830-1880 | Increases | Height declines | | Declines |
| 1860-1915 | Declines | Height increases | Increases | Stable |
| 1915-1940 | | Age Declines | Declines | Declines |

*Conclusions*

These data suggest that there are several major periods over which marked shifts in reproductive function occur: 1800-1830; 1830-1880; 1880-1915; 1915-1940 (see Table 1). Reductions in DZ twinning and menarche occur in the same cohorts of women. Periods of decline are separated by hiatuses in the decline in menarcheal age that also tend to be periods in which DZ twinning increases. In Scandinavia, the age of menarche declines in women born between 1830-1880 and 1915-1940. DZ twinning also declines during the latter period and increases in the intervening period when menarcheal age is stable. In the US, the same changes occur but begin earlier. DZ twinning declines in women born between 1800-1830 and 1880-1915. In the US, a hiatus in the decline in DZ twinning occurs in cohorts born from 1830-1880. Data on age of menarche is not available for cohorts born before 1900. However, data on height for US males born in the nineteenth century indicate that the period from 1830-1890 was a period of reversal in the historical trend for greater male height, a developmental parameter associated with earlier puberty (Fogel, 1986).

The conjunction of the observed trends is curious in light of the different causative factors to which they have been attributed. Declining age of menarche has been taken as an index of improved nutrition and public health and accompanying acceleration in growth (Tanner, 1973; Marshall and Tanner, 1986). Norwegian data, in fact, demonstrate a good correlation between gross domestic production in the year of birth and menarcheal age (Liestol, 1982). Declining twinning rates, on the other hand, have been taken as an index of declining fecundity and perhaps toxic exposure (James, 1982). If both are developmental effects, it is necessary to explain how one factor could produce such divergent endpoints. A generalized improvement in nutrition does not easily explain both, nor does broad based toxicity. Only an organizational change in gonadotropin function, like the changes known to be induced by sex steroids in rodents, can readily explain these coordinated changes.

## USING SEXUAL BEHAVIOR TO ASSESS SEXUAL DEVELOPMENT

*Sex Typical and Heterotypical Sexual Behaviors*

Human sexual behavior is another area worth examining since the organization of sexual behavior has been well studied in rodents. Perinatal androgens and estrogens suppress female behavior and enhance male behavior in rodents while antiestrogens and aromatase inhibitors prevent the suppression of female behavior (Baum, 1979). Suppression and enhancement are expressed in altered thresholds of response to gonadal steroids in adulthood.

Primate sexual behavior, however, is less stereotypic and less subject to hormonal control than rodent sexual behavior. Anatomical differences allow primates to copulate in the absence of female assumption of a receptive posture (lordosis); therefore, hormonal regulation of primate sexual behavior is expressed primarily in fluctuations in motivation rather than the presence or absence of behaviors (Wallen, 1990). Consequently, hormonal effects are highly situation-dependent, and thus organizational effects are far more difficult to detect in primates (and humans) than in rodents. The early discovery that nonaromatizable androgens induce masculinization of sexual behavior in nonhuman primates (Goy and Resko, 1972; Eaton et al., 1973) focussed experimental work almost exclusively on the role of androgens in primate development. These studies suggest that androgens defeminize the behavior of genetic females primarily by reducing sexual solicitations (Thornton and Goy, 1986; Pomerantz et al., 1988) and masculinize behavior by increasing mounting behavior in juveniles (Goy et al, 1988; Eaton et al., 1990) and adults (Pomerantz et al., 1986; 1988). Thus organizational effects of steroids are observed primarily in changes in rates, rather than the presence or absence, of sex-typical behaviors.

The data on human exposure to diethylstilbestrol suggest that defeminization is the major effect in human women. *In utero* exposure to DES is associated with an increased incidence of hyposexuality in heterosexual relationships, characterized by lower levels of sexual desire and excitability and coital orgasmic dysfunction (Meyer-Bahlberg et al., 1984).

*Sexual Orientation*
Recent experiments have shown that perinatal androgen treatment of rodents enhances sexual orientation to females and suppresses orientation to males (DeJonge et al., 1986; Vega Matuszczyk et al., 1988). These changes are expressed as increased responsiveness to same-sex individuals following castration and treatment with sex steroids. Sexual orientation *per se* has not been examined in nonhuman primates, but a male-typical trait of expressing preference for one female over others has been shown to be induced by perinatal androgen treatment (Pomerantz et al., 1988). An increased incidence of homosexuality and bisexuality is evident among DES-exposed women, suggesting some influence of this estrogen on the development of human sexual orientation (Ehrhardt et al., 1985). No studies have observed significant effects of prenatal DES exposure on the sexual orientation or behavior of human males (Meyer-Bahlburg, 1984).

*Significance For Human Sexual Behavior*
There are a number of difficulties in attempting to extrapolate these experimental studies to human behavior. For example, gonadal steroids in intact individuals

may obscure the presence of heterotypical sexual behaviors. Another complexity lies in the biocultural nature of human social behavior. Cultural anthropologists, in fact, have argued that sexuality itself is a cultural construct that has no reality apart from its own cultural context (Stein, 1990). An example of the influence of culture is seen in the consequences of 5-alpha reductase deficiency, a metabolic disorder that results in ambiguous genitalia at birth but a physically male appearance at puberty. In the Dominican Republic, males with this disorder assume a male sexual identity upon puberty (Imperato-McGinley et al., 1979) while among the Sambia of Papua New Guinea, males assume the identity of a third sex (Herdt, 1990). This example demonstrates that culture plays an important role in the construction of gender identity, but it also indicates that biology influences the construction of cultural categories. Consequently, cultural changes may often accompany biological changes, making it difficult to separate cause and effect.

An additional obstacle to assessing human sexual development is the difficulty of distinguishing sexual orientation from intrasexual affiliation (Rosenblum, 1990), a distinction that is not an issue in experimental studies of asocial rodents but can be significant in social primates. The majority of the anthropoid primates are "female-bonded", characterized by high rates of female-female association and social interaction (Wrangham, 1980). Male bonding, however, is more characteristic of the Hominoidea, with the exception of the bonobo (*Pan paniscus*) where female-bonding is expressed in homosexual behavior as well as female-female association (Kuroda, 1980). This primate propensity for within-sex bonding confounds homosexual orientation with preference for association with liked-sex individuals, making it more difficult to identify sex-linked changes in sexual orientation.

## HISTORICAL CHANGES IN SEXUAL BEHAVIOR

*Patterning of Sexual Behavior*
The most evident changes in human sexual behavior over the past few decades in America have been 1) a reduction in the age of first intercourse, 2) an increase in the incidence of sexual intercourse and, 3) the disappearance of sex differences in coital behavior (DeFries, 1985). Beginning in the mid 1940s, rates of premarital intercourse increased steadily and the age of first intercourse declined (Colp, 1985). Convergence in male and female behavior accompanied sexual liberalization (Christensen and Gregg, 1970). The age of first intercourse declined steadily in female cohorts born after 1920 while male proportions changed little (see Fig. 2). Prior to the publication of the Kinsey reports in 1948 and 1953, five surveys between 1929-1947 reported rates of premarital intercourse that were twice as high for males as females (DeFries, 1985). Kinsey found a similar difference: 49 percent of males had engaged in premarital intercourse but only 20-27% of females (Kinsey, 1948, 1953). Fig. 2 shows that this sex difference began to disappear in generations of the 1950s and was nearly nonexistent among Americans born after 1965 (DeFries, 1985).

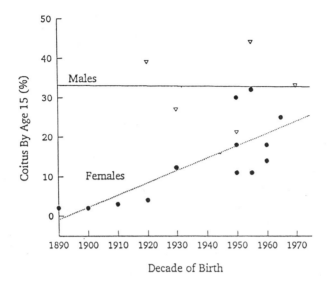

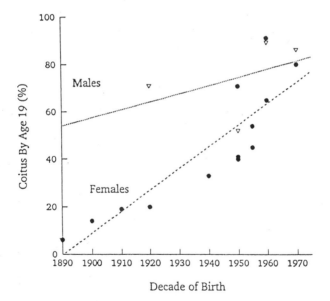

**FIGURE 2.** Secular changes in age of first coitus. Percentages of males and females who experience intercourse by age 15 (a) or 19 (b) according to decade of birth. Data from Kinsey, 1953; Bell and Chaskes, 1970; Gebhardt, 1980; Sorenson et al., 1973; Vener et al., 1971; Wyatt et al., 1988, Miller and Moore, 1990.

Along with the revolution in sexual behavior came a revolution in attitudes about the appropriate standards for premarital sexual behavior and a demise of the double standard (Colp, 1985). The major changes in the post-War period were 1) increasing approval of premarital sex; 2) a reduction in sex differences in approval of premarital sex; and 3) a reduction in the level of affection needed to justify involvement in a sexual relationship (Walsh, 1989). Men and women born before the second World War can be considered the generations of the "double standard" (Walsh, 1989). These standards changed among generations born after the second World War. A majority of college and high school students born in the 1940s espoused sexual abstinence (DeFries, 1985), but were more accepting of premarital sexuality for males (see Fig. 3). The period from 1955-1970, was an era of "permissiveness with affection" (Walsh, 1989). Beginning at the end of the 1950s, premarital intercourse was increasingly considered appropriate within the context of a love relationship (Christensen and Gregg, 1970; Luckey and Nass, 1969). After 1970, intercourse was increasingly regarded as a natural response and there was greater acceptance of intercourse without affection (Walsh, 1989).

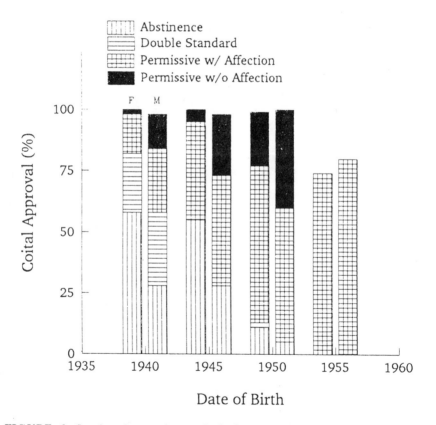

**FIGURE 3.** Secular changes in standards for premarital coitus. Proportions of females (left bar) and males (right bar) espousing abstinence, double standard (female abstinence), coitus within an affectionate relationship, or coitus in the absence of an affectionate relationship. Data from DeLamater and MacCorquodale, 1979.

These changes accompany reductions in sex differences in attitudes about sexual behavior (see Fig. 3). Initially, males were more approving of all reasons for premarital intercourse than females, but this sex difference had virtually disappeared by the end of the 70s (Hunt, 1970; DeLamater and MacCorquodale, 1979). These trends were also evident in other industrialized countries, beginning somewhat earlier in Scandinavia than in the US (Christensen and Gregg, 1970; Luckey and Nass, 1969).

*Trends in Sexual Orientation*
Most authors assert that the incidence of homosexual behavior has not changed in the past few decades. However, there are few surveys of the actual incidence of homosexual behavior. The Kinsey reports remain the largest studies to have examined rates of homosexual behavior. A recent comparison of a 1970 survey by the Kinsey Institute (N=3018) and a national survey conducted in 1988 (N=1450) indicate that the overall incidence of homosexual contact in males has not changed markedly over the last several decades (Fay et al., 1989). Fig. 4a shows that the proportions of males and females with at least one homosexual experience have not changed, nor has the sex difference in homosexual experience. There is some suggestion of increased frequency of homosexual interaction, however. Fig. 4b shows an increased proportion of males engaging in frequent homosexual behavior and a reduced proportion for whom homosexual interaction is rare. Fewer data are available for women, but a comparison of the sexual behavior of women in 1970 and 1988 found a higher proportion of women had engaged in homosexual behavior in the late teens in 1988 than in 1970 (Wyatt et al., 1988).

Although the proportions of individuals engaging in homosexual behavior may not have changed, the public awareness of homosexuality has increased. Changes in public awareness are primarily a consequence of gay political movements which reflect changes in sexual identity. The development of homosexual awareness and a gay sexual identity followed World War II and the post World War II purges of homosexuals in the military and industry (Berube, 1989). Increasing gay political activity in the 1960s culminated in a political movement in the 1970s (D'Emilio, 1989). Political activism was accompanied by identification with gay and lesbian lifestyles as separate sexual identities (D'Emilio, 1989). In the lesbian community, the political movement was accompanied by a change in sexual identity within lesbian couples. In the forties and fifties, partners in lesbian relationships traditionally assumed stereotyped masculine (butch) and feminine (femme) roles (Davis and Kennedy, 1989). These roles, then considered normative behavior in the lesbian community, were played out in dress and mannerism and in sexual behaviors. In the sixties and seventies, these stereotyped roles gave way to more varied and mutual relationships (Davis and Kennedy, 1989). These changes in sexual identity within lesbian relationships parallel the contemporaneous reductions in sex differences in sexual behavior and sexual standards within heterosexual relationships.

*Summary of Behavioral Trends*
These behavioral changes indicate that the period from the late-fifties to the

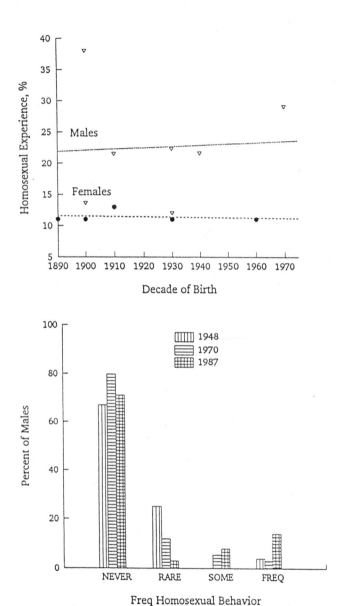

**FIGURE 4.** Frequency of homosexual experience and interactions (a) Prevalence of males and females with at least one homosexual experience by decade of birth (b). Frequencies of male homosexual behavior in 1948, 1970, and 1987. Data from Fay *et al.*, Wyatt *et al.*, 1988.

eighties was truly a sexual revolution in which both traditional standards and patterns of sexual behavior were overturned. No major changes in sexual orientation are evident over this period, nor are there major changes in the sexual behavior of males. Instead, these changes occurred primarily through the loss of those patterns of behavior traditionally considered feminine in Western culture:

delayed sexual experience, a reluctance to engage in coital behavior outside of a pair bond, and a lower incidence of sexual behavior. These changes appear to have occurred within lesbian as well as heterosexual communities.

These trends are not inconsistent with defeminization of sexual behavior. The conjunction of the earlier described changes in age of menarche and DZ twinning suggest that some biological changes preceded these events. However, there are a number of more compelling sociological explanations. Some behavior changes could be an indirect result of earlier menarche. Age of menarche is associated with age at first intercourse (Udry and Cliquet, 1982; Sandler et al., 1984; Komlos, 1989), and precocious pubertal development is associated with early onset of sexual activity (Udry, 1988; Miller and Moore, 1990). In addition, there are a number of alternative, social explanations. For example, the observed changes in sexual behavior and attitudes about sexual behavior have occurred in the context of increasing equality in sex roles and employment and postponement of marriage and family (DeFries, 1985). Technological advances such as the development of contraceptives in the 1960s and the legalization of abortion and contraceptives in the 1970s also have contributed to changes in sexual behavior and perceived sex roles of women (Colp, 1985).

The diversity of alternative explanations for these behavioral changes point out the difficulty of demonstrating subtle changes in behavioral tendencies in a species whose behavior is so heavily influenced by social factors and suggests a need for more rigorous bio-markers of human behavioral differentiation. One solution would be the use of species-specific sexual behaviors, similar to behaviors used in experimental studies of sexual differentiation in rodents and primates (Vega Matuszczyk et al., 1988; Pomerantz et al., 1986). Ethological studies suggest that species-specific postures and behaviors do play a role in human courtship and sexual behavior (Eibl-Eibesfeldt, 1989; Grammer, 1989) and might prove to be more useful indices of human behavioral differentiation than the crude measures of sexual activity and preference detected in sociological surveys. For the present, however, measures of sexual behavior would appear to be less satisfactory indices of human sexual development than are the measures of reproductive function available through demographic data.

## CONCLUSIONS

Over the last two centuries, rates of DZ twinning and ages of menarche have varied with a periodicity of 25-50 years in western countries. Reductions in DZ twinning accompany earlier menarche while elevations in DZ twinning occur when menarcheal age stabilizes. The surprising conjunction of these changes, the former taken as an index of falling fecundity and latter traditionally seen as an index of improving nutrition and fecundity, suggests a more fundamental change in the organization of gonadotropin function. Gonadal steroids and other substances with steroid-like action are known to alter both the timing of sexual maturation and adult gonadotropin secretion when provided to rodents perinatally.

Although the data are less clear in primates, they suggest that some changes in gonadotropin function follow prenatal exposure.

Whatever factors precipitated these changes appeared in the US at the turn of the century and in Scandinavia about 30 years later. In America, this period coincides with a period of upward shift in male growth and is followed by a period of decline in adult male height that coincides with the period of increase in DZ twinning (Fogel, 1986). These changes occur in rural as well as urban families and so are not simply a response to urban life, and may reflect increasing inequities in wealth during this period (Fogel, 1986). In Scandinavia, the decline in menarcheal age parallels a secular trend for increasing gross national product; the hiatus in the menarcheal trend is a period when the gross national product plateaus (Liestol, 1982). These changes in economic conditions are likely to be reflected in changes in dietary composition as well as nutrition, with potentially significant effects on developmental processes.

There are also a number of industrial developments during this time. The first periods coincide with the early development of the gas and the chemical industries (Aftalion, 1991). Commercial use of gas and gas production from coal occurred with the introduction of gas street lamps in America and Europe at the turn of the century. The first gas lamps appeared in the US, England, France, and Germany around 1820 and in Scandinavia and Australia between 1840-1850 (Peebles, 1980). The aromatic by-products of this industry and the dye industry that developed as an offshoot would have been early sources of environmental pollution that might have influenced sexual development.

The worldwide decline in menarche and DZ twinning that occurs in women born between 1915-1940 suggests a more marked and global effect, which might be related to industrial production or social disruption ensuing from the First and Second World Wars, but might also reflect the continuation of the century-long trend for increasing domestic production, improved nutrition and replacement of whole grain products with animal fat and protein (Fogel, 1986; Adlercreutz, 1990). Declining sex differences in sexual behavior during the final phase of menarcheal decline in the US suggest the provocative possibility that these changes, too, might have been mediated by biological events, although here the evidence is much less compelling.

What is the significance of these data to the problem of chemically induced alterations in sexual development? First, these findings indicate that demographic data can provide some insights into neuroendocrine development and might prove a useful tool in the survey of populations for chemical effects. Second, comparison of historical patterns of change in DZ twinning rates and age of menarche shows that these variables change in a coordinated fashion, a novel result given the markedly different interpretations that have been attached to these two trends. Third, these changes are consistent with altered sexual differentiation and suggest that some fundamental shifts in the human reproductive development have occurred over the last century. Finally, these trends coincide with changes in diet and chemical production, both of which have the potential to influence developmental processes. These considerations add weight to our current concern by showing that far smaller shifts in environmental factors are associated with prolonged and far-reaching changes in human development.

## REFERENCES

Aftalion, F. (1991). *A History of the International Chemical Industry*, translated by O. T. Benfey. University of Pennsylvania Press, Philadelphia.

Adlercreutz, H. (1990). Western diet and Western diseases: some hormonal and biochemical mechanisms and associations. *Scand. J. Clin. Lab. Invest.* **50**, Suppl. 201: 3-23.

Barbarino, A., De Marinis, L, Lafuenti, G., Mscatell, P., and Matteucci, B. (1979). Presence of positive feedback between oestrogen and LH in patients with Klinefelter's syndrome, and Sertoli-cell-only syndrome. *Clin. Endocrinol.* (Oxf.) **10**, 235-242.

Baum, M. J. (1979). Differentiation of coital behavior in mammals: a comparative analysis. *Neurosci. Biobehav. Rev.* **3**, 265-284.

Bell, R. R. and Chaskkes, J. B. (1970). Premarital sexual experience among coeds, 1958 and 1968. *Jr. Marr. Fam.* **32**, 81-84.

Bern, H.A. (1991). Diethylstilbestrol (DES) syndrome: present status of animal and human studies. In *Hormonal Carcinogenesis*, ed. J. Li, S.A. Li, and S. Nandi. Springer-Verlag, New York, pp. 1-8.

Berube, A. (1989). Marching to a different drummer: Lesbian and gay GIs in World War II. In *Hidden From History: Reclaiming the Gay and Lesbian Past*, ed. M. B. Duberman, M. Vicinus, and G. Chauncey, Jr. New American Library/Penguin Books, New York, pp. 383-394.

Billiar, R. B., Richardson, D., Anderson, E., Mahajan, D., and Little, J. B. (1985). The effect of chronic and acyclic elevaton of circulating androstenedione or estrone concentrations on ovarian function in the rhesus monkey. *Endocrinol.* **116**, 2209-2220.

Blair, P. (1981) Immunologic consequences of early exposure of experimental rodents to diethylstilbestrol and steroid hormones. In *Developmental Effects of Diethylstilbestrol (DES) in Pregnancy*, ed. A. L. Herbst and H. Bern. Thieme-Stratton Inc, New York, pp 167-178.

Bonnelykke, B. (1989). Menstrual characteristics of mothers of twins. *J. Biosoc. Sci.* **21**, 329-334.

Boyar, R.M., Finkelstein, J., Roffwarg, H., Kapen, S., Weitzman, and E. Hellman, L. (1972). Synchronization of augmented luteinizing hormone secretion with sleep during puberty. *New Eng. J. Med* **287**, 582-586.

Brown, M. (1981). *Laying Waste: The Poisoning of America by Toxic Chemicals*. Washington Square Press, Simon and Schuster, Inc, New York.

Brudevall, J. E., Liestol, K., and Walloe, L. (1979). Menarcheal age in Oslo during the last 140 years. *Ann. Hum. Biol.* **9**, 35-43.

Burroughs, C.S., Mills, K.T., and Bern, H.A. (1990). Reproductive abnormalities in female mice exposed neonatally to various doses of coumestrol. *J. Toxicol. Environ. Health* **30**, 105-122.

Caplan, R. (1990). *Our Earth, Ourselves*. Bantam Books, New York.

Carmelli, D., Hasstedt, S., and Andersen, S. (1981). Demography and genetics of human twinning in the Utah Morman geneology. *Twin Res.* **3**, 81-93.

Carson, R. (1962). *Silent Spring*. Houghton-Mifflin, Boston.

Christensen, H.T. and Gregg, C.F. (1970). Changing sex norms in America and Scandinavia. *J. Marr. Fam.* **32**, 616-627.

Colp Jr., R. (1985) Changes in American sexual attitudes during the past century. In *Sexuality. New Perspectives*, ed. Z. DeFries, R. C. Friedman, and R. Corn. Greenwood Press, Westport, CT. pp. 313-329.

Davis, M. and Kennedy, E.L. (1989). Oral history and the study of sexuality in the lesbian community: Buffalo, New York, 1940-1960. In *Hidden From History: Reclaiming the Gay and Lesbian Past*, ed. M. B. Duberman, M. Vicinus, and G. Chauncey, Jr. New American Library/Penguin Books, New York. pp. 426-440.

DeFries Z. (1985). New sex codes in adolescence. In *Sexuality. New Perspectives*, ed. Z. DeFries, R. C. Friedman and R. Corn. Greenwood Press, Westport, CT. pp. 89-98.

De Jonge, F.H., Meyerson, B.J., and van de Poll, N.E. (1986). Attractivity of male and female rats which are hormonally manipulated during early development and in adulthood. *Horm. Behav.* **20**, 379-389.

DeLamater, J. and MacCorquodale, P. (1979). *Premaritial Sexuality*. University of Wisconsin Press, Madison, WI.

D'Emilio, J. (1989). Gay politics and community in San Francisco since World War II. In *Hidden From History: Reclaiming the Gay and Lesbian Past*, ed. M. B. Duberman, M. Vicinus, and G. Chauncey, Jr. New American Library/Penguin Books, New York, pp. 456-473.

Doherty, J.D.H. and Lancaster, P.A.L. (1986). The secular trend of twinning in Australia, 1853-1982. *Acta Genet. Med. Gemellol.* **35**, 61-76.

Dohler, K.D., Hancke, J.L., Srivastava, S.S., Hofmann, D., Shryne, J.E., and Gorski, R.A. (1984). Participation of estrogens in female sexual differentiation of the brain; neuroanatomical, neuroendocrine and behavioral evidence. *Prog. Brain Res.* **61**, 99-117.

Dunlap, T.R. (1981). *DDT. Scientists, Citizens, and Public Policy*. Princeton University Press, Princeton, NJ.

Eaton, G.G., Goy, R.W., and Phoenix, C.H. (1973). Effects of testosterone treatment in adulthood on sexual behavior of female pseudohermaphroditic rhesus monkeys. *Nature* (New Biol.) **242**, 119-120.

Eaton, G.G., Worlein, J.M., and Glick, B.B. (1990). Sex differences in Japanese macaques (*Macaca fuscata*): Effects of prenatal testosterone on juvenile social behavior. *Horm. Behav.* **24**, 270-283.

Ehrhardt, A.A., Meyer-Bahlburg, H.F.L., Risen, L.R., Feldman, J.F., Veridiano, N.P., Zimmerman, I., and McEwen, B.S. (1985) Sexual orientation after prenatal exposure to exogenous estrogens. *Arch. Sex. Behav.* **14**, 57-77.

Eibl-Eibesfeldt, I. (1989). *Human Ethology*. Aldine de Gruyter, New York.

Fay, R.E., Turner, C.J.F., Klassen, A.D., and Gagnon, J.H. (1989). Prevalence and patterns of same-gender sexual contact among men. *Science* **243**, 338-348.

Fogel, R.W. (1986). Physical growth as a measure of the economic well-being of populations: The eighteenth and nineteenth centuries. In *Human Growth. A Comprehensive Treatise*. Volume 3. Methodology. Ecological, Genetic, and Nutritional Effects on Growth, ed. F. Falkner and I J. M. Tanner. Plenum, New York, 2nd Edition, pp. 263-282.

Fuller, G.B., Yates, D.E., Helton, E.D., and Hobson, W.C. (1981). Diethylstilbestrol reversal of gonadotropin patterns in infant rhesus monkeys. *J. Steroid Biochem.* **15**, 497-500.

Gebhard, P.H. (1980). Sexuality in the post-Kinsey era. In *Changing Patterns of Sexual Behaviour*, ed. W. H. G Armytage, R. Chester, and J. Peel. Academic Press, New York, pp. 45-57.

Goodman, M.J. (1983). Secular changes in recalled age at menarche. *Ann. Hum. Biol.* **10**, 585.

Gorski, R.A. (1968). Influence of age on the response to perinatal administration of a low dose of androgen. *Endocrinology* **82**, 1001-1004.

Goy, R.W. and Resko, J.A. (1972). Gonadal hormones and behavior of normal and pseudohermaphroditic nonhuman female primates. *Rec. Progress Hormone Res.* **28**, 707-733.

Goy, R.W., Bercovithc, F.B., and McBrair, M.C. (1988). Behavioral masculinization is independent of genital masculinization in prenatally androgenized female rhesus monkeys. *Horm. Behav.* **22**, 552-571.

Grammer, K. (1989). Human courtship behaviour: biological basis and cognitive processing. In *Sociobiology of Sexual and Reproductive Strategies*, ed. A. E. Rasa, C. Vogel, and E. Voland. Chapman and Hall, New York, pp. 147-169.

Herdt, G. (1990). Mistaken gender: 5-alpha reductase hermaphroditism and biological reductionism in sexual identity reconsidered. *American Anthropologist* **92**, 433-446.

Hines, M., Alsum, P., Roy, M., Gorski, R.A., and Goy, R.W. (1987). Estrogenic contributions to sexual differentiation in the female guinea pig: Influences of diethylstilbestrol and tamoxifen on neural, behavioral, and ovarian development. *Horm. Behav.* **21**, 402-417.

Hunt, M. (1974). *Sexual Behavior in the 1970s.* Playboy Press, Chicago.

Imperato-McGinley, J., Peterson, R.E., Gautier, T., and Sturla, E. (1979). Male pseudoheramaphroditism secondary to 5a-reductase—a model for the role of androgens in both the development of the male phenotype and the evolution of a male gender identity. *J. Steroid Biochem.* **11**, 637-745.

Inouye, E. and Imaizumi, Y. (1981). Analysis of twinning rates in Japan. *Twin Res.* **3**, 21-33.

James, W.H. (1972) Secular changes in dizygotic twinning rates. *J. Biosoc. Sci.* **4**, 427-434.

James, W.H. (1975). The secular decline in dizygotic twinning rates in Italy. *Acta Genet. Med. Gemell.* **24**, 9.

James, W.H. (1982). Second survey of secular trends in twinning rates. *J. Biosoc. Sci.* **14**, 481-497.

James, W.H. (1986). Recent secular trends in dizygotic twinning rates in Europe. *J. Biosoc. Sci.* **18**, 497-504.

Jeanneret, O. and MacMahon, B. (1962). Secular changes in rates of multiple births in the United States. *Am. J. Hum. Genet.* **14**,410-425.

Jost, A. and Magre, S. (1984). Testicular developmental phases and dual hormonal control of sexual organogenesis. In *Sexual Differentiation: Basic and Clinical Aspects*, ed. M. Serio, M. Zanisis, M. Motta, and L. Martini. Raven Press, New York.

Karsch, F.J., Weick, R.F., Hotchkiss, D.J., Dierschke, D.J., and Knobil, E. (1973). An analysis of the negative feedback control of gonadotropin secretion utilizing chronic implantation of ovarian steroids in ovariectomized rhesus monkeys. *Endocrinology* **93**, 478.

Kellis, J.T. and Vickery, L.E. (1984). Inhibition of human estrogen synthetase (aromatase) by flavones. *Science* **225**, 1032-1034.

Kinsey, A.C., Pomeroy, W.B., and Martin, C.E. (1948). Sexual Behavior in the Human Male. W.B. Saunders, Philadelphia.

Kinsey, A.C., Pomeroy, W.R., Martin, C.E., and Gebhard, P.H. (1953). *Sexual Behavior in the Human Female.* W. B. Saunders, Philadelphia.

Komlos, J. (1989). The age at menarche and age at first birth in an undernourished population. *Ann. Hum. Biol.* **16**, 463-466.

Kuroda, S. (1980). Social behavior of pygmy chimpanzees. *Primates* **21**, 181-197.

Laing, L.M. (1980). Declining fertility in a religious isolate: the Hutterite population of Alberta, Canada, 1951-71. *Hum. Biol.* **52**, 288.

Lephart, E.D., Mathews, D., Noble, J.F., and Ojeda, S.R. (1989). The vaginal epithelium of immature rats metabolizes androgens through an aromatase-like reaction: Changes through the time of puberty. *Biol. Reprod.* **40**, 259-267.

Liestol, K. (1982). Social conditions and menarcheal age: the importance of early years of life. *Ann. Hum. Biol.* **9**, 521-537.

Lu, J.K.H., Hooper, B.R., Vargo, T.M., and Yen, S.S.C. (1979). Chronological changes in sex steroid, gonadotropin and prolactin secretion in female rats displaying different reproductive states. *Biol. Reprod.* **21**, 193-203.

Luckey, E.B. and Nass, G.D. (1969). A comparison of sexual attitudes and behavior in an international sample. *J. Marr. Fam.* **31**, 364-379.

McGillivray, I. (1979). The changing incidence of twinning in Scotland, 1939-68. *Acta Gen. Med. Gemell.* **19**, 26.

McLachlan, J.A. (1985). *Estrogens in the Environment II: Influences on Development.* Elsevier North Holland, New York.

McLachlan, J.A. and Newbold, R.R. (1987). Estrogens and development. *Envir. Hlth. Perspect.* **75**, 25-27.

McLarin, A. (1990). What makes a man a man? *Nature* **346**, 216-217.

MacLusky, N.J. and Naftolin, F. (1981). Sexual differentiation of the central nervous system. *Science* **211**, 1294-1302.

Marshall, W.A. and Tanner, J.M. (1986). Puberty. In *Human Growth. A Comprehensive Treatise.* Volume 2. Postnatal Growth, Neurobiology, ed. F. Falkner and J. M. Tanner. Plenum, New York, 2nd Edition. pp. 171-209.

Matsumoto A., Arai, Y. (1978) Sexual dimorphism in 'wiring pattern' in the hypothalamic arcuate nucleus and its modification by neonatal hormonal environment. *Brain Res.* **190**, 238-242.

Matsumoto A., Arai, Y, (1977) Precocious puberty and synaptogenesis in the hypothalamic arcuate nucleus in pregnant mare serum gonadotropin (PMSG) treated immature female rats. *Brain Res.* **129**, 375-378.

Meyer-Bahlburg, H.F.L. (1984). Psychoendocrine research on sexual orientation. Current status and future options. *Prog. Brain Res.* **61**, 375-398.

Milham, S. (1964). Pituitary gonadotropin and dizygotic twinning. *Lancet* **2**, 566.

Miller, B.C. and Moore, K.A. (1990). Adolescent sexual behavior, pregnancy, and parenting: Research through the 1980s. *J. Marr. Fam.* **52**, 1025-1044.

Mosher, W.D. (1982). Infertility trends among U.S. couples: 1965-1976. *Fam. Plann. Perspect.* **14**, 22-27.

Mosteller, M., Townsend, J.I., Corey, L.A., and Nance, W.E. (1981). Twinning rates in Virginia: Secular trends and the effects of maternal age and parity. *Twin Res.* **3**, 57-69.

Naftolin, F., Garcia-Segura, L.M., Keefe, D., Leranth, C., MacLusky, N.J., and Brawer, J.R. (1990). Estrogen effects on the synaptology and neural membranes of the rat hypothalamic arcuate nucleus. *Biol. Reprod.* **42**, 21-28.

Newbold, R.R. and McLachlan, J.A. (1985). Diethylstilbestrol assoicated defects in murine genital tract development. In *Estrogens in the Environment*, ed. J. McLachlan. Elsevier, New York, pp. 288-315.

Noller, K.L, Blair, P.B., O'Brien, P.C., Mellton II, L.J., Offord, J.R., Kaufman, R.H., and Colton, T. (1988). Increased incidence of autoimmune disease among women exposed *in utero* to diethylstilbestrol. *Fertil. Steril.* **49**, 1080-1082.

Nylander, W.H. (1973). Serum levels of gonadotropins in relation to multiple births in Nigeria. *J. Obstet. Gynaec. Br. Commonw.* **80**, 651-653.

Peebles, M.W.H. (1980). Evolution of the gas industry. New York University Press, New York.

Peress, M.R., Tsai, C.C., Mathur, R.S., and Williamson, H.O. (1982). Hirsutism and menstrual patterns in women exposed to diethylstilbestrol *in utero*. *Am. J. Obstet. Gynecol.* **144**, 135-138.

Pomerantz, S.M., Goy, R.W. and Roy, M.M. (1986) Expression of male-typical behavior in adult female pseudohermaphroditic rhesus: comparisons with normal males and neonatally gonadectomized males and females. *Horm. Behav.* **20**, 483-500.

Pomerantz, S.M., Roy, M.M., and Goy, R.W. (1988) Social and hormonal influences on behavior of adult male, female, and pseudohermaphroditic rhesus monkeys. *Horm. Behav.* **22**, 219-230.

Plant, T.M., Gay, V.L., Marshall, G.R., and Arslan, M. (1987). Chronic intermittent chemical excitation of the hypothalamic GnRH system of the prepubertal monkey with N-methyl-DL-aspartate prematurely reactivates the pituitary-Leydig cell axis. *Endocr. Soc. Abstr.* **1987**, 37.

Ramirez, V.D., Sawyer, C.H. (1965). Advancement of puberty in the female rat by estrogen. *Endocrinology* **76**, 1158-1168.

Rosenberg, M. (1991). Menarcheal age of Norwegian women born 1830-1960. *Ann. Hum. Biol.* **18**, 207-219.

Rosenblum, L.A. (1990). Primates, *Homo sapiens*, and homosexuality. In *Homosexuality/Heterosexuality*, ed. D. P. McWhirter, S. A. Sanders, and J. M. Reinisch. Oxford University Press, New York, pp. 171-174.

Sandler, D.P., Wilcox, A.J., and Horney, L.F. (1984). Age at menarche and subsequent reproductive events. *Am. J. Epidemiol.* **119**, 765-774.

Sorensen, R.C. (1973). *Adolescent Sexuality in Contemporary America.* World Publishing, New York.

Smith, L.M., Schwartz, T.R., Feltz, K., and Kubiak, T.J. (1990). Determination and occurrence of AHH-active polychlorinated biphenyls, 2,3,7,8-tetrachloro-p-dioxin and 2,3,7,8-tetrachlorodibenzofuran in Lake Michigan sediment and biota. The question of their relative toxicological significance. *Chemosphere* **21**, 1063-1085.

Spector, I.P. and Carey, M.P. (1990). Incidence and prevalence of the sexual dysfunctions: a critical review of the empirical literature. *Arch. Sex. Behav.* **19**, 389-408.

Stein, E. (1990). *Forms of Desire. Sexual Orientation and the Social Constructionist Controversy.* Garland Publishing, New York.

Tanner, J.M. (1973) Trend towards earlier menarche in London, Oslo, Copenhagen, the Netherlands and Hungary. *Nature (London)* **243**, 95-96.

Taylor, G.D. and Sudnik, P.E. (1984). *Du Pont and the International Chemical Industry.* Twayne Publishers (G. K. Hall and Co), Boston.

Terasawa, E., Bridson, W.E., Nass, T.E., Noonan, J.J., and Dierschke, D.J. (1984). Developmental changes in the luteinizing hormone secretory pattern in peripubertal female rhesus monkeys: comparisons between gonadally intact and ovariectomized animals. *Endocrinology* **115**, 2233-2240.

Thornton, J. and Goy, R.W. (1986). Female-typical sexual behavior of rhesus and defeminization by androgens given prenatally. *Horm. Behav.* **20**, 129-147.

Trowell, H.C. and Burkitt, D.P. (1983). *Western Diseases: their emergence and prevention.* Edward Arnold, London.

Udry, J. R. (1988) Biological predispositions and social control in adolescent sexual behavior. *Am. Sociol. Rev.* **53**, 709-722.

Udry, J.R. and Cliquet, R.L. (1982). A cross-cultural examination of the relationship between ages at menarche, marriage, and first birth. *Demography* **19**, 53-63.

Urbanski, J.F. and Ojeda, S.R. (1987). Activation of luteinizing hormone-releasing hormone release advances the onset of female puberty. *Neuorendocrinology* **46**, 273-276.

Vega Matuszczyk, J. V., Fernandez-Guasti, A., and Larsson, K. (1988). Sexual orientation, proceptivity, and receptivity in the male rat as a function of neonatal hormonal manipulation. *Horm. Behav.* **22**, 362-378.

Vener, A. M., Steward, C. S., and Hager, D. L. (1971). The sexual behavior of adolescents in middle-America: Generational and American-British comparisons. *J. Marr. Fam.* **34**, 696-705.

Wallen, K. (1990). Desire and ability: Hormones and the regulation of female sexual behavior. *Neurosci. Biobehav Rev.* **14**, 233-241.

Walsh, R.H. (1989). Premarital sex among teenagers and young adults. In *Human Sexuality: The Societal and Interpersonal Context*, ed. K. McKinney and S. Sprecher. Ablex Publishing Co., Norwood, NJ. pp. 162-186.

Whitten, P.L. (1992) Phytochemical endocrinology: new paradigms for the evolution and ontogeny of alternative reproductive strategies. *Am. J. Phys. Anth. Suppl.* **14**,172-173.

Whitten P.L. and Naftolin, F. (1991). Dietary plant estrogens: A biologically active background for estrogen action. In *The New Biology of Steroid Hormones*, ed. R. Hochberg and F. Naftolin. Raven Press, New York. pp. 155-167.

Whitten, P. and Naftolin, F. (in press). Xenoestrogens and neuroendocrine development. In *Prenatal Exposure to Environmental Toxicants: Developmental Consequences*, ed. H. L. Needleman and D. Bellinger. Johns Hopkins University Press, Baltimore, MD.

van Wieringen, J.C. (1986). Secular growth changes. In *Human Growth. A Comprehensive Treatise*. Volume 3. Methodology. Ecological, Genetic, and Nutritional Effects on Growth, ed. F. Falkner and I. J. M. Tanner. Plenum, New York, 2nd Edition. pp. 307-331.

Wildt, L., Marshall, G., and Knobil, E. (1980). Experimental induction of puberty in the infantile female rhesus monkey. *Science* **207**, 1373-1375.

Williams, B.A., Mills, K.T., Burroughs, C.D., and Bern, H.A. (1989). Reproductive alterations in female C57BL/Crgl mice exposed neonatally to zearalenone, an estrogenic mycotoxin. *Cancer Lett.* **46**, 225-230.

Williamson, H.O. and Satteerfield, R.G. (1976). Diethylstilbestrol adenosis and dysfunctional uterine bleeding. *JAMA* **235**, 1687.

Wilson, J.D., George, F.W., and Griffin, J.E. (1981). The hormonal control of sexual development. *Science* **211**, 1278-1284.

Worldwatch Institute (1988). *State of the World, 1988*. W. W. Norton and Co, New York.

Wrangham, R. (1980). An ecological model of female bonded groups. *Behaviour* **75**, 262-300.

Wu, C.H., Mangan, C.E., Burtnett, M.M., and Mikhail, G. (1980). Plasma hormones in DES-exposed females. *Obstet. Gynecol.* **55**, 157-162.

Wyatt, G.E., Peters, S.D., and Guthrie, D. (1988). Kinsey revisited, part I: Comparisons of the sexual socialization and sexual behavior of white women over 33 years. *Arch. Sex. Behav.* **17**, 201-239.

Wyshak, G. (1981). Reproductive and menstrual characteristics of mothers of multiple births and mothers of singletons only: a discriminant analysis. *Twin. Res.* **3**, 95.

Wyshak, G. (1983). Secular changes in age at menarche in a sample of US women. *Ann. Hum. Biol.* **10**, 69-74.

Wyshak, G. and White, C. (1965). Geneological study of human twinning. *Am. J. publ. Hlth.* **55**, 1586.

# US APPLICATION AND DISTRIBUTION OF PESTICIDES AND INDUSTRIAL CHEMICALS CAPABLE OF DISRUPTING ENDOCRINE AND IMMUNE SYSTEMS

**Carol W. Bason**
World Wildlife Fund, Toxics and Wildlife Program, Washington, DC

**Theo Colborn**
World Wildlife Fund, Toxics and Wildlife Program, Washington, DC, and
W. Alton Jones Foundation, Charlottesville, Virginia

*Data were obtained from a number of sources to determine US application and distribution of pesticides which are capable of effecting changes in endocrine and immune systems. National annual use of conventional pesticides, measured by volume of active ingredients (A.I.) applied, has remained relatively constant for the last ten years even though product potency has increased. Acres treated has risen as more selective, narrow spectrum materials replace older, broad spectrum toxic compounds. Herbicides were the most used type of pesticide in 1989 with the largest quantity (by weight) attributed to atrazine and alachlor. Over the last ten years, herbicide use has increased, insecticide use has decreased, and fungicide use has remained constant. Of 1.1 billion pounds (A.I.) of conventional pesticides available for use in the US in 1989, 800 million pounds were used for agriculture. Exports of products identified as health or endocrine disrupters were estimated at over 66 million pounds in 1990 and included products which have been canceled for use in the US (such as chlordane and mirex). A proper assessment of potential exposure to pesticides by wildlife and humans is limited due to inaccessibility of production data.*

## INTRODUCTION

This survey focuses on application and distribution of pesticides capable of effecting changes in endocrine and immune systems. Endocrine and reproductive changes have been associated with all pesticide types: insecticides (carbaryl, DDT, methoxychlor, aldrin, chlordane, dieldrin, and kepone); herbicides (2,4-D, 2,4,5-T); and fungicides (thiocarbamates such as zineb and maneb) (Casarett and Doull, 1991). Immunosuppressive effects have been associated with organochlorines (chlordane, dieldrin, DDT, mirex, aldrin, lindane); carbamates (carbaryl and aldicarb); organophosphates (parathion, malathion, methyl-parathion); and organotins (Casarett and Doull, 1991). These substances are effective as pesticides because of all or some of the following characteristics: persistence, low volatility, low water solubility, high lipid solubility, or low

---

1. Corresponding Author: Theo Colborn, World Wildlife Fund, Toxics and Wildlife Program, 1250 Twenty-Fourth St., NW, Washington, DC 20037.

rate of biodegradation to more active compounds. These same characteristics may lead to bioaccumulation and biomagnification with resultant toxicity in secondary targets, such as wildlife and humans (see Fox, chapter 8; Thomas and Colborn, chapter 21).

In order to provide some estimate of potential wildlife and human exposure to pesticides, a review of historical trends in application and distribution is presented in this chapter, as well as a commentary on access to the information. Estimates of annual market use and import/export quantities for pesticide types are discussed. Where available, estimates of use for selected individual pesticides of each type which have been associated with affecting endocrine or immune system action are presented. Individual pesticides cited in this document were selected based on their known effects and/or structural chemical similarity to known endocrine system and immune system disrupters. Industrial contaminants are also discussed because of their known endocrine disruptive and immunosuppressive effects.

## MATERIALS AND METHODS

Several approaches were used to acquire information for this chapter. Computer searches of environmental data bases were undertaken and personal and/or telephone interviews were conducted with appropriate agencies. The Toxic Release Inventory (TRI) and the Hazardous Substance Data Base (HSDB) were among the data bases searched.

The TRI has facility estimates of toxics released into the environment in 1987, 1988, and 1989. Information was obtained from TRI for 2,4-D, Carbaryl, Chlordane, Hexachlorobenzene (HCB), Lindane, Parathion, Polyram, and Toxaphene. Data from TRI represent the "Total Environmental Release" quantity or the sum of air, water, and land release by those facilities which manufacture, process, or use the chemicals (USEPA, 1989b). Historical manufacturing information for production, importation, and exportation were found in the HSDB. This data base is updated regularly, with the exception of manufacturing information, which is of a proprietary nature. The HSDB was particularly useful in obtaining information on products which are canceled for production in the US, but are imported or exported.

In addition to data bases, a number of sources were contacted for information on the production and/or use of the substances of interest for this study with little success. The organizations contacted included the US Environmental Protection Agency's (USEPA) Public Information Office, Office of Pesticide Programs (OPP), and Office of Toxic Substances (OTS). The OPP Economic Analysis Branch was helpful in providing a draft of its 1989 Market Estimates Report (USEPA, 1991). In addition to the USEPA, the US Trade Commission, the Chemical Manufacturers Association (CMA), and the SRI International Specialty, Agricultural, and Inorganic Chemicals Center were contacted. Most of these queries resulted in inaccessibility of data because of the proprietary nature of the information, and with one exception, requests were referred back to USEPA. The US Trade Commission offered the use of its library facilities for further information at the chemical class level, but distribution data were not available by product.

Two other sources, the US Department of Agriculture's (USDA) Yearly Fiscal Reports for the US Forest Service (USFS) (USDA, 1988, 1989) and a Summary Report on Herbicide Use in the US by Resources for the Future (RFF) (Gianessi and Puffer, 1991), provided a more complete perspective on pesticide use in the US. USFS applications were summarized by pesticide and year. Applications were classified as aquatic, general, noxious, and nursery weed control; poisonous plant control; conifer and hardwood release; range management; rights-of-way; site preparation; and wildlife habitat improvement. RFF provided both state and nationwide estimates of distribution by pesticide and crop.

All pesticide amounts cited in this document are in "pounds active ingredient" unless otherwise stated. The term "conventional" pesticide includes herbicides, fungicides, insecticides, rodenticides, fumigants, and molluscicides. "Total pesticides" refers to conventional pesticides as well as wood preservatives, disinfectants, and sulfur. "Agricultural pesticides" are pesticides used on crops. "Non-agricultural pesticides" include all non-crop uses, such as lawn care products.

## FINDINGS

*Pesticides*
In its annual marketing estimates report, the US Environmental Protection Agency (USEPA) stated that of a total supply of 1.5 billion pounds conventional pesticides, 1.3 billion pounds were produced in the US in 1989 and 0.2 billion pounds were imported. Of that amount, 0.4 billion pounds were exported, resulting in 1.1 billion pounds net supply in the US (USEPA, 1991). USEPA estimated the 1989 world market for conventional pesticides to be 4 billion pounds, of which 46% are herbicides, 35% are insecticides, 14% are fungicides, and 5% other. Total 1989 pesticide use in the US was estimated at 2.1 billion pounds (USEPA, 1989a).

In 1989, the breakdown of national conventional pesticide use by class was as follows: herbicides (655 million pounds), insecticides (226 million pounds), fungicides (111 million pounds), and other (78 million pounds) (USEPA, 1991). Analysis of the USEPA estimates of total pesticide use from 1979 to 1989 indicates that herbicide use has increased from 50% to 62%, whereas insecticide use has decreased from 34% to 21%. Fungicide use has remained relatively constant, averaging 10% during this timeframe. Figure 1 presents conventional pesticide use by class.

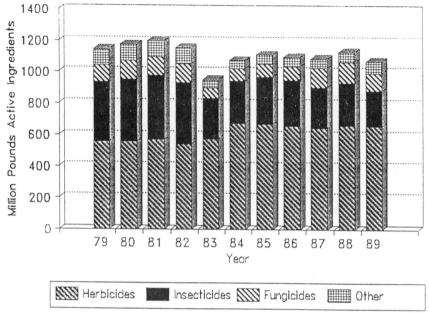

**FIGURE 1.** U.S. Use of Pesticides by Class. (Source: USEPA 1989 Market Estimates.)

The 1989 USEPA market survey characterized the use of pesticides as follows:
- US use was one-third of world pesticide market by sales and one-half on a weight basis.
- Agricultural use was three-quarters of total US volume.
- 900,000 farms and over 70 million households used pesticides.
- Herbicides were the most used pesticide type (based on weight and expenditure).
- The herbicides, atrazine and alachlor, represented the largest quantity used among all pesticides.
- Based on the 1989 US population of 250 million, 4.28 pounds per capita could be equated to all conventional pesticides; 1.1 pounds per capita could be equated to non-agricultural pesticides.

USEPA's 1991 market estimate report reveals that there was no significant change in the quantity of pesticides used nationally for the last ten years except for a decline in 1983. Figure 2 represents the national use of pesticides over a ten-year period, indicating total amount of conventional pesticides used, amount of agricultural use, and total sales (USEPA, 1989a, 1991). USEPA attributed the stability in use to "the application of more potent pesticides, a greater efficiency of use, and lower farm commodity prices" forcing reduction of use (USEPA, 1991). RFF attributed the 1983 decline in pesticide use to fewer acres planted (Gianessi, 1991, pers. comm.).

Atrazine, the most used agricultural pesticide in 1989, provided a 20% lower cost alternative to phenoxy herbicides (2,4-D) in the treatment of weeds in corn

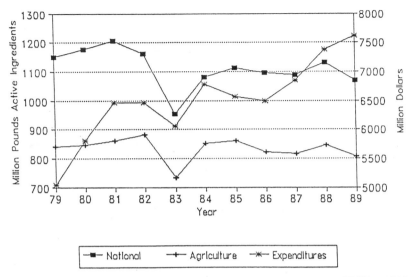

**FIGURE 2.** U.S. Pesticides: Annual Use and Expenditures. (Source: USEPA 1989 Market Estimates.)

(Ammon and Irla, 1984). Agricultural use of atrazine was over 64 million pounds for 1990 (Gianessi and Puffer, 1991). Potential problems from the increased use of the herbicide, atrazine, are similar to those that became evident after continued use of insecticides. These are evidenced by the following:

- increased weed resistance resulting in increased costs (Slife, 1986),
- presence in drinking water wells with concentrations above the minimum reporting limits in 1.7% of community wells and 0.7% rural wells (USEPA, 1990), and
- persistence in 89% of the prior year-treated soils and 98% of post-runoff tested cropland samples (USGS, 1991).

Analyzing the USDA data for forestry application of pesticides, a general increase is seen between 1988 and 1990 in pounds A.I. per acre by unit treated (USDA, 1990). The ratio of pounds A.I. per acre to units treated increased from 0.51 in 1988 to 0.77 in 1989 and to 0.79 in 1990. This ratio increased between 1988 and 1990 for insecticides, while the ratio decreased for fungicides and herbicides. The total volume of pesticides used per year for forest applications decreased from 352,659 pounds in 1988 to 266,789 pounds in 1990. Of the pesticides cited in this report, 2,4-D was the most used pesticide for forest application.

Although some pesticides have been banned by USEPA or discontinued voluntarily by producers, US manufacture of some of these pesticides continued for export to other countries. Of 465 million pounds of pesticides exported in 1990, 52 million pounds were pesticides which have been banned, unregistered, or designated for restricted use; 66 million pounds were pesticides which have been associated with health and endocrine effects (S. Beckmann, 1991, unpubl. data). The Foundation For Advancements in Science and Education (FASE) reports that export data based on US Customs shipping records underestimated actual amounts by 70% due to inadequate labelling (S. Beckmann, 1991, unpubl. data). The largest importers were Chile (6050 tons), Colombia (2512 tons), Thailand (2305 tons), Taiwan (1648 tons), and the Philippines (1532 tons). Another independent estimate of US export of banned pesticides is reported at 250,000 tons per year, close to the estimate provided by FASE (Newstab, 1991). Individual exportation amounts are noted in Table 1 of this report. Of the top 20 importers, most were Third World Nations.

Exported pesticides included US discontinued or restricted products such as chlordane, heptachlor, and mirex (USEPA, 1985b). Chlordane and mirex exportation during a 1990 FASE three-month study were almost 600,000 and 250,000 pounds, respectively (S. Beckmann, 1991, unpubl. data). Export of DDT continued in large amounts through 1978 (over 30 million pounds A.I.) (HSDB, 1991). Individual amounts of DDT exported in recent years could not be determined from the HSDB because the volume exported was combined with other chlorinated hydrocarbon preparations.

Fugitive emissions from the manufacture of chlordane decreased between 1987 and 1989 from 22,443 pounds in 1987, to 4841 in 1988, and 3757 pounds in 1989 (USEPA, 1987b, 1988, 1989b). Even as late as 1981, national urban application of chlordane exceeded other urban pesticide applications with over 3.6 million pounds distributed (USEPA, 1985a). Like many of the insecticides, the continued use of chlordane worldwide has led to the discovery of its metabolites in Antarctic Adelie penguins and Dall's porpoises (Kawano et al., 1988), in Sargasso Sea sediments (Knap et al., 1986), and in Canadian Arctic air, snow, seawater, and invertebrates (Bidleman et al., 1989).

The USEPA survey of pesticide content of drinking water wells conducted between 1988 and 1990 found that 10.4% of the community wells and 4.2% of the rural wells were contaminated with at least one pesticide "at or above minimum reporting level" (USEPA, 1990). Analysts estimated that nationally 9,850 community and 446,000 rural drinking water wells were contaminated. (This study did not include drinking water wells at the city, county, and state level.) Counties in the survey were categorized based on level of pesticide use, groundwater vulnerability, and "cropping" level. Regrouping the counties into high risk or "cropped and vulnerable" categories indicated that 5.5% of the rural wells were now at risk of containing "at least one pesticide". With regard to the USEPA Lifetime Health Advisory Levels (HAL) and Maximum Contaminant Levels (MCL), only 0.8% community and 0.6% rural wells had pesticides over these quantities (USEPA, 1990). In most instances, HALs and MCLs are based solely on cancer risk.

**TABLE 1.**   **Pesticide Summary Information (thousand pounds active ingredients)**

| PESTICIDE | 1989 ANNUAL USE (Rank) | 1989/1990 AGRICULTURE USE | 1990 EXPORT (3-months) | 1989 FORESTRY USE | 1981 URBAN APPLICATION | 1989 TRI |
|---|---|---|---|---|---|---|
| Herbicides: | | | | | | |
| 1,3-D | 35000-45000 (5) | - | - | - | - | - |
| 2,4-D | 40000-65000 (3) | 33000-45000 | 760 | 17 | - | 11 |
| Alachlor | 60000-75000 (2) | 55000-91000 | 1520 | - | 140 | - |
| Atrazine | 70000-90000 (1) | 64000-84000 | - | < 1 | 1058 | - |
| Cyanazine | 20000-30000 (8) | 23000-29000 | - | - | - | - |
| Metolachlor | 40000-55000 (4) | 46000-50000 | 5 | < 1 | 143 | - |
| | | | | | | |
| Insecticides: | | | | | | |
| Carbamate Pesticide | - | - | 11780 | - | - | - |
| Carbaryl (SEVIN) | 10000-15000 (12) | 10000 | 1215 | 4 | 853 | 45 |
| Chlordane | - | - | 600 | - | 3626 | 4 |
| Lindane (gamma-HCH) | - | - | - | < 1 | 2 | 1 |
| Mirex | - | - | 247 | - | - | - |
| Malathion | - | 3000 | 2312 | < 1 | 649 | - |
| | | | | | | |
| Fungicides: | | | | | | |
| Hexachlorobenzene (HCB) | - | - | - | - | - | 6 |
| Mancozeb/Maneb | 8000-12000 (16) | - | 250/840 | < 1 | 32 | 1 |
| Methyl Parathion | 8000-12000 (17) | 9000 | 25 | - | - | - |
| Parathion | - | 6000 | - | - | 164 | 2 |
| | | | | | | |
| TOTALS BY CLASS | | | | | | |
| | | | | | | |
| Fungicides | 111000 | 65000 | - | 148 | 1037 | - |
| Herbicides | 655000 | 520000 | - | 145 | 8918 | - |
| Insecticides | 226000 | 151000 | - | 8 | 37002 | - |
| Other Pesticides | 78000 | 70000 | - | - | 177 | - |
| 1989 Total | 1070000 | 806000 | 465339 | 301 | 47134 | - |

CITATIONS:

| | |
|---|---|
| 1989 Annual Use | USEPA, 1991 |
| 1989 Agriculture Use | Gianessi & Puffer, 1991 |
| 1990 Export | Beckmann, 1991 (Unpubl.Data) |
| 1989 Forestry | USDA, 1990 |
| 1981 Urban Application | USEPA, 1985a |
| 1989 TRI | USEPA, 1989b |
| HSDB | Hazardous Substances Data Bank, 1991 |

Information regarding the quantity of specific pesticides produced or used is proprietary and is therefore difficult to access. Although federal agencies were asked for specific information, only limited and disjointed information could be gathered. Table 1 summarizes the obtainable information for individual pesticides and totals within applications by type. For comparative purposes and information timeliness, data from 1989 or 1990 were used where available.

*Industrial Contaminants*
Dioxins, including 2,3,7,8-tetrachlorodibenzo-p-dioxin (2,3,7,8-TCDD) and furans, such as 2,3,7,8-tetrachlorodibenzofuran (2,3,7,8-TCDF) are unintentional by-products of pesticide processing. Furans have the same biological effects as dioxins but are less potent. Besides being present as contaminants in pesticides, dioxins and furans are found in: technical products; emissions from municipal, hospital, and industrial waste incineration; emissions from iron, steel, and other metal production; emissions from automobiles; and in material associated with bleaching pulp and other uses of chlorine (Rappe, 1991; USEPA, 1987a). Distribution and exposure varies considerably depending upon geographical location and human activity in the area.

In 1987, USEPA conducted the National Dioxin Study to determine 2,3,7,8-TCDD concentrations in the environment. Chemical production sites were investigated using soil, sediment, fish, water, and animal or plant tissue. Samples from sites suspected of contamination had 2,3,7,8-TCDD levels at 0.2-6623 ppt (soil), 0.7-200 ppt (sediments), and 9-47 ppt (fish). As a result of this study, USEPA is further evaluating large production sites (greater than 100,000 pounds of pesticide production) for dioxin contamination (USEPA, 1987a). This study found elevated concentrations of TCDD in fish which were linked to chemical industry activity and the paper and pulp industry. TCDD was found in 23 of 29 composite samples of Great Lakes fish and in a number of major rivers nationwide.

Of the 75 dioxin and 115 furan congeners, the dioxin congener, 2,3,7,8-TCDD (TCDD) exhibits the most toxicity when measured as enzyme induction activity. Using TCDD as the standard, toxicity equivalent factors have been derived for the other dioxin congeners and furan congeners, as well. Recently, when considering the risks from exposure to these compounds, the concentration is often reported as dioxin toxicity equivalents (TEQs) rather than the amount of compound present. However, the dioxin-like (enzyme induction) effects that are used to determine TEQs may not be related to the hormonal activity of TCDD (See Peterson, Chapter 10).

Polychlorinated biphenyl (PCB) mixtures were used industrially in electrical equipment as fire retardants, plastics, preservatives, varnishes, and waxes (Hooper et al., 1990). World PCB production (excluding USSR) was estimated at $1.53 \times 10^9$ kg (over 3.4 billion pounds) since use began in 1929 (Marquenie and Reijnders, 1989). US sales of PCBs were estimated at $5.08 \times 10^6$ kg (11.2

million pounds) during this time period (Hooper et al., 1990). Annual world production was cited at 16.5 x $10^6$ kg (36.3 million pounds) from 1980-1984 and 10.0 x $10^6$ kg (22 million pounds) from 1984-1990 (Marquenie and Reijnders, 1989). Estimates of the fate of PCBs vary, with 30% in lake or estuarine sediments, storage, or landfills; 30% unknown; and 30%-70% still in use (Marquenie and Reijnders, 1989; Hooper et al., 1990). Marquenie and Reijnders (1989) estimate that about 1% of all PCBs produced have reached the oceans thus far.

Recent investigations have led to the discovery that a mixture of tetrachlorobenzyltoluenes (TCBTs), known commercially as Ugilec 141, a PCB substitute used in Germany, has the same toxic profile as Aroclor 1254, a commercial PCB product whose production ceased in the US in 1969. Qualitatively and quantitatively Ugilec-141 induced CP-450 and EROD activity, and reduced plasma retinol and thyroxin levels, similar to Aroclor 1254 and 3,3',4,4'-tetrachlorobiphenyl (PCB 77). Ugilec-141 has been found in edible parts of fish in Western Germany at 25 ppm and downstream in the Netherlands where Ugilec 141 was never used, at 4.8 ppm in red eels (Murk et al., 1991).

## DISCUSSION

Based on the minimal change seen in pesticide use over the last ten years, there is little data available to suggest that pesticide distribution in the US will change significantly in the next decade. In 1987, expenditures for pesticides began to increase whereas the quantity of pesticides in use remained about the same (Figure 1). Different economic factors (such as increased costs between 1979 and 1982) may have driven use down in 1983. With the accompanying decrease in cost, use increased in 1984 to the level it held until 1988. It should also be noted that although higher potency products were introduced, the amount of pesticides by weight in use in 1988 did not significantly differ from previous years. In contrast to the current data trends, RFF predicts that future herbicide use will decline because of new technologies in lower rate compounds (e.g., use of 0.03 lb A.I./acre versus 3.0 lb. A.I./acre), greater specificity in mode of action in controlling weeds, and herbicide resistant crops (L.P. Gianessi, 1991, pers. comm.).

The objective of this review was to determine the US application and distribution of substances which are known to have the potential to be disrupters of endocrine or immune systems. Accessibility to the data required for this study was limited. Except for world totals, production information could not be obtained readily. Production/use data is proprietary due to the need to keep "confidential business information" secure for marketing purposes. Other than the USEPA market estimates, the major source of information was through private correspondence.

Evaluating the hazards from exposure to hormonally active chemicals in the environment will continue to be impossible unless data regarding production and distribution of chemicals of this nature are made public information. The difficulties associated with determining exposure are exacerbated by the large number of products on the market, the large quantities used, the number of possible exposure pathways and events, the seasonality of use, and the global distribution of many of the products. Persistence and long range atmospheric and aquatic transport of exported banned/restricted/unregistered pesticides also contribute to the difficulty of assessing hazard. When all of the above are taken into consideration, it is apparent that widespread exposure exists, that exposure can be sporadic and uncontrollable, and that exposure will continue to occur in the future. This provides an argument for new approaches by regulatory agencies to eliminate the release of substances of this nature in the environment.

## REFERENCES

Ammon, H.U. and Irla, E. (1984). In *Pesticide Resistance, Strategies and Tactics for Management*, ed. Committee on Strategies for the Management of Pesticide Resistant Pest Populations, Board on Agriculture and National Research Council. (1986). National Academy Press, Washington, DC.

Bidleman, T.F., Patton, G.W., Walla, M.D., Hargrave, B.T., Vass, W.P., Erickson, P., Fowler, B., Scott, V., and Gregor, D.J. (1989). Toxaphene and other organochlorines in Arctic Ocean fauna: evidence for atmospheric delivery. *Arctic*, **42**(4), 307-313.

*Casarett and Doull's Toxicology, The Basic Science of Poisons*. (1991). Pergammon Press, New York. Amdur, M.O., Doull, J., Klaassen, C.D., eds. pp. 314, 505-506, 565-622.

Gianessi, L.P. and Puffer, C. (1991). *Herbicide Use in the United States: National Summary Report*. Resources for the Future.

Hazardous Substances Data Bank (HSDB). (1991). National Library of Medicine. Toxicology Data Network (TOXNET).

Hooper, W.S., Pettigrew, C.A., and Sayler, G.S. (1990). Ecological fate, effects, and prospects for the elimination of environmental polychlorinated biphenyls (PCBs). *Environmental Toxicology and Chemistry*, **9**, 655-667.

Knap, A.H., Binkley, K.S., and Deuser, W.G. (1986). Synthetic organic chemicals in the deep Sargasso Sea. *Nature*, **319**, 572-574.

Kawano, M., Inoue, T., Wada, T., Hidaka, H., and Tatsukawa, R. (1988). Bioconcentration and residue patterns of chlordane compounds in marine animals: invertebrates, fish, mammals, and seabirds. *Environ. Sci. Technol.*, **22**, 792-797.

Marquenie, J.M. and Reijnders, P.J.H. (1989). PCBs, an increasing concern for the marine environment. ICES: CM, 1989/N:12, 5pp.

Murk, A J., van der Berg, J.H.J., Koeman, J.H., and Brouwer, A. (1991). The toxicity of tetrachlorobenzyltoluenes (Ugilec 141) and polychlorobiphenyls (Aroclor 1254 and PCB-77) compared with Ah-responsive and Ah-nonresponsive mice. *Environmental Pollution*, **72**, 57-67.

Newstab. (1991). Banned pesticides detected in coral reefs. May 13.

Rappe, C. (1991). Introduction, level, profiles, and patterns. Paper presented at 11th International Symposium on Chlorinated Dioxins and Related Compounds, Dioxin '91. Research Triangle Park, North Carolina, USA. September 23-27.

Slife, F.W. (1986). Resistance in Weeds. In *Pesticide Resistance, Strategies and Tactics for Management*. Committee on Strategies for the Management of Pesticide Resistant Pest Populations, Board on Agriculture and National Research Council. National Academy Press, Washington, D.C., 1986.

TRI, Toxic Chemical Release Inventory. (1989). National Library of Medicine Fact Sheet. June.

United States Department of Agriculture (USDA). (1988). Report of the Forest Service Fiscal Year 1988. Table 44—Pesticide Use Report, pp. 162-170.

United States Department of Agriculture (USDA). (1989). Report of the Forest Service Fiscal Year 1989. Table 47—Pesticide Use Report, pp. 186-194.

United States Department of Agriculture (USDA). (1990). Report of the Forest Service Fiscal Year 1990. Table 49—Pesticide Use Report, pp. 184-192.

United States Environmental Protection Agency. (USEPA). (1985a). National Urban Pesticide Applicator Survey: Final Report -Overview and Results. July.

United States Environmental Protection Agency. (USEPA). (1985b). Suspended, Canceled and Restricted Pesticides. January.

United States Environmental Protection Agency. (USEPA). (1987a). The National Dioxin Study, Tiers 3, 5, 6, and 7. February.

United States Environmental Protection Agency. (USEPA). (1987b). Toxic Release Inventory.

United States Environmental Protection Agency. (USEPA). (1988). Toxic Release Inventory.

United States Environmental Protection Agency. (USEPA). (1989a). Pesticide Industry Sales and Usage: 1988 Market Estimates. December, pp. 1-21.

United States Environmental Protection Agency. (USEPA). (1989b). Toxic Release Inventory.

United States Environmental Protection Agency. (USEPA). (1990). National Pesticide Survey: Summary Results of EPA's National Survey of Pesticides in Drinking Water Wells. pp. 1-16.

United States Environmental Protection Agency. (USEPA). (1991). Pesticide Industry Sales and Usage: 1989 Market Estimates. Draft, pp. 1-17.

United States Geological Survey (USGS). (1991). Atrazine in Stream Water, Post-1989 Application. Unpublished.

United States International Trade Commission. (1984). *Synthetic Organic Chemicals: US Production and Sales, 1984.*

# HERBICIDES AND FUNGICIDES: A PERSPECTIVE ON POTENTIAL HUMAN EXPOSURE

**Coralie R. Clement**
World Wildlife Fund, Washington, DC

**Theo Colborn**
World Wildlife Fund, Washington, DC
W. Alton Jones Foundation, Charlottesville, Virginia

## INTRODUCTION

It is difficult to ascertain measures of human exposure and developmental risks to herbicides and fungicides because of their widespread distribution and the limited information concerning their health effects. Studies of these products primarily focus on carcinogenicity, acute toxicity, genotoxicity, and irritation, whereas long-term, multigenerational studies exploring functionality are rare. Despite the paucity of information from which wildlife and human health safety statements can be made, herbicides continue to be used in increasing quantities according to usage data on large-acreage commodities (see Bason and Colborn, Chapter 19). Efforts to assemble information on small acreage crops have only recently been initiated by the US Department of Agriculture (Gianessi and Puffer, 1991b).

Herbicides and fungicides provide a convenient means to control pesky weeds and facilitate reduced tillage farming systems. Such systems have been developed and are encouraged by public policy because of the need to reduce soil erosion rates on cropland. Herbicides also meet the public's demand for lawns and gardens with limited maintenance requirements, flawless golf courses, and weed-free roadsides. Since herbicides are now used in rural, urban, and suburban areas nationwide, the possibility of wildlife and human exposure has increased. While herbicides are efficient weed control agents, the safety of continuous and/or sporadic human and animal exposure to low-dose concentrations of these chemicals has not been clearly demonstrated.

This paper discusses herbicide and fungicide use, the composition of the products on the market, and expands on the general knowledge concerning exposure to these products. We were not able to find daily intake estimates that considered multiple exposure to a number of herbicides and fungicides at one time, as well as information that considered simultaneous exposure via a number of pathways, such as dermal, inhalation, and dietary exposure. As a result, this paper provides a perspective on potential human exposure to herbicides and fungicides based on available statewide herbicide and fungicide use data. In order to translate state data into meaningful expressions of exposure, we related this data to federal tolerance

1. Corresponding Author: Theo Colborn, World Wildlife Fund, 1250 24th Street, N.W., Washington, DC  20037.

levels and reference doses per person for high-use products. The data were reduced to the increments of daily release over acceptable federal tolerance levels per person on a statewide basis. To complement this information, we provide an overview of the literature on animal and human reproductive and endocrine disruption effects of herbicides and fungicides. The paper closes with a review of the federal regulatory procedures governing the use of herbicides with a case study of the herbicide, Dacthal (DCPA). Dacthal was found more frequently in a 1990 nationwide survey of well-water contamination than any other pesticide (USEPA, 1990). The term "pesticides" in this paper includes insecticides, herbicides, and fungicides. In many instances herbicide and fungicide data are not separated from total pesticide data. Occupational exposure is not included in the analysis.

The data reviewed and analyzed in this paper were acquired through retrospective and current literature searches. Retrospective documents were revealed through computer databases including Chemical Abstracts, TOXLINE, and the Hazardous Substance Data Base (HSDB). Current documents were acquired through the Institute for Scientific Information's (ISI) database, FOCUSON, and by screening colleague publications and magazines such as *Chemical and Engineering News* and the *Chemical Regulation Reporter*. Government criteria documents, primarily reregistration documents from the Environmental Protection Agency's (EPA) Office of Pesticides and Toxic Substances, were used. Reports from the U.S. Fish and Wildlife Service, the Agency for Toxic Substances and Disease Registry (ATSDR), and the USGAO/RCED (U.S. General Accounting Office/Resources, Community, and Economic Development Division) were also used.

## HERBICIDE AND FUNGICIDE APPLICATIONS

*Agricultural Use*

Herbicides are registered for both crop and non-crop (e.g., lawn and garden care) use thereby increasing the chances of exposure of target and non-target species in almost every type of habitat in the US. Herbicides are currently used on approximately 90 million hectares in the US (Pimentel et al., 1991), and since most fruit, grain, and vegetable crops are treated with herbicides, it is reasonable to assume that almost every individual residing in the US is exposed to herbicides at one time or another throughout the year. Although pesticide use patterns vary with crop type, soil, and climate, "nearly all cultivated cropland in the United States is treated annually with at least one herbicide" (National Research Council, 1987). Of the estimated 955 million pounds (434 million kg) of pesticides applied annually for both agricultural and non-agricultural uses in the US, 69% are herbicides and 12% are fungicides (Pimentel et al., 1991). Corn and soybeans account for two-thirds of the total national agricultural use of herbicides (Gianessi and Puffer, 1991a). Field corn, where more than 90% of the hectarage is treated, accounts for 53% of agricultural herbicide use, with more than 6.6 pounds (3 kg) of herbicide applied per hectare (2.6 pounds (1.2 kg) per acre). The second largest amount is applied to soybeans with approximately 96% of soybean hectarage receiving treatment (Pimentel et al., 1991).

Fungicide use is generally limited to fruit and vegetable crops and for seed treatment. Apples and potatoes account for 26% of all the fungicides used in agriculture, with about 97% of potato hectarage treated with fungicides (Pimentel et al., 1991).

*Domestic Use*
Although the above figures represent a large component of herbicide and fungicide use, they do not include an important source of relatively high-dose exposure--lawn and garden care. The "perfect lawn" has become a national obsession with associated health hazards not yet fully understood. According to 1988 sales estimates from the US Environmental Protection Agency (USEPA), 67 million pounds (30 million kg) of active ingredients are applied as lawn care pesticides (insecticides as well as herbicides and fungicides), about 8% of the 814 million pounds (370 million kg) of active ingredients applied annually for agricultural purposes (USGAO/RCED, 1990). According to the Professional Lawn Care Association, 53 million homeowners maintain their own lawns while 9 million hire a professional service (Brown, 1991). The National Academy of Sciences estimates that homeowners use four to eight times more chemical pesticides per acre than farmers, resulting in 1990 expenditures of $1.2 billion on home-use pesticides (Brown, 1991). Although efforts have been made to encourage natural lawn care, 2,4-D (an herbicide) is applied annually at the rate of 4 million pounds (1.8 million kg) to residential lawns (USGAO/RCED, 1990).

*Factors Driving Increased Use of Herbicides*
In addition to their ease of application and their effectiveness as weed deterrents, two other factors are driving the increased use of herbicides: (1) resistance of weeds to herbicides leading to applications of additional products; and (2) the sensitivity of non-target plants requiring the application of herbicide safeners to protect non-target species. Kits are now available to test weed resistance to six triazine herbicides; atrazine, cyanazine, metribuzin, prometryne, propazine, and simazine (Pesticide News, 1991).

Despite the increasing selectivity of new herbicides to specific weeds, certain crops require the application of herbicide safeners to avoid herbicide injury to botanically related crop plants. In other words, safeners are compounds with antidotal activity to herbicides. In general, safeners act as either "bioregulators" regulating the amount of herbicide which reaches target areas within the plant or as "antagonists" of herbicidal action at target areas (Hatzios, 1989a).

Herbicide safening was first discovered in 1947 when 2,4-D vapors were accidentally applied to tomato plants concurrently treated with the analog 2,4,6-T without causing the expected injuries (Hatzios, 1989b). Since then the safening potential of several growth regulating substances, fungicides, and other agrochemicals have been researched. Generally, crop safeners are growth regulators (such as auxins, CCC, and daminozide), fungicides (such as fenaminosulf), and herbicides (such as the s-triazines combined with urea) with antagonistic activity (Phatak and Vavrina, 1989). Safeners are marketed as prepackaged tank mixtures with a herbicide, or as components of pre-treated crop seeds. The use of safeners increases the number of active ingredients applied to a crop, and thus increases risks to wildlife and humans.

## INERT INGREDIENTS

Little is known about the inert ingredients which may constitute as much as 99% of a pesticide product, because state and federal laws protect confidentiality concerning pesticide statements of formula. Inert ingredients preserve or enhance the action of the active ingredient and serve as diluents for powerful active ingredients. Producers are not required to list the names of inert ingredients on product labels; they need only indicate their presence as combined percentage of total weight as a lumped figure. Approximately 50,000 pesticide products on the market today are composed of different mixtures of nearly 600 active ingredients and 1200 inert ingredients (Krewski et al., 1991). In some instances, active pesticide ingredients are listed as inert ingredients when they are not the primary active ingredient in a product.

## EXPOSURE PATHWAYS

In the past, the primary exposure pathways to herbicides and fungicides were considered to be via the consumption of treated foods and contaminated groundwater. Of the total "worst case" risk of pesticide exposure from food intake, about 80% is from fresh foods and 20% is from processed foods. Fungicides alone constitute 55% of the 80% of pesticide risk in fresh foods and 78% of the 20% of pesticide risk in processed foods (Benbrook, C., 1991, pers. comm.). Nearly 300 pesticide active ingredients used in commercial agricultural products are tolerated as food residues under USEPA regulations (Krewski et al., 1991).

According to a USEPA survey conducted between 1988 and 1990, 10.4% of the nation's community water supply wells and 4.2% of its rural domestic water supply wells contain detectable levels of one or more pesticides (USEPA, 1990). The two most commonly detected pesticides were the herbicides Dacthal, as DCPA acid metabolites, and atrazine. The herbicides alachlor, atrazine, and simazine, as well as some insecticides, were detected in rural domestic water supply wells at levels which exceeded health-based limits (USEPA, 1990). The EBDC (ethylenebisdithiocarbamate) fungicide metabolite, ethylene thiourea (ETU), was also detected in rural domestic wells and the banned fungicide, hexachlorobenzene (HCB), was detected in community public drinking water wells at levels exceeding health based limits (USEPA, 1990). The use of active ingredients on fields in areas of high groundwater vulnerability, combined with the solubility of herbicides, exacerbates the problem of human and animal exposure to contaminated drinking water. A study of the distribution of the herbicides atrazine, simazine, alachlor, and metolachlor in Connecticut showed that although the concentrations of the surface samples were much higher than those in the deeper samples, the herbicides were detected continuously in the soil from the surface to the water table at 7.5 ft (Huang and Frink, 1989). Since herbicide degradation is reduced in deeper soil, the herbicides detected in deep soils can leach into groundwater over several years, without the addition of newer applications. For this reason, surface water contamination is seasonal in accordance with herbicide application periods because chemicals are in contact with the degradation processes of air, sun, and bacteria, but contaminated groundwater, removed from these degradation factors, is a constant source of exposure.

Recent data, however, provides evidence of contamination beyond food residues and contaminated water. The US Geologic Survey reports the finding of herbicides in rainwater samples in 23 states. Its data suggest that the triazine and acetanilide herbicides volatilize in large quantities to the atmosphere after application, with the greatest volatilization occurring "...during a 1- or 2-month period after spring application of the chemicals." (SETAC News, 1991, p.9). Precipitation inputs of herbicides into the Great Lakes include methoxychlor and hexachlorobenzene (Murphy, 1984). Atrazine was reported in rainwater as early as 1977 (Wu, 1981) and the herbicides atrazine, simazine, alachlor, metolachlor, and pendimethalin have also been detected in fog (Glotfelty et al., 1987).

The occurrence of this "pesticide rain" supports similar reports of long-range at-mospheric migration of chemicals such as toxaphene, HCB, hexachlorocyclo-hexanes (HCHs), polychlorinated biphenyls (PCBs), chlordanes, DDT, alkylben-zenes, polycyclic aromatic hydrocarbons and other chlorinated hydrocarbons, and technical chlordane constituents (Hites et al., 1980; Smith and Bomberger, 1980; Rapaport et al., 1985; Andersson et al., 1988; Bidleman et al., 1989; Czuczwa et al., 1988; Rapaport and Eisenreich, 1988; Swackhamer and Hites, 1988; Gregor and Gummer, 1989). Although no such data were found for herbicides or fungi-cides (except hexachlorobenzene (HCB)), quantifiable levels of polycyclic aro-matic hydrocarbons, polychlorinated biphenyls, and other chlorinated hydrocar-bons were found in rain and snow samples in the Great Lakes Region, the Canadian Arctic, and Switzerland (Gregor and Gummer, 1989; Czuczwa et al., 1988; Strachan et al., 1980). There are no federal standards for rainwater contam-ination.

A 1991 USEPA House Dust/Infant Pesticides Exposure Study, which checked for residues of 30 common household pesticides in house dust and yard soil of nine homes, suggests that the ingestion of house dust by small children may be more of a problem than their respiratory exposure to pesticides (Lewis et al., 1991). The pesticides were found in carpet dust and indoor air. The herbicides detected during the study included Dacthal, and the fungicides, captan, chlorothalonil, and folpet. Researchers concluded that "For the most prevalent pesticides, house dust levels tended to be higher than those found in outdoor soil." (Lewis et al., 1991, p.8). The study also noted that residues of many pesticides were found on residential property even when there had been no known use of them on the premises. Since children spend more time on the floor than the average individual, one estimate noted that children under age five swallow 2.5 times more soil around the home than do adults, but only have about 20% of the body weight of an adult (Hawley, 1985). More general exposure pathways including dermal absorption and inhalation, and the accumulation of residues from processed foods and soils, are not well researched. In addition, increased exposure may result from recreational experiences in areas such as national forests where large quantities of herbicides are used by the Forest Service (see Bason and Colborn, Chapter 19). No studies considering cumulative exposure from all pathways could be found. Studies considering exposure to herbicide mixtures were also not available.

## INDICES OF EXCEEDANCE OF RELEASE OVER RECOMMENDED DAILY DOSES

It is evident that exposure involves many pathways, some of which could result in greater exposure during a short period of time than dietary intake. However, exposure data are scarce and are often limited to a single exposure pathway. In lieu of the necessary information to provide multiple exposure estimates, we turned to the information that was available and converted annual use figures into a crude estimate of exceedances of release over recommended doses based on a daily per capita basis (Table 1). Exceedances of recommended daily exposure to an herbicide active ingredient were calculated for the average 70 kg (154 pound) adult male on a daily basis using estimates of the total annual amount of a particular active ingredient used in a particular state (Gianessi and Puffer, 1991a); the 1988 population estimates of that state (US Bureau of the Census, 1990); and the suggested advisory levels (mg/kg/body weight/day) of human exposure to the particular herbicide (Eisler, 1989; USEPA, 1987b; USEPA, 1988a,c,f). Advisory levels, such as ADI (Acceptable Daily Intake, also known as the reference dose or RfD) and PADI (Provisional Acceptable Daily Intake) represent a daily dose that is presumed to present no appreciable health risk over a lifetime exposure of 70 years based on currently available toxicological data and risk assessment methods. To reach the most realistic figures possible, daily exceedances were not only calculated on a yearly basis (365 days of exposure) but also for 60 days out of the year, since herbicides are used primarily in the spring over a two month period and, more specifically, during the planting period (USGS, 1990).

Herbicides used annually in large amounts and for which Federal health advisories have been issued, were chosen for this exercise. Fungicides were not used for this analysis since annual use per state were not available. States using

**TABLE 1.**   **Indices of exceedance of selected herbicides on a statewide basis**

| HERBICIDE | PADI | STATE<br>Pounds used | INDEX<br>(70 kg adult) |
|---|---|---|---|
| 2,4-D | 0.003 | Texas<br>3,854,826 | 1356*<br>8248** |
| | | Iowa<br>1,223,237 | 2557*<br>15552** |
| Atrazine | 0.0375 | Illinois<br>8,503,397 | 347*<br>2111** |
| | | Iowa<br>5,583,992 | 934*<br>5680** |
| Hexazinone | 0.033 | California<br>55,974 | 1.1*<br>6.5** |
| | | Wisconsin<br>53,751 | 6*<br>36** |
| Picloram | 0.07 | Texas<br>904,969 | 14*<br>83** |
| | | New Mexico<br>541,250 | 91*<br>555** |
| Trifluralin | 0.01 | Texas<br>3,818,844 | 403*<br>2451** |
| | | Iowa<br>3,673,498 | 2303*<br>14012** |

Index of Exceedance =  $\dfrac{X \times 454g \times 1000}{365(\text{or } 60) \times Y \times 70kg \times PADI}$

X = number of pounds of active ingredient used per year/state.
Y = 1988 state population estimates (US Bureau of the Census, 1990).

Provisional Acceptable Daily Intake (PADI) is in mg/kg body weight per day and is based on a 70 kg adult. The amounts used are 1989-1990 figures in pounds of active ingredient (Gianessi & Puffer, 1991a).

(*) ratio based on the assumption that herbicides are applied evenly over 365 days. For 365 days of the year, recommended exposure(PADI) is exceeded by this amount.

(**) ratio based on a more realistic assumption that herbicides are applied over a 60 day planting period. For 60 days of the year, recommended exposure (PADI) is exceeded by this amount.

the largest quantities of a chosen herbicide (Texas for 2,4-D, picloram, and trifluralin; Illinois for atrazine; California for hexazinone) were selected for this analysis. Since these states have large metropolitan centers whose dense populations can bias exceedance estimates per person, several states with more evenly distributed populations were also chosen (Iowa, Wisconsin, and New Mexico). Based on releases evenly distributed over the year (365 days), hexazinone releases exceed the suggested advisory levels 1.1 times per individual in California whereas 2,4-D exceeds it 2557 times per individual in Iowa. Based on a more realistic release schedule where the chemicals are used only over a 60 day period, calculations suggest that 6.5, in California, to 15,552 times, in Iowa, the suggested health advisory levels of hexazinone and 2,4-D, respectively, are released per individual (Table 1).

The calculated daily exceedance estimates should be viewed with the following caveats in mind: herbicide use is not evenly distributed throughout the state and release is not necessarily equivalent to exposure; the suggested advisory levels are based on cancer risk and do not consider developmental effects; the calculated exceedances are for a single herbicide and do not reflect concomitant releases of various herbicides. In addition, this methodology is limited to a single herbicide and a single exposure pathway (oral intake) because the ADI does not take into account that individual exposure differs with age, lifestyle, type and quantity of food consumed, and location of occupation and residence.

Additionally, advisory levels cannot represent continuous and simultaneous exposure to low doses of numerous toxicants through various exposure pathways. Nor do they consider the possibility of bioaccumulation in both animal and human tissues. Because tolerance levels and reference doses are based on the average 70 kg (154 pound) adult male, they do not offer adequate protection to infants and children who tend to have a less diverse diet while consuming larger quantities of a particular food type. A review of the 1977-78 and the 1987-88 Nationwide Food Consumption Survey revealed that the inadequate sampling of subpopulations such as infants and pregnant women prohibited the precise estimation of their dietary exposure to pesticide residues thereby invalidating tolerance levels for this population group (USGAO/RCED, 1991). Furthermore, as noted earlier, children under five years of age swallow 2.5 times more soil around the home than do adults—soil and dust which could contain pesticide residues (Hawley, 1985). Thus it seems reasonable to assume that tolerance levels and reference doses do not adequately protect developing children as they do not incorporate all exposure pathways into their estimates and do not take into consideration that children ingest more pesticides per pound of body weight than the average adult.

It could be argued that the half life of some of the chemicals mentioned in this paper reduces their hazard to wildlife and humans. However, timing of exposure during a vulnerable window of time can have a profound effect on an embryo (see Peterson et al., Chapter 10). Peterson demonstrated that neither long term exposure nor preconception bioaccumulation were necessary to change the course of sexual development of male rats exposed *in utero* to dioxin.

## KNOWN HEALTH EFFECTS

The human health effects of herbicide and fungicide exposure generally are not well known because of the proprietary nature of health effects information and the shortage of publications in the peer reviewed literature. An extensive literature search yielded studies designed to determine the carcinogenicity and acute toxicity of herbicides and fungicides and few studies exploring multigenerational developmental effects resulting from hormonal activity. Several herbicides and fungicides have been associated in a number of laboratory species with reproductive and endocrinological changes in the offspring of parental animals exposed before and/or during pregnancy (Table 2). Although the majority of the studies were animal based, several observations of effects in humans following occupational or accidental exposure were found.

**TABLE 2**  Reproductive and endocrinological effects associated with herbicides and fungicides in the literature

| PESTICIDES | REPRODUCTIVE IMPAIRMENT** | TARGET ORGAN DYSFUNCTION | REFERENCES*** |
|---|---|---|---|
| | | | |
| **HERBICIDES** | | | |
| | | | |
| 2,4-D* | ◊4, 5, 7, 9      Δ12 | ◊ thyroid | 4, 11, 32 |
| Alachlor* | ◊12 | ◊ testes (possible) | 8, 11 |
| Amitrole | ◊1, 3, 5, 7, 10, 11 | ◊ thyroid | 16, 20, 22, 27 |
| Atrazine* | ◊1, 3, 7, 10 | ◊ ovaries, pituitary, prostate | 2, 11, 17, 25 |
| Trifluralin* | ◊1, 2, 5, 7, 11 | ◊ pituitary, testes, thyroid | 5, 6, 7, 30, 34 |
| | | | |
| **FUNGICIDES** | | | |
| | | | |
| Hexachlorobenzene | ◊1, 2, 3, 5, 7, 9, 11   Δ1 | ◊ testes, thyroid   Δ thyroid | 1, 9, 11, 15, 21, 26, 28 |
| Mancozeb (ETU) | ◊1, 3, 6, 10, 11 | ◊ Δ   prostate, thyroid | 11, 19, 29 |
| Maneb (ETU) | ◊1, 2, 3, 4, 6, 7, 10, 11 | ◊ ovaries, testes, thyroid | 3, 11, 13, 14, 18, 19, 23, 24, 32 |
| Metiram-Complex (ETU) | ◊8, 12 | ◊ Δ   thyroid | 33 |
| Zineb (ETU) | ◊1, 2, 6, 10 | ◊ thyroid | 3, 11, 14, 18 |
| Ziram | ◊1, 6, 7, 10 | ◊ testes, thyroid | 11, 12 |
| Ethylene thiourea (ETU) | ◊1, 8, 12 | ◊ Δ   pituitary, thyroid | 18, 29, 32 |

◊ = laboratory animal      Δ = human

** 
| 1 | Abnormal Development | 7 | Reduced Growth |
| 2 | Abortion/Stillbirths | 8 | Reduced Litter Size |
| 3 | Hormone Disruption | 9 | Reduced Survival to Weaning |
| 4 | Postimplantation Mortality | 10 | Resorption |
| 5 | Reduced Birth Weight | 11 | Retardation of Development |
| 6 | Reduced Fertility | 12 | Temporary Loss of Sexual Potency/Performance |

Cells not marked do not necessarily mean there is no effects; only that no citation was found. Products with an asterisk (*) were among the top ten herbicides in highest use, by weight, from 1989-1990 (Gianessi & Puffer, 1991a). No citations for endocrinological and reproductive effects were found for high-use products not on the list.

*** High dose studies except for atrazine, metiram-complex, and ziram. High and low dose studies for amitrole and hexachlorobenzene.

We were unable to find many citations related to the endocrine effects of herbicides and fungicides. Most of what we found was published between the early 1950s to mid-1970s, probably about the time when these ingredients were first introduced. Most studies used a high-dose regimen to determine obvious, gross end points, such as cancer or mortality. High mortality in the studies and insufficient description of methodology preclude reaching a conclusion concerning the endocrine disruptive effect of these chemicals. However, several of these reports inferred possible endocrine disruptive effects such as thyroid and testicular damage, gross fetal abnormalities, and delayed or impaired growth. The studies were not designed to look for these effects specifically but the effects were reported as observations. With few exceptions no recent citations could be found other than USEPA reregistration documents that focused on cancer, genotoxicity, acute toxicity, and gross reproductive and developmental effects, functional deficits in offspring were not addressed. A few lower-dose studies were found for the herbicides atrazine and molinate, and the fungicides hexachlorobenzene, metiram-complex, and ziram (see Table 2).

A summary of the reproductive and endocrinological effects associated with herbicides and fungicides in laboratory animals include impairments prior to birth such as abortion, resorption of fetuses, postimplantation mortality, and gross abnormal development (Table 2). Others include impairments during early life which can affect survival and reproductive potential, such as reduced birth weight, reduced survival to weaning, retardation of development, reduced fertility, hormone disruption, and temporary loss of sexual potency. Other effects on reproductive potential in both parental animals and offspring include lesions, hemorrhage, atrophy, hyperplasia, and changes in morphology of the reproductive organs.

Documented human effects of exposure to a herbicide include the temporary loss of sexual potency following 2,4-D exposure (Berwick, 1970). The effects of EBDC (ethylenebisdithiocarbamate) fungicides such as mancozeb, maneb, metiram-complex, and zineb probably result from their common metabolite, ethylene thiourea (ETU) (USEPA 1987a, 1988d,e).

In addition to the above reproductive and endocrinological effects, weight loss, decreased food consumption, depressed growth, and immune system effects have been reported in laboratory animals exposed to herbicides (Hodge et al., 1956; Tjalve, 1974). Others, like alachlor, amitrole, and hexachlorobenzene, cause dose related alterations in cytochrome P-450 activity (Leslie et al., 1989; Raisfeld et al., 1970; Stenger and Johnson, 1972; Grant et al., 1974).

Only in the case of HCB, banned as a fungicide in 1985, were we able to locate an appreciable amount of information concerning human health effects because of a severe poisoning incident in Turkey. HCB is a ubiquitous unwanted by-product of the manufacture of approximately 135 pesticide ingredients, and other manufacturing processes that use chlorine (Tobin, 1986). It was found in 100% of human adipose tissue samples nationwide in the US in 1983 (Robinson et al., 1986) and in 100% of breast milk samples nationwide in Canada (Davies and Mes, 1987; see Thomas and Colborn, Chapter 21).

HCB can cause porphyria cutanea tarda (PCT), manifested by hepatic disease, photosensitivity, vesicular or bullous skin rash, and skin fragility (Jones and Chelsky, 1986). A condition called "pink sore" was noted in Turkey in children under the age of 1 year whose mothers had unknowingly ingested HCB-treated seed wheat during gestation and lactation, and in most instances developed PCT (Peters et al., 1987). The children suffered weakness and convulsions leading to 95% mortality. This was accompanied by a large number of stillbirths. Twenty years after the incident (1955-1959) about half the exposed offspring exhibited hyperpigmentation, scarring, pinched faces, hypertrichosis, enlarged thyroid, and arthritis, as well as continued porphyria.

HCB, like Zineb (Kvitnitskaya et al., 1971), poses a direct risk to developing embryos and fetuses by crossing both laboratory animal and human placentae (Ando et al., 1985; ATSDR, 1990). In humans it is preferentially transferred from maternal blood to fetal cord blood (ratio 0.5) (Bush et al., 1984). Postmenopausal women, the geriatric population, and the developing fetus and neonate are also at increased risk because HCB compromises the mechanisms that maintain calcium homeostasis (Andrews et al., 1988).

## A CASE STUDY: THE GOVERNMENT'S ROLE

Under the Federal Insecticide, Fungicide, and Rodenticide (FIFRA) Amendments of 1988, USEPA must conduct the reregistration of older pesticide products using newer evaluation techniques within 9 years. Of the 32 most widely used lawn care products requiring reregistration, not one had been completely reassessed as of 1990 (USGAO/RCED, 1990). A study conducted by the United States General Accounting Office showed that professional pesticide applicators make false and misleading claims that the products they use are safe and nontoxic (USGAO/RCED, 1990). Yet USEPA has no authority over pesticide applicator claims.

The potential dangers of false claims are almost inconsequential when one considers that some chemicals are registered for use despite a lack of basic health and safety data. A case in point is the active ingredient DCPA, dimethyl tetrachloroterephthalate, otherwise known as Dacthal. First registered under FIFRA in 1958 for use on turf grasses, Dacthal was next registered for food-crop use in 1962. As of 1988, with 162 DCPA products registered under FIFRA and 15 pending registration, the total annual usage of the active ingredient was approximately 3.2-4.7 million pounds (1.5-2.1 million kg). Also as of 1988, no multigenerational or developmental studies had been conducted on DCPA. Information regarding possible exposure pathways was lacking (i.e., dermal, inhalation) and no sufficient environmental fate and bioaccumulation studies existed. As a result, the USEPA Reregistration Guide to DCPA (1988b) states that because of the "...numerous data gaps..." (p.8) that existed for DCPA, "...few definitive conclusions..." (p.8) could be made and "...only a hazard assessment will be presented for DCPA." (p.8). It further stated that "Because this assessment is based on the data available, it is subject to change." (p.8) (USEPA, 1988b). Despite these limitations, USEPA continued to allow the use of DCPA for all formerly registered uses of the pesticide with the precautions delineated in the statement.

Dacthal is only one example of how chemicals are released into the environment without adequate safety review that requires multigenerational, reproductive, and environmental fate studies. Not only is it important to rule out possible hormonal activity and developmental effects of Dacthal, but to also factor in the effects of 2,3,7,8-TCDD (dioxin) and HCB, both compounds known to cause developmental problems in laboratory animals. 2,3,7,8-TCDD and HCB are formed during the manufacture of technical Dacthal and remain as impurities at levels up to 0.1 ppb and 0.3% respectively (USEPA, 1988b).

This lack of basic information becomes more urgent when studies such as the 1990 USEPA survey of the nation's water-supply wells find Dacthal acid metabolites to be the most commonly detected pesticide in the nation's groundwater (USEPA, 1990). Since the 1988 USEPA review, Dacthal has been found in the tissues of trout and whitefish from Siskiwit Lake on Isle Royale in Lake Superior (Swackhamer and Hites, 1988). The discovery that Dacthal bioaccumulates in fish tissue at this remote site is in keeping with reports of herbicides and other pesticides being transported via the atmosphere.

Rather than a strong health and safety statement fully supported by multidisciplinary research, many registration and reregistration documents are merely a list of missing data and research needs. As with Dacthal, the process of reregistration falls short of its purpose—to acquire complete studies of a pesticide before its release into the environment and before it becomes widely dispersed and potentially detrimental to human, animal, and environmental health.

## CONCLUSION

In the past, a great deal of attention has focused on food residues and farm labour contact as the major sources of exposure to agricultural chemicals. Recent discoveries of frequent contamination of groundwater, surface water, and rain water with herbicides should prompt new concerns over exposure to wildlife and humans. In addition, the new knowledge of risk associated with transgenerational exposure via the mother, as described by Peterson and co-workers (Chapter 10), should become part of these considerations as well. For in this case, a female needs only one exposure "hit" at a critical stage during gestation or the egg laying period and her offspring can be severely affected. The large quantities of agricultural chemicals in production and use (see Bason and Colborn, Chapter 19) also support the argument that multigeneration studies must become a part of the pesticide registration process.

The lack of information concerning reproductive and endocrinological effects encountered during this study reiterates the need for an open-book policy when dealing with chemicals that have the potential for widespread distribution in the biosphere. Although limited information is available on the health effects of herbicides and fungicides, enough data exist to raise questions concerning their potential to disrupt the endocrine system.

For this reason, it is imperative to upgrade testing protocols for all pesticides, including herbicides and fungicides, beyond traditional cancer and mortality studies. Broader pesticide management must include multigenerational reproductive and developmental testing for hormonal activity to assure the safety of a pesticide product. As the number of potential exposure pathways increases with increased use, the establishment of cumulative daily estimates of exposure becomes necessary. Future research should not only consider continual low-dose exposure which could result in bioaccumulation, but also continual low-dose exposure to a large number of products simultaneously, taking additivity, antagonism, and synergy into consideration. Other parameters of concern beyond food residues must be considered when assessing exposure during application and use, and following inadvertent release into the environment. And most important, as described by Peterson et al., Chapter 10, there must be an assurance that a single low- or/high-dose exposure "hit" during a critical window of time throughout embryo and fetal development will have no effect on the quality of life and future potential of *in utero* exposed offspring.

## REFERENCES

Andersson, O., Linder, C., Olsson, M., Reutergardh, L., Uvemo, U., and Wideqvist, U. (1988). Spatial differences and temporal trends of organochlorine compounds in biota from the northwestern hemisphere. *Arch. Environ. Contam. Toxicol.*, **17**, 755-765.

Ando, M., Hirano, S. and Itoh, Y. (1985). Transfer of hexachlorobenzene (HCB) from mother to new-born baby through placenta and milk. *Arch. Toxicol.*, **56**, 195-200.

Andrews, J., Courtney, K., and Donaldson, W. (1988). Impairment of calcium homeostasis by hexachlorobenzene (HCB) exposure in Fischer 344 rats. *J. Toxicol. and Environ. Health*, **23**, 311-320.

ATSDR (Agency for Toxic Substances and Disease Registry). (1990). *Toxicological Profile for Hexachlorobenzene*. US Public Health Service. TP-90-17.

Bidleman, T.F., Patton, G.W., Walla, M.D., Hargrave, B.T., Vass, W.P., Erickson, P., Fowler, B., Scott, V., and Gregor, D.J. (1989). Toxaphene and other organochlorines in arctic ocean fauna: evidence for atmospheric delivery. *Arctic*, **42**(4), 307-313.

Brown, E.A. (1991). Fertile market for organic lawn-care products. *Christian Science Monitor*, May 23, 1991.

Bush, B., Snow, J., and Koblintz, R. (1984). Polychlorobiphenyl (PCB) congeners, p,p'-DDE, and hexachlorobenzene in maternal and fetal cord blood from mothers in upstate New York. *Arch. Environ. Contam. Toxicol.*, **13**, 517-527.

Czuczwa, J., Leuenberger, C., and Giger, W. (1988). Seasonal and temporal changes of organic compounds in rain and snow. *Atmospheric Environment*, **22**(5), 907-916.

Davies, D. and Mes, J. (1987). Comparison of the residue levels of some organochlorine compounds in breast milk of the general and indigenous Canadian populations. *Bull. Environ. Contam. Toxicol.*, **39**, 743-749.

Eisler, R. (1989). *Atrazine Hazards to Fish, Wildlife, and Invertebrates: A Synoptic Review*. US Fish and Wildlife Service, Biological Report 85(1.18), Contaminant Hazard Reviews Report No. 18.

Gianessi, L.P. and Puffer, C.A. (1991a). *Herbicide Use in the United States: National Summary Report*. Quality of the Environment Division, Resources for the Future, Inc., pp. 1-128.

Gianessi, L.P. and Puffer, C.A. (1991b). Inadequacy of scientific and economic data in pesticide benefits analyses. *Resources*, Resources for the Future, Inc., Summer 1991, No. 104, pp. 14-17.

Glotfelty, D.E., Seiber, J.N., and Liljedahl, L.A. (1987). Pesticides in Fog. *Nature*(Lond.), **325**, 602-605.

Grant, D.L., Iverson, F., Hatina, G.V., and Villeneuve, D.C. (1974). Effects of hexachlorobenzene on liver porphyrin levels and microsomal enzymes in the rat. *Environ. Physiol. Biochem.*, **4**, 159-165.

Gregor, D.J. and Gummer, W.D. (1989). Evidence of atmospheric transport and deposition of organochlorine pesticides and polychlorinated biphenyls in canadian arctic snow. *Environ. Sci. Technol.*, **23**(5), 561-565.

Hatzios, K.K. (1989a). Mechanisms of action of herbicide safeners: an overview. In *Crop Safeners for Herbicides*, ed. K.K. Hatzios and R.E. Hoagland. Academic Press, Inc., San Diego, CA., pp. 65-93.

Hatzios, K.K. (1989b). Development of herbicide safeners: industrial and university perspectives. In *Crop Safeners for Herbicides*, ed. K.K. Hatzios and R.E. Hoagland. Academic Press, Inc., San Diego, CA., pp. 3-38.

Hawley, J.K. (1985). Assessment of health risk from exposure to contaminated soil. *Risk Analysis*, **5**, 289.

Hites, R.A., Laflamme, R.E., and Windsor, J.G. (1980). Polycyclic aromatic hydrocarbons in the marine environment: gulf of Maine sediments and nova Scotia soils. In *Hydrocarbons and Halogenated Hydrocarbons in the Aquatic Environment*, ed. B.K. Afghan and D. Mackay. Plenum Press, New York, pp. 397-404.

Hodge, H.C., Maynard, E.A., Downs, W., Coye, R.D., and Steadman, L.T. (1956). Chronic oral toxicity of ferric dimethyldithiocarbamate (ferbam) and zinc dimethyldithiocarbamate (ziram). *J. Pharmacol. Exp. Ther.*, **118**(2), 174-181.

Huang, L.Q. and Frink, C.R. (1989). Distribution of atrazine, simazine, alachlor, and metolachlor in soil profiles in Connecticut. *Bull. Environ. Contam. Toxicol.*, **43**, 159-164.

Jones, R. and Chelsky, M. (1986). Further discussion concerning porphyria cutanea tarda and TCDD exposure. *Arch. Environ. Health*, **41**(2), 100-103.

Krewski, D., Wargo, J., and Rizek, R. (1991). Risks of dietary exposure to pesticides in infants and children. In *Monitoring Dietary Intakes*, ed. I. Macdonald. Springer-Verlag, Berlin Heidelberg, pp. 75-89.

Leslie, C., Reidy, G.F., and Stacey, N.H. (1989). Effect of ofurace, oxadixyl, and alachlor on xenobiotic biotransformation in the rat liver. *Arch. Environ. Contam. Toxicol.*, **18**, 876-880.

Lewis, R.G., Bond, A.E., Fortmann, R.C., Sheldon, L.S., and Camann, D.E. (1991). Determination of routes of exposure of infants and toddlers to household pesticides: A pilot study to test methods. Paper presented at the 84th Annual Meeting and Exhibition, Vancouver, British Columbia, 16-21 June.

Murphy, T.J. (1984). Atmospheric inputs of chlorinated hydrocarbons to the Great Lakes. In *Toxic Contaminants in the Great Lakes*, ed. J.O. Nriagu and M.S. Simmons. John Wiley and Sons, New York, pp.53-76.

Peters, H., Cripps, D., Gocmen, A., Bryan, G., Erturk, E., and Morris, C. (1987). Turkish epidemic hexachlorobenzene porphyria, a 30 year study. *Ann. New York Acad. Sci.*, **514**, 183-190.

*Pesticide and Toxic Chemical News.* (1991). Pesticides in house dust hazard described in USEPA-er's study. May 1, 1991, pp. 11-12.

*Pesticide News.* (1991). Small doses. October, p. 14.

Phatak, S.C. and Vavrina, C.S. (1989). Growth regulators, fungicides, and other agrochemicals as herbicide safeners. In *Crop Safeners for Herbicides*, ed. K.K. Hatzios and R.E. Hoagland. Academic Press, Inc., San Diego, CA., pp. 299-313.

Pimentel, D., McLaughlin, L., Zepp, A., Lakitan, B., Kraus, T., Kleinman, P., Vancini, F., Roach, W.J., Graap, E., Keeton, W.S., and Selig, G. (1991). Environmental and economic effects of reducing pesticide use. *Bioscience*, 41(6), 402-409.

Raisfeld, I.H., Bacchin, P., Hutterer, F., and Schaffner, F. (1970). The effect of 3-amino-1,2,4-triazole on the phenobarbital-induced formation of hepatic microsomal membranes. *Molecular Pharmacology*, 6, 231-239.

Rapaport, R.A., Urban, N.R., Capel, P.D., Baker, J.E., Looney, B.B., Eisenreich, S.J., and Gorham, E. (1985). "New" DDT inputs to north America: atmospheric deposition. *Chemosphere*, 14(9), 1167-1173.

Rapaport, R.A. and Eisenreich, S.J. (1988). Historical atmospheric inputs of high molecular weight chlorinated hydrocarbons to eastern north America. *Environ. Sci. Technol.*, 22, 931-941.

Robinson, P.E., Leczynski, B.A., Kutz, F.W., and Remmers, J.C. (1986). An evaluation of hexachlorobenzene body-burden levels in the general population of the USA. In *Hexachlorobenzene: Proceedings of an International Symposium*, ed. C. Morris and J. Cabral. IARC, Lyon, France, pp. 183-192.

SETAC News (The Society of Environmental Toxicology and Chemistry News). (1991). Government and regulatory affairs committee. Vol. 11, No. 4, pp. 9.

Smith, J.H. and Bomberger, D.C. (1980). Prediction of volatilization rates of chemicals in water. In *Hydrocarbons and Halogenated Hydrocarbons in the Aquatic Environment*, ed. B.K. Afghan and D. Mackay. Plenum Press, New York, pp. 445-452.

Stenger and Johnson. (1972). Modifying effects of 3 amino 1,2,4-triazole on phenobarbitol changes in rat liver. *Exp. Mol. Pathol.*, 16, 147-157.

Strachan, W.M.J., Huneault, H., Schertzer, W.M., and Elder, F.C. (1980). Organochlorines in precipitation in the great lakes region. In *Hydrocarbons and Halogenated Hydrocarbons in the Aquatic Environment*, ed. B.K. Afghan and D. Mackay. Plenum Press, New York, pp. 387-396.

Swackhamer, D.L. and Hites, R.A. (1988). Occurrence and bioaccumulation of organochlorine compounds in fishes from Siskiwit Lake, Isle Royale, Lake Superior. *Environ. Sci. Technol.*, 22(5), 543-548.

Tjalve, H. (1974). Fetal uptake and embryogenetic effects of aminotriazole in mice. *Arch. Toxicol.*, 33, 41-48.

Tobin, P. (1986). Known and potential sources of hexachlorobenzene. In *Hexachlorobenzene: Proceedings of an International Symposium*, ed. C.R. Morris and J.R.P. Cabral. International Agency for Research on Cancer, Lyon, pp. 3-11.

US Bureau of the Census. (1990). *Statistical Abstract of the United States: 1990 (110th edition).* Washington, DC.

USEPA (United States Environmental Protection Agency). (1987a). *Guidance for the Reregistration of Pesticide Products Containing Mancozeb as the Active Ingredient.* Office of Pesticides and Toxic Substances, Washington, DC.

USEPA (United States Environmental Protection Agency). (1987b). *Guidance for the Reregistration of Pesticide Products Containing Trifluralin as the Active Ingredient.* Office of Pesticides and Toxic Substances, Washington, DC.

USEPA (United States Environmental Protection Agency). (1988a). *Guidance for the Reregistration of Pesticide Products Containing 2,4-dichlorophenoxyacetic acid (2,4-D) as the Active Ingredient.* Office of Pesticides and Toxic Substances, Washington, DC, 540/RS-88-115.

USEPA (United States Environmental Protection Agency). (1988b). *Guidance for the Reregistration of Pesticide Products Containing Dimethyl Tetrachloro-terephthalate (DCPA) as the Active Ingredient.* Office of Pesticides and Toxic Substances, Washington, DC, 540/RS-88-084.

USEPA (United States Environmental Protection Agency). (1988c). *Guidance for the Reregistration of Pesticide Products Containing Hexazinone as the Active Ingredient.* Office of Pesticides and Toxic Substances, Washington, DC, 540/RS-88-081.

USEPA (United States Environmental Protection Agency). (1988d). *Guidance for the Reregistration of Pesticide Products Containing Maneb as the Active Ingredient.* Office of Pesticides and Toxic Substances, Washington, DC.

USEPA (United States Environmental Protection Agency). (1988e). *Guidance for the Reregistration of Pesticide Products Containing Metiram-Complex as the Active Ingredient.* Office of Pesticides and Toxic Substances, Washington, DC.

USEPA (United States Environmental Protection Agency). (1988f). *Guidance for the Reregistration of Pesticide Products Containing Picloram as the Active Ingredient.* Office of Pesticides and Toxic Substances, Washington, DC, 540/RS-88-132.

USEPA (United States Environmental Protection Agency). (1990). *National Pesticide Survey: Summary Results of EPA's National Survey of Pesticides in Drinking Water Wells.* Office of Water, Office of Pesticides and Toxic Substances, Washington, DC.

USGAO/RCED (United States General Accounting Office, Resources, Community, and Economic Development Division). (1990). *Lawn Care Pesticides, Risks Remain Uncertain While Prohibited Safety Claims Continue.* GAO/RCED-90-134, pp. 1-24.

USGAO/RCED (United States General Accounting Office, Resources, Community, and Economic Development Division). (1991). *Pesticides, Food Consumption Data of Little Value to Estimate Some Exposures.* GAO/RCED-91-125, pp. 1-20.

USGS (United States Geological Survey). (1990). Atrazine in stream water post 1989 application. Briefing Sheet to Accompany Exhibit No. W-401-90. unpublished.

Wu, T.L. (1981). Atrazine in estuarine water and the aerial deposition of atrazine into Rhode River, Maryland. *Water Air Soil Pollut.*, **15**, 173-184.

## REFERENCES FOR TABLE 2

1. Arnold, D., Moodie, C., Charbonneau, S., Grice, H., McGuire, P., Bryce, F., Collins, B., Zawidzka, Z., Krewski, D., Nera, E., and Munro, I. (1985). Long-term toxicity of hexachlorobenzene in the rat and the effect of dietary vitamin A. *Fd. Chem. Toxic.*, **23**(9), 779-793.

2. Babic-Gojmerac, T., Kniewald, Z. and Kniewald, J. (1989). Testosterone metabolism in neuroendocrine organs in male rats under atrazine and deethylatrazine influence. *J. Steroid Biochem.*, **33**(1), 141-146.

3. Bankowska, J., Bojanowska, A., Komorowska-Malewska, W., Krawcynski, K., Majle, T., Syrowatka, T., and Wiakrowska, B. (1970). The studies on the influence of zineb and maneb on the functional state of the thyroid gland and some related enzymatic systems. *Rocz. Panstw. Zakl. Hig.*, **21**, 117-127. (in Polish).

4. Berwick, P. (1970). 2,4-Dichlorophenoxyacetic acid poisoning in man. *Jama*, **214**(6), 1114-1117.

5. Couch, J.A. (1984). Histopathology and enlargement of the pituitary of a teleost exposed to the herbicide trifluralin. *J. of Fish Diseases*, **7**, 157-163.
6. Couch, J.A., Courtney, L.A., and Foss, S.S. (1981). Laboratory evaluation of marine fishes as carcinogen assay subjects. In *Phyletic Approaches to Cancer*, ed. C.J. Dawe et al., Japan Sci. Soc. Press, Tokyo, pp. 125-139.
7. Couch, J.A., Winstead, J.T., Hansen, D.J., and Goodman, L.R. (1979). Vertebral dysplasia in young fish exposed to the herbicide trifluralin. *J. of Fish Diseases*, **2**, 35-42.
8. Diamond, D.W., Scott, L.K, Forward, R.B., and Kirby-Smith, W. (1989). Respiration and osmoregulation of the estuarine crab, *Rhithropanopeus harrisii* (Gould): Effects of the herbicide, alachlor. *Comp. Biochem. Physiol.*, **93**A(2), 313-318.
9. Gocmen, A., Peters, H.A., Cripps, D.J., Bryan, G.T., and Morris, C.R. (1989). Hexachlorobenzene episode in Turkey. *Biomedical and Environ. Sci.*, **2**, 36-43.
10. Grant, D.L., Iverson, F., Hatina, G.V., and Villeneuve, D.C. (1974). Effects of hexachlorobenzene on liver porphyrin levels and microsomal enzymes in the rat. *Environ. Physiol. Biochem.*, **4**, 159-165.
11. Hayes, W.J. and Laws, E.R. (eds.). (1991). *Handbook of Pesticide Toxicology*, Vol. 1-3. Academic Press, Inc., San Diego, CA.
12. Hodge, H.C., Maynard, E.A., Downs, W., Coye, R.D., and Steadman, L.T. (1956). Chronic oral toxicity of ferric dimethyldithiocarbamate (ferbam) and zinc dimethyldithiocarbamate (ziram). *J. Pharmacol. Exp. Ther.*, **118**(2), 174-181.
13. Ivanova-Tchemischanska, L, Markov, D.V., and Dashev, G. (1971). Light and electron microscopic observations on rat thyroid after administration of some dithiocarbamates. *Environ. Res.*, **4**, 201-212.
14. Izmirova, N., Ismirov, I., and Ivanova, L. (1969). The effect of zineb and maneb on the isoenzymes of lactate dehydrogenase in the testes of rats. *C.R. Acad. Bulg. Sci.*, **22**, 225-227.
15. Jones, R. and Chelsky, M. (1986). Further discussion concerning porphyria cutanea tarda and TCDD exposure. *Arch. Environ. Health*, **41**(2), 100-103.
16. Jukes, T.H. and Shaffer, C.B. (1960). Antithyroid effects of aminotriazole. *Science*, **132**, 296.
17. Kniewald, J., Peruzovic, M., Gojmerac, T., Milkovic, K., and Kniewald, Z. (1987). Indirect influence of *s*-triazines on rat gonadotropic mechanism at early postnatal period. *J. Steroid Biochem.*, **27**, 1095-1100.
18. Laisi, A., Tuominen, R., Mannisto, P., Savolainen, K., and Mattila, J. (1985). The effect of maneb, zineb, and ethylenethiourea on the humoral activity of the pituitary- thyroid axis in rat. *Arch. Toxicol., Suppl.*, **8**, 253-258.
19. Larsson, K.S., Arnander, C., Cekanova, E., and Kjellberg, M. (1976). Studies of teratogenic effects of the dithiocarbamates maneb, mancozeb, and propineb. *Teratology*, **14**, 171-184.
20. Mayberry, W.E. (1968). Antithyroid effects of 3-amino-1, 2, 4-triazole (33367). *Proc. Soc. Exp. Biol. Med.*, **129**, 551-556.
21. Peters, H., Cripps, D., Gocmen, A., Bryan, G., Erturk, E., and Morris, C. (1987). Turkish epidemic hexachlorobenzene porphyria, a 30 year study. *Ann. New York Acad. Sci.*, **514**, 183-190.
22. Raisfeld, I.H., Bacchin, P., Hutterer, F., and Schaffner, F. (1970). The effect of 3-amino-1,2,4-triazole on the phenobarbital-induced formation of hepatic microsomal membranes. *Molecular Pharmacology*, **6**, 231-239.
23. Seidler, H., Hartig, M., and Lewerenz, H.J. (1975). The control of the function of the thyroid gland by means of radioactive iodine in the toxicological investigation of foreign substances. *Nahrung*, **19**, 715-726. (in German).

24. Shtenberg, A.I., Kirlich, A.E., and Orlova, N.V. (1969). Toxicological characteristics of maneb used in treatment of food crops. *Vopr. Pitan*, **28**, 66-72. (in Russian).

25. Simic, B., Kniewald, Z., Davies, J.E., and Kniewald, J. (1991). Reversibility of the inhibitory effect of atrazine and lindane on cytosol 5alpha-Dihydrotestosterone receptor complex formation in rat prostate. *Bull. Environ. Contam. Toxicol.*, **46**, 92-99.

26. Smith, A., Dinsdale, D., Cabral, J., and Wright, A. (1987). Goitre and wasting induced in hamsters by hexachlorobenzene. *Toxicology*, **60**(5), 343-349.

27. Tjalve, H. (1974). Fetal uptake and embryogenetic effects of aminotriazole in mice. *Arch. Toxicol.*, **33**, 41-48.

28. USEPA (United States Environmental Protection Agency). (1987a). *Hexachlorobenzene. Health Advisory Draft*. Office of Drinking Water, Washington, DC.

29. USEPA (United States Environmental Protection Agency). (1987b). *Guidance for the Reregistration of Pesticide Products Containing Mancozeb as the Active Ingredient*. Office of Pesticides and Toxic Substances, Washington, DC.

30. USEPA (United States Environmental Protection Agency). (1987c). *Guidance for the Reregistration of Pesticide Products Containing Trifluralin as the Active Ingredient*. Office of Pesticides and Toxic Substances, Washington, DC.

31. USEPA (United States Environmental Protection Agency). (1988a). *Guidance for the Reregistration of Pesticide Products Containing 2,4-dichloro-phenoxyacetic acid (2,4-D) as the Active Ingredient*. Office of Pesticides and Toxic Substances, Washington, DC, 540/RS-88-115.

32. USEPA (United States Environmental Protection Agency). (1988b). *Guidance for the Reregistration of Pesticide Products Containing Maneb as the Active Ingredient*. Office of Pesticides and Toxic Substances, Washington, DC.

33. USEPA (United States Environmental Protection Agency). (1988c). *Guidance for the Reregistration of Pesticide Products Containing Metiram-Complex as the Active Ingredient*. Office of Pesticides and Toxic Substances, Washington, DC.

34. Wells, D.E. and Cowan, A.A. (1982). Vertebral dysplasia in salmonids caused by the herbicide trifluralin. *Environmental Pollution (Series A)*, **29**, 249-260.

# ORGANOCHLORINE ENDOCRINE DISRUPTORS IN HUMAN TISSUE

**Kristin Bryan Thomas**
World Wildlife Fund, Washington, DC

**Theo Colborn**
World Wildlife Fund, Washington, DC
W. Alton Jones Foundation, Charlottesville, Virginia

## INTRODUCTION

Measurable residues of organochlorine pesticides, polychlorinated biphenyls (PCBs), polybrominated biphenyls (PBBs), polychlorinated dibenzodioxins (PCDDs), and polychlorinated dibenzofurans (PCDFs) are present in human tissues worldwide (Mes et al., 1982, 1986; Ahmad et al., 1988; Patterson et al., 1988; Thoma et al., 1990; Schecter, 1991; Sasaki et al., 1991). These contaminants share similar physical and chemical properties such as low vapor pressure, chemical stability, lipid solubility, and a slow rate of biotransformation and degradation. Because of these same properties, they also persist in the environment, bioaccumulate, and biomagnify within various food chains and food webs to eventually reach measurable concentrations in human tissue.

This chapter is a synthesis of reports from the last decade on concentrations of organochlorine contaminants in human reproductive tissues, adipose tissue, and blood from the general population worldwide, excluding industrial exposure (Table 1). Special consideration is given to human breast milk fat concentrations of those chemicals that have been shown to disrupt the endocrine system *in vivo* (Table 2). This chapter also focuses on recent findings of transgenerational health effects, expressed as loss of function that are not obvious and are difficult to measure in offspring of exposed adult animals and humans.

The purpose of this chapter is threefold: first to provide evidence that humans are exposed to chemicals capable of disrupting the endocrine system; second to demonstrate that each endocrine disrupting chemical appears to have its own mix of mechanism(s) of action and unique target sites; and third to provide insight into the difficulty of interpreting what exposure to these chemicals means. Only recently have researchers begun to understand the effects of these chemicals on functionality and have begun to develop parameters for measuring the results of parental exposure in offspring. It is this literature that this chapter reviews.

## BACKGROUND

A number of factors hinder comparisons between and among studies reporting on concentrations of contaminants in human tissue. For example, sample

1. Corresponding Author: Theo Colborn, World Wildlife Fund, 1250 Twenty Fourth Street, NW, Washington, DC 20037.

collection, storage, preparation (extraction and cleanup), chemical analyses, statistical, and mathematical analyses, and data interpretation vary among reports world wide. Consideration must be given to whether concentrations are reported on a whole weight or lipid basis; whether isomer- or congener-specific analyses were performed for components of complex mixtures; and whether the same analytical method was used in each study. For example, DDT can be analyzed colorimetrically as opposed to the more sensitive gas-liquid chromatography (GLC) multi-residue screening technique which yields very different results (Jensen and Slorach, 1991). Table 1 includes the various quantitative analyses used to measure human tissue concentrations from a number of geographical locations. In most instances, the more recent studies cited in this paper provide complete descriptions of the technology used, thereby making comparisons between reports feasible.

Recently, a number of generalities concerning the bioaccumulation and compartmentalization of organochlorine contaminants in human tissues have emerged as the result of new technologies capable of detecting chemicals at parts per trillion or less. With rare exceptions, levels of persistent organohalogens are about the same in milk, blood, adipose, and muscle tissue, when calculated on an extractable fat basis. Blood concentrations of these compounds, however, will vary depending on the mobilization from body fat and recent intake of the compounds (Humphrey, 1988; Jensen and Slorach, 1991). Mobilization of stored contaminants from adipose tissue takes place during starvation and lactation and as a result of disease. In general, individuals from many third world countries still using DDT have higher concentrations in their tissues than individuals in countries where DDT has been banned or restricted. Individuals in industrialized nations have higher levels of the industrial chemicals, PCBs, PCDDs, and PCDFs in their tissues than individuals in developing nations (Jensen and Slorach, 1991).

Long-term exposure to relatively small amounts of the organochlorine contaminants in Table 1 leads to the accumulation of considerable deposits in animal and human tissues (Calabrese, 1982; Humphrey, 1987, 1988; Subramanian et al., 1987; Norstrom et al., 1988). These contaminants have been associated with an array of harmful effects in laboratory animals, such as endocrine disruption (Table 2), immunotoxicity, neurotoxicity, carcinogenicity, metabolic disorders, and reproductive disorders (Street and Sharma, 1975; Rattner et al., 1984; Skene et al., 1989; Safe, 1990). In some instances, the disorders are expressed as loss of function in offspring resulting from maternal exposure (Kubiak et al., 1989; Sager et al., 1991; Peterson et al., Chapter 10). In humans, the transfer of organochlorine chemicals across the placenta to the fetus has been well documented, as has the transfer via breast milk to the new born (Ando et al., 1985; Roncevic et al., 1987; Rao and Banerji, 1988; Ron et al., 1988; Jacobson et al., 1989). The effects of chemicals in the developing offspring may be entirely different than the effects noted in mature individuals. In addition, what may be con

**TABLE 1.   Concentrations of organochlorine contaminants in human reproductive tissue, adipose tissue, and blood from the general population worldwide (See legend at end.)**

| Geographic Location Year of Sample Chemical | Number of Samples (% Positive) | Units Mean/SD | Standard Deviation | Range | Tissue | Case Information * | Quantification ** Analysis & Detection Limits | Reference |
|---|---|---|---|---|---|---|---|---|
| India, Bombay (1987) | | ppm | | | amniotic fluid | No history of exposure | GC-ECD | Rao, C.V., & S. Banerji (1988) |
| PCBs | 26 (100%) | 0.131 | 0.026 | 0.001-1.162 | | | | |
| Norway, Oslo (1981-82) | | ppb (ug/kg) | | | | No history of exposure | GLC-ECD | Skaare, J.U. et al. (1988) |
| HCB | 15 (100%) | 2 | 2 | | maternal serum/wet | | | |
| | 20 (90%) | 1 | 1 | | " " | Caesarean | 0.001 mg/kg (HCH) | |
| PCBs | 15 (93.3%) | 10 | 4 | | " " | Normal delivery | 0.002 mg/kg (PCBs) | |
| | 20 (100%) | 10 | 7 | | " " | Caesarean | | |
| p,p'-DDE | 15 (100%) | 19 | 21 | | " " | Normal delivery | 0.002 mg/kg (DDE) | |
| | 20 (100%) | 10 | 8 | | " " | Caesarean | | |
| beta-HCH | 15 (73.3%) | <1 | | | " " | Normal delivery | 0.001 mg/kg (b-HCH) | |
| | 20 (30%) | <1 | | | " " | Caesarean | | |
| HCB | 12 (83.3%) | 2 | 1 | | umbilical cord serum | Normal delivery | | |
| | 20 (85%) | 1 | 2 | | " " | Caesarean | | |
| PCBs | 12 (75%) | 5 | 4 | | " " | Normal delivery | | |
| | 20 (65%) | 3 | 1 | | " " | Caesarean | | |
| p,p'-DDE | 12 (100%) | 10 | 9 | | " " | Normal delivery | | |
| | 20 (100%) | 3 | 2 | | " " | Caesarean | | |
| beta-HCH | 12 (16.6%) | <1 | | | " " | Normal delivery | | |
| | 20 (10%) | <1 | | | " " | Caesarean | | |

**TABLE 1.   (Continued)**

| Geographic Location Year of Sample Chemical | Number of Samples (% Positive) | Units Mean/SD | Standard Deviation | Range | Tissue | Case Information * | Quantification ** Analysis & Detection Limits | Reference |
|---|---|---|---|---|---|---|---|---|
| Yugoslavia (1985-86) | | ppb (ug/l) Geometric | | | maternal serum | No history of exposure | GLC-ECD | Roncevic, N. et al. (1987) |
| beta-HCH | 14 (100%) | 1.69 | | 1.0- 3.6 | " " | Nonpregnant | | |
| | 14 (100%) | 1.45 | | 1.1- 2.8 | " " | At delivery | | |
| gamma-HCH | 14 (100%) | 1.77 | | 1.2- 3.6 | " " | Nonpregnant | | |
| | 14 (100%) | 2.72 | | 0.9- 5.4 | " " | At delivery | | |
| p,p'-DDE | 14 (100%) | 9.31 | | 6.1-14.4 | " " | Nonpregnant | | |
| | 14 (100%) | 7.57 | | 2.8-11.7 | " " | At delivery | | |
| p,p'-DDT | 14 (100%) | 5.87 | | 3.2- 9.7 | " " | Nonpregnant | | |
| | 14 (100%) | 3.62 | | 1.0- 8.2 | " " | At delivery | | |
| PCBs | 14 (100%) | 2.86 | | 1.8- 3.9 | " " | Nonpregnant | | |
| | 14 (100%) | 2.01 | | 1.1- 4.65 | " " | At delivery | | |
| India, Lucknow (1979-80) | | ppb | | | placental tissue | No history of exposure | GLC-ECD | Saxena, M.C. et al. (1983) |
| HCH | 27 (100%) | 39.9 | | 10.7- 97.9 | " " | Live-Born | | |
| | 9 (100%) | 35.7 | | 17.2- 62.4 | " " | Stillborn | | |
| gamma-HCH (lindane) | 27 (100%) | 17.1 | | 4.1- 95.6 | " " | Live-Born | | |
| | 9 (100%) | 13.4 | | 5.5- 26.1 | " " | Stillborn | | |
| Aldrin | 27 (<100%) | 8 | | 0.0- 83.3 | " " | Live-Born | | |
| | 9 (<100%) | 31.7 | | 0.0- 83.3 | " " | Stillborn | | |
| p,p'-DDE | 27 (100%) | 18.3 | | 2.8- 93.0 | " " | Live-Born | | |
| | 9 (100%) | 12.4 | | 4.7- 22.3 | " " | Stillborn | | |
| p,p'-DDT | 27 (100%) | 13.8 | | 2.0- 46.3 | " " | Live-Born | | |
| | 9 (100%) | 38.5 | | 5.4- 80.0 | " " | Stillborn | | |
| DDT Total | 27 (100%) | 39.8 | | 7.6-162.2 | " " | Live-Born | | |
| | 9 (100%) | 60.8 | | 21.9- 93.2 | " " | Stillborn | | |

**TABLE 1.** (Continued)

| Geographic Location Year of Sample Chemical | Number of Samples (% Positive) | Units Mean/SD | Standard Deviation | Range | Tissue | Case Information * | Quantification ** Analysis & Detection Limits | Reference |
|---|---|---|---|---|---|---|---|---|
| Poland, Pozna'n (1981) | | ppm (ug/g) | | | | No history of exposure | GC-ECD | Szymczynsk, G.A., & S.M. Waliszewski (1983) |
| HCB | 36 (86.1%) | 0.029 | 0.025 | 0.004-0.117 | testicular | | | |
| alpha-HCH | 36 (100%) | 0.018 | 0.014 | 0.004-0.058 | " | | | |
| beta-HCH | 36 (72.2%) | 0.124 | 0.09 | 0.049-0.571 | " | | | |
| gamma-HCH | 36 (69.4%) | 0.022 | 0.02 | 0.004-0.083 | " | | | |
| delta-HCH | 36 (97.2%) | 0.055 | 0.053 | 0.011-0.254 | " | | | |
| epsilon-HCH | 36 (38.8%) | 0.094 | 0.045 | 0.039-0.177 | " | | | |
| p,p'-DDE | 36 (97.2%) | 0.072 | 0.045 | 0.015-0.216 | " | | | |
| heptachlor epoxide | 36 (8.3%) | 0.131 | 0.047 | 0.083-0.194 | " | | | |
| Yugoslavia, Labin North Adriatic Area (1989) | | ppb (ug/l) Median | | | | No history of exposure | GC-ECD (Krauthacker et al. 1980) | Krauthacker, B. (1991) |
| HCB | 10 (100%) | 2 | | 1.0-4 | blood | | | |
| alpha-HCH | 10 (80%) | 2 | | 1.0-2 | " | (Samples taken | | |
| beta-HCH | 10 (80%) | 18 | | 13.0-31 | " | from lactating | | |
| p,p'-DDE | 10 (100%) | 6 | | 4.0-13 | " | mothers) | | |
| PCB | 10 (100%) | 7 | | 6.0? | " | | | |
| Japan (1986-88) | | ppm | | | | No history of exposure | GC-ECD | Sasaki, K. et al. (1991) |
| beta-HCH | 23 (100%) | 0.84 | 0.44 | 0.37-2.02 | adipose/fat | | | |
| p,p'-DDE | 23 (100%) | 2.4 | 2.5 | 11.04-0.52 | " | | | |
| heptachlor epoxide | 23 (91.3%) | 0.07 | 0.06 | 0.00-0.25 | " | | | |
| chlordane | 23 (100%) | 0.67 | 0.48 | 0.13-2.16 | " | | | |
| dieldrin | 20 (85%) | 0.08 | 0.08 | 0.00-0.27 | " | | | |

**TABLE 1.** (Continued)

| Geographic Location Year of Sample Chemical | Number of Samples (% Positive) | Units Mean/SD | Standard Deviation | Range | Tissue | Case Information * | Quantification ** Analysis & Detection Limits | Reference |
|---|---|---|---|---|---|---|---|---|
| USA, Massachusetts, New Bedford (1985-86) | | ppb | | | | No history of exposure | (Needham, undated) (Burse et al. 1963a) | Miller, D.T. et al. (1991) |
| PCB | 391 | 5.9 | | 0.0- 60.9 | blood | Males | | |
|  | 449 | 5.7 | | 0.0-154.2 | " | Females | | |
| Germany, Munich | | ppt | | | | No history of exposure | HRGC/HRMS | Thoma, H. et al. (1990) |
| T4CDD | 28 (100%) | 8 | | 2.6- 18.0 | adipose | | | |
| P5CDD | 28 (100%) | 16.4 | | 7.7- 40.4 | " | | | |
| H6CDD | 28 (100%) | 94.7 | | 35.7-178.2 | " | | | |
| H7CDD | 28 (100%) | 106.7 | | 35.1-246.0 | " | | | |
| OCDD | 28 (100%) | 373.2 | | 116.5-789.1 | " | | | |
| T4CDF | 28 (100%) | 2.5 | | 0.7- 12.8 | " | | | |
| P5CDF | 28 (100%) | 35.2 | | 7.6- 93.3 | " | | | |
| H6CDF | 28 (100%) | 41.5 | | 15.8-146.0 | " | | | |
| H7CDF | 28 (100%) | 14.2 | | 3.8- 45.6 | " | | | |
| OCDF | 28 (100%) | 4 | | 1.2- 13.5 | " | | | |
| T4CDD | 28 (100%) | 16.4 | | 1.0- 88.9 | liver/fat | | | |
| P5CDD | 28 (100%) | 20.1 | | 7.3- 58.7 | " | | | |
| H6CDD | 28 (100%) | 166.8 | | 56.4- 615.1 | " | | | |
| H7CDD | 28 (100%) | 1002.4 | | 95.5- 3463.1 | " | | | |
| OCDD | 28 (100%) | 4416.2 | | 472.7-15259.2 | " | | | |
| T4CDF | 28 (100%) | 5.5 | | 0.9- 45.3 | " | | | |
| P5CDF | 28 (100%) | 173.7 | | 36.7- 643.0 | " | | | |
| H6CDF | 28 (100%) | 389.5 | | 40.8- 1800.7 | " | | | |
| H7CDF | 28 (100%) | 218.9 | | 12.2- 757.0 | " | | | |
| OCDF | 28 (100%) | 29.7 | | 4.3- 65.8 | " | | | |

**TABLE 1. (Continued)**

| Geographic Location Year of Sample Chemical | Number of Samples (% Positive) | Units Mean/SD | Standard Deviation | Range | Tissue | Case Information * | Quantification ** Analysis & Detection Limits | Reference |
|---|---|---|---|---|---|---|---|---|
| Pakistan, Quetta (1987) | | ppb (ug/l) | | | | No history of exposure | GC/MS | Krawinkel, M.B. et al. (1989) |
| alpha-HCH | 21 (66.6%) | 0.396 | | 0 - 1.88 | blood | | (Specht & Tillkes 1985) | |
| beta-HCH | 21 (90%) | 1.99 | | 0 - 7.16 | " " | | | |
| 4,4'-DDE | 21 (100%) | 9.26 | | 0.53-18.98 | " " | | | |
| 4,4'-DDT | 21 (76.2%) | 0.94 | | 0 - 4.83 | " " | | | |
| India 1. Delhi 2. Faridabad (1987) | 7 (42.9%) | ppb (ng/g) 12.19 | 8 | 0- 64 | adipose/wet | No history of exposure | GLC-ECD | Nair, A. & M.K.K. Pillai (1989) |
| 1. HCB | | | | | | | | |
| 2. HCB | 4 (100%) | 280 | 180 | 59-830 | " " | | (EPA Manual 1980) | |
| India, Bombay (1986-87) | | ppm | | | | Male Professionals | (Heeshane et al. 1983) (Vaman Rao & Savtri 1988) | Rao, C.V. & S. Banerji (1989) |
| PCBs | 60 (100%) | 0.837 | 0.1 | 0.005-3.33 | blood | | | |
| Spain, Agrarian Area (1985-87) | | ppm (mg/kg) | | | adipose/ext. lipid | No history of exposure | GLC-ECD | Camps, M. et al. (1989) |
| HCB | 87 (100%) | 2.99 | 2.24 | | " " | | | |
| p,p'-DDE | 87 (100%) | 6.27 | 5.67 | | " " | | | |
| lindane | 87 (100%) | 0.083 | 0.05 | | " " | | | |
| beta-HCH | 87 (100%) | 3.06 | 5.18 | | " " | | | |
| p,p'-DDD | 87 (62%) | 0.079 | 0.079 | | " " | | | |
| p,p'-DDT | 87 (100%) | 1.5 | 0.89 | | " " | | | |
| dieldrin | 87 (100%) | 0.072 | 0.068 | | | | | |

**TABLE 1.  (Continued)**

| Geographic Location Year of Sample Chemical | Number of Samples (% Positive) | Units Mean/SD | Standard Deviation | Range | Tissue | Case Information * | Quantification ** Analysis & Detection Limits | Reference |
|---|---|---|---|---|---|---|---|---|
| USA, Michigan (1980-81) | | ppb (ng/ml) | | | | (Children 4 yrs. old) | GLC-ECD (Webb-McCall method) | Jacobson, J.L. et al. (1989) |
| PCBs | 205 (52.2%) | 4.18 | 3.29 | 1.00-19.40 | blood | No history of exposure | 3.0 ng/mL | |
| | 80 (48.8%) | 4.82 | 4.81 | 1.00-23.30 | " " | Fish exposure | " " | |
| PBBs | 205 (12.7%) | 2.44 | 1.5 | 1.00-6.40 | " " | Farm exposure | 1.0 ng/mL | |
| | 80 (21.3%) | 2.95 | 2.66 | 1.00-9.50 | " " | Fish exposure | " " | |
| DDT | 202 (69.8%) | 4.36 | 3.87 | 1.00-21.40 | " " | Farm exposure | " " | |
| | 79 (77.2%) | 4.24 | 4.47 | 1.00-143.2 | " " | Fish exposure Farm exposure | " " | |
| USA, Missouri (1987) | | ppt | | | | No history of exposure | HRGC-HRMS | Patterson, D.G. et al. (1988) |
| 2,3,7,8-TCDD | 50 (100%) | 54.4 | 125.8 | 2 -.745 | adipose/whol | | | |
| | 50 (100%) | 0.519 | 1.314 | 0.013-8.290 | serum/whole | | | |
| Australia, Sydney (1985-86) | | ppm (ug/g) | | | | No history of exposure | GLC-ECD (Ahmad & Marolt 1986) | Ahmad, N. et al. (1988) |
| DDT | 292 (99.3%) | 3.72 | | 0.0-26.30 | adipose/wet | | 0.001 ppm (81%) | |
| dieldrin | 292 (99.3%) | 0.13 | | 0.0-00.16 | " " | | 0.001 ppm (81-102%) | |
| Canada, Ontario (1984) | | ppb (ng/g) | | | | No history of exposure | GC/MS (LeBell & Williams 1986) | Williams, D.T. et al. (1988) |
| HCB | 141 (100%) | 84 | 56 | 18- 373 | adipose | | 1.4 ng/g | |
| beta-HCH | 141 (100%) | 84 | 82 | 14- 530 | " " | | 3.0 ng/g | |
| Heptachlor epoxide | 141 (100%) | 33 | 27 | 2- 107 | " " | | 1.1 ng/g | |
| p,p'-DDE | 141 (100%) | 3237 | 2602 | 138-12167 | " " | | 1.2 ng/g | |
| dieldrin | 141 (99.3%) | 47 | 41 | 0- 235 | " " | | 0.9 ng/g | |
| p,p'-DDT | 141 (100%) | 84 | 80 | 7- 369 | " " | | 1.7 ng/g | |
| mirex | 141 (92.2%) | 11 | 13 | 0- 98 | " " | | 1.8 ng/g | |
| PCB | 141 (100%) | 2136 | 1473 | 197-11209 | " " | | 100 ng/g | |

## TABLE 1. (Continued)

| Geographic Location / Year of Sample / Chemical | Number of Samples (% Positive) | Units Mean/SD | Standard Deviation | Range | Tissue | Case Information * | Quantification ** Analysis & Detection Limits | Reference |
|---|---|---|---|---|---|---|---|---|
| Israel, Jerusalem (1984-85) | | ppb (ng/g) | | | | No history of exposure (Males-5 yr. history of infertility = | GC-MS (Greichus et al. 1974) | Pines, A. et al. (1987) |
| p,p'-DDT | 29 | 3.09 | 6.81 | 0.0-28.8 | blood | Study group | | |
| | 14 | 0.4 | 0.99 | 0.0-3.5 | " | Control group | | |
| p,p'-DDE | 29 (100%) | 16.1 | 11.82 | 2.9-43.4 | " | Study group | | |
| | 14 (100%) | 10.55 | 8.17 | 2.1-32.1 | " | Control group | | |
| o,p'-DDT | 29 | 7.11 | 6 | 0.0-21.6 | " | Study group | | |
| | 14 | 5.83 | 8.6 | 0.0-32.2 | " | Control group | | |
| o,p'-DDE | 29 | 2.61 | 3.51 | 0.0-15.4 | " | Study group | | |
| | 14 | 1.27 | 2.04 | 0.0-6.4 | " | Control group | | |
| lindane | 29 | 2.28 | 2.42 | 0.0-9.8 | " | Study group | | |
| | 14 | 1.13 | 0.67 | 0.0-3.0 | " | Control group | | |
| Dieldrin | 29 | 3.65 | 3.71 | 0.0-15.9 | " | Study group | | |
| | 14 | 2.69 | 2.47 | 0.0-7.1 | " | Control group | | |
| heptachlor epoxide | 29 (100%) | 8.31 | 3.83 | 3.0-15.8 | " | Study group | | |
| | 14 (100%) | 11.64 | 3.67 | 7.0-21.7 | " | Control group | | |
| total PCBs | 29 | 11.21 | 13.48 | 0.0-64.2 | " | Study group | | |
| | 14 | 7.94 | 14.69 | 0.0-47.3 | " | Control group | | |

| Geographic Location / Year of Sample / Chemical | Number of Samples (% Positive) | Units Mean/SD | Standard Deviation | Range | Tissue | Case Information * | Quantification ** Analysis & Detection Limits | Reference |
|---|---|---|---|---|---|---|---|---|
| USA, Texas, Gulf Coast (1979-80) | | ppm | | | | No history of exposure | GLC-ECD | Ansari, G.A.S. et al. (1986) |
| HCB | 7 (85.7%) | 0.021 | | 0.0 -0.043 | adipose | | 0.005 ppm (86%) | |
| p,p'-DDE | 7 (100%) | 3.849 | | 0.843-6.527 | " | | 0.004 ppm (96%) | |
| 2,4,5,2',4',5'-HCBP | 7 (100%) | 0.184 | | 0.098-0.267 | " | | 0.005 ppm (92%) | |
| 2,3,4,2',4',5'-HCBP | 7 (100%) | 0.645 | | 0.211-1.625 | " | | 0.005 ppm (95%) | |

**TABLE 1. (Continued)**

| Geographic Location / Year of Sample / Chemical | Number of Samples (% Positive) | Units Mean/SD | Standard Deviation | Range | Tissue | Case Information* | Quantification** Analysis & Detection Limits | Reference |
|---|---|---|---|---|---|---|---|---|
| Japan (1985) | | ppt (pg/g) | | | | No history of exposure (Cancer patients) | GC-MS | Ono, M. et al (1986) |
| 2,3,7,8-T4CDD | 13 (92.3%) | 9 | | 6 - 18 | adipose/wet | | | |
| 1,2,3,7,8-P5CDD | 13 (100%) | 15 | | 3 - 36 | " " | | | |
| 1,2,3,4,7,8-H6CDD | 13 (69.2%) | 8 | | 5 - 14 | " " | | | |
| 1,2,3,6,7,8-H6CDD | 13 (92.3%) | 70 | | 26 - 220 | " " | | | |
| 1,2,3,7,8,9-H6CDD | 13 (76.9%) | 12 | | 4 - 44 | " " | | | |
| 1,2,3,4,6,7,9-H7CDD | 13 (69.2%) | 28 | | 14 - 53 | " " | | | |
| 1,2,3,4,6,7,8-H7CDD | 13 (92.3%) | 77 | | 29 - 180 | " " | | | |
| O8CDD | 13 (92.3%) | 230 | | 25 -1100 | " " | | | |
| PCDDs Total | | 410 | | 160-1400 | " " | | | |
| 2,4,7,8-T4CDF | 13 (100%) | 9 | | 3 - 12 | " " | | | |
| 2,3,4,7,8-P5CDF | 13 (100%) | 25 | | 4 - 71 | " " | | | |
| 1,2,3,4,7,8/ 1,2,3,4,7,9-H6CDF | 13 (84.6%) | 15 | | 4 - 24 | " " | | | |
| 1,2,3,6,7,8-H6CDF | 13 (84.6%) | 14 | | 3 - 28 | " " | | | |
| 2,3,4,6,7,8-H6CDF | 13 (23.1%) | 8 | | 4 - 16 | " " | | | |
| PCDFs Total | | 63 | | 7 - 120 | " " | | | |
| Japan, Tokushima Cit (1984-85) | | ppb (ng/g) Geometric | | | | No history of exposure | GC-ECD (Warishi et al 1984) 0.01 ppb | Warishi, M. et al (1986) |
| chlordane | 22 (100%) | 0.51 | 1.6 | 0.18-1.16 | blood | Male subjects | | |
| | 21 (100%) | 0.46 | 1.7 | 0.12-1.12 | " " | Female subjects | | |
| USA, Texas, El Paso (1982-83) | | ppb | | | | No history of exposure | EPA (1974) Manual of Analytical Methods | Mossing, M.L. et al (1985) |
| Aldrin | 112 (34%) | 4.6 | 8.6 | 0.0-46.8 | blood | | | |
| BHC | 112 (24%) | 2.5 | 2 | 0.0-16.5 | " " | | | |
| p,p'DDE | 112 (99%) | 7.1 | 4.3 | 0.0-34.6 | " " | | | |
| Heptachlor | 112 (19%) | 3.1 | 3 | 0.0- 9.9 | " " | | | |

GC-ECD   = Gas Chromatography - Electron Capture Detector
GLC-ECD  = Gas Liquid Chromatography - Electron Capture Detector
GC-MS    = Gas Chromatography - Mass Spectrometry
HRGC-HRMS = High Resolution....

\* General information regarding the subjects analyzed
\*\* Methodology cited in paper

sidered "safe levels" for human adults may be detrimental to the developing embryo, fetus, and newborn (Calabrese, 1982; Tilson et al., 1990).

Historically, research on the health effects of organochlorine chemicals has focused primarily on carcinogenicity and acute toxicity. It is now realized that many of these contaminants are probably weak carcinogens at concentrations currently found in human tissue. However, wildlife and laboratory studies reveal that at ambient concentrations these contaminants may have other less obvious, but equally devastating effects, depending upon timing of exposure, especially during the prenatal period (Fry et al., 1987; Peterson et al., Chapter 10). Recent human studies suggest that the contaminants are functional teratogens at contemporary concentrations found in cord blood and breast milk (Rogan et al., 1985; Jacobson and Jacobson, 1988). Since most of these xenobiotic compounds are transported across the placenta and via breast milk to the progeny, simultaneous exposure to a number of them takes place during this most sensitive period of development (Wasserman et al., 1982; Rogan and Gladen, 1985; Rogan et al., 1986).

A number of *in vivo* studies were undertaken to address the unknowns associated with simultaneous exposure to large numbers of chemical contaminants. Contaminated Great Lakes fish were fed to rats (Villenueve et al., 1981; Chu et al., 1984; Daly et al., 1989; Daly, 1991, 1992) to coho salmon (*Oncorhynchus kisutch*) (Leatherland and Sonstegard, 1982), to ranch mink (Heaton et al., 1991), and to white leghorn chickens (Summer et al., 1991). In each case, significant measurable changes in either functionality or survivability were reported in the animals, lending support to the hypothesis that compounds that bioaccumulate in fish were responsible.

Several human epidemiological studies provide clues and raise a number of questions concerning the effects of concomitant exposure to a number of organochlorine contaminants on the well being of individuals as a result of intrauterine and breast feeding exposure. For example, prenatal exposure to contaminants in Lake Michigan fish has been associated with deficits in birth size and gestational age (Fein et al., 1984), postnatal growth (Jacobson and Jacobson, 1988), motor development (Gladen et al., 1988), and short-term memory in infancy and childhood (Jacobson et al., 1985, 1990a,b). These effects are reported in children whose mothers consumed contaminated Lake Michigan fish two to three times a month for at least six years preceding their pregnancies. A noteworthy conclusion from this series of reports is that the functional deficits detected in the children were not associated with what their mothers ate during pregnancy, but with what their mothers ate in their lifetime prior to conception. In these studies, significant associations were reported between PCB concentrations in maternal serum and breast milk and mother's fish consumption. Associations were also reported between cord blood PCB concentrations and children's lowered weight and loss of verbal and quantitative function; and between breast milk PCB concentrations and children's activity deficits. The children's deficits, in this case, could represent the integrated toxicity of the antagonistic, agonistic, additive, and synergistic effects of all the other contaminants in the fish, and not PCB alone.

## PESTICIDES COMMONLY REPORTED IN HUMAN TISSUE

### Cyclodienes

Chlorinated cyclodienes are now recognized as environmentally persistent and among the more toxic pesticides. As a result, in recent years their production and use have been restricted in the US and Canada, yet they continue to be reported as residues in human tissue (Table 1). The cyclodienes most often found in human tissue are chlordane, oxychlordane, trans-nonachlor, heptachlor, heptachlor epoxide (HE), aldrin and dieldrin. All of these pesticides induce hepatic microsomal cytochrome P-450 activity, and induce the monooxygenases which hydroxylate testosterone (Haake et al., 1987).

*Animal Data*
Adult male and female rats fed 0.31 ppm dieldrin, approximately 0.015 mg/kg/body weight (15 ppb), for 300 days experienced reduced fertility when mated. In a later study, it took twenty times the dose to produce the same effect when dosing females alone. Whether this indicates a male-dependent effect needs to be explored (ATSDR, 1987a). Three-week old rats were administered 20 mg/kg/body weight dieldrin in a corn oil vehicle and sacrificed 5 days later, at which time hepatic 16-alpha- and beta-hydroxytestosterone hydroxylases were significantly increased (Haake et al., 1987).

Chlordane had a damaging effect on spermatogenesis and caused dose-related degenerative changes in testicular tissue in mice fed by stomach tube the equivalent of 0.08 mg, or 0.25 mg active ingredient per day for 30 days (Balash et al., 1987). Lundholm (1988) reported that $110 \times 10^{-6}$ M of chlordane reduced progesterone binding in rabbit uterine mucosa *in vitro* and $1.1 \times 10^{-6}$ M of chlordane significantly inhibited progesterone binding in the mucosa of the shell gland of egg-laying ducks. Prenatal chlordane exposure at 0.16 mg/kg/maternal body weight/day throughout gestation effected alterations in plasma corticosterone concentrations in murine offspring which varied according to sex at days 101 and 400 (Cranmer et al., 1984).

*Human Data*
The average background levels of cyclodienes in breast milk world wide are presented in Table 2. In recent years, the levels of dieldrin in human milk have decreased, although relatively high levels are still reported in the Middle East, South America, and Australia. Heptachlor epoxide (HE) is found in elevated concentrations in breast milk in Belgium, Italy, Israel, and Guatemala. Heptachlor levels in milk from Italy and Spain are also elevated. Chlordane and its isomers are found more frequently in human milk in the US than elsewhere. The highest levels of chlordane in breast milk have been found in Mexico and Iraq (Table 2).

**TABLE 2.** Human breast milk fat concentrations worldwide compared with the lowest observed endocrine or reproductive effect levels in animal studies

| HUMAN DATA (Adapted from DeWailly et al, 1989*; Jensen & Slorach, 1991.) | | | ANIMAL DATA | | |
|---|---|---|---|---|---|
| Chemical & Units | Avg. Levels in Human Breast Milk Fat | High Levels & Location | Dose & Exposure Route | Impairment | Reference |
| Dieldrin | 0.05 ppm | 1.78 ppm Australia 1.00 ppm Iraq 1.00 ppm Urugary | 20 mg/kg/bw. Single injection to 3-week old rats. | Induced testosterone 16-alpha-and 16-beta-hydroxylases. | Haake et al., 1987 |
| Heptachlor & its Epoxide | 0.05 ppm | 2.50 ppm Spain 0.48 ppm Italy | 250 umol/kg/bw. Single injection to 3-week old rats | Induced testosterone 16-alpha-and 16-beta-hydroxylases. | Haake et al., 1987 |
| Chlordane (Oxychlordane & Trans-nonachlor) | 0.08 ppm | > 2.00 ppm Mexico & Iraq | 0.16 mg/kg wt/day Dietary exposure to pregnant mice throughout gestation. | Elevation of plasma corticosterone concentrations, when measured on day 400 in both male & female offspring. | Cranmer et al., 1984 |
| Total DDT | 1.00 ppm | > 100 ppm Guatemala | | | |
| o,p'-DDT | 0.25 ppm | | 2 ppm Dissolved in corn oil and injected into yolk of gull embryos. | Caused feminization (a thickened ovary-like cortex in left testis). | Fry & Toone, 1981 |

**TABLE 2.** (Continued)

| HUMAN DATA Adapted from DeWailly et al, 1989*; Jensen & Slorach, 1991. | | | ANIMAL DATA | | |
|---|---|---|---|---|---|
| Chemical & Units | Avg. Levels in Human Breast Milk Fat | High Levels & Location | Dose & Exposure Route | Impairment | Reference |
| HCB | 0.10 ppm | 7.00 ppm Greece | 300 umol/kg/bw. Single injection to 3-week old rats | Induced testosterone 16-alpha-and 16-beta-hydroxylases. | Haake et al., 1987 |
| Beta-HCH | 1.00 ppm | 6.50 ppm Chile | 50 mg/kg/bw. (ppm) Dietary exposure to weaned rats for for 13 weeks. | Caused a reduction in testes weight. | Van Velsen et al., 1986 |
| Gamma-HCH | 0.06 ppm | 0.89 ppm Italy | 8 mg/kg (ppm) i.p. daily in glycerine suspension to adult male rats for 10 days. | Caused a reduction in testes wt., degeneration of seminiferous lumens, & affected both spermatocytes & spermatids. | Chowdhury et al., 1987 |
| Total PCB | 1.00 ppm | * 3.6 ppm Canada (Hudson Bay) | 8 mg Aroclor 1254/kg (ppm) Dissolved in 0.2 ml peanut oil, Lactating dam's were exposed via their diet on days 1,3,5,7, & 9 of lactation. | Males exposed only during lactation exhibited reduced fertility as adults. Specifically, decreased # of implants and decreased # of embryos when mated with normal females. | Sager et al., 1987 |
| 2,3,7,8-TCDD | 2.00 ppt | 1.45 ppb Vietnam (1970's) | 0.064 ug/kg (ppb) Dietary exposure to pregnant rat on day 15 of gestation. | Male offspring had decreased sperm counts when exposed perinatally in utero & via lactation. | Peterson, Chapter 10 1991 |

## Dichlorodiphenylethanes

The dichlorodiphenylethanes include DDT, DDD, DDE, dicofol, perthane, and methoxychlor (Amdur et al., 1991). DDT and its metabolites are commonly found in human tissue samples, and are the most widespread contaminant in human milk (Jensen and Slorach, 1991). A newer analogue of DDT, methoxychlor, used extensively in urban areas of the Eastern United States for elm bark beetle control, breaks down readily to an estrogenic-like compound (Gray et al., 1989), but is not monitored in human tissue.

*Animal Data*
Commercial DDT consists of 10% to 25% o,p'-DDT, an estrogenic isomer of DDT (Fry and Toone, 1981; Jensen and Slorach, 1991). Following a 0.5 mg intravenous injection of p,p'-DDT, rat uteri exhibited myometrial hypertrophy and endometrial edema, evidence that p,p'-DDT also has estrogenic activity (Bustos et al., 1988).

Fry and Toone (1981) induced feminization in male California gulls (*Larus californicus*) and western gulls (*Larus occidentalis*) by injecting fertilized eggs with 2-100 ppm of commercial DDT. Following a single 2 ppm injection of o,p'-DDT into eggs, seven of eight male embryos developed a thickened ovary-like cortex in the left testis, a sensitive indicator of feminization requiring histopathological examination to detect. (Normal gull testes have a thin fibrous cortex surrounding the seminiferous tubules and interstitial cells.) Male gulls treated embryonically via egg injections with 5 ppm of o,p'-DDT developed both left and right oviducts. The concentrations of DDT which caused feminization in the gulls was the same as those found in seabird eggs in southern California in the late 1960s (Fry and Toone, 1981).

In an effort to determine the underlying cause of the abnormal sex ratio skew and breeding patterns of Western and California gulls in the 1970s, Fry et al., (1987) considered both toxicological, demographic, and behavioral variables. They injected fertile eggs of both species with 2, 5, 20, 50, or 100 µg/g of o,p'-DDT, p,p'-DDT, p,p'-DDE, and methoxychlor, reflecting the range of pollutant concentrations found in pelican and gull eggs in southern California in 1970 and 1973. Administration of o,p'-DDT (5> ppm) and methoxychlor (20, 50, or 100 ppm) caused feminization (modification of the reproductive organs), demasculinization (modification of the developing brain) of male embryos, and development of right oviductal tissue in surviving female embryos (ordinarily females have only a left oviduct). A 4:1 mixture of p,p'-DDE and p,p'-DDT at 50 ppm caused feminization of both male and female embryos via increased development of oviductal tissue.

Fry and co-workers also reported female-female pairing in two demographic situations. One in newly formed or rapidly expanding colonies of ring-billed gulls (*Larus delawarensis*) and western gulls where the gulls shifted nesting sites from year to year. The second in situations where populations of herring gulls (*Larus argentatus*), western gulls, and glaucous-winged gulls (*Larus glaucescens*) were breeding in areas polluted with organochlorines and exhibiting declines in numbers. An incidence of 14% supernormal clutches attended by two females was reported in the Santa Barbara Island colony of western gulls. The authors concluded that the increased number of female gulls in the second situation might be the result of: (1) a reflection of the decreased fitness of male gulls hatched from contaminated eggs, and (2) juvenile and/or adult male gulls exposed to organochlorine chemicals in their food base.

Lundholm (1988) studied the effects of o,p'-DDE and p,p'-DDE *in vitro* on the progesterone receptor in the eggshell gland mucosa of egg-laying ducks and domestic fowl, and in the endometrium of the rabbit uterus. At a range of 1.1 to $110 \times 10^{-6}$ M, both isomers inhibited the binding of progesterone to its receptor in a dose-dependent fashion in the tissue of the three species. The most potent inhibitor was the o,p'-DDE isomer. He also noted that p,p'-DDE was a partial agonist to progesterone. He reached this conclusion because p,p'-DDE *in vivo* acted similarly to chronic administration of progesterone, reducing ovulation and effecting atrophy of uterine mucosa.

*Human Data*

Levels of total hexachlorocyclohexane (HCH) isomers, lindane, aldrin, p,p'-DDT, p,p'-DDD, p,p'-DDE, and total DDT were measured in maternal blood, placentae, and umbilical-cord blood from women experiencing stillbirth and live births (Saxena et al., 1983). The levels of aldrin and p,p'-DDT in all samples of stillbirth cases were significantly higher than the controls (Table 1). The authors concluded that since the samples taken from stillborn cases held considerably higher concentrations of the above chemicals than those associated with live births, a possible association with the fetal deaths existed. The additive effects of these compounds may be more toxic than the individual compounds alone, but was impossible to determine in the study.

Jacobson et al., (1989) analyzed serum from 285 Michigan children at age 4 for environmental contaminants. The children who were exposed *in utero* and during breast feeding were divided into two cohorts: those whose mothers consumed Lake Michigan fish and those whose mothers consumed food contaminated with PBBs or PCBs as a result of farm incidents. DDT was present in more than 70% of the samples tested. Factors such as duration of nursing, having older mothers, and residing in a rural area were reflected in significantly elevated children's serum DDT levels. The authors concluded that breast feeding was the principal source of exposure for DDT, PCBs, and PBBs in these children.

Large differences in tissue levels of DDT are not unusual from country to country. The concentration of total DDT found in breast milk did not change noticeably in the United States from 1970 to 1982, although in the last two decades concentrations have decreased gradually in several European countries

(Calabrese, 1982; Jensen and Slorach, 1991). Since the 1973 ban of DDT in Ontario, Canada, there has been no significant change in total DDT or DDE levels in milk fat in that province, and since 1985 the DDE levels in human breast milk appear to have reached an "equilibrium" with DDE levels in the Ontario environment (Gobas, 1990). Jensen and Slorach (1991) report elevated concentrations in human tissue in southeastern US, southern and eastern Europe, and in third world countries. DDT use has been restricted in North America and Europe, but it is used extensively in Third-world countries because it is considered the least expensive alternative to control insects which devastate crops and affect human health (Amdur et al., 1991; Jensen and Slorach, 1991).

## Hexachlorobenzene (HCB)

HCB was used as a fungicide in the US until 1985. Until recently, a large component of HCB in the US environment was derived as a by-product from the production of three chlorinated solvents (Holliday, 1988). However, the main source in the environment today is from the manufacture of pesticides in which it is an unwanted by-product (Ando et al., 1985; ATSDR, 1990). It has been reported as a contaminant in approximately 135 pesticides ingredients (Nair and Pillai, 1989). It is estimated that in the US 10,000 kg HCB per year are released through the use of the pesticides, dacthal (DCPA), picloram, and pentachlorophenol alone (ATSDR, 1990). It was detected in human fat and breast milk samples from residents in India, where it was never used as a fungicide, and where the highest HCB concentrations were found in samples collected from industrial areas (Nair and Pillai, 1989). A mass-intoxication resulting from the consumption of HCB-treated wheat in Turkey in the late 1950s generated global concern over HCB and led to its banning.

*Animal Data*
At a dose of 300 µM/kg intraperitoneal HCB induces hepatic 6-beta-, 16-alpha-, and 16-beta-hydroxytestosterone and androstenedione hydroxylases in rats (Haake et al., 1987). Rat pups were fed HCB at 0.32, 1.6, 8.0, or 40.0 ppm from weaning to 90 days (Arnold et al., 1985). At the end of the 90 days these rats (the $F_0$ generation) were bred. Following weaning, the $F_1$ generation were also fed the same diet as their parents for 130 weeks. At 130 weeks the $F_1$ animals displayed linear trends in parathyroid adenomas and phaeochromocytomas in both sexes, and sex-specific liver and kidney anomalies, however fertility was not affected (Arnold et al., 1985).

*Human Data*
The average worldwide background concentration of HCB in human milk fat is approximately 0.1 ppm (100 ppb) (Jensen and Slorach, 1991). Mes et al., (1986) found HCB in 100% of human milk samples from Canada with a mean concentration of 54.0 ng/g (ppb) and a maximum of 256.0 ng/g (ppb) in milk fat. HCB was present in all 50 human milk samples from a town in Croatia, Yugoslavia (median concentration of 0.21 mg/kg (210 ppb) milk fat)

(Krauthacker et al., 1986). Mes et al., (1984) measured a significant drop in Canadian breast milk HCB concentrations throughout 98 days of lactation. This is in agreement with the findings of Ando and coworkers (1985).

HCB was detected in all samples of maternal blood from 36 healthy women from rural Japan in the seventh month of pregnancy (Ando et al., 1985). It was also detected in all samples of placentae, cord blood, and breast milk following parturition, confirming that HCB is transferred from mother to fetus through the placenta and breast milk. A significant correlation was discovered between placental HCB and cord blood. It was concluded that the main sources of HCB exposure in the general population in Japan are from the use of pentachloronitrobenzene (PCNB) and pentachlorophenol (PCP), two commercial pesticides (Ando et al., 1985).

Based on Canadian data, HCB intake is two to three times higher for toddlers and infants than it is for adults (Holliday, 1988). The breast-fed baby is the most highly exposed, taking in 10 times as much as the mother. This is equivalent to 200 - 300 times the adult intake on a bodyweight basis.

The US Environmental Protection Agency (EPA) Office of Water Regulation and Standards (OWRS, 1986), reported that HCB was found in 98% of human fat samples in a nationwide survey at levels between 50 and 100 ppb. It also reported that during the preceding 10 years [1975 to 1985] the level of HCB remained the same or possibly increased in human tissue. This is confirmed by a more recent survey that found HCB levels in adipose tissue increasing in the US, UK, and Canada (Jensen and Slorach, 1991).

### Hexachlorocyclohexanes

Technical hexachlorocyclohexane is a mixture of isomeric hexachlorocyclohexanes (HCHs), and is also referred to as benzene hexachloride (BHC). The approximate isomer content of the insecticide is *alpha*-HCH (53-70%), *beta*-HCH (3-14%), *gamma*-HCH (11-18%), *delta*-HCH (6-10%), others (3-10%). The International Organization for Standardization (IOS) recognizes *gamma*-BHC, *gamma*-HCH, and lindane as common names for the gamma isomer. The pure isomer is not less than 99% pure *gamma*-BHC (Smith, 1991). The pure isomer (lindane) is the most acutely toxic with an $LD_{50}$ in rats of approximately 200 mg/kg/body weight, while the $LD_{50}$ for *alpha* and *beta*-HCH are in the range of 500 to 2000 mg/kg/body weight (Jensen and Slorach, 1991). However, *beta*-HCH is the most persistent, bioaccumulating isomer and is often 90% of the total HCH found in human milk samples. It has also been reported to exhibit estrogenic activity in rodents (Jensen and Slorach, 1991; Van Velsen et al., 1986).

*Animal Data*

Both estrogen and anti-estrogen effects of lindane (gamma-HCH) were demonstrated in a two-phased study in which vaginal opening was delayed and ovarian cyclicity was disrupted up to 110 days of age in female rats when chronically exposed to lindane (5, 10, 20, and 40 mg/kg). In the second phase, 21-day-old prepubertal female rats were gavaged with lindane (30 mg/kg) for 7 days and then administered estradiol (Cooper et al., 1989). Reduced serum luteinizing hormone (LH) and increased pituitary LH, follicle-stimulating hormone (FSH), and prolactin levels suggested that lindane interfered with target tissue responding to the estradiol. The authors admit that interpretation of the results is difficult.

Weanling rats were fed *beta*-HCH (purity > 98%), at 0, 2, 10, 50, or 250 mg/kg (ppm) in their feed for 13 weeks (Van Velsen et al., 1986). Doses of 2> mg/kg induced liver enzyme induction and at 50> mg/kg significantly reduced testes and thymus weights. Males dosed with 250 mg/kg beta-HCH experienced atrophied testes, which involved reduced size of the seminiferous tubules and decreased number of interstitial cells in association with spermatogenic arrest. In females the 250 mg/kg dose caused atrophy of the ovaries, impaired oogenesis, and focal hyperplasia.

*Human Data*

Concentrations of HCH reported in human breast milk for most of the European countries average around 0.2 ppm in milk fat, with higher concentrations found in Czechoslovakia, France, and Italy. In Italy, a high ratio of total-HCH/*beta*-HCH is reported, indicating possible ongoing use of technical HCH or lindane. In India and the People's Republic of China the average concentration is 6 ppm in milk fat. Concentrations of the *gamma*-HCH isomer alone average around 0.05 ppm in human milk fat worldwide (Jensen and Slorach, 1991).

## INDUSTRIAL POLLUTANTS COMMONLY REPORTED IN HUMAN TISSUE

### Polychlorinated Biphenyls (PCBs)

Polychlorinated biphenyls are industrial chemicals which have been used as heat transfer fluids, adhesives, dielectric fluids for capacitors and transformers, fire retardants, and waxes (Safe, 1990). PCBs consist of 209 different congeners or permutations, depending upon the number of chlorine atoms present and their position on two benzene rings. Each of the congeners has its own chemical and toxicity profile. Fifteen coplanar PCBs, including the non-*ortho* chlorine substituted 3,3',4,4'-tetrachlorobiphenyl, 3,3',4,4',5-pentachlorobiphenyl, and 3,3',4,4',5,5'-hexachlorobiphenyl, elicit the same receptor binding avidity as the highly toxic 2,3,7,8-tetrachlorodibenzo-p-dioxin, but with less potency (Safe, 1986, 1990). These congeners have been associated with immune suppression, dermal abnormalities, porphyria, "wasting", and teratogenicity in laboratory animals. However, endocrine disruption, neurotoxicity, respiratory problems, and male fertility have been associated with other PCB congeners that are not among the 15 dioxin-like congeners (Dieringer et al., 1979; Bush et al., 1986; USEPA, 1991; Seegal and Shain, 1992).

*Animal Data*

Sager (1983) observed the reproductive success of male rats exposed to PCB (Aroclor 1254) postnatally via dam's milk. Lactating mothers received 8, 32, or 64 mg/kg (ppm) Aroclor 1254 in 0.2 ml peanut oil on days 1, 3, 5, 7, and 9 of lactation. At maturity the males at the two highest doses when mated with unexposed females displayed reduced incidence of implantations and embryonic loss following implantation in a dose response manner. In a more recent study using the same methodology with an additional dose of 16 mg/kg added to the dosing regime, Sager and coworkers (1991) found PCB affected the ability of sperm to fertilize eggs. Other parameters such as epididymal sperm production, morphology, and motility, were not affected.

Shain et al., (1986) measured the accumulation of PCB congeners in perinatally exposed rat pups. The dams' diet contained 0, 3, 30, and 300 µg/gm (ppm) Aroclor 1254 from the time of fertilization to the time the pups were weaned. Tissue samples from both the dams and pups were analyzed for 67 PCB congeners at birth and weaning, allowing the description of PCB congener compartmentalization during gestation and lactation. Exposure to pups was greater during breast feeding than during gestation. The more highly chlorinated PCB congeners accumulated in breast milk and at concentrations that correlated with those in the feed. In other words, they were not readily metabolized by the dams, but stored in maternal fat. At weaning, the pups of the dams exposed to 30 µg/gm PCB accumulated PCBs 3.5 times greater than that found in the feed. The authors concluded that the increase could be due to the additional time of exposure during lactation, or could be partially due to dietary PCBs bypassing the liver and moving directly to the mammary glands in the nursing rats.

Schantz et al., (1991) found that low-level PCB (Aroclor 1016 or 1248) perinatal exposure in rhesus monkeys (*Macaca mulatta*) alters cognitive function. Learning deficits were recorded at four to six years of age, even though the four and six year olds had not been exposed to PCBs since they were weaned at four months of age. PCB concentrations of maternal milk ranged 0.5 to 4.0 µg/g (ppm) on a fat basis, which is in the range of the human population.

A cross-fostering study using virgin rats on a diet of 0 and 30 mg/kg (30 ppm) lower-chlorinated PCBs in their diet for 60 days preceding mating revealed that "active avoidance learning" and "retention of a visual discrimination task" deficits occurred only in the prenatally exposed pups (Lilienthal and Winneke, 1991). Brain tissue analysis revealed that the lower chlorinated PCB congeners were more readily transferred across the placenta and the blood brain barrier than the higher chlorinated biphenyls. Exposure to the lesser chlorinated PCBs was greater prenatally, whereas exposure to the more highly chlorinated PCBs increased during breast feeding.

*Human Data*

The average concentration of PCBs in human breast milk is approximately 1 ppm on a fat basis in industrialized nations. This is equivalent to a dose of approximately 5 µg/kg/body weight/day for the suckling infant based on the infant consuming 130 g milk/body weight/day and breast milk consisting of 3.7% fat (Jensen and Slorach, 1991). This is well above the Allowable Daily Intake (ADI) for PCBs set by the Food and Agriculture Organization, at 1 µg/kg/body weight/day based on a 70 kg adult (ATSDR, 1987b).

At birth, the baby and mother are at equilibrium in respect to PCB concentrations. On a fat basis, PCB is the same in maternal blood, breast milk, and baby cord blood. Eventually an infant will exhibit a 4 fold increase in blood PCB after 6 to 9 months of breast feeding, whereas the mother's blood PCB will drop 2.5 fold during the same time period (Gobas, 1990). A survey of breast milk fat from 24 Inuit women from Hudson Bay in 1987 and 1988 revealed a mean of 3.6 ppm PCB, reflecting the mothers' diets of marine mammals and fish and freshwater fish (Dewailly et al., 1989). At 6 to 9 months, the Inuit infants could carry 14.4 ppm PCB in their blood fat if the above increases are also true for Inuit populations.

Tilson et al., (1990) found that children exposed to PCBs transplacentally at concentrations considered to be background in the U.S. experienced hypotonia and hyporeflexia at birth, delays in psychomotor development at 6 and 12 months, and poorer visual recognition memory at 7 months. Using EPA's risk assessment model (USEPA, 1989) for the determination of a PCB reference dose (RfD) for humans based on neurotoxicological endpoints, Tilson et al., (1990) reexamined the results of the above studies that measured standard development in infants and young children. They arrived at a no-observed-adverse-effect-level (NOAEL) of 93 µg/kg/body weight/day for hypotonicity based on the results of the Brazelton Neonatal Behavioral Assessment Scale; 93 µg/kg/body weight/day based on a decreased Bayley Psychomotor Scale Index (motor and language development) measured at 12 months of age; and 27 µg/kg/body weight/day for Impaired Visual Recognition Memory. Introducing a safety factor of ten, they arrived at RfDs of 9.3, 9.3, and 2.7 µg/kg PCB/body weight/day, respectively for PCBs. This places suckling infants consuming breast milk at the nationwide average of 5 µg/kg PCB/body weight/day (1 ppm PCB on a fat basis in the breast milk) at the margin of safety for neurotoxicological effects. Using the USEPA (1989) risk assessment model mentioned earlier, Tilson and co-workers also compared PCB NOAELs between rodents, rhesus monkeys, and humans and found that the human fetus is 4 orders of magnitude more sensitive than the rodent to the neurological effects mentioned above.

Levels of PCBs in human breast milk from the Great Lakes Basin have remained constant from 1969 to 1985 with a range of 0.5 to 1.5 ppm (Gobas, 1990). PCB concentrations in breast milk doubled in Norway between 1970 and 1976 from 11 to 24 µg/kg (ppb) whole milk; and between 1976 and 1982 (mean = 0.8 ppm on a fat basis), no change was noted (Skaare et al., 1988).

## Dioxins and Furans

Polychlorinated dibenzo-p-dioxins (PCDDs) and polychlorinated dibenzofurans (PCDFs) consisting of 75 and 135 PCDF congeners respectively (Safe, 1986). Of the 75 dioxin congeners, 2,3,7,8-tetrachlorodibenzo-p-dioxin (TCDD), also referred to as dioxin, is considered most toxic. All other 2,3,7,8-substituted congeners have the same toxicological profiles as 2,3,7,8-TCDD, but are less potent. Both PCDDs and PCDFs are by-products or unwanted components from the manufacture of many industrial and agricultural chemicals. They are formed during the processing of intermediate chlorophenols in the manufacture of, for example, 2,4,5-T and 2,4-DCPB (dacthal), which are widely used herbicides. Other sources include the emissions from steel foundries, municipal waste and hospital incinerators, paper and pulp bleaching, and exhaust emissions from vehicles (Skene et al., 1989; Rappe, 1991). PCDFs are by-products in the manufacture and combustion of polychlorinated biphenyls and naphthalenes (Safe, 1986).

*Animal Data*

The endocrine disrupting toxicity of TCDD varies from species to species and is expressed in a number of ways depending on how it interacts with a number of hormones and hormone receptors, e.g., epidermal growth factor, estrogens, glucocorticoids, low density lipids, prolactin, and thyroxine (Umbreit and Gallo, 1988). In addition, timing of exposure to TCDD plays a significant role in the development of the embryo, fetus, and neonate. For example, a single meal of TCDD administered to a female rat on day 15 of gestation can adversely affect the sexual maturation of the male rats she is bearing. Male rats are highly sensitive to intrauterine and lactational TCDD exposure at a single dose as low as 0.064 µg TCDD/kg to the mother (See Chapter 10, Peterson et al., for a description of TCDD effects in male offspring).

The male reproductive system is more sensitive to TCDD when exposure occurs early in development than at maturity. Androgenic deficiency was reported in mature male rats when exposed to 15 µg/kg TCDD (Moore et al., 1985). Deficiencies were reported in *in utero* exposed male rats whose mothers were exposed to 0.064 µg/kg TCDD, which signifies much greater sensitivity between rats exposed perinatally and those exposed after sexual maturation. The effects on the female offspring were not determined in these studies (Peterson et al., Chapter 10).

*Human Data*

In industrialized countries the background concentration of the most toxic dioxin congener (TCDD) in human milk fat is approximately 2 ppt (Jensen and Slorach, 1991). TCDD serum levels reported on a lipid basis in children from Seveso, Italy were from 1770 to 56,660 ppt (ng/kg). The exposure was the result of an explosion in a factory during the production of 2,4,5-trichlorophenol (Kimbrough, 1990).

A number of schemes to compare the toxic potency of the various PCDD and PCDF congeners and the dioxin-like PCB congeners have been developed. TCDD-equivalency factors (TEFs) based on enzyme induction activity using the most potent compound, 2,3,7,8-TCDD, as the standard compared with the other structurally related compounds are currently under evaluation in the US (Safe, 1990; USEPA, 1991). The 1988 Nordic International Toxicity Equivalency Factors (I-TEF) are used in the data that follows concerning congeners present in milk fat (Slorach and Jensen, 1991).

The PCDDs that have been detected in human milk samples are all 2,3,7,8-chlorine substituted, considered the most toxic of the PCDD congeners. One of the relatively toxic congeners, 1,2,3,7,8-PentaCDD, (I-TEF = 0.5), is found in human milk at concentrations averaging 50 ppt; three hexa substituted PCDDs concentrations are found between 20-300 ppt (I-TEF = 0.1); and only one of the two hepta-substituted PCDDs is found at concentrations between 30 and 150 ppt (I-TEF = 0.01) (Slorach and Jensen, 1991).

The total background concentrations for PCDF (two having the 2,3,7,8-substitution) in human milk fat is 20-50 ppt (I-TEF = 0.01). Three hexa substituted isomers, all with 2,3,7,8-substitution have been detected in milk fat at concentrations ranging from 10-100 ppt (I-TEF = 0.1). The concentration of 2,3,7,8-TCDF in human milk fat ranges between 2-5 ppt (I-TEF = 0.1) (Jensen and Slorach, 1991). On an equivalency basis, it is estimated that the breast fed infant takes in 70 pg TCDD equivalents for each kilogram of body weight each day compared with 1.2 pg for an adult (Jensen and Slorach, 1991).

TCDD induced carcinogenicity, immunosuppression, reproductive and behavioral effects, and enzyme induction have been reported in laboratory animals at exposure levels equal to or only one or two orders of magnitude higher than the concentrations normally found in human milk in industrialized countries (Jensen and Slorach, 1991).

## DISCUSSION

It was not within the scope of this paper to report on every study concerning bioaccumulative chemicals in human tissue. This review, however, reveals that many of the chemicals of concern were and are still found in human tissue at concentrations that can have untoward effects on wildlife and humans. Data are accumulating across a number of wildlife and laboratory animal species as well as in humans that these chemicals can disrupt the organization and progressive development of the endocrine system via transfer of the chemicals to the offspring. This information has been slow coming to light because of the indirect pathway of exposure and the delayed manifestation of the functional deficits. In addition, it is difficult to measure loss or change of function and in many instances researchers have not known what to measure or when. The delayed effects in the offspring often are not fully manifested until adulthood, and are therefore the most difficult to trace. For example, the current epidemiological approach of screening exposed adults (the initial targets of exposure) for cancer and other obvious clinical symptoms has not revealed significant associations with the chemical(s), e.g., symptoms such as cancer, fertility, or even gross birth defects in offspring. Epidemiological surveys of exposed individuals must transcend the initial target individual and include functional decrements expressed in the offspring of the targeted adult.

In theory, a woman who suspects that she has experienced excessive exposure to bioaccumulative chemicals could have her blood tested before she decided to get pregnant or during her pregnancy to determine the risks posed to her baby. The equilibrium between blood fat, adipose tissue, and breast milk fat makes this possible and could be used to determine whether to breast feed or not. However, the cost involved, the shortage of qualified laboratories, the long turn-around-time between sample collection and final analyses, and the shortage of properly informed physicians make this an option to only a few women. In addition, interpretation of the quantitative results would be difficult using current knowledge.

Recent reports continue to support the practice of breast feeding despite the knowledge that (1) infants are exposed to elevated concentrations of certain chemicals through breast milk and (2) associations have been made with untoward effects in exceptionally exposed infants and these chemicals (IJC, 1991). This support for breast feeding is based on the advantages associated with breast feeding, such as mother-child bonding, immunological benefits transferred from mother to child, nutritional values, and reduced risk of sepsis from poorly prepared formulas. It is also based on the results of studies revealing that prenatal intrauterine exposure is the source of the greatest neurological effects, compared with postnatal breast feeding exposure. On the other hand, it does not consider the exceptional early dose to a female child who can someday, in turn, expose her own embryonic, fetal, and breast feeding offspring to the chemicals in her body. Until long-term studies surveying the results of delayed onset endocrine disruption in adults exposed in the womb have been completed, questions of this nature will not be answered. Future research must be directed toward developing end points that signal endocrine disruption in its early stages in order to remove the anxieties associated with the decision of whether or not to breast feed.

## REFERENCES

Ahmad, N., Harsas, W., Marolt, R.S., Morton, M., and Pollack, J.K. (1988). Total DDT and dieldrin content of human adipose tissue. *Bull. Environ. Contam. Toxicol.*, **41**, 802-808.

Amdur, M.O., Doull, J., and Klaassen, C.D. (1991). In *Casarett and Doull's Toxicology: The basic science of poisons: Fourth Edition*, ed. Casarett and Doull, Pergamon Press, New York.

Ando, M., Hirano, S., and Itoh, Y. (1985). Transfer of hexachlorobenzene (HCB) from mother to new-born baby through placenta and milk. *Arch. Toxicol.,* **56**, 196-200.

Ansari, G.A.S., James, G.P., Hu, L.A., and Reynolds, E.S. (1986). Organochlorine residues in adipose tissue of residents of the Texas Gulf coast. *Bull. Environ. Contam. Toxicol.*, **36**, 311-316.

Arnold, D.L., Moodie, C.A., Charbonneau, S.M., Grice, H.C., McGuire, P.F., Bryce, F.R., Collins, B.T., Zawidzka, Z.Z., Krewski, D.R., Nera, E.A., and Munro, I.C. (1985). Long-term toxicity of hexachlorobenzene in the rat and the effect of dietary vitamin A. *Fd. Chem. Toxic.*, **23**(9), 779-793.

ATSDR. (1987a). Toxicological Profile for Aldrin/Dieldrin. US Department of Health and Human Services. pp. 120.

ATSDR. (1987b). Toxicological Profile for Selected PCBs (Aroclor-1260, -1254, -1248, -1242, -1232, -1221, and 1016). U.S. Department of Health and Human Services. pp. 121.

ATSDR. (1990). Toxicological Profile for Hexachlorobenzene. U.S. Department of Health and Human Services. TP-90-17. pp. 97.

Balash, K.J., Al-Omar, M.A., and Latif, B.M.A. (1987). Effect of chlordane on testicular tissues of Swiss mice. *Bull. Environ. Contam. Toxicol.*, **39**, 434-442.

Bush, B., Bennett, A., and Snow, J. (1986). Polychlorinated biphenyl congeners, p,p'-DDE, and sperm function in humans. *Arch. Environ. Contam. Toxicol.*, **15**, 333-341.

Bustos, S., Denegri, J.C., Diaz, F., and Tchernitchin, A.N. (1988). p,p'-DDT is an estrogenic compound. *Bull. Environ. Contam. Toxicol.*, **41**, 496-501.

Calabrese, E.J. (1982). Human breast milk contamination in the United States and Canada by chlorinated hydrocarbon insecticides and industrial pollutants: Current status. *J. Am. College of Toxicol.*, **1**(3), 91-98.

Camps, M., Planas, J., Gomez-Catalan, J., Sabroso, M., To-Figueras, J., and Corbella, J. (1989). Organochlorine residues in human adipose tissue in Spain: study of an agrarian area. *Bull. Environ. Contam. Toxicol.*, **42**, 195-201.

Chowdhury, A.R., Venkatakrishna-Bhatt, H. and Gautam, A.K. (1987). India testicular changes in rats under lindane treatment. *Bull. Environ. Contam. Toxicol.*, **38**, 154-156.

Chu, I., Villeneuve, D.C., Valli, V.E., Ritter, L., Norstrom, R.J., Ryan, J.J., and Becking, G.C. (1984). Toxicological response and its reversibility in rats fed Lake Ontario or Pacific coho salmon for 13 weeks. *J. Environ. Sci. Health*, **B19**(8 and 9), 713-131.

Cooper, R.L., Chadwick, R.W., Rehnberg, G.L., Goldman, J.M., Booth, K.C., Hein, J.F., and McElroy, W.K. (1989). Effect of lindane on hormonal control of reproductive function in the female rat. *Toxicol. Appl. Pharmacol.*, **99**, 384-394.

Cranmer, J.M., Cranmer, M.F., and Goad, P.T. (1984). Prenatal chlordane exposure: Effects on plasma corticosterone concentrations over the lifespan of mice. *Environ. Res.*, **35**, 204-210.

Daly, H.B. (1992). The evaluation of behavioral changes produced by consumption of environmentally contaminated fish. In *The Vulnerable Brain and Environmental Risks, Vol. 1: Malnutrition and Hazard Assessment*, eds. R.L. Isaacson and K.F. Jensen. Plenum Press, New York, NY. (in press).

Daly, H.B. (1991). Reward reductions found more aversive by rats fed environmentally contaminated salmon. *Neurotoxicology and Teratology*, **13**, 449-453. (in press).

Daly, H.B., Hertzler, D.R., and Sargent, D.M. (1989). Ingestion of environmentally contaminated Lake Ontario salmon by laboratory rats increases avoidance of unpredictable aversive nonreward and mild electric shock. *Behavioral Neuroscience*, **103**(6), 1356-1365.

Dieringer, C.S., Lamartiniere, C.A., Schiller, C.M., and Lucier, G.W. (1979). Altered ontogeny of hepatic steroid-metabolizing enzymes by pure polychlorinated biphenyl congeners. *Biochem. Pharmacol.*, **28**, 2511-2514.

Dewailly, E., Nantel, A., Weber, J., and Meyer, F. (1989). High levels of PCBs in breast milk of Inuit women from arctic Quebec. *Bull. Environ. Contam. Toxicol.*, **43**, 641-646.

Fein, G.G., Jacobson, J.L., Jacobson, S.W., Schwartz, P.M., and Dowler, J.K. (1984). Prenatal exposure to polychlorinated biphenyls. Effects on birth size and gestational age. *J. Pediatr.*, **105**, 315-320.

Fry, M.D., Toone, K.C., Speich, S.M., and Peard, J.R. (1987). Sex ratio skew and breeding patterns of gulls: Demographic and toxicological considerations. *Studies in Avian Biology*, **10**, 26-43.

Fry, M.D. and Toone, K.C. (1981). DDT-induced feminization of gull embryos. *Science*, **213**, 992-924.

Gladen, B.C., Rogan, W.J., Hardy, P., Thullen, J., Tinglestad, J., and Tully, M. (1988). Development after exposure to polychlorinated biphenyls and dichlorophenyl dichloroethene transplacentally and through human milk. *J. Pediatr.*, **113**, 991-995.

Gobas, F.A.P.C. (1990). *Selected persistent toxic substances in human breast milk in the Great Lakes Basin.* Contract for The Great Lakes Institute, University of Windsor, Windsor, Ontario Canada. International Joint Commission.

Gray, Jr., L.E., Ostby, J., Ferrell, J., Rehnberg, G., Linder, R., Cooper, R., Goldman, J., Slott, V., and Laskey, J. (1989). A dose-response analysis of methoxychlor-induced alterations of reproductive development and function in the rat. *Fund. Appl. Toxicol.*, **12**, 92-108.

Haake, J., Kelley, M., Keys, B., and Safe, S. (1987). The effects of organochlorine pesticides as inducers of testosterone and benzo[a]pyrene hydroxylases. *Gen. Pharmac.*, **18**(2), 165-169.

Heaton, S.N., Aulerich, R.J., and Bursian, S.J. (1991). Reproductive effects of feeding Saginaw Bay source fish to ranch mink. In *Cause-Effect Linkages II Symposium Abstracts*, eds. S. Schneider and R. Campbell. Michigan Audubon Society, Ann Arbor, MI. pp. 24-25.

Holliday, M.G. (1988). *Intake of Hexachlorobenzene by Canadians.* Contract Reference No. 1688, Monitoring and Criteria Division, Health and Welfare Canada, Ottawa, Ontario.

Humphrey, H.E.B. (1988). Chemical contaminants in the Great Lakes: The human health aspect. In *Toxics Contaminants and Ecosystem Health: A Great Lakes Focus*, ed. M.S. Evans. Wiley and Sons, New York. pp. 153-156.

Humphrey, H.E.B. (1987). The human population—An ultimate receptor for aquatic contaminants. *Hydrobiologia*, **149**, 75-80.

IJC. International Joint Commission, Science Advisory Board. (1991). *Report to the International Joint Commission.* Canada.

Jacobson, J.L., Jacobson, S.W., and H.E.B. Humphrey. (1990a). Effects of exposure to PCBs and related compounds on growth and activity in children. *Neurotox. Terat.*, **12**, 319-326.

Jacobson, J.L., Jacobson, S.W., and Humphrey, H.E.B. (1990b). Effects of *in utero* exposure to polychlorinated biphenyls and other contaminants on cognitive functioning in young children. *J. Pediatr.*, **116**, 38-45.

Jacobson, J.L., Humphrey, H.E.B., Jacobson, S.W., Schantz, S.L., Mullin, M.D., and Welch, R.W. (1989). Determinants of polychlorinated biphenyls (PCBs), polybrominated biphenyls (PBBs), and dichlorodiphenyl trichloroethane (DDT) levels in the sera of young children. *AJPH*, **79**(10), 1401-1404.

Jacobson, J.L. and Jacobson, S.W. (1988). New methodologies for assessing the effects of prenatal toxic exposure on cognitive functioning in humans. In *Toxic Contaminants and Ecosystem Health: A Great Lakes Focus*, ed. M. Evans. John Wiley and Sons, New York. pp. 374-388.

Jacobson, S.W., Fein, G.G., Jacobson, J.L., Schwartz, P.M., and Dowler, J.K. (1985). The effects of PCB exposure on visual recognition memory. *Child Dev.*, **56**, 853-860.

Jensen, A.A. and Slorach, S.A. (1991). *Chemical Contaminants in Human Milk*. CRC Press, Boston, MA. pp. 298.

Kimbrough, R.D. (1990). How toxic is 2,3,7,8-tetrachlorodibenzodioxin to humans? *J. Toxicol. Environ. Health*, **30**, 261-271.

Krauthacker, B. (1991). Levels of organochlorine pesticides and polychlorinated biphenyls (PCBs) in human milk and serum collected from lactating mothers in the northern Adriatic area of Yugoslavia. *Bull. Environ. Contam. Toxicol.*, **46**, 797-802.

Krauthacker, B., Kralj, M., Tkalcevic, B. and Reiner, E. (1986). Levels of *B*-HCH, HCH, p,p'-DDE, p,p'-DDT and PCBs in human milk from a continental town of Croatia, Yugoslavia. *Int. Arch. Occup. Environ. Health*, **58**, 69-74.

Krawinkel, M.B., Plehn, G., Kruse, H., and Kasi, A.M. (1989). Organochlorine residues in Baluchistan/Pakistan: Blood and fat concentrations in humans. *Bull. Environ. Contam. Toxicol.*, **43**, 821-826.

Kubiak, T.J., Harris, H.J., Smith, L.M., Schwartz, T.R., Stalling, D.L., Trick, J.A., Sileo, L., Docherty, D.E., and Erdman, T.C. (1989). Microcontaminants and reproductive impairment of the Forster's Tern on Green Bay, Lake Michigan-1983. *Arch. Environ. Contam. Toxicol.*, **18**, 706-727.

Leatherland, J.F. and Sonstegard, R.A. (1982). Bioaccumulation of organochlorines by yearling coho salmon (*Oncorhynchus kisutch walbaum*) fed diets containing Great Lakes coho salmon, and the pathophysiological responses of the recipients. *Comp. Biochem. Physiol.*, **72**C(1), 91-99.

Lilienthal, H. and Winneke, G. (1991). Sensitive periods for behavioral toxicity of polychlorinated biphenyls: Determination by cross-fostering in rats. *Fundamental and Applied Toxicol.*, **17**, 368-375.

Lundholm, C.E. (1988). The effects of DDE, PCB and chlordane on the binding of progesterone to its cytoplasmic receptor in the eggshell gland mucosa of birds and the endometrium of mammalian uterus. *Comp. Biochem. Physiol.*, **89**C(2), 361-368.

Mes, J., Davies, D.J., Turton, D., and Sun, W.F. (1986). Levels and trends of chlorinated hydrocarbon contaminants in the breast milk of Canadian women. *Food Additives and Contam.*, **3**(4), 313-322.

Mes, J., Davies, D.J., and Turton, D. (1982). Polychlorinated biphenyl and other chlorinated hydrocarbon residues in adipose tissue of Canadians. *Bull. Environ. Contam. Toxicol.*, **28**, 97-104.

Mes, J., Doyle, J.A., Barrett, R.A., Davies, D.J., and Turton, D. (1984). Polychlorinated biphenyls and organochlorine pesticides in milk and blood of Canadian women during lactation. *Arch. Environ. Contam. Toxicol.*, **13**, 217-223.

Miller, D.T., Condon, S.K., Kutzner, S., Phillips, D.L., Krueger, E., Timperi, R., Burse, V.W., Cutler, J., and Gute, D.M. (1991). Human exposure to polychlorinated biphenyls in Greater New Bedford, Massachusetts: A prevalence study. *Arch. Environ. Contam. Toxicol.*, **20**, 410-416.

Moore, R.W., Potter, C.L., Theobald, H.M., Robinson, J.A., and Peterson, R.E. (1985). Androgenic deficiency in males rats treated with 2,3,7,8-tetrachlorodibenzo-p-dioxin. *Toxicol. Appl. Pharmacol.*, **79**, 99-111.

Mossing, M.L., Redetzke, K.A., and Applegate, H.G. (1985). Organochlorine pesticides in blood of persons from El Paso, Texas. *J. Environ. Health,* **47**(6), 312-313.

Nair, A. and Pillai, M.K.K. (1989). Monitoring of hexachlorobenzene residues in Delhi and Faridabad, India. *Bull. Environ. Contam. Toxicol.*, **42**, 682-686.

Norstrom, R.J., Simon, M., Muir, D.C.G., and Schweisburg, R.E.. (1988). Organochlorine contaminants in Arctic marine food chains: Indentification, geographical distribution, and temporal trends in polar bears. *Environ. Sci. Technol.*, **22**(**9**), 1063-1071.

Ono, M., Wakimoto, T., Tatsukawa, R., and Masuda, Y. (1986). Polychlorinated dibenzo-p-dioxins and dibenzofurans in human adipose tissue of Japan. *Chemosphere,* **15**(9-12), 1629-1634.

OWRS. Office of Water Regulations and Standards. USEPA. (1986). *Work Quality Assurance Project Plan for the Bioaccumulation Study.* p. 49.

Patterson, D.G., Needham, L.L., Pirkle, J.L., Roberts, D.W., Bagby, J., Garrett, W.A., Andrews, J.S., Falk, H., Bernert, J.T., Sampson, E.J., and Houk, V.N. (1988). Correlation between serum and adipose tissue levels of 2,3,7,8-tetrachlorodibenzo-p-dioxin in 50 persons from Missouri. *Arch. Environ. Contam. Toxicol.*, **17**, 139-143.

Pines, A., Cucos, S., Ever-Hadani, P., and Ron, M. (1987). Some organochlorine insecticide and polychlorinated biphenyl blood residues in infertile males in the general Israeli population of the middle 1980's. *Arch. Environ. Contam. Toxicol.*, **16**, 587-597.

Rao, C.V. and Banerji, S. (1988). Polychlorinated biphenyls in human amniotic fluid. *Bull. Environ. Contam. Toxicol.*, **41**, 798-801.

Rao, C.V. and Banerji, S. (1989). Polychlorinated biphenyls in human blood samples of Bombay. *Bull. Environ. Contam. Toxicol.*, **43**, 656-659.

Rappe, C. (1991). Introduction, levels, profiles, and patterns. Paper presented at the 11th International Symposium on Chlorinated Dioxins and Related Compounds: DIOXIN '91. Research Triangle Park, NC, USA. September 23-27. p. 17.

Rattner, B.A., Eroschenko, V.P., Fox, G.A., Fry, D.M. and Gosline, J. (1984). Avian endocrine responses to environmental pollutants. *J. Exp. Zool.*, **232**, 683-689.

Rogan, W.J., and Gladen, B.C. (1985). Study of human lactation for effects of environmental contaminants: The North Carolina breast milk and formula project and some other ideas. *Environ. Health Perspectives*, **60**, 215-221.

Rogan, W.J., Gladen, B.C., and Wilcox, A.J. (1986). Potential reproductive and postnatal morbidity from exposure to polychlorinated biphenyls: Epidemiologic considerations. *Environ. Health Perspectives*, **60**, 233-239.

Ron, M., Cucos, B. Rosenn, B., Hochner-Celnikier, D., Ever-Hadani, P., and Pines, A. (1988). Maternal and fetal serum levels of organochlorine compounds in cases of premature rupture of membranes. *Acta. Obstet. Gynecol. Scand.*, **67**, 695-697.

Roncevic, N., Pavkov, S., Galetin-Smith, R., Vukavic, T., Vojinovic, M., and Djordjevic, M. (1987). Serum concentrations of organochlorine compounds during pregnancy and in the newborn. *Bull. Environ. Contam. Toxicol.*, **38**, 117-124.

Safe, S.H. (1990). Polychlorinated biphenyls (PCBs), dibenzo-p-dioxins (PCDDs), dibenzofurans (PCDFs), and related compounds: Environmental and mechanistic considerations which support the development of toxic equivalency factors (TEFs). *Critical Reviews in Toxicology*, **21**(1), 51-88.

Safe, S.H. (1986). Comparative toxicology and mechanism of action of polychlorinated dibenzo-p-dioxins and dibenzofurans. *Ann. Rev. Pharmacol. Toxicol.*, **26**, 371-399.

Sager, D., Girard, D., and Nelson, D. (1991). Early postnatal exposure to PCBs: sperm function in rats. *Environ. Toxicol. Chem.*, **10**, 737-746.

Sager, D.B. (1983). Effect of postnatal exposure to polychlorinated biphenyls on adult male reproductive function. *Environ. Res.*, **31**, 76-94.

Sager, D.B., Shih-Schroeder, W., and Girard, D. (1987). Effects of early postnatal exposure to polychlorinated biphenyls (PCBs) on fertility in male rats. *Bull. Environ. Contam. Toxicol.*, **38**, 946-953.

Sasaki, K., Ishizaka, T., Suzuki, T., Takeda, M. and Uchiyama, M. (1991). Accumulation levels of organochlorine pesticides in human adipose tissue and blood. *Bull. Environ. Contam. Toxicol.*, **46**, 662-669.

Saxena, M.C., Siddiqui, M.K.J., Agarwal, V., and Kuuty, D. (1983). A comparison of organochlorine insecticide contents in specimens of maternal blood, placenta, and umbilical cord-blood from stillborn and live-born cases. *J. Toxicol. Environ. Health.*, **11**, 71-79.

Schantz, S.L., Levin, E.D., and Bowman, R.E. (1991). Review: Long-term neurobehavioral effects of perinatal polychlorinated biphenyl (PCB) exposure in monkeys. *Environ. Toxicol. Chem.*, **10**, 747-756.

Schecter, A. (1991). Dioxins and related chemical in humans and the environment. In *Banbury Reports 35: Biological Basis for Risk Assessment of Dioxins and Related Compounds*. Cold Springs Harbor Laboratory Press, Cold Springs Harbor, NY. (in press).

Seegal, R.F. and Shain. (1992). Neurotoxicity of polychlorinated biphenyls: The role of ortho-substituted congeners in altering neurochemical function. In *The Vulnerable Brain: Nutritional and Toxicological Influences*. (in press).

Shain, W., Overmann, S.R., Wilson, L.R., Kostas, J., and Bush, B. (1986). A congener analysis of polychlorinated biphenyls accumulating in rat pups after perinatal exposure. *Arch. Environ. Contam. Toxicol.*, **15**, 687-707.

Skaare, J.U., Tuveng, J.M., and Sande, H.A. (1988). Organochlorine pesticides and polychlorinated biphenyls in maternal adipose tissue, blood, milk, and cord blood from mothers and their infants living in Norway. *Arch. Environ. Contam. Toxicol.*, **17**, 55-63.

Skene, S.A., Dewhurst, I.C., and Greenberg, M. (1989). Polychlorinated dibenzo-p-dioxins and polychlorinated dibenzofurans: The risks to human health. A Review. *Human Toxicol.*, **8**, 173-203.

Smith, A.G. (1991). Chlorinated hydrocarbon insecticides. In *Handbook of Pesticide Toxicology*, ed. Hayes, W.J. and Laws, E.R. Academic Press, New York. p. 791.

Street, J.C. and Sharma, R.P. (1975). Alteration of induced cellular and humoral immune responses by pesticides and chemicals of environmental concern: Quantitative studies of immunosuppression by DDT, Aroclor 1254, Carbaryl, Carbofuran, and Methylparathion. *Toxicol. Appl. Pharmacol.*, **32**, 587-602.

Subramanian, A., Tanabe, S., Tatsukawa, R., Saitao, S., and Miyazaki, N. (1987). Reduction in the testosterone levels by PCBs and DDE in Dall's porpoises of northwestern North Pacific. *Mar. Poll. Bull.*, **18**, 643-646.

Summer, C.L., Aulerich, R.J., and Bursian, S.J. (1991). Preliminary analysis of reproductive effects from feeding white leghorn chickens Saginaw Bay source fish. In *Cause-Effect Linkages II Symposium Abstracts.* Michigan Audubon Society, Ann Arbor, MI. pp. 28-29.

Szymczynsk, G.A. and Waliszewski, S.M. (1983). Chlorinated pesticide residues in testicular tissue samples: Pesticides in human testicles. *Andrologia,* **15(6)**, 696-698.

Tilson, H.A., Jacobson, J.L., and Rogan, W.J. (1990). Polychlorinated biphenyls and the developing nervous system: Cross-species comparisons. *Neurotoxicol. Teratol.,* **12,** 239-248.

Thoma, H., Mucke, W., and Kauert, G. (1990). Comparison of the polychlorinated dibenzo-p-dioxin and dibenzofuran in human tissue and human liver. *Chemosphere,* **20**(3/4), 433-442.

Umbreit, T.H. and Gallo, M.A. (1988). Review: Physiological implications of estrogen receptor modulation by 2,3,7,8-tetrachlorodibenzo-p-dioxin. *Toxicology Letters,* **42,** 5-14.

USEPA. (1989). Proposed amendments to the guidelines for health assessment of suspect developmental toxicants. Federal Regulations, **54,** 9386-9403.

USEPA. (1991). Workshop Report on Toxicity Equivalency Factors for Polychlorinated Biphenyl Congeners. Risk Assessment Forum. Eastern Research Group, Inc. EPA/625/3-91/020. pp. 71.

Van Velsen, F.L., Danse, L.H.J.C., Van Leeuwen, F.X.R., Dormans, J.A.M.A., and Van Logten, M.J. (1986). The subchronic oral toxicity of the B-isomer of hexachlorocyclohexane in rats. *Fund. Appl. Toxicol.,* **6,** 697-712.

Villeneuve, D.C., Villi, V.E., Norstrom, R.J., Freeman, H., Sanglang, G.B., Ritter, L., and Becking, G.C. (1981). Toxicological response of rats fed Lake Ontario or Pacific coho salmon for 28 days. *J. Environ. Sci. Health,* **B16**(6), 649-689.

Wariishi, M., Suzuki, Y., and Nishiyama, K. (1986). Chlordane residues in normal human blood. *Bull. Environ. Contam. Toxicol.,* **36,** 635-643.

Wasserman, M., Ron, M., Bercovici, B., Wassermann, D., Cucos, S., and Pines, A. (1982). Premature delivery and oganochlorine compounds: Polychlorinated biphenyls and some organochlorine insecticides. *Environ. Res.,* **28,** 106-112.

Williams, D.T., LeBel, G.L., and Junkins, E. (1988). Organohalogen residues in human adipose autopsy samples from six Ontario municipalities. *J. Assoc. Off. Anal. Chem.,* **71**(2), 410-414.

Advances in Modern Environmental Toxicology • Volume XX

# PREDICTING ECOSYSTEM RISK

*edited by*
John Cairns, Jr., B.R. Niederlehner, David R. Orvos

Most ecosystems are experiencing anthropogenic changes. Global atmosphere, oceans, forests, agricultural lands, and surface and ground water are all at risk from diverse human activities. The recognition and quantification of these risks are the first steps in sustaining a healthy environment.

Two major factors must be considered in predicting ecosystem risk: the probability of deleterious effects and the resilience or ability to recover following anthropogenic and/or natural disturbance. Predicting the probability of deleterious effects should depend upon a comparison of an estimate of a safe concentration that does not damage biological integrity to an independent estimate of the expected environmental concentration. In addition to predicting the probability of adverse effects, ecosystem resiliency must also be estimated.

Much attention has been given in recent years to the problem of restoring damaged ecosystems. Evidence is mounting that some ecosystems recover quite rapidly from pollutional effects (although recovery is not to their predisturbance condition), but others do not recover for tens, hundreds, or perhaps even thousands of years. Risk and resilience should be considered together because an ecosystem unlikely to recover or to be restored in time spans of interest to humans should be subjected to much less risk than those with considerably higher resiliency. Ideally, the purpose of predicting ecosystem risk is to prevent damage, i.e., effective prediction of risk is far superior to reacting to oil spills, environmental pollution, and the like *after* damage has occurred.

Of course, all ecosystem risk estimation must consider various cost and benefit factors, and this volume does not intend to be an exhaustive methodological book; rather, its purpose is to furnish illustrative examples to introduce more detailed explanations of this fascinating topic of predicting ecosystem risk.

## • TABLE OF CONTENTS •

*Pages:* approx. 400; *Size:* 6 x 9 inches, hard cover     *Publication Date:* April 1992
*Price:* US $65.00 + $3.00 shipping & handling          *ISBN:* 0-911131-27-2

• to order PREDICTING ECOSYSTEM RISK send $68.00 prepayment to•
Princeton Scientific Publishing Co., Inc. • P.O. Box 2155 • Princeton, NJ 08543
• or fax your order to• (609) 683-0838 •

P R O C E E D I N G S   O F
## The IXth UOEH International Symposium and
## The First Pan Pacific Cooperative Symposium

## Industrialization and Emerging Environmental Health Issues: Risk Assessment and Risk Management

*edited by:*
Takesumi Yoshimura • Kenzaburo Tsuchiya • S.D. Lee • L.D. Grant • M. A. Mehlman

In Kitakyushu, Japan, October 2-6, 1989, an international symposium on "Industrialization and Emerging Environmental Health Issues: Risk Assessment and Risk Management" was held. This five-day symposium addressed problems related to the impact of industrialization on the environment and human health. The symposium brought together internationally-recognized experts and scholars from around the world. The topics covered a wide range of interests and concerns for both industrialized and developing nations.

This volume documents the meeting by publishing the papers presented in Kitakyushu. These papers are valuable reading material for anyone involved in, or interested in, the scientific and medical fields addressing environmental health issues, and in particular the risk assessment and risk management of those issues in developing nations. The volume contains over 60 articles by internationally-known scientists and professionals, including:

ENVIRONMENTAL PROBLEMS: PAST, PRESENT, AND FUTURE K. Fuwa

CURRENT ISSUES IN THE EPIDEMIOLOGY AND TOXICOLOGY OF OCCUPATIONAL EXPOSURE TO LEAD P.J. Landrigan

GLOBAL POLLUTION E. Bingham

THE DISTRIBUTION, CYCLING, AND POTENTIAL HAZARDS OF INDUSTRIAL CHEMICALS IN MARINE ENVIRONMENTS M. Morita

COMPREHENSIVE ASSESSMENT OF OCCUPATIONAL AND ENVIRONMENTAL HEALTH PROBLEMS: AN OVERVIEW - A PROPOSAL OF MACRO APPROACH: INDUSTRIAL ECOLOGICAL SCIENCES K. Tsuchiya

SEMICONDUCTOR INDUSTRIES J. LaDou

LONG-TERM CARCINOGENICITY BIOASSAYS ON INDUSTRIAL CHEMICALS AND MAN-MADE MINERAL FIBERS : PREMISES, PROGRAMS, AND RESULTS  C. Maltoni, F. Minardi, M. Soffritti, and G. Lefemine

INFORMATION AND MANAGEMENT SYSTEM TO REDUCE CHEMICAL RISKS N. Htun

ROAD TRANSPORT IMPACT ON THE ENVIRONMENTAL HEALTH M. Murakami, M. Ono, and K. Tamura

ASBESTOS DISEASE-1990-2020: THE RISKS OF ASBESTOS RISK ASSESSMENT I.J. Selikoff

HEALTH RISK ASSESSMENT OF RADIATION T. Sugahara

TOXIC EVALUATION OF CHLORINATED AROMATIC HYDROCARBONS IN HUMAN ENVIRONMENTS Y. Masuda

CARCINOGENICITY OF MOTOR FUELS: GASOLINE M.A. Mehlman

INDUSTRIALIZATION AND EMERGING ENVIRONMENTAL HEALTH ISSUES: LESSONS FROM THE BHOPAL DISASTER C.R. Krishna Murti

MUNICIPAL AND INDUSTRIAL HAZARDOUS WASTE MANAGEMENT: AN OVERVIEW L. Fishbein

THE EXPORT OF HAZARDOUS WASTE TO THE CARIBBEAN BASIN REGION W.H.E. Suite

WASTE MANAGEMENT IN *ASEAN* COUNTRIES F.A. Uriarte, Jr.

THE CURRENT STATUS OF SOLID WASTE MANAGMENT IN P.R. CHINA Shi Qing

MANAGMENT OF INDUSTRIAL WASTE - A EUROPEAN PERSPECTIVE T. Schneider

RISK REDUCTION MANAGEMENT FOR HAZARDOUS WASTE IN JAPAN M. Tanaka and K. Ueda

MANAGING THE RISK TRANSITION K.R. Smith

MULTIMEDIA RISK ASSESSMENT FOR ENVIRONMENTAL RISK MANAGEMENT S.D. Lee

RISK ASSESSMENT AND RISK MANAGEMENT IN JAPAN J. Kagawa

RISK ASSESSMENT/RISK MANAGEMENT OF MOTOR VEHICLE EMISSIONS M.P. Walsh

RISK ASSESSMENT AND RISK MANAGEMENT IN JAPAN E. Yokoyama

THE ROLE OF EPIDEMIOLOGY IN RISK ASSESSMENT T. Yoshimura

ENVIRONMENTAL AND OCCUPATIONAL HAZARDS IN EXPORT PROCESSING ZONES IN SOUTH AND EAST ASIA M. Thorborg

plus the many more papers by international authorities such as: J.J. Convery, E. L. Anderson , N.A. Ashford, A. Koizumi , D.J. Ehreth , B.D. Goldstein , D.G. Hoel , J. Higginson

### Princeton Scientific Publishing Co., Inc.
**P.O. Box 2155 • Princeton, New Jersey 08543 • (609) 683-4750 • fax: (609) 683-0838**
Price: $65 + $5 shipping and handling.                    Prepayment required on all orders.

ADVANCES IN MODERN ENVIRONMENTAL TOXICOLOGY

## VOLUME XVIII

# THE EFFECT OF PESTICIDES ON HUMAN HEALTH

Edited by Scott R. Baker and Chris F. Wilkinson

## CONTENTS

INTRODUCTION AND OVERVIEW: Current Pesticide Production and Use • Types of Pesticides • Risks and Benefits of Pesticide Use • Pesticide Exposure Levels • Adverse Health Effects of Pesticides • Assessing Chronic Human Health Risks • Pesticides Versus Other Health Risks

EXPOSURE TO PESTICIDES: Routes of Exposure to Pesticides and Their Disposition in the Body • Occupational Exposure to Pesticides • Exposure of the General Population to Pesticides • Exposure of Bystanders to Pesticides • Methods of Assessing Exposure to Pesticides

NEUROTOXIC EFFECTS OF PESTICIDES: Epidemiology of Neurotoxic Effects • Potential for Neurotoxic Effects • Developmental Neurotoxicity After Perinatal Pesticide Exposure • Current Regulatory Status of Neurotoxic Chemicals • Assessment of Neurotoxic Effects • Future Directions

CARCINOGENIC EFFECTS OF PESTICIDES: The Carcinogenic Potential of Pesticides Based on Epidemiologic Studies • The Carcinogenic Potential of Pesticides as Based on Animal Studies • Mechanisms of Action of Carcinogenesis

IMMUNOLOGIC EFFECTS OF PESTICIDES: Potential for Adverse Effect of Pesticides on the Immune System • Regulatory Status on Immunotoxicology of Pesticides • Specific Concerns of the Chronic Effects of Pesticides on the Immune System

REPRODUCTIVE EFFECTS OF PESTICIDES: Mechanisms of Action of Reproductive Toxicants • Clinical Manifestations Suggesting Human Reproductive Toxicity • Male Reproductive Toxicants • Dibromochloropropane • Chlordecone • Ethylene Dibromide • Carbaryl • Female Reproductive Toxicants • Female Toxicity Due to Estrogenicity • Reproductive Effects Associated with Organophosphates • Carbamates • Reproductive Toxicity of Kepone and Hexachlorobenzene • Mathematical Models for Reproductive Toxicology • Methods for Risk Assessment in Reproductive Toxicology

DEVELOPMENTAL EFFECTS OF PESTICIDES: Relationship of Pesticide Exposure and Human Development • Predictability of Animal Tests • Evaluating Human Epidemiologic Studies • Basic Epidemiologic Concepts in Developmental Toxicology • Confounding Factors • Comparison of Human and Animal Data • Risk Assessment for Developmental Toxicity

*$65.00 + $3.00 shipping and handling*

**Princeton Scientific Publishing Co., Inc.**

P.O. Box 2155 • Princeton, New Jersey 08543 • Tel: 609-683-4750 • Fax: 609-683-0838

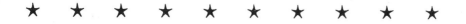

Agency for Toxic Substances and Disease Registry
Conference Announcement

# International Congress

## *on the*

# HEALTH EFFECTS OF HAZARDOUS WASTE

The Agency for Toxic Substances and Disease Registry (ATSDR), in collaboration with the Emory University School of Public Health and the Association of Occupational and Environmental Clinics, announces the First International Congress on the Health Effects of Hazardous Waste. The Congress, which will be co-sponsored by the National Institute of Environmental Health Sciences and the Environmental Protection Agency, will be held May 3-6, 1993, at the Atlanta Marriott Marquis.

This Congress will provide an opportunity for international-recognized scientific experts from various technical disciplines (biomedical and environmental scientists, epidemiologists, physicians, risk assessors, and toxicologists) to evaluate and disseminate state-of-the-art information concerning the human health effects associated with exposure to hazardous waste. Topics to be addressed at the Congress include: the magnitude of health problems associated with hazardous waste, exposure assessment (including routes of exposure to toxic substances, environmental measurements, modeling, and use of biological markers), populations at risk, health effects resulting from exposure to toxic substances (including toxicologic studies, health effects studies, diagnostics strategies, and risk analysis), mitigation strategies, risk communication, technology, and information transfer, emerging technologies, gaps in data, and research needs.

*For further information, contact :*
John S. Andrews, Jr., M.D., M.P.H.
Associate Administrator for Science
ATSDR, 1600 Clifton Road, NE
Mailstop E-28, Atlanta, GA 30333
Tel: (404) 639-0708, FTS 236-0708.

# GASOLINE: ASSESSMENT OF HUMAN EXPOSURE

## The Proceedings of the Workshop on General Population Exposure to Gasoline

a special issue of the *Journal of Exposure Analysis and Environmental Epidemiology (Vol. 2, No. 1, 1992)*

The estimated exposures and risks associated with gasoline constituents for the general population is of concern because regulations traditionally have been formulated or considered for various sources and uncontrolled emission situations. This regulatory response to the risk posed by gasoline appears to suffer from the lack of adequate data bases on human exposure. In addition, many types and routes of exposure have not been considered in the overall prioritizing of concerns about gasoline. The issues are magnified by the fact that gasoline is a commercial product to which at least 110 million people in the U.S. may be exposed.

The American Petroleum Institute and other organizations co-sponsored a workshop, held on December 12-14, 1990, in Annapolis, Maryland, to address these issues. The workshop featured four parallel Work Group sessions, addressing the following areas of study: 1) the methods used in exposure assessment, 2) current and anticipated measurement techniques, 3) the use of exposure data in assessments, and 4) the application of exposure assessment to risk characterization. Presentations were given by scientists and professionals from government, industry, and universities in both workshop sessions and in formal presentations on the current status of research on gasoline exposure.

Specific topics addressed during the three-day conference included gasoline exposures resulting from automobile refueling, vehicular emissions, ground-water contamination through gasoline spills and leaking underground storage tanks, and home appliances and equipment. The peer-reviewed manuscripts derived from the presentations are published in this important 150-page volume.

## • Table of Contents •

*Pages:* approx. 150; *Size:* 6 x 9 in., soft cover
*Price:* US $65.00 + $3.00 shipping & handling

*Publication Date:* January 1992
*ISSN:* 1053-4245; Vol. 2, No. 1

• send order and prepayment of $68.00 to •
Princeton Scientific Publishing Co., Inc. • P.O. Box 2155 • Princeton, NJ 08543
• or fax your credit card order to • 609-683-0838 •

ADVANCES IN MODERN ENVIRONMENTAL TOXICOLOGY

# VOLUME III
# ASSESSMENT OF REPRODUCTIVE AND TERATOGENIC HAZARDS

Edited by M.S. CHRISTIAN, Argus Research Laboratories, Inc.
W.M. GALBRAITH, U.S. Environmental Protection Agency
P. VOYTEK, U.S. Environmental Protection Agency
and M.A. MEHLMAN, Mobil Oil Corporation

## SECTION I

The 1980s: An Era of Reproductive Confrontation, *J.E. Gocke*
Statement of Problem: Reproductive Hazard, *M.S. Christian*
The Teratologist as a Consultant, *E.M. Johnson*
Pharmaceuticals, Drugs, and Birth Defects, *R.M. Hoar*
Food, Food Additives, and Natural Products, *G. Nolan*
Practical Applications of Systems for Rapid Detection of Potential Teratogenic Hazards, *E.M. Johnson*
Reproductive Toxicology: Radiation Effects, *R.P. Jensh*
Assessment of Reproductivity Toxicity - State of the Art, *M.S. Christian*
Petroleum and Petroleum Products: A Brief Review of Studies to Evaluate Reproductive Effects, *C.A. Schreiner*

## SECTION II

*Assessment of Risks to Human Reproduction and to Development of the Human Conceptus from Exposure to Environmental Substances. Proceedings of U.S Environmental Protection Agency - 1982. Documented information by over 100 noted experts in the fields of developmental biology and teratology.*

Chapter 1: Introduction
Chapter 2: Female Reproduction
General Reproductive Toxicity Screen
Qualitative Reproductive Toxicity Tests
Quantitative Reproductive Toxicity Tests
Risk Assessment
Research Needed
   Extrapolation of animal data to humans
Details of Test Protocols and Glossary of Terms for Female Risk Assessments
Description and Discussion of Tests Useful in Assessing Risk to the Female Reproductive System
Ovarian Toxicity

Chapter 3: Male Reproduction
Aspects of the Problem
Selection of an Animal Model
Tests for Evaluating Reproductive Damage
Evaluation of Reproductive Damage in Exposed or Potentially Exposed Men
Protocols for Testing Compounds with Animal Models - Research Needed
Details of Test Protocols and Glossary of Terms for Male Risk Assessment
Description and Discussion of Tests Useful in Animals Models or Man
Testicular Characteristics
Epididymal Characteristics
Assessment of Male Reproductive Toxicity Using Endocrinological Methods
Examinations of Known Toxic Exposure
   Humans • Animal Models
Fertility Testing
   Tests available
Sperm Nucleus Integrity
   Spermatozoal morphology
   Karyotyping of human spermatozoa by the denuded-hamster-egg technique
Dose Response
Chapter 4:
Current Status of, and Consideration for, Estimation of Risk to the Human Conceptus from Environmental Chemicals
Definition and Scope
Impact of Developmental Abnormalities on Humans
Causes of Congenital Malformations
Qualitative Evaluation of Risk Potential
Chapter 5:
Other Considerations: Epidemiology, Pharmacokinetics, and Sexual Behavior
Epidemiology: Methods and Limitations
   Possible data sources and useful approaches
Pharmacokinetics
Sexual Behavior
   Qualitative evaluation of risk potential
   Animal studies
   Assessment of human sexual behavior: surveillance and epidemiological studies

*$58.00 + $3.00 shipping and handling*

**Princeton Scientific Publishing Co., Inc.**
P.O. Box 2155 • Princeton, New Jersey 08543 • Tel: 609-683-4750 • Fax: 609-683-0838

ADVANCES IN MODERN ENVIRONMENTAL TOXICOLOGY

## VOLUME XVII

# ENVIRONMENTAL AND OCCUPATIONAL CANCER: SCIENTIFIC UPDATE

Edited by M.A. Mehlman

## CONTENTS

*$65.00 + $3.00 shipping and handling*

**Princeton Scientific Publishing Co., Inc.**
P.O. Box 2155 • Princeton, New Jersey 08543 • Tel: 609-683-4750 • Fax: 609-683-0838